Management of Blistering Diseases

Management of Blistering Diseases

EDITED BY

Fenella Wojnarowska

The Slade Hospital, Oxford, UK

AND

Robert A. Briggaman

University of North Carolina School of Medicine
Chapel Hill, USA

SPRINGER-SCIENCE+BUSINESS MEDIA, B.V.

Typeset in 10/12pt Sabon by
EJS Chemical Composition
Midsomer Norton, Bath

British Library Cataloguing in Publication Data

Management of blistering diseases.
1. Man. Skin. Diseases
I. Wojnarowska, Fenella II. Briggaman, Robert
616.5

ISBN 978-0-412-28990-3

ISBN 978-0-412-28990-3 ISBN 978-1-4899-7190-6 (eBook)
DOI 10.1007/978-1-4899-7190-6

Originally published by Chapman and Hall Ltd in 1990
Softcover reprint of the hardcover 1st edition 1990

Contents

PART TWO *The genetically determined bullous diseases*

PART THREE *Blistering as a reaction pattern*

Contributors

Grant J. Anhalt	Immunodermatology Unit, The Johns Hopkins University School of Medicine, Baltimore, MD, USA
David J. Atherton	Department of Dermatology, The Hospital for Sick Children, Great Ormond Street, London, UK
Eugene A. Bauer	Department of Dermatology, Stanford University, Stanford, CA, USA
B.S. Bhogal	Institute of Dermatology, United Medical and Dental Schools, Guys and St Thomas's Hospitals, London, UK
David R. Bickers	Department of Dermatology, Case Western Reserve University School of Medicine, Cleveland, Ohio, USA
Martin M. Black	Institute of Dermatology, United Medical and Dental Schools, Guys and St Thomas's Hospitals, London, UK
Stephen Michael Breathnach	Department of Medicine, Charing Cross and Westminster Medical School, London, UK
Robert A. Briggaman	Department of Dermatology, University of North Carolina School of Medicine, Chapel Hill, NC, USA
Robert Charles-Holmes	Warneford Hospital, Leamington Spa, Warwickshire, UK
Luis A. Diaz	Immunodermatology Unit, The Johns Hopkins University School of Medicine, Baltimore, MD, USA
Robin A.J. Eady	Department of Cell Pathology, Institute of Dermatology, United Medical and Dental Schools of Guys and St Thomas's Hospitals, London, UK

Jo-David Fine — Department of Dermatology, University of Alabama at Birmingham, Birmingham, AL, USA

Lionel Fry — Department of Dermatology, St Mary's Hospital, London, UK

W. Ray Gammon — Department of Dermatology, University of North Carolina School of Medicine, Chapel Hill, NC, USA

Tobias Gedde-Dahl Jr — Polar Institute of Medical Genetics, Regional Hospital and University of Tromso, Tromso, Norway

Karl Holubar — Department of Dermatology and Institute for the History of Medicine, University of Vienna, Vienna, Austria

G.M. Levene — St John's Hospital for Diseases of the Skin and Bloomsbury Skin Unit, Middlesex Hospital, London, UK

R.A. Marsden — Department of Dermatology, St George's Hospital, London, UK

Lynne H. Morrison — Immunodermatology Unit, The Johns Hopkins University School of Medicine, Baltimore, MD, USA

Stephan Müller — Dermatology Branch, National Cancer Institute, NIH, Bethesda, MD, USA

Jean-Claude Roujeau — Service de Dermatologie, Hôpital Henri Mondor, 94010 Creteil, France

John R. Stanley — Dermatology Branch, National Cancer Institute, NIH, Bethesda, MD, USA

Michael J. Tidman — University Department of Dermatology, The Royal Infirmary, Edinburgh, UK

Vanessa A. Venning — Department of Dermatology, The Slade Hospital, Headington, Oxford, UK

Fenella Wojnarowska — Department of Dermatology, The Slade Hospital, Headington, Oxford, UK

David T. Woodley — Department of Dermatology, University of North Carolina School of Medicine, Chapel Hill, NC, USA

Preface

The blistering (bullous) diseases, although relatively uncommon, are of major clinical and scientific importance. Patients with bullous diseases can present great difficulties in diagnosis and management. The bullous diseases are life-threatening and many patients perish either from their disease or from complications of therapy. They may present to dermatologists, general physicians, paediatricians, oral surgeons, dentists, otolaryngologists and ophthalmologists. All of these specialities may be involved in their management.

The acquired bullous diseases, pemphigus, bullous and cicatricial pemphigoid, epidermolysis bullosa acquisita, herpes gestationis, linear IgA disease of adults, chronic bullous disease of childhood and dermatitis herpetiformis are autoimmune diseases whose target organ is the skin. Current research on these conditions has shed light on both autoimmune phenomena and pathogenic mechanisms, and the structure and functioning of the skin. The antigen has been identified in some of these conditions.

The genetically determined mechanobullous diseases, epidermolysis bullosa simplex, junctional epidermolysis bullosa and dystrophic epidermolysis bullosa require recognition and diagnosis for management, prognosis and genetic counselling.

The elucidation of the structural and functional defects in these diseases is expanding our knowledge of the skin.

In this book, emphasis has been placed on both practical management, i.e. diagnosis and therapy, and summarizing the major advances of the past decade. It is hoped that it will prove to be of practical value and stimulate scientific interest in these conditions.

Preface

Introduction

Blistering diseases often have a very dramatic clinical presentation and their occurrence in a neonate or sudden onset in a child or adult causes panic in both the patient and their relatives. Although the autoimmune and genetic blistering diseases are regarded as rare, an estimate from our local population (Oxfordshire and Buckinghamshire, England) suggests that approximately 1 in 5000 of the population may suffer from one of the bullous diseases.

The significance of these diseases is twofold: firstly clinical management is complex and challenging; secondly, the immense amount of research into them has contributed to our understanding of not only the diseases themselves but also the biology of normal skin.

CLINICAL MANAGEMENT

Blistering diseases are often abrupt in onset and very symptomatic. There is an appreciable morbidity and mortality from the diseases both in the acute and chronic stages, and although modern treatment has lessened the mortality it is still considerable. Accurate diagnosis is essential, and although each disease has a characteristic clinical presentation, many patients have misleading presentations. The technique that has made the greatest contribution to both diagnosis and research has been immunofluorescence, which has both clarified and complicated diagnosis by creating new entities. This has enabled dermatitis herpetiformis to be distinguished from linear IgA disease, and chronic bullous disease of childhood from childhood bullous pemphigoid. Immunofluorescence is currently being extended to the diagnosis of epidermolysis bullosa. The newer techniques of immunoelectron microscopy and immunoblotting or immunoprecipitation are not in routine use but are invaluable in certain cases and may eventually become routine.

The problems of clinical management do not end with diagnosis. Treatment is often difficult and dangerous; immunosuppression is associated with many problems both in the short and long term. There is a significant acute and chronic morbidity and mortality from the treatment. This is compounded by a rising elderly population who are susceptible to pemphigoid and also particularly prone to the side effects of treatment. Topical treatment is often neglected and the search for improved systemic treatments has been disappointing.

Treatment of epidermolysis bullosa (EB) is still unavailable, but practical management is greatly improved. The outlook for parents of children with epidermolysis bullosa has been revolutionized by the development of prenatal diagnosis.

RECENT ADVANCES

The most exciting devlopments in the understanding of the genetic bullous diseases is the identification of the abnormal or absent molecules in certain types of epidermolysis bullosa, e.g. the absence of GB3/AA3 in junctional epidermolysis bullosa and of type VII collagen in recessive dystrophic epidermolysis bullosa, in which the collagenase is also abnormal.

The autoimmune bullous diseases have undergone major advances in the past decade. The target antigens have been identified in bullous pemphigoid (Chapter 5), epidermolysis bullosa acquisita (Chapter 10) and pemphigus (Chapter 4), and others are near to identification. The ultrastructural localization of these molecules has been identified. In pemphigus and pemphigoid the antibody has been demonstrated to be pathogenic. The mechanisms by which the antibody–antigen reaction triggers the inflammatory cascade which results in blister formation is currently being investigated in many centres.

THE CONTRIBUTION TO SKIN BIOLOGY

The identification of the target molecules in both the genetic and autoimmue bullous diseases, and the availability of both monoclonal and polyvalent antibodies to them makes them useful probes in studying normal biology, embryology and phylogeny of skin. They have shown similarities between stratified squamous epithelium of all types and also amnion epithelium. They have also shown that many of these molecules are common not only to all mammals but also to birds and possibly reptiles. These probes have also been used to study wound healing and invasion by skin and other carcinomas. They may also be relevant to dermo-epidermal adhesion.

The increasing development and use of these antibodies should greatly increase our understanding of both skin diseases and skin biology.

One
Historical background

Karl Holubar

'Non illa pro simplici habenda est involucro,
sed organum constituit,'...

(Anne-Charles Lorry, 1726–1783) [1]

1.1 INTRODUCTION

Blisters have always attracted the physicians' attention and have been considered distinctive skin lesions worthy of specific designation. The Greeks used words such as pemphix (πέμφιξ), pomphos (πομφός), pompholyx (πομφόλυξ), phlyctaina (φλύκταινα) and phlyzakion (φλυζάκιον) [2]. The Old Testament spoke of ababuʿoth (buʿah) אֲבַעְבֻּעֹת (בועה) [3, 4]. Preuss [4] also referred to mazor (מָזוֹר) when checked under blisters; the Arabic literature cites many synonyms not unlike the Greek, for example nuffākha (نُفَّاخَة) by 'Alī ibn al-'Abbās (Haly Abbas), nuffāṭa (نُفَّاطَة) by Ibn Sīnā (Avicenna) and nafṭa (نَفْطَة) in the Murshid of at-Tamīmī from Jerusalem [5–8]. Old Chinese texts write of pào (Pinyin) (pauh according to Guoryuu Romatzyh) 疱 皰 [9, 10] or tiān pào (tianpauh) 天疱 [11, 12]. Modern dictionaries translate the expression tiān-pàochuāng (tianpauh chuang) 天疱疮 into pemphigus [5, 6]. In Latin the most common terms are *vesica*, *vesicula* and *bulla*. These terms in the various languages relate to air or liquid to insufflation or boiling, gargling.

There has been much speculation as to what ancient terms stand for, e.g. the biblical shechin (שְׁחִין) or ababuʿoth [4, 13, 14] and the Greek terms. Many were used interchangeably by various authors. Pemphigus is the only one that has developed into a modern word.

It is not much more than 250 years since systematization of diseases in a modern sense was attempted by Sauvages (the system used in botany) [15, 16]), and it is about 200 years since Plenck tried (1776), and Willan succeeded (1798), in establishing a workable system for dermatology [17, 18]. In the past, a variety of terms have been applied to ill-characterized clinical syndromes hallmarked by blisters. Today some three dozen diagnoses have to be considered when a patient presents with a blistering disorder, the exact diagnosis of which may require the most sophisticated laboratory techniques.

1.2 PEMPHIGUS AS AN ALL-ENCOMPASSING TERM FOR BLISTERING DISEASES

The term pemphigus was introduced by François Boissier de la Croix de Sauvages (1706–1767) [15, 19]. It had already been used by Hippocrates as febris pemphigodes (πυρετοὶ ... πεμφιγώδεες) [20]. This designation constitutes a hapax legomenon, i.e. it is only mentioned once in the whole Corpus Hippocraticum [21]. The corresponding noun is pemphix, pomphos (apophony) or pompholyx [22]. These forms, along with the terms phlyctaina and phlyzakion, have been applied over the centuries to bullous conditions. Pemphigus was used at first as an all-encompassing designation for blistering disorders.

Sauvages described five forms of pemphigus: maior, castrensis, helveticus, indicus and brasiliensis [19]. These forms cannot be identified with modern variants of pemphigus, even when they sound identical, e.g. pemphigus brasiliensis. This does not exclude the possibility that individual cases of the past may well have been true pemphigus. However, the majority of cases represented feverish infectious bullous eruptions. A brief biography of Sauvages is given below.

Sauvages was a pioneer of classification and order in medicine. He was born on May 12, 1706 (the day of a total eclipse [23]) in the town of Alais, Southern France. He graduated from the Medical School of Montpellier in 1725 (March 10). His thesis was entitled 'Si l'amour peut être guéri par des remedes tirés des plantes'; he became an MD on March 9, 1726 [16]. In 1731, he published his first work on classification entitled 'Nouvelles classes des maladies dans un ordre semblable à celui des botanistes, comprenant les genres et les espèces' [16]. At the age of 28 he became a professor at his Alma Mater. He was in touch with the scholars of the time, Herman Boerhaave in the Low Countries, Albrecht von Haller in Germany, and, in particular, with Carl Linnaeus (1707–1778), the Swede. Linnaeus' term 'Sauvagesia' for a plant from Cayenne, was a token of his esteem for his French colleague (Figure 1.1) [24, 25]. His main work on the classification of diseases produced 10 classes, 295 genera and more than 2400 species, a formidable array. This system did not survive but it was a forerunner of later more down-to-earth attempts, notably, those of Plenck [17] and Willan [18] in dermatology. De Ratte [23] eulogized him thus: 'M. de Sauvages, dans sa patrie plus qu'ailleurs, fut le médecin de l'amour: il eut dans sa jeunesse, ou parut avoir le coeur tendre; il faisoit de vers,'... obviously an educated and passionate young gentleman. He died on February 20, 1767 [16].

Gilibert in 1813 [26] published his monograph of cases he considered pemphigus; in 1825, Sachse [27] had collected 124 cases of pemphigus from the literature. Two authors deserve mention here – Wichmann of Erfurt and Devergie of Paris – because their descriptions illustrate the exactness of their observations. Wichmann in 1791 [28] wrote: 'die ganze Epidermis ... (war) ... so lose und runzlig, dass sie sich schieben liess und so allmählig ... die Haut sich entblösste' (the patient, a 60-year-old man died after a little more than 1 year). Devergie [29], over half a century later, gives a very similar description in his book, under the heading of pemphigus diutinus. He describes the stepwise appearance of bullae, some of which dry up, others not, ...'dans un autre point, cet épiderme s'ouvre, se détache en lamelles larges, moitié flottantes, moitié adhérentes, laissant à nu le corps muqueux ... Dans ces conditions, il s'exhale de la surface du corps un odeur fade, nauséabonde et tout spéciale au pemphigus.' Both texts describe the detachment of the epidermis (by shearing forces), a distinguishing phenomenon described by Nikolski (see page 4).

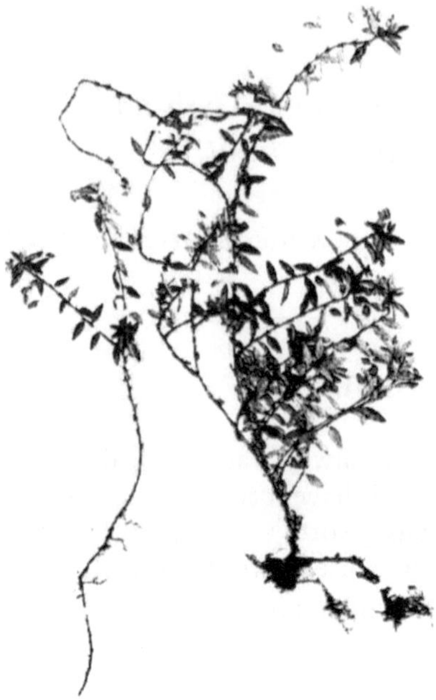

Figure 1.1 Sauvagesia erecta L. (dried). This tropical plant has been named by Linnaeus (Linné) in honour of F. Boissier de la Croix de Sauvages. There are some 12 species, most of which occur in South America (Brazil). This one is from the island of Zanzibar and belongs to the herbarium of the Naturhistorische Museum Wien, Vienna. Reproduced with permission.

In 1880, the first step in establishing the entity of

pemphigus was made. Heinrich Auspitz (1835–1886) [30, 31] coined the term *acantholysis* and described the histopathology of a pemphigus blister, stating for the first time that the stratum basale, at places, remained at the floor of the blister [32, 33]. All previous authors had only spoken of separation of the epidermis from the dermis. Unfortunately, the importance of this discovery was not recognized for another half century, possibly because of the short life and tragic career of Auspitz [34].

Lever and Talbott [35] have already tabulated the early descriptions of pemphigus and evaluated them in modern terms. The history of the various forms of modern pemphigus will be summarized.

Semantically, *pemphigus brasiliensis* is the oldest [19]. Sauvages wrote about it and referred to earlier authors, commenting 'tactus colubri bicephali apud Brasilienses, etiam mortui, excitat hanc speciem,...'. There appears to be no relation to fogo selvagem (see below) [36, 37].

Pemphigus foliaceus, historically, is the next. Cazenave coined the term in 1844. Writing in volume 1 of the first dermatological periodical (*Annales des Maladies de la Peau*, 1844–1852), he says 'Le pemphigus est une des maladies de la peau qui méritent le plus de fixer l'attention des médecins,'... and later on continues, 'cette observation offre l'éxample d'une forme rare de pemphigus chronique, forme que l'on trouve à peine indiquée dans les auteurs;... [38]. He did not claim to have observed something entirely new; de la Motte, in 1773 [39], may have described an earlier example.

Pemphigus vularis was introduced by Hebra in 1860 [40]. Discussing pemphigus in his treatise, he wrote, 'Wir wollen diese Form *Pemphigus vulgaris* nennen' [40], as opposed to pemphigus foliaceus described by Cazenave 18 years earlier.

Pemphigus vegetans was described later. Usually it carries the eponym Neumann (Isidor Neumann 1832–1906) and the year 1886 [41]. Actually, Neumann had described it 10 years earlier in 1876 [42] and he referred to even earlier descriptions of similar cases by Kaposi in 1869 (then still Kohn) [43], and by Auspitz [44], who referred back to Alibert, Willan and Bateman, Plenck and, ultimately, Sauvages.

There are even earlier reports of pemphigus, e.g. the reports by König in 1681 [45], de la Motte in 1773 [39], MacBride in 1777 [46] and Wichmann in 1791 [28].

1.3 THE IDENTIFICATION OF PEMPHIGUS AND THE ACQUIRED BULLOUS DISEASES

The eighties of the last century were the beginning of a new era in pemphigus research. Auspitz created a new system of skin diseases in 1880–1885 [30–33]. There were nine classes, the seventh of which was subdivided into the families of keratonoses, chromatoses and akanthoses (spelt with a 'k'). The latter were subdivided further into hyperakanthoses, parakanthoses and akantholyses. Pemphigus was listed under acantholyses (the modern spelling) and the blister formation in pemphigus was called acantholytic, as opposed to spongiotic, blister formation in inflammatory conditions of the skin. Loss of the intercellular bridges and loss of cohesion between the epidermal cells was considered by Auspitz to be responsible for blister formation. He described, part of the cylindrical basal layer of cells remaining on the floor of the blister, i.e. suprabasal blister formation, and he gave it a separate name, *acantholysis*. For this reason Auspitz's description must be considered a landmark in pemphigus research. Unfortunately, his system did not appeal to the dermatological world of the time and nor did acantholysis – both were buried with him.

There were earlier equivocal reports on intra-epithelial blister formation, e.g. Haight's in 1868 [47].

Louis Adolphus Duhring from Philadelphia described a new entity in 1884 and called it dermatitis herpetiformis [48]. Heinrich Köbner of Breslau (now Wroclaw), one of Hebra's Jewish pupils, created the term epidermolysis bullosa hereditaria in litteral allusion to Auspitz's acantholysis in 1886 [49]. Both terms were not immediately accepted, and one can easily imagine how confusing the whole field appeared at this point.

At the beginning of the following decade, in 1891, Ernest Besnier and Adrien Doyon, two famous French dermatologists translated Kaposi's textbook into French from German, with an extensive commentary. This is an invaluable source of critical evaluation of the state of the art: the chapter on bullous dermatoses alone makes up more than 30 pages of small print! Therein the confusion of terms and clinical syndromes is stressed: 'Dans le sens traditionel, le terme de "pemphigus" sert à designer radicalement la presque totalité des affections bulleuses, que l'on specific ensuite par des qualificatifs rariés, mais ces affections sont si nombreuses, si profondément diverses, que cette unité nominale est devenue l'occasion de la plus grande confusion dans la nomenclature ...' [50].

A decade later, Brocq [51] used more than 100 printed pages to deal with 'les pemphigus', 30 of which are devoted to the intricacies of terminology and differences in perception by individual authors. He writes 'La question du pemphigus est encore à l'heure actuelle une des plus discutées de dermatologie'. The following forms of pemphigus were still grouped together; acute febrile; true chronic; vegetans; foliaceus; des jeunes filles et des hystériques; traumatic; epidemic, of child and adult. Brocq elaborated two important points hitherto only expressed in the original studies: the histopathology of true pemphigus and the Nikolski sign. He described three types of blisters: subcorneal, suprabsal and subepidermal [51].

Piotr Vasilievitch Nikolski (1858–1940) had written his first observation of the Nikolski sign in a case report of a 44-year-old Jewish woman, from Professor Stoukovenkoff's department in Kiev [52]. His thesis on the subject appeared in Kiev in 1895. The phenomenon was originally considered only to represent the shearing off of the stratum corneum from the underlying layers of the skin by pressure, e.g. with the fingertip. Nowadays it includes sliding off of all layers above the basal layer. In 1900 and 1901 this phenomenon was made internationally known by Danlos and Dubreuilh [53, 54].

As a result of the First World War, no pertinent developments were recorded in the following decade. Therefore let us move on to the twenties and consider another grand master – Ferdinand-Jean Darier (1856–1938) – and the third edition of his *Précis de dermatologie*, 1923 [55]. The chapter on bullous dermatoses bears the heading 'Phlyctènes et dermatoses bulleuses', and his subdivisions are acute pemphigus, congenital pemphigus (epidermolysis hereditaria), pemphigus hystérique and chronic true pemphigus. It is notable that Darier describes the types of blisters as superficial (or subcorneal), subepithelial or acantholytic (without reference to Auspitz). According to him all three types may be observed in true pemphigus (pemphigoid and dermatitis herpetiformis were not separated). Darier considered the Nikolski sign to be a consequence of acantholysis [55], the importance of which he emphasized. A biographical sketch of Darier is given below.

As described above, Sauvages was born in Alais (now known as Alès) in the south of France. In this city, King Louis XIII partially revoked the Edict of Hantes in 1629. Originally this edict also granted rights to Protestants (Henri IV, 1598), and it was completely revoked by Louis XIV, in 1685. In the aftermath of this act, the ancestors of F.J. Darier left their native country and turned to Geneva, where they became citizens a century later. Jules Darier, born 1817, made a journey to Vienna where he met another Genèvoise Jean-Justin Rey, director of the First Danube Steamship Company of Vienna [the oldest (1829) and biggest of its kind]. Jules Darier was persuaded to stop painting and become a (successful) businessman. He moved to Trieste, then Austria's main port, but frequently returned to Vienna where he married Anne (Annette) Rey in 1847. Shortly after, the couple moved to Hungary. Ferdinand Jean, their second son, was born on April 26, 1856, in Budapest. In 1864 the family moved to Geneva, where Jean attended the gymnasium and the first year of university. In 1877 Darier went to Paris university in the country of his ancestors. The remainder of Darier's life is too well known to be repeated here. He died on June 4, 1938, in Longpont-sur-Orge, where he had been mayor for many years. See the beautiful treatise on his life by Marie-Paule and Gérard Ledoux [56, 56a].

1.3.1 Pemphigus erythematosus

In 1926 Francis Eugene Senear and Barney Usher described a new form of pemphigus [57], calling it an 'unusual type of pemphigus'. The name *pemphigus erythematosus* was not proposed until 1933 by Ormsby [58]. Earlier cases had been presented by Ormsby and Mitchell in 1921 [59] and the Haileys in 1925 [60, 61]. Pemphigus erythematosus and pemphigus foliaceus are considered to be related, comprising superficial pemphigus (a question that remains controversial). One wonders whether the case described by Cazenave in 1844, which stimulated him to create the foliaceus type of pemphigus, may not originally have presented as pemphigus erythematosus: 'A woman with a four-year history of alleged facial erysipelas, slowly extending over neck and body with subsequent appearance of features of pemphigus just within this area' [38].

1.3.2 Pemphigus vulgaris

In the 1930s, Auspitz's findings and terminology had gained recognition [62, 63]. But it was Achille Civatte in 1943 who eventually continued what his teacher and friend Darier had initiated, i.e. emphasizing the importance of acantholysis for the histopathological diagnosis of pemphigus, again without reference to Auspitz, despite many allusions to the École de Vienne, to Hebra and Kaposi, etc. [64]. Civatte's paper was a landmark. He wrote 'there are no intraepidermal ("intra-malpighiennes") bullae in dermatitis herpetiformis ... the bullae are always subepidermal' or 'C'est *cette acantholyse*, très facile à reconnaître, *qui constitute la lésion élémentaire histologique du pemphigus*'. His illustrations unmistakably depict intraepithelial, partly suprabasal, split formation and acantholytic cells [64]. By this time Lever's extensive work (historical and histopathological) was already under way [65]. Another crucial period in pemphigus research had begun.

Lever himself reports how he and his collaborators started to recheck all the cases of bullous disorders of the Massachusetts General Hospital in Boston 1936. The results of their work were published in 1951 [65] in the classical study on the histopathology of pemphigus. Acantholysis is described and the Nikolski phenomenon explained on its basis, thereby confirming and expanding Civatte's studies of 1943. 'Pemphigus vulgaris...has a *characteristic* diagnostic histologic appearance... The essential histologic feature... is the loss of intercellular bridges and other degenerative changes in the cells of the lower epidermis leading to acantholysis and formation of clefts within the lower epidermis, predominantly located in suprabasal position with only the basal layer remaining adherent to the corium' [65]. Lever credits acantholysis to Civatte; Auspitz is not mentioned.

In this study by Lever [65], there is still only a 'pemphigus vulgaris acutus' or true malignant pemphigus vulgaris and a 'pemphigus vulgaris chronicus', the former with, the latter without, acantholysis.

1.3.3 Pemphigus brasiliensis

Pemphigus brasiliensis, more frequently called Brazilian pemphigus, had been described in the meantime by Joao Paulo Viera from Brazil. Not surprisingly, he refers to reports from earlier in this century; he mentions various names but does not give specific references [36]. He also introduces the synonym of fogo selvagem (wild fire) and tabulates three acute and nine chronic clinical forms. Nevertheless, pemphigus brasiliensis is commonly conceived as a foliaceus-type of pemphigus with an initial bullous phase. From this time, foci of outbreaks of pemphigus brasiliensis were noticed and theories about vectors and a possible infectious origin were established.

1.3.4 Pemphigoid and cicatricial pemphigoid

In his 1953 monograph, Lever introduces the term pemphigoid [60]. The alternative term, parapemphigus, of Prakken and Woerdeman did not appeal to the dermatological world [66].

Benign mucous membrane pemphigoid or *cicatricial pemphigoid* (ocular pemphigus, pemphigus mucosae, etc.) was also classified by Lever in 1953 [60]. Earlier reports of this disease are available, e.g. Thost [67,68] and Wichmann [69]. A special variant of mucosal pemphigoid was reported by Brunsting and Perry in 1957 [70]; it has borne their name as an eponym ever since.

1.3.5 Herpes gestationis

This was named by Milton in 1872 [71]. Again, several previous reports are known describing patients with gestational blistering dermatoses. Bunel, in his thesis of 1811, reports such an observation [72]. Chausit in 1852 beautifully describes cases as pemphigus aigu pruriginosus [73] as does Köbner in 1869 [74] and Hebra in 1860 [40]. In 1884, Duhring considers this dermatosis to constitute a variant of his dermatitis herpetiformis. Riecke, in 1931, mentions more than a dozen synonyms [75]. No clarification was possible before immunopathological methods were introduced. Thereafter, it was clear that herpes gestationis belonged to the group of bullous pemphigoid (see Chapter 5) [76].

1.3.6 Immunopathology and its contribution

Beutner, Jordon and collaborators reported their revolutionary findings of pemphigus antibodies in 1964/65 [77, 78]. Antibodies to antigens of the intercellular area of stratified squamous epithelium had been detected, which bind *in vivo* and *in vitro* to pemphigus skin or to substrate tissue. Two years later (1967) complementary results regarding bullous pemphigoid followed from the same laboratory. This time, antigens of the basement membrane zone were involved. In the same year, Rudi Cormane of Amsterdam reported his preliminary findings of immunoglobulin deposition in the skin in dermatitis herpetiformis [79]. In 1969 van der Meer, Cormane's pupil, published the first study on dermatitis herpetiformis, proving the deposition of IgA in the skin of these patients [80]. Soon after, the deposition of C3 was also detected [81]. In only 5 years the pathogenetic concepts of most of the major bullous diseases had been revolutionized.

Confirmatory results obtained with immuno-electron microscopic techniques followed [82, 83]. There was no longer any doubt that the reactions actually took place in the intercellular area in pemphigus, in the basement membrane zone in pemphigoid, cicatricial pemphigoid and herpes gestationis, and differently in dermatitis herpetiformis. And there was more confirmatory evidence to come: tissue culture studies and antibody-transfer experiments were performed; *in vivo* and *in vitro* models were designed and antigens started to be isolated from the various diseases in question (see Part One) [77, 78, 83–85]. However, the prospects for certain fields of dermatology appeared brighter than they really were. Some of the most disputed diseases, for instance pemphigus and pemphigoid, could soon be explained with regard to their pathogenesis, but less well so dermatitis herpetiformis. However, new 'entities' were described and soon several more diseases had been discovered as a result of the introduction of immunofluorescence techniques, e.g. *chronic bullous disease of childhood acquisita* (Chapter 9) [86], *linear IgA disease* (Chapter 8), *epidermolysis bullosa acquisita* (Chapter 10) and *bullous lupus erythematosus* (Chapter 18) [87–89].

1.3.7 Pemphigus herpetiformis (herpetiform pemphigus)

This is the most recent form of pemphigus to be described by Jabłońska *et al.* in 1975 [90]. Their studies were based on earlier reports [91–93]. This form of pemphigus, with the clinical picture of a herpetiform papulo-vesiculo-bullous eruption, cannot be recognized as pemphigus on purely clinical or histological grounds [91], without immunopathological work up. This form must have been encountered earlier as the designations of pemphigus circinatus or serpiginosus demonstrate [94].

Lever in 1979 [83] outlined the concepts of the major bullous disorders valid then. Subsequent reviews have updated pemphigus [95, 96], pemphigoid [84] and dermatitis herpetiformis [85].

Unfortunately, Rudi Cormane of Amsterdam met his untimely death recently. Because of his substantial contributions to the field, I hope the reader will permit a few lines as an epitaph. Born in the then Dutch East Indies, in Bandung on Java, in 1925 on the 7th of April (the anniversary of Robert Willan's in 1812), his youth was marred by internment in the war and by poliomyelitis during medical school. He was of noble ancestry and lived up to noble standards, bravely facing these adversities in life. Undeterred by physical handicap he made his mark as a human being, a physician and a dermatologist. A believer in an ecumenical format, a man of gentle character, he passed away on February 18, 1987. He will not be forgotten by those who knew him.

1.4 THE GENETICALLY DETERMINED MECHANOBULLOUS DISEASES

1.4.1 Pemphigus familiaris chronicus benignus (Hailey–Hailey)

In April of 1939 the Hailey brothers described four patients with the above diagnosis [97]. Ayres and Anderson reported five other cases in the same year and acknowledged them to be 'of exactly the same nature' as the Haileys' cases [98]. One had been under their care since 1921. For a number of years, there was an animated discussion in the literature as to whether it is justified to consider this disease as a separate entity or whether it was rather a variant of Darier's disease [99, 100]. The negative immunofluorescence results definitively excluded Hailey–Hailey's disease from the pemphigus group, and today it is considered a separate entity, a genodermatosis [101].

1.4.2 Epidermolysis bullosa hereditaria

As has been mentioned above, the term was created and introduced by Köbner in 1886 in an explicit allusion to Auspitz's acantholysis [49]. In today's terminology the hereditaria is dropped and another term added to specify the form under consideration. For the purpose of a historical review the original terminology will be adhered to. Köbner's paper was printed only about 20 years after the trail-blazing work by Johann Gregor Mendel (1822–1884) in the 1860s and no differentiation between autosomal and X-linked, recessive and dominant was possible then. Köbner himself alluded to earlier reports, e.g. Goldscheider, 1882 [102], Fox, 1879 [103] and Hebra, 1860 [104]. Riecke in 1931 [105] listed 30 synonyms for the condition. This makes superfluous any comment about the confusion which must have existed at one time or other [106]. The advent of electron microscopy, with the elucidation of the fine structural morphology of the epidermis and the junctional zone and advances in molecular biology and genetics have permitted a better insight and the differentiation of a series of variants (see Part Two). Gedde-Dahl and Anton-Lamprecht [107,108] speak of at least 16 genetic loci responsible for the expression of the many variants known today. Their papers also nicely depict the micromorphology of the basement membrane area, a prerequisite for the interested reader. The only 'withdrawal' from the group of epidermolysis bullosa hereditaria, is epidermolysis bullosa acquisita (see Chapter 10).

1.5 BLISTERING AS A REACTION PATTERN

Pompholyx has, since ancient times, been used as a synonym for many a bullous disorder. Willan preferred it as a term for pemphigus [18]. Today, however, pompholyx is a morphological rather than a nosological designation, customarily reserved for dyshidrotic constitutional eczema, restricted to hands and feet.

Herpes is another age-old term, used even by the ancient Greek physicians. *Sensu strictiori*, the term herpes should be reserved for diseases of viral origin presenting with grouped blisters or vesicles (save herpes gestationis).

Dermatitis exfoliativa neonatorum was described originally by Gottfried Ritter von Rittershain in 1878 in Prague [109]. In today's terminology, the disease is staphylococcal scalded-skin syndrome (SSSS) [110].

Toxic epidermal necrolysis (Lyell, 1956) [111] should probably be considered to be related, or identical with, *butcher's pemphigus* and severe erythema exsudativum multiforme (see Chapter 17). Butcher's pemphigus was described by George Pernet and William Bulloch in 1896 [112]. A series of cases of acute pemphigus are reported: 'There is a group of rare cases of acute bullous eruption, accompanied by severe constitutional symptoms, and generally terminating fatally, which affects butchers.' Pernet had reported seven cases (four of his own) the year before [113]. In this latter paper, Pernet refers to Sir George Burrows, who had seen a similar case in a butcher in 1856, and another one in 1854. Further references in Pernet's paper of 1895 [113] are not followed up, because the evidence presented is weak. It does not always relate to butchers and cannot be evaluated in today's terms.

Porphyria cutanea tarda will be the last subject to receive attention from a medicohistorical point of view. Porphyrias are complex and, in part, genetically mediated disorders with many clinically and biologically different manifestations. The following will refer only to porphyria cutanea tarda. The term was introduced by Waldenström in 1937 [114]. Reports from the last century are available. Johann Heinrich Schultz, of Frankenhagen (West-Prussia) wrote a thesis in 1874 (University of Greifswald), in which he presented a case with porphyria and a bullous eruption. Reading the report, one is convinced that photosensitivity was the cause of the blisters [115]. Baumstark, working up the same case, reported the detection of porphyric compounds in the urine [116]. The diagnosis of porphyria cutanea tarda is possible but not certain.

Bullous lichen planus, pyoderma gangraenosum, bullous amyloidosis, bullous mycosis fungoides, bullosis diabeticorum, UV-induced blisters, friction blisters, blisters after insect bites or after contact or ingestion of toxic substances are representatives of an endless variety of blistering conditions, a historical perspective of which would be impossible.

1.6 CONCLUSIONS

In all too many cases we are unable to identify the aetiology and pathogenesis of blister formation. On the other hand, there are conditions (diseases), the nature of which we are reasonably sure. Certain of these diseases carry a name which is hallowed by medical tradition. Pemphigus is such a term and such a disease. Historical evaluation is performed by posterity, and only then, when medical reasoning may have become more refined, does identification of diseases become possible [117]. The world literature abounds with examples.

ACKNOWLEDGEMENTS

Professor Arne A. Ambros (Vienna), Dr Roberto Doglia Azambuja (Brasilia), Professor Albert Dietrich (Göttingen), Dr Louis Dulieu (Montpellier), Professor John A.A. Hunter (Edinburgh), Professor Samuel Kottek (Jerusalem), Professor Charles Lapière (Liège), Mme Dolores Liret (Paris), Professor Ma. Kanwen (Beijing), Herr M.A. Jian (Vienna), Dr Roger Meyer (Geneva), Dr Lawrence Charles Parish (Philadelphia), Dozent Dr Harald Riedl (Vienna), Professor Leonid S. Rosenstrauch (Moscow), Professor Manfred Ullmann (Tübingen), Professor Vladimir Vladimirow (Moscow), Dr Daniel Wallach (Paris), Dr Franz Wawrik (Vienna).

REFERENCES

1. Lorry, Anne-Charles (1777) *Tractatus de Morbis Cutaneis*, P.G. Cavelier, Paris, p. 2.
2. Liddell, H.G. and Scott, R. (1968) *A Greek–English Lexicon.* Revised and augmented throughout by Sir H.S. Jones *et al.* with a supplement. Clarendon Press, Oxford.
3. Mandelkern, S. (1896, 1985) *Veteris Testamenti Concordantiae Hebraicae Atque Chaldaicae*, Veit et Comp, Leipzig (Feldheim, Jerusalem), p. 180.
4. Preuss, J. (1911, reprinted 1978) *Biblisch–talmudische Medizin (Biblical and Talmudic Medicine)*, translated and edited by F. Rosner, Sanhedrin Press, New York, pp. 630, 343, 194.
5. Wehr, H. (1971) *A Dictionary of Modern Written Arabic* (ed. M. Cowan), Harrassowitz, Wiesbaden, pp. 982, 987.
6. Ullmann, M. (1987) Personal communication.
7. Ullmann, M. (1970) *Die Medizin im Islam*, in *Handbuch der Orientalistik* (Ergänzungsband VI) (ed. B. Spuler) Brill, Leiden, pp. 140ff, 152ff.
8. Sezgin, F. (1970) *Die Geschichte des arabischen Schrifttums*, vol. III, Medizin-Pharmazie-Zoologie-Tierheilkunde bis ca 430 H, Brill, Leiden, p. 317ff.
9. *A Chinese–English Dictionary* (1979) Commercial Publishers, Beijing, pp. 511, 677.
10. *Lin Yutang's Chinese–English Dictionary of Modern Usage* (1972) The Chinese University of Hongkong, Hongkong, pp. 909, 475.
11. Chén Shígōng (1617) *Wèi Kē Zhèng Zōng (Orthodox Manual of Surgery)* Courtesy of Professor M.A. Kanwen, Beijing.
12. *Yī Zōng Jīh Jiàn (Golden Mirror of Medicine)* (1742) Vol. 74, Courtesy of Professor Ma. Kanwen, Beijing.
13. Ingber, A. (1987) What is really the biblical 'shechin'? Letter to the editor. *Amer. J. Dermatopathol.*, 9, 81.

14. Hoenig, L. (1987) Letter to the editor (reply to the former). *Amer. J. Dermatopathol.*, **9**, 82.
15. Sauvages, François Boissier de la Croix de (1731) *Nouvelles Classes des Maladies dans un Ordre Semblable à celui des Botanistes, Comprenant les Genres et les Espèces*, d'Avanville, Avignon.
16. Dulieu, L. (1969) François Boissier de Sauvages (1706–1767) *Revue d'histoire des Sciences et de leurs Applications*, Presses universitaires de France, Vendôme, pp. 303–322.
17. Plenck, J.J. (1776) *Doctrina de Morbis Cutaneis qua hi Morbi in suas Classes, Genera et Species Rediguntur*, R. Graeffer, Vienna.
18. Willan, R. (1798) *Description and Treatment of Cutaneous Diseases. Order I. Papulous Eruptions on the Skin*, J. Johnson, London.
19. Sauvages, François Boissier de la Croix de (1768) *Nosologia Methodica Sistens Morborum Classes juxta Sydenhami Mentem et Botanicorum Ordinem*, de Tournes, Amsterdam, p. 430.
20. van der Linden, J. (1665) *Magni Hippocratis Coi Opera Omnia. Graece et latine*, Vol. I, Gaasbeeck, Leiden, p. 798, 47–51.
21. Manetti, D. and Roselli, A. (1982) *Ippocrate: Epidemie Libro Sexto. Introduzione, Testo Critico, Commentario e Traduzione.* (*Biblioteca di Studi Superiori* LXVI), La nuova Italia ed, Firenze, p. 17.
22. Frisk, H. (1973) *Griechisches etymologisches Wörterbuch*, 2nd edn, Vol II, C. Winter, Heidelberg, pp. 503, 1030.
23. de Ratte, E.-H. (1768) Eloge de Monsieur de Sauvages, in *Nosologia methodica. Sistens Morborum Classes juxta Sydenhami Mentem et Bolanicorum Ordinem*, de Tournes, Amsterdam, pp. 3–21.
24. Farr, E.R., Leussink, J.A. and Stafleu, F.A. (eds) (1979) *Index Nominorum Genericorum (Plantarum), Vol. II, Pegaeophyton-Zyzygium*, Bohn, Scheltema and Holkema, Utrecht and Junk, The Hague, p. 1560.
25. Moeller, J. and Thoms, H. (eds) (1908) *Real-Enzyklopädie der gesamten Pharmazie, Vol. XI, S-Szutor*, 2nd edn, Urban and Schwarzenberg, Berlin, Vienna, p. 153.
26. Gilibert, S. (1813) *Monographie du Pemphigus ou Traité de la Maladie Vesiculaire*, Panckoucke, Paris.
27. Sachse, J.D.W. (1825) *Nosologisch-ätiologische Abhandlung über den Pemphigus* (eds C.W. Hufel and E. Osann), *Journal der praktischen Heilkunde*, 4 (Oktober), pp. 3–53, 5 (November), pp. 28–63.
28. Wichmann, J.E. (1791) *Beytrag zur Kenntniss des Pemphigus*, G.A. Keyser, Erfurt.
29. Devergie, A. (1854) *Traité Pratique des Maladies de la Peau*, Masson, Paris, pp. 296–309.
30. Auspitz, H. (1880) System der Hautkrankheiten. *Arch. Derm. Syph.*, **12**, 293–305.
31. Auspitz, H. (1881) *System der Hautkrankheiten*, Braumüller, Vienna, pp. 143–62.
32. Auspitz, H. (1883) Allgemeine Nosolgie der Haut, in *Handbuch der speciellen Pathologie und Therapie* (ed. H.V. Ziemssen). Vol. 14, Part 1, F.C.W. Vogel, Leipzig, pp. 208–12.
33. Auspitz, H. (1885) Pathology and therapeutics of the skin, in *Handbook of Diseases of the Skin* (ed. H.V. Ziemssen), Wood & Company, New York, pp. 108–9.
34. Holubar, K. (1986) Remembering Heinrich Auspitz. *Amer. J. Dermatopathol.*, **8**, 83–5.
35. Lever, W.F. and Talbott, J.H. (1942) Pemphigus. A historical study. *Arch. Dermatol.*, **46**, 800–23.
36. Vieira, J.P. (1940) Pemphigus foliaceus (fogo selvagem). *Arch. Dermatol.*, **41**, 858–63.
37. Martins-Castro, R., Roscoe, J.T. and Sampaio, S.A.P. (1983) Brazilian pemphigus foliaceus, in *Clinics in Dermatology* Vol. 1, No. 2. (Pemphigus) (ed. L.C. Parish) Lippincott, Philadelphia, pp. 23–41.
38. Cazenave, P.L.A. (1844) Pemphigus chronique, général; forme rare de pemphigus foliacé; mort; autopsie; altération du foie. *Annales des Maladies de la Peau et de la Syphilis*, **1**, 208–10.
39. de la Motte, G.M. (1773) Sur une maladie singulière de l'epiderme, communiquée à M. Banaud, docteur en médecine, in *Observations sur la Physique, sur l'Histoire Naturelle et sur les Arts*, M. l'Abbé Rozier, Hôtel de Thou Paris, pp. 22–4.
40. Hebra, F. (1860) Acute Exantheme und Hautkrankheiten, in *Handbuch der speciellen Pathologie und Therapie*, Vol. 3, (ed. R. Virchow), F. Enke, Erlangen, pp. 572–601.
41. Neumann, I. (1886) Ueber Pemphigus vegetans (frambosioides). *Arch. Derm. Syph.*, **18**, 157–78.
42. Neumann, I. (1876) Beitrag zur Kenntniss des Pemphigus, in *Medizinische Jahrbücher* (ed. S. Stricker), Braumüller, Vienna, pp. 409–16.
43. Kohn, M. (Kaposi) (1869) Ueber die sogenannte Framboesia und mehrere andere Arten von papillären Neubildungen der Haut. *Arch. Derm. Syph.*, **1**, 382–423.
44. Auspitz, H. (1869) Herpes vegetans. *Arch. Derm. Syph.*, **1**, 246–252.
45. König, S. (1681) *Disputationes Morborum Historiam et Curationem Facientes*, Vol. 3, (ed. A. Haller), Lausanne 1757, pp. 476–81 (reference to Berne 1685 and 1681).
46. MacBride, D. (1787) Introduction méthodique à la théorie et à la pratique de la médecine (originally in English, Dublin 1777, translated by M. Petit-Radel), Vol. II, P.J. Duplain, Paris, pp. 541–42.
47. Haight, D. (1868) Über Blasenbildung bei einigen Hautkrankheiten. Sitzungsberichte der kaiserlichen Akademie der Wissenschaften, mathe-

matisch-naturwissenschaftliche Classe, Vol. 57, k.k.Hof- und Staatsdruckerei, Vienna, pp. 633–40.
48. Duhring, L.A. (1884) Dermatitis herpetiformis. *J. Amer. Med. Assoc.*, 3, 225–9.
49. Köbner, H. (1886) II. Hereditäre Anlage zur Blasenbildung (Epidermolysis bullosa hereditaria). *Dtsch. Med. Wochenschr.*, **12**, 21–2.
50. Besnier, E. and Doyon, A. (1891) Appendice des traducteurs, in M. Kaposi's *Pathologie et Traitement des Maladies de la Peau* (translated from German), 2nd edn, Vol. II, Masson, Paris, pp. 822–54.
51. Brocq, L. (1902) Les pemphigus, in Besnier E., Brocq L., Jacquet L, *La pratique Dermatologique*, Vol. I (eds E. Besnier, L. Brocq and L. Jacquet), Masson, Paris, pp. 721–838.
52. Nikolski, P.V. (1894) Case of pemphigus foliaceus Cazenave. *Medizinskoye Obosrenye*, 1894, No. 2, 126–30 (in Russian).
53. Danlos, H.A. (1900) Societé Française de Dermatologie et de Syphiligraphie, séance du 8 novembre 1900: Dermatite herpétiforme avec diminuition au niveau des parties saines et de l'adhérence de la couche cornée (signe de Nikolsky). *Annal. Derm. Syph. 4th Ser.*, **2**, 1164–6.
54. Dubreuilh, W. (1901) Societé Francaise de Dermatologie et de Syphiligraphie, séance du 10 janvier 1901: Le signe de Nikolsky dans le pemphigus. *Annal. Derm. Syph. 4th Ser.*, **1**, 72–4.
55. Darier, F.J. (1923) *Précis de Dermatologie*, Masson et Cie, Paris, pp. 198–223.
56. Ledoux, M.P. and Ledoux, G. (1987) *Ferdinand-Jean Darier (1856–1938)*, Société historique de Longpont-sur-Orge.
56a. Holubar, K. (1988) Epidermolysis bullosa acquisita, *Am. J. Dermatopathol.*, **10**, 375.
57. Senear, F.E. and Usher, B. (1926) An unusual type of pemphigus, *Arch. Dermatol.*, **13**, 761–81.
58. Ormsby, O. (1934) Discussion of a case presentation by H. Ebert and B.B. Beeson, Chicago Dermatological Society, November 15, 1933 (pemphigus erythematodes). *Arch. Dermatol.*, **29**, 772–3.
59. Ormsby, O. and Mitchell, J.H. (1921) Case presentation at the Chicago Dermatological Society, May 18, 1921 (case for diagnosis). *Arch. Dermatol.*, **4**, 284.
60. Lever, W.F. (1953) Pemphigus. *Medicine*, **32**, 2–123.
61. Lever, W.F. (1965) *Pemphigus and Bullous Pemphigoid*, C.C. Thomas, Springfield.
62. Lapière, M. (1939) A propos du diagnostic différential du pemphigus chronique vulgaire et de la dermatite polymorphe de Duhring–Brocq. *Arch. Belges Derm. Syph.*, **1**, 216–22.
63. Pawlow, S.T. (1933) Zur Frage des Wesens des Nikolskyphänomens bei Pemphigus foliaceus. *Arch. Derm. Syph.*, **168**, 116–24.
64. Civatte, A. (1943) Diagnostic histopathologique de la dermatite polymorphe douloureuse ou maladie de Duhring–Brocq. *Annal. Derm. Syph. 8th Ser.*, **3**, 1–30.
65. Lever, W.F. (1951) Pemphigus. A histopathologic study. *Arch. Dermatol.*, **64**, 727–53.
66. Prakken, J.R. and Woerdeman, M.J. (1955) "Pemphigoid" (parapemphigus): its relationship to other bullous dermatoses. *Brit. J. Dermatol.*, **67**, 92–7.
67. Thost, A. (1911) Ueber Schleimhautpemphigus. *Arch. Laryngol. Rhinol.*, **25**, 459–78.
68. Thost, A. (1918) Der chronische Schleimhautpemphigus der oberen Luftwege. *Arch. Laryngol. Rhinol.*, **31**, 599–631.
69. Wichmann, J.E. (1798) *Ideen zur Diagnostik* (*on pemphigus and on febris bullosa*, p. 46), *mit van Ghelenschen Schriften* (no publisher mentioned), Vienna (a later edition under the same title appeared in Hanover, Helwigsche Hofbuchhandlung, 1800, pp. 88–90).
70. Brunsting, L.A. and Perry, H.O. (1957) Benign pemphigoid? A report of seven cases with chronic, scarring herpetiform plaques about the head and neck. *Arch. Dermatol.*, **75**, 489–501.
71. Milton, J.L. (1872) *Pathology and Treatment of Diseases of the Skin*, Hardwicke, London, pp. 202–6.
72. Bunel, J.H.B. (1811) Essai sur le pemphigus, Thesis, Paris.
73. Chausit, M. (1851/52) Pemphigus aigu prurginosus. *Annales des Maladies de la Peau*, **4**, 141–7.
74. Köbner, H. (1869) Zur Streitfrage über die Existenz eines Pemphigus acutus. *Arch. Derm. Syph.*, **1**, 209–18.
75. Riecke, E. (1931) Pemphigus (including herpes gestationis), in *Handbuch für Haut- und Geschlechtskrankheiten*, Vol. VII, Part 2 (ed. J. Jadassohn), Springer, Berlin, pp. 358–759 (herpes gestationis: pp. 637–759).
76. Holmes, R.C. and Black, M.M. (1983) The specific dermatoses of pregnancy. *J. Amer. Acad. Dermatol.*, 8, 405–12.
77. Beutner, E.H., Chorzelski, T.P. and Jordon, R.E. (1970) *Autosensitization in Pemphigus and Bullous Pemphigoid*, C.C. Thomas, Springfield.
78. Beutner, E.H., Chorzelski, T.P. and Kumar, V. (eds) (1987) *Immunopathology of the Skin*, 3rd edn, J Wiley & Sons, New York.
79. Cormane, R.H. (1967) Immunofluroescent studies of the skin in lupus erythematosus and other diseases. *Pathol. Eur.*, **2**, 170–80.
80. van der Meer, J.B. (1969) Granular deposits of immunoglobulins in the skin of patients with

dermatitis herpetiformis. An immunofluorescent study. *Brit. J. Dermatol.*, **81**, 493–503.
81. Holubar, K., Doralt, M. and Eggerth, G. (1971) Immunofluorescence patterns in dermatitis herpetiformis. Investigations on skin and intestinal mucosa. *Brit. J. Dermatol.*, **85**, 505–10.
82. Hönigsmann, H., Stingl, G., Holubar, K. *et al.* (1976) Antibodies and immune complexes in immunodermatology. Mapping of fine structural binding sites. *J. Invest. Dermatol.*, **66**, 263 (abstr.).
83. Lever, W.F. (1979) Pemphigus and pemphigoid. A review of the advances made since 1964. *J. Amer. Acad. Dermatol.*, **1**, 2–31.
84. Korman, N. (1987) Bullous pemphigoid. *J. Amer. Acad. Dermatol.*, **16**, 907–24.
85. Hall, R.P. (1987) The pathogenesis of dermatitis herpetiformis. Recent advances. *J. Amer. Acad. Dermatol.*, **16**, 1129–44.
86. Jordon, R.E., Bean, S.F., Triftshauser, C.T. and Winkelmann, R.K. (1970) Childhood bullous dermatitis herpetiformis. *Arch. Dermatol.*, **101**, 629–34.
87. Gammon, W.R., Woodley, D.T., Dole, K.C. and Briggaman, R.A. (1985) Evidence that anti-basement membrane zone antibodies in bullous eruption of systemic lupus erythematosus recognize epidermolysis bullosa acquisita autoantigen. *J. Invest. Dermatol.*, **84**, 472–6.
88. Briggaman, R.A., Gammon, W.R. and Woodley, D.T. (1985) Epidermolysis bullosa acquisita of the immunopathological type (dermolytic pemphigoid). *J. Invest. Dermatol.*, **85**, 79s–84s.
89. Woodley, D.T. (1987) Importance of the dermal–epidermal junction. Recent advances. *Dermatologica*, **174**, 1–10.
90. Jablońska, S., Chorzelski, T.P., Beutner, E.H. and Jarzabek-Chorzelska, M. (1975) Herpetiform pemphigus, a variable pattern of pemphigus. *Int. J. Dermatol.*, **14**, 353–9.
91. Emmerson, R.W. and Wilson-Jones, E. (1968) Eosinophilic spongiosis in pemphigus. A report of an unusual histological change in pemphigus. *Arch. Dermatol.*, **97**, 252–7.
92. Winkelmann, R.K. and Roth, H.L. (1960) Dermatitis herpetiformis with acantholysis or pemphigus with response to sulfonamides. *Arch. Dermatol.*, **82**, 385–90.
93. Doepfmer, R. (1961) Über eine nosologisch ungeklärte bullöse Dermatose (Pemphigus chronicus vulgaris oder Dermatitis herpetiformis Duhring). *Hautarzt*, **12**, 452–6.
94. Hebra, F. (1866) *On Diseases of the Skin, including the Exanthemata*, Vol. II (edited and translated by C.H. Fagge and P.H. Pye-Smith), The New Sydenham Society, London, pp. 361–98.
95. Stanley, J.R., Klaus-Votun, V. and Sampaio, S.A.P. (1986) Antigenic specificity of fogo selvagem autoantibodies is similar to North American pemphigus foliaceus and distinct from pemphigus vulgaris autoantibodies. *J. Invest. Dermatol.*, **87**, 197–201.
96. Brautbar, C., Szafer, F., Tzfoni, E. *et al.* (1988) Disease-specific polymorphisms associated with HLA-DQ and DR in pemphigus vulgaris. Proc. 17th World Congr. Dermatol., Berlin, 1987. In *Dermatology in Five Continents* (eds C.E. Orfanos *et al.*), Springer, Berlin, pp. 377–9.
97. Hailey, H. and Hailey, H. (1939) Familial benign chronic pemphigus. *Arch. Dermatol.*, **39**, 679–85.
98. Ayres, Jr., S. and Anderson, N.P. (1939) Recurrent herpetiform dermatitis repens. *Arch. Dermatol.*, **40**, 402–13.
99. Pels, I.R. and Goodman, M.H. (1939) Criteria for the histologic diagnosis of keratosis follicularis (Darier). *Arch. Dermatol.*, **39**, 438–55.
100. Jablońska, S. and Chorzelski, T. (1958) Zur Klassifikation des Pemphigus Hailey–Hailey. *Dermatologica*, **117**, 24–38.
101. Steffen, C.G. (1987) Familial benign chronic pemphigus. *Amer. J. Dermatopathol.*, **9**, 58–73.
102. Goldscheider, A. (1882) Hereditäre Neigung zur Blasenbildung. *Monatsh. prakt. Dermatol.*, **1**, 163–4. (This journal has become "Dermatologica" of today.)
103. Fox, T. (1879) Notes on unusual or rare forms of skin disease. *Lancet*, **i**, 766–7.
104. Hebra, F. (1870) Bericht der Klinik und Abtheilung für Hautkranke, in *Aerztlicher Bericht des k.k.allgemeinen Krankenhauses zu Wien im Jahre 1870*, Sommer und Comp, Vienna, pp. 362–3.
105. Riecke, E. (1931) Epidermolysis bullosa, in *Handbuch für Haut- und Geschlectskrankheiten*, Vol. VII, Part 2 (ed. J. Jadassohn), Springer, Berlin, pp. 222–97.
106. Siemens, W. (1922) Über die Differentialdiagnose der mechanisch bedingten Blasenausschläge, mit Beiträgen zur Kasuistik der sog. Epidermolysis bullosa (Bullosis mechanica symptomatica und Bullosis spontanea congenita) und der hereditären Dermatitis herpetiformis. *Arch. Derm. Syph.*, **139**, 80–112.
107. Gedde-Dahl, T. and Anton-Lamprecht, I. (1983) Epidermolysis bullosa, in *Principles and Practice of Medical Genetics*, Vol. I (eds A.E.H. Emery and D.L. Rimoin), Churchill Livingstone, Edinburgh, pp. 672–87.
108. Anton-Lamprecht, I. (1984) Prenatal diagnosis of epidermolysis bullosa hereditaria: a review. *Semin. Dermatol.*, **3**, 231–40.
109. Ritter von Rittershain, G. (1878) I. Die exfoliative Dermatitis jüngerer Säuglinge. *Central-Zeit. Kinderheilk.*, **2**, 3–23.
110. Melish, M.E. and Glasgow, L.A. (1970) The

staphylococcal scalded-skin syndrome. *New Engl. J. Med.*, **282**, 114–19.
111. Lyell, A. (1956) Toxic epidermal necrolysis. An eruption resembling scalding of the skin. *Brit. J. Dermatol.*, **68**, 355–61.
112. Pernet, G. and Bulloch, W. (1896) Acute pemphigus: a contribution to the aetiology of the acute bullous eruptions. *Brit. J. Dermatol.*, 8, 157–71, 205–17.
113. Pernet, G. (1895) The aetiology of acute pemphigus. *Brit. Med. J.*, ii, 1554–5.
114. Waldenström, J. (1937) Studien über Porphyrie. *Acta Med. Scand. Suppl.*, **82**, 1–254.
115. Schultz, J.H. (1874) Ein Fall von Pemphigus leprosus complicirt durch Lepra visceralis. Inaugural Dissertation (public defence of this April 25, 1874), F.W. Kunike, Greifswald.
116. Baumstark, F. (1874) Zwei pathologische Harnfarbstoffe. *Pflüger's Arch. Ges. Physiol. Menschen Tieren*, **9**, 568–84.
117. Dirckx, J.H. (1986) Julius Cesar and the Julian emperors. A family cluster with Hartnup disease. *Amer. J. Dermatopathol.*, **8**, 351–7.

PART ONE

The immunological bullous diseases

Two
Diagnosis, diagnostic and research techniques

B. S. Bhogal and Martin M. Black

2.1 INTRODUCTION

The diagnosis of acquired bullous diseases is always important, as some of these disorders can be life-threatening. Although they often have definitive clinical features, the diagnosis of an acquired bullous disease is positively made both histologically and particularly by immunofluorescence (IF) techniques. However, at all times the correct diagnosis is ensured by correlating the clinical, histological and IF findings. This in turn requires a close co-operation between the clinician and the laboratory staff. Depending on the blistering condition under investigation, the clinician should biopsy a representative site which should then be properly handled and processed accordingly. Also at the time of biopsy, serum should be obtained to detect the presence or absence of circulating antibodies by the indirect immunofluorescence (IIF) method. The value of positive or negative IF findings is greatly dependent on the reliability, skill and experience of the laboratory staff carrying out these techniques and also on the knowledge of dermatopathology of the observer who reports them.

Immunofluorescence techniques together with immunoperoxidase techniques are also employed as research tools. Studies involving these techniques have enabled dermatologists to categorize blistering disease processes and have given some insight into the underlying pathological mechanisms especially when complemented by immunoelectron microscopy. This chapter outlines and details those diagnostic techniques we consider important in differentiating the acquired bullous dermatoses. The findings on the major acquired blistering diseases are summarized in Table 2.1.

2.2 METHODS AND TECHNIQUES

2.2.1 Specimen collection and handling of skin biopsy

(a) *Skin biopsy*

Skin biopsies are required for both histological examination and immunofluorescence studies. The biopsy should be taken from a fresh blister not older than 24–48 h. Biopsies of older blisters are not satisfactory as changes such as regeneration, degeneration or secondary infection may occur. These changes in turn make the microscopic interpretation of the initial events difficult if not impossible.

When a lesion has been selected for biopsy for histological studies, an elliptical excision is preferred to a punch procedure. Punch biopsies are not recommended in blistering disorders as these cause crushing which may lead to disintegration of the blister. However, a punch biopsy is adequate for immunofluorescence studies of uninvolved skin or mucosa.

Histology Whenever possible a single biopsy including both edges of a small blister and the adjacent clinically uninvolved skin should be performed. If only large blisters are present, the edge of the blister and the adjacent uninvolved skin

Table 2.1 Diagnostic histology features and immunological findings in acquired blistering diseases

Disease	*Key histology features*	*Immunofluorescence findings* — *Direct (biopsy)*	*Immunofluorescence findings* — *Indirect (serum)*	*Immunofluorescence findings* — *Indirect (split-skin technique)*	*Immunoelectron microscopy*
Pemphigus					
foliaceus	High epidermal blister Subgranular or intragranular Acantholysis				
vulgaris	Intraepidermal blister Suprabasal Acantholysis Isolated papillae lined by basal cells producing 'tombstone effect'	Intercellular immunoglobulins and complement IgG = 100% IgA/IgM = 20% C3 present when disease is active, usually in lower epidermis	Intercellular (IC) IgG antibodies = 90% Antibody titre frequently reflects disease activity Generally falling with treatment and increasing with relapse 30% IC antibodies bind complement	Not applicable	Immunoreactants on glycocalyx (intercellular substance) coating the membrane on the outside of keratinocytes
vegetans	Vegetating intra-epidermal eosinophilic abscesses, often extending into hair follicles				
erythematosus	Intraepidermal blister, often in granular cell layer Acantholysis	Mixed IF pattern Intercellular IgG/C3 associated with granular BMZ = 80%	IC IgG antibodies = 100% Antinuclear antibodies (ANA) = 20%		
Pemphigoid					
bullous	Subepidermal blister No acantholysis Eosinophil-rich dermal infiltrate	Linear BMZ immunoglobulins and complement IgG/C3 = 80% IgA/IgM = 27%	Linear BMZ IgG antibodies = 75% The correlation between antibody titre and severity of disease is not significant 50% pemphigoid antibodies (anti-BMZ) bind complement	Antibodies bind to the epidermal side of the split	Immunoreactants in lamina lucida
cicatricial	Subepidermal blister granulation tissue in dermis Eosinophil-rich dermal infiltrate	Linear BMZ IgG/C3 = 80% IgA = 40%	Anti-BMZ IgG antibodies = 10%	Antibodies bind to the epidermal side of the split	Immunoreactants in lower lamina lucida

Herpes (pemphigoid) gestationis	Focal necrosis of basal cell layer Spongiosis in mid and lower epidermis Exocytosis of eosinophils	Linear BMZ C3 = 100% IgG = 40%	Anti-BMZ antibodies IgG = 10% Complement binding anti-BMZ antibodies = 100%	Antibodies bind to the epidermal side of the split	Immunoreactants in lamina lucida
Linear IgA bullous dermatosis					
Linear IgA disease of adults (LAD)	Subepidermal blister	Linear BMZ IgA = 80% IgG/IgM/C3 = 10%	Anti-BMZ IgA antibodies = 20%	Antibodies bind to the epidermal side of the split	Immunoreactants in either sublamina densa or in lamina lucida
Chronic bullous disease of childhood (CBDC)	Neutrophil-rich dermal infiltrate		Anti-BMZ IgA antibodies = 75%		
Epidermolysis bullosa acquisita	Subepidermal blister No acantholysis Eosinophils absent in the dermal infiltrate	Linear BMZ IgG = 100%	Anti-BMZ IgG antibodies = 25%	Antibodies bind to the dermal side of the split	Immunoreactants in sublamina densa
Dermatitis herpetiforms	Subepidermal blister Papillary neutrophilic abscesses	Granular deposits of IgA in dermal papillae = 100% C3/Fibrinogen = 40%	Absent	Not applicable	Immunoreactants associated with micro-fibrillous part of the elastic fibres

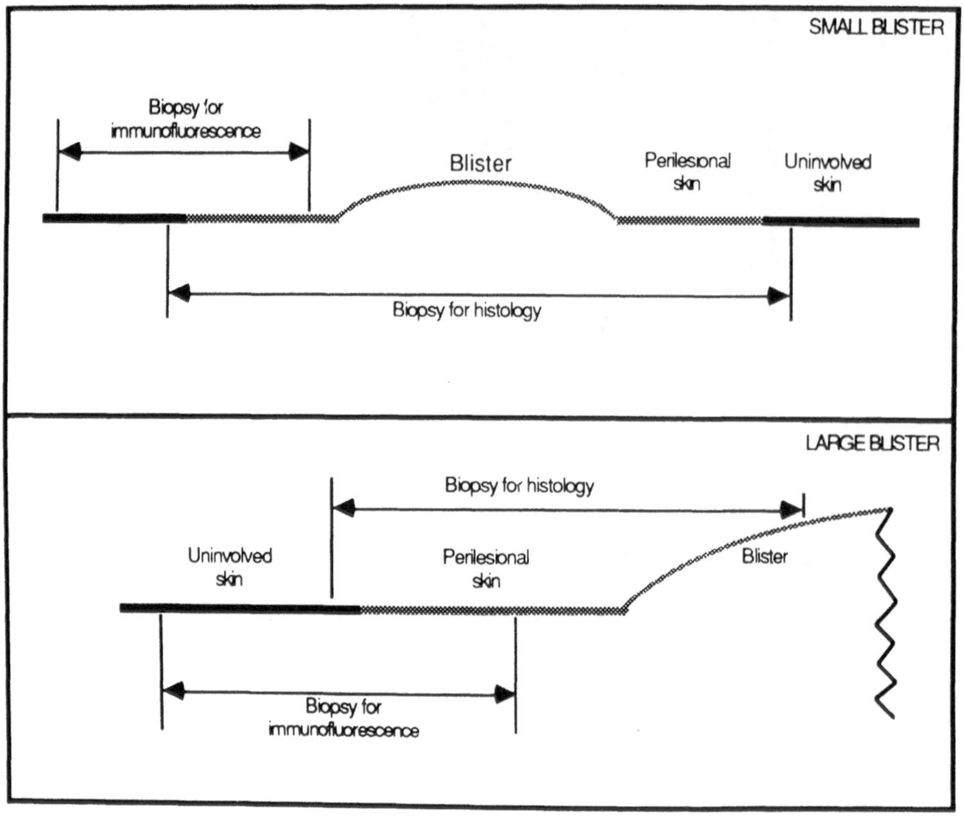

Figure 2.1 Biopsy sites for blistering disorders (histology and immunofluorescence studies).

should be biopsied (Figure 2.1). The biopsy is then placed with the epidermis upward on a small piece of blotting paper and immersed in a jar of tissue fixative (formal saline). The fixative being a protein coagulant helps to stick the biopsy on the blotting paper, thus preventing the tissue from curling.

Immunofluorescence Ideally, two biopsies should be taken for immunofluorescence studies, the first and most important from the clinically uninvolved skin, the second from an edge of a blister which should include adjacent cutaneous tissue. A single biopsy alone is not suitable for immunofluorescence investigation. Blistered skin often gives negative results because the bound immunoreactants and tissue structures are destroyed, especially in pemphigoid and dermatitis herpetiformis. Subsequently, the biopsy sent for immunofluorescence is briefly washed in phosphate-buffered saline (PBS) (see Appendix A) to remove blood and serum proteins, snap-frozen and stored at −70° C until used.

Several methods for snap-freezing are available [1]. The most commonly used method is to place the biopsy in a labelled plastic tube which is then immersed in liquid nitrogen until frozen. Unfortunately, this method may induce freezing artefacts causing distortion of the tissue architecture. The method routinely used in our laboratory and which has proven to be consistently satisfactory was originally described by Chayen *et al.* [2]. This involves the use of n-hexane which is cooled in a bath of carbon dioxide snow pellets and alcohol mixture (Figure 2.2). A drop of OCT embedding compound is placed on a small piece of cork which is then briefly immersed in the cold

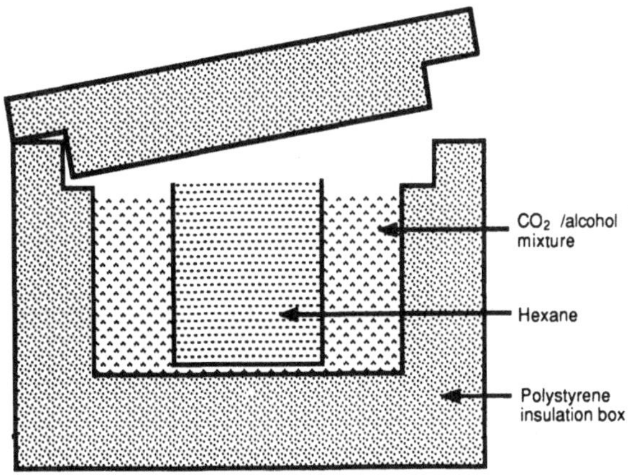

Figure 2.2 Apparatus for freezing biopsies.

n-hexane until the edges are frozen whilst the central part remains fluid. The skin biopsy is then orientated in the fluid central part, covered with more OCT compound and reimmersed in the cold n-hexane leaving the skin biopsy frozen in a shell of OCT compound (Figure 2.3).

This method of freezing greatly reduces the degree of artefacts. A further advantage is that the biopsy is properly orientated ready for sectioning. Freezing is the preferred method for handling and processing immunofluorescence biopsy specimens. However, when skin biopsies need to be transported and liquid nitrogen or carbon dioxide snow is not available, the biopsies can then be transported in Michel's liquid fixative (see Appendix B) at ambient temperature [3]. This liquid fixative prevents degradation of tissue and immunoreactants by inhibiting tissue enzymes. The results of studies of tissues processed by snap-freezing and those kept in Michel's liquid fixative for a period of several days are largely comparable [4]. This was confirmed by studies done in our laboratory evaluating the liquid fixative [5]. The results of our study indicate that the pH of the liquid fixative is of primary importance and should be maintained above 7.0. This is best achieved by prior washing of the biopsy in normal saline or PBS buffer to remove blood and serum proteins.

The biopsy received in Michel's liquid fixative should be washed in buffer (see Appendix B) for 30 min and subsequently frozen and stored at −70° C until used.

(b) Blood specimens

Serum samples are required for the detection of circulating autoantibodies by indirect immunofluorescence. At least 10 ml of blood without anticoagulant should be collected and incubated at 37° C for 1 hour to isolate the serum. This is then removed from the blood clot

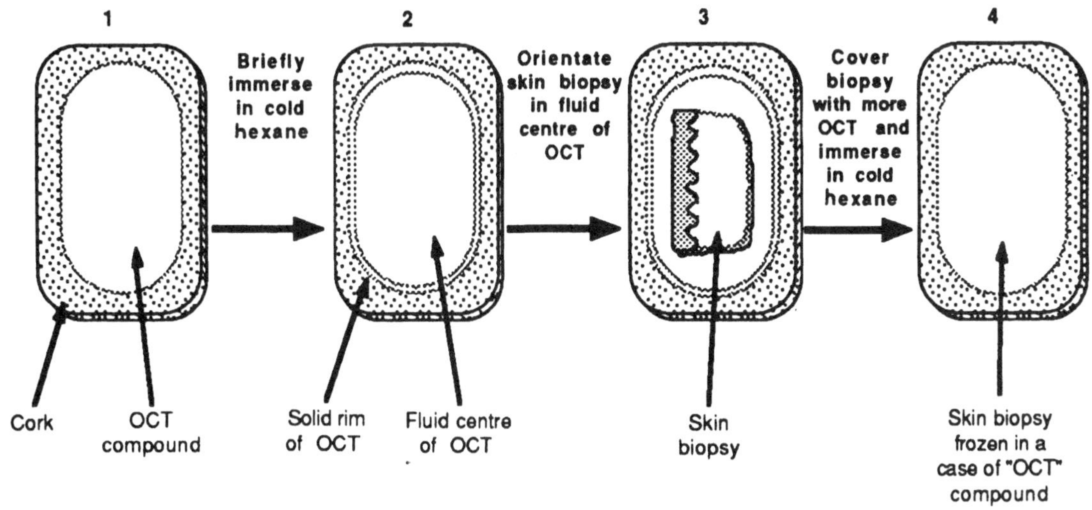

Figure 2.3 Freezing the skin biopsy for immunofluorescence.

by centrifuging; it is then pipetted into a sterile container and stored at −25° C until analysed. Serum and not clotted blood samples should be frozen as this causes massive haemolysis which in turn causes destruction of autoantibodies.

2.2.2 Techniques

(a) Histology

The best results for histology processing are achieved by fixing the biopsy specimen in neutral buffered formal saline, although various other fixatives are also available. As the fixation progresses from the periphery of the tissue into the middle, the time of fixation depends on the size of the specimen. Therefore, larger biopsies should be trimmed to reduce the thickness of the specimen. This is achieved by either cutting a 4 mm strip from the middle of the specimen or by dividing it into two halves through the centre which also produces a flat surface for embedding (Figure 2.4). The procedures for subsequent processing and staining can be found in several major textbooks [6, 7].

(b) Immunofluorescence

Immunofluorescence techniques were introduced by Coons who successfully coupled the fluorochrome (fluorescein) to the antibodies without destroying their immunological properties. This molecule could then be combined with an antigen in the tissue to form an antigen–antibody complex which could then be visualized by fluorescence microscopy. These techniques are simple to perform and are both reliable and reproducible.

Immunofluorescence techniques in our laboratories are performed on coverslips rather than microslides. The advantages of working with coverslips are that they both save space and require smaller volumes of washing buffer. Two or more 4 μm-thick frozen sections are picked up on to prelabelled coverslips and placed in coverslip racks.

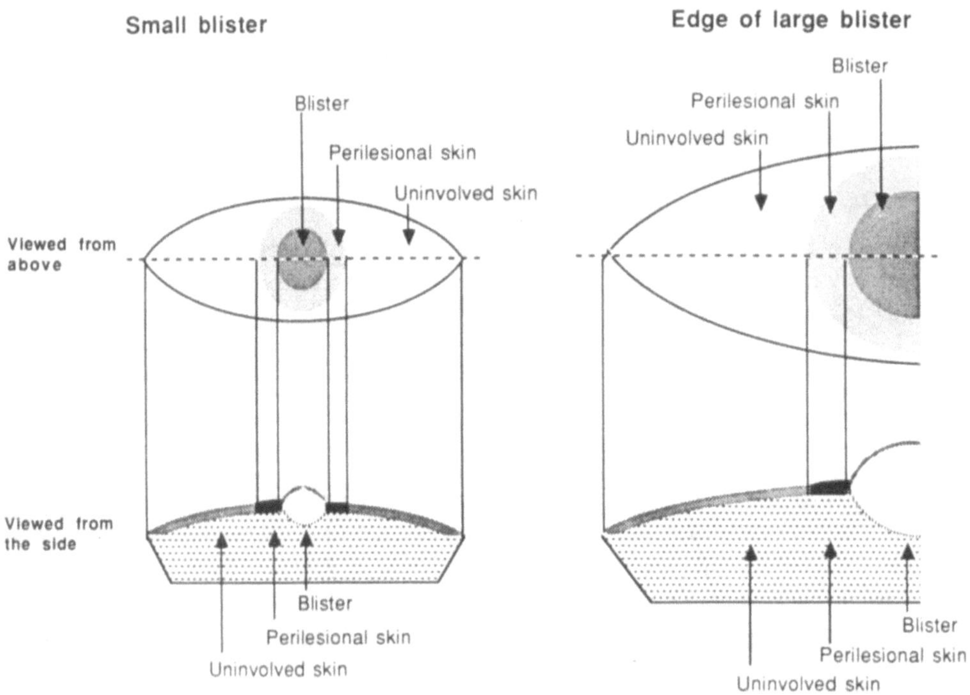

Figure 2.4 Trimming the biopsy for histology processing.

The initial and subsequent drying of sections between washing is achieved by an ordinary electric fan. Inadequate drying of sections may cause them to detach from the coverslips during washing. Washing of sections is performed by the immersion of the coverslip racks into a bath of buffer with continued stirring using a magnetic stirrer. The incubation of sections with antisera are carried out in a moist chamber (closed plastic container) in an incubator at 37° C. After the final wash the sections are fan-dried, mounted on to glass slides using a drop of buffered glycerol as mounting medium (see Appendix C) and viewed through a fluorescence microscope.

For the differential diagnosis of blistering diseases three immunofluorescence techniques used routinely in our laboratory are:

1. the direct immunofluorescence method (DIF)
2. the indirect immunofluorescence method (IIF)
3. the complement-binding indirect immunofluorescence method (C3 method)

Direct immunofluorescence (Appendix E) This is a one-step procedure for the detection *in vivo* of deposition of immunoglobulins, complement components and fibrinogen in a patient's skin. Frozen sections are incubated with monospecific fluorescein isothiocyanate (FITC)-labelled antisera. To obtain maximum tissue-specific fluorescence with minimum background fluorescence the optimum dilution of the conjugates should be used. Thsis is achieved by utilizing a chess-board titration procedure using a known positive tissue specimen [8].

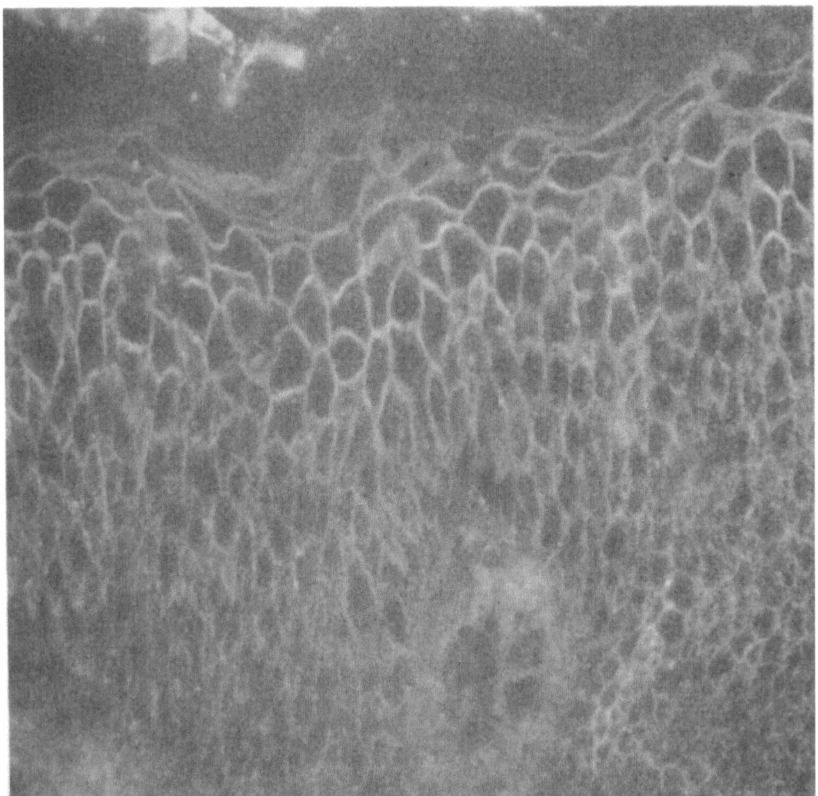

Figure 2.5 DIF of pemphigus showing deposition of intercellular IgG.

For routine DIF screening, five coverslips with at least two or more 4 μm-thick sections are required for each biopsy. These are then fan-dried for 10 min and washed in PBS at pH 7.4 for a further 10 min. This initial washing removes the surrounding OCT compound in which the biopsy is embedded and also any non-specific proteins in the sections. The sections are fan-dried again, covered with one of the following FITC-labelled antisera – anti-human IgM; IgG; IgA; complement 3 (C3); fibrinogen – and incubated for 30 min at 37° C. The unreacted antiserum is washed off in PBS for 30 min (three 10-min changes). The coverslips are fan-dried once again, mounted on to microslides using a drop of buffered glycerol as mounting medium and examined with a fluorescence microscope. Examples of the use of DIF are shown in Figures 2.5–2.9.

Indirect immunofluorescence (Appendix F) This is a two-step procedure for demonstrating circulating autoantibodies in a patient's serum. Frozen sections of the tissue substrate (tissue–antigen) are incubated with serially diluted patient's serum followed by FITC-labelled anti-human IgG. A large number of tissue substrates

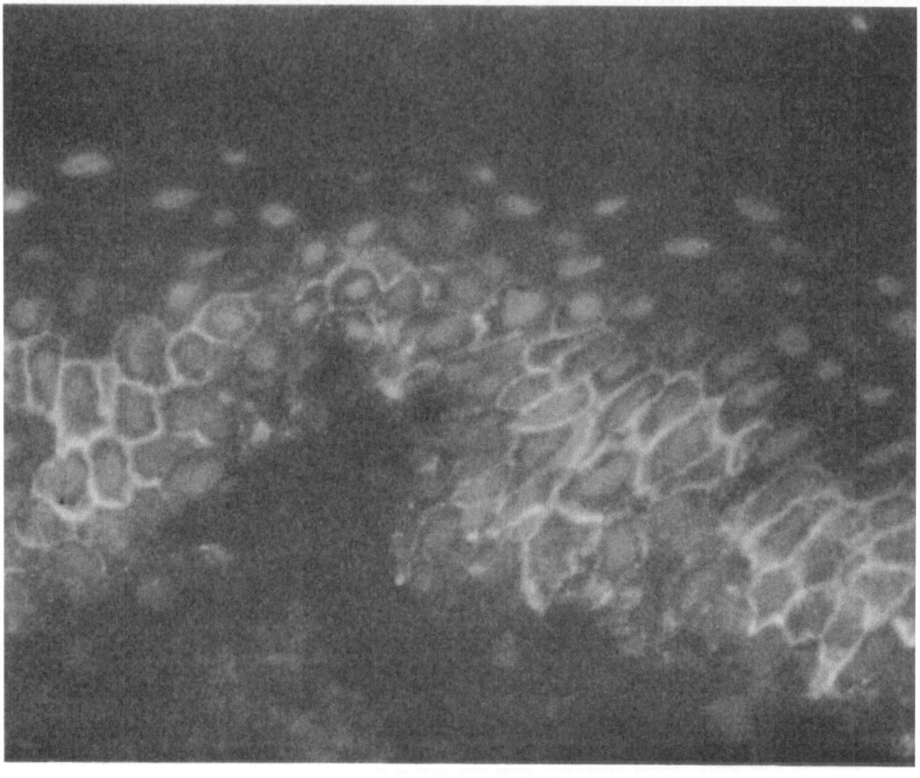

Figure 2.6 DIF of pemphigus showing intercellular C3 staining in lower epidermis only.

Figure 2.7 Pemphigus erythematosus showing mixed IF staining pattern. Intercellular and granular BMZ immunofluorescence with IgG (DIF).

Figure 2.8 DIF of bullous pemphigoid showing linear deposition of IgG in the BMZ.

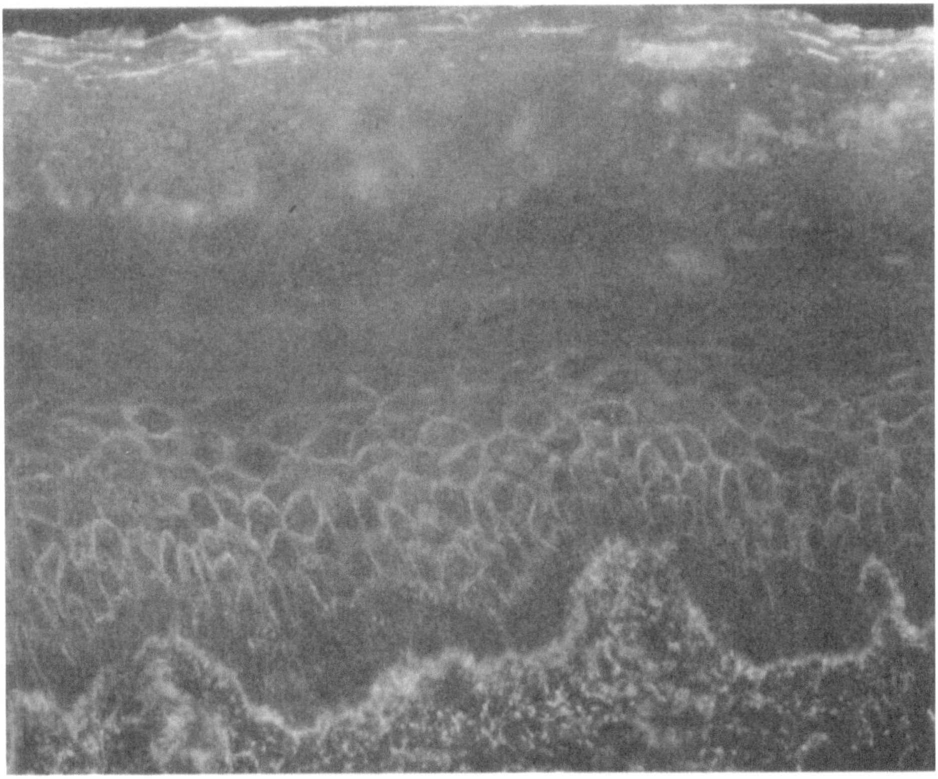

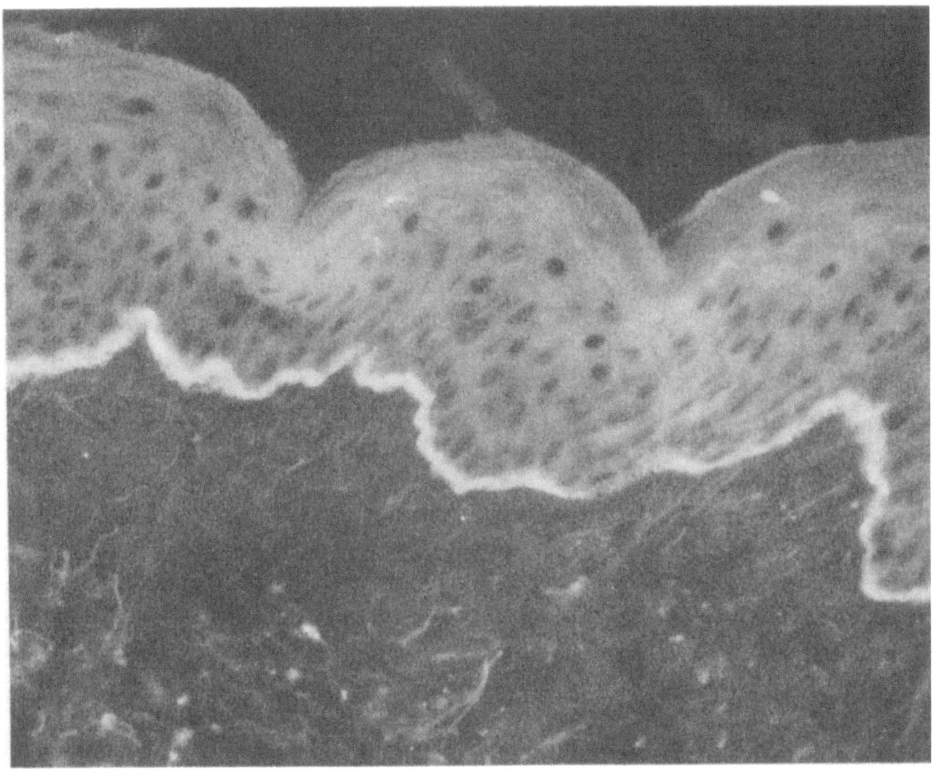

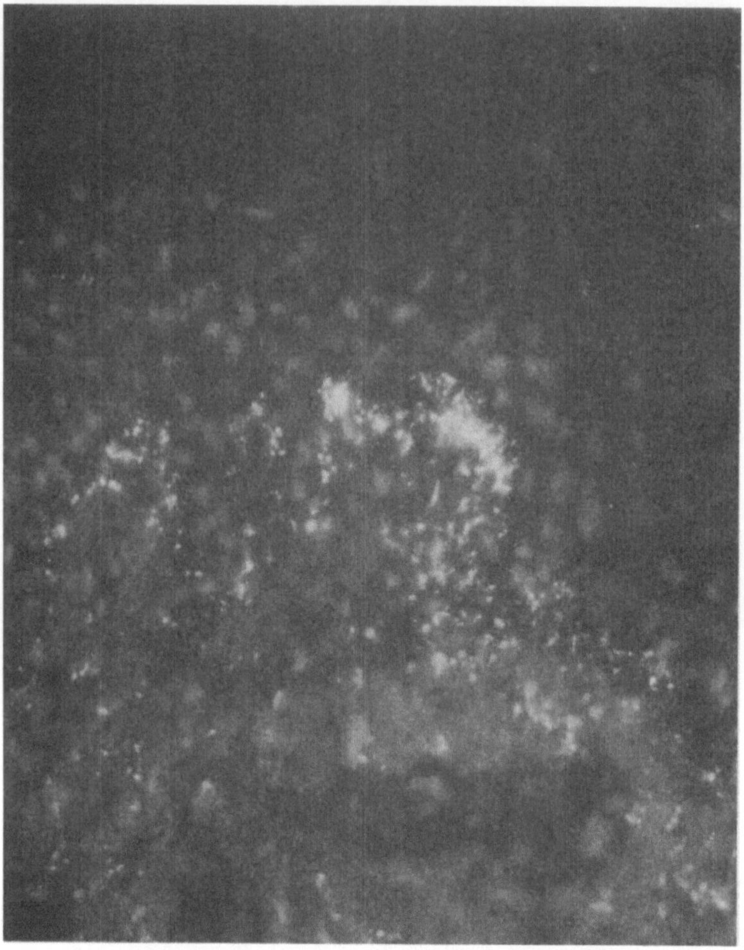

Figure 2.9 DIF. Granular IgA deposition in dermal papillae in dermatitis herpetiformis.

have been used in this technique. These include monkey oesophagus, guinea-pig lip/oesophagus, rabbit lip/oesophagus and normal human skin. Guinea-pig and rabbit tissues have been shown to give an unacceptably high rate of false negative results and are not recommended (Figure 2.10). However, a recent study suggests the use of several different substrates simultaneously for the optimum results for detecting intercellular antibodies in various clinical types of pemphigus [9]. Also the use of Tris–acetate-buffered saline supplemented with calcium chloride is reported to increase the sensitivity of IIF assay for detecting pemphigus antibodies on human skin [10].

Although monkey oesophagus has been advocated to be the best substrate, we find that human skin from the abdomen, the flexor surfaces of the arms, legs and thighs to be the most suitable and reliable source of substrate for detecting circulating pemphigus, pemphigoid and IgA anti-basement membrane zone (BMZ) antibodies. Neonatal foreskin or skin from scalp or face should not be used as substrate for IIF procedures as they also yield high rates of false negative results [11, 12].

For routine screening of patient's serum two coverslips with at least two or more 4 μm-thick frozen sections of the tissue substrate (normal

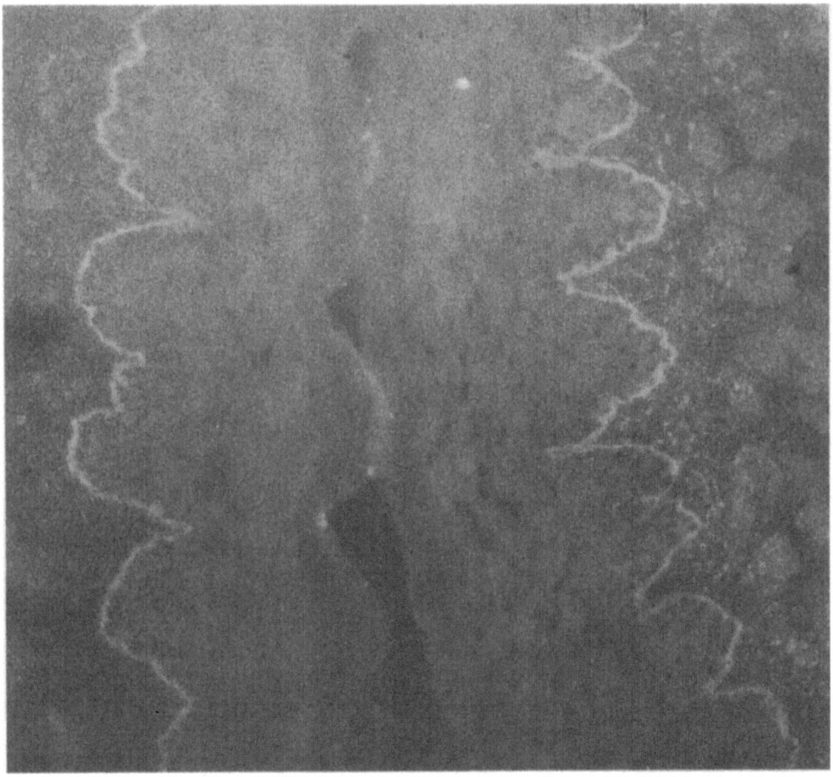

Figure 2.10 IIF showing IgA anti-BMZ antibodies binding to BMZ of rabbit oesophagus.

human skin) are required. The sections are fan-dried for 10 min, washed in PBS for 10 min and fan-dried again for 10 min. Each coverslip is then covered by one of two dilutions of the patient's serum [1 : 10 or 1 : 80] and incubated for 30 min at 37° C. The excess serum is washed off in PBS for 30 min (three 10-min changes), fan-dried and incubated with FITC-labelled anti-human IgG at 37° C for another 30 min. After the final three washes (10 min each wash) in PBS, the sections are fan-dried and mounted on to microslides using a drop of buffered glycerol and examined with a fluorescence microscope.

For negative controls additional sections are incubated with normal human serum instead of patient's serum and other sections are incubated with the fluorescein-conjugated anti-human IgG only. This provides information about non-specific binding of the immunoglobulins in the tissue substrate and also warns of the possible presence of non-specific heterophilic antibodies in the conjugate.

The complement-binding indirect method (C3 method) (Appendix G) This is a method for demonstrating whether circulating antibodies in the patient's serum are capable of binding complement. The information in turn may provide some clue as to the immunopathological mechanisms involved in the disease. The indirect C3 method is a three-stage procedure which amplifies the staining obtained by the IIF technique when complement-binding antibodies are present. It is used particularly in the differential diagnosis of herpes (pemphigoid) gestationis (Figure 2.11). In this condition the circulating antibodies are

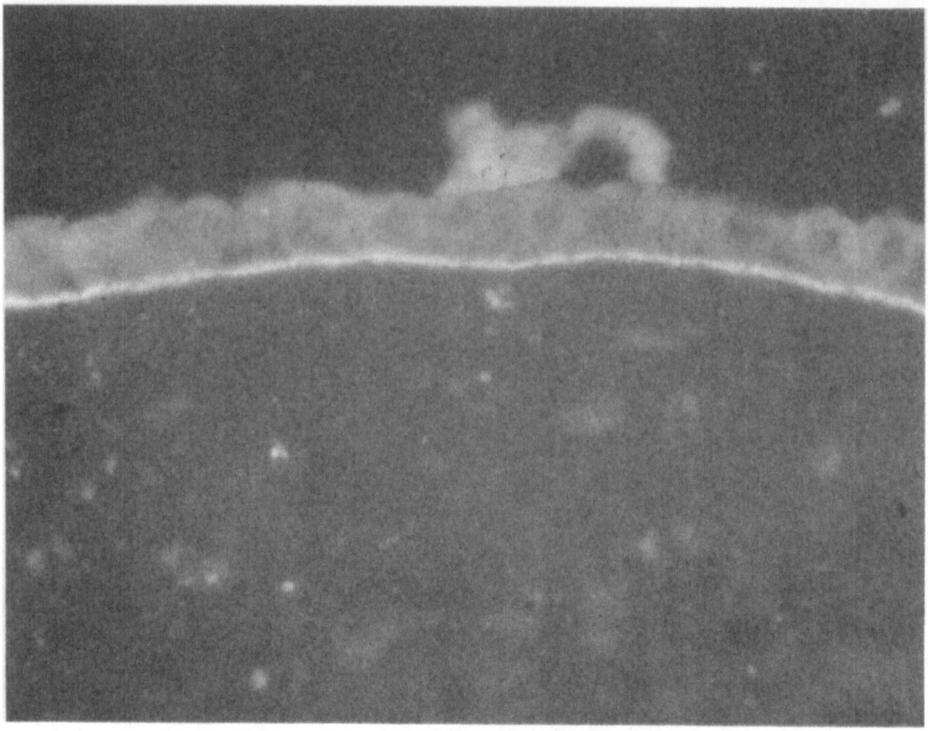

Figure 2.11 Indirect C3 IF method showing herpes (pemphigoid) gestationis antibodies binding to the BMZ of placenta amnion (C3).

difficult to detect by the conventional IIF method, but are known to bind complement avidly and therefore can be detected by this technique.

For routine screening, two coverslips with 4 μm-thick cryostat sections of normal human skin (substrate) are required for each serum. The sections are fan-dried for 10 min, washed in PBS for a further 10 min and fan-dried again. Each coverslip is then overlaid with one of two dilutions of the patient's serum made in PBS [1 : 2 or 1 : 4], and incubated for 30 min at 37° C. The sections are then washed in PBS for 30 min (three 10-min changes), fan-dried and incubated with complement for a further 30 min at 37° C. The source of complement we use is normal human serum diluted 1 in 5 with complement diluting buffer (see Appendix D). After the second incubation the sections are washed in PBS for 30 min (three 10-min changes), fan-dried and covered with optimum diluted fluoroscein conjugated anti-C3 and incubated for 30 min at 37° C. After the final three washes of 10 min each in PBS the sections are fan-dried, mounted on to microslides using a drop of buffered glycerol as mounting medium and examined with a fluorescence microscope.

2.2.3 Split-skin indirect technique

Circulating IgG anti-BMZ antibodies are characteristic features in a number of acquired bullous dermatoses. Immunoelectron microscopy (IEM) divides these antibodies into two groups based on their ultrastructural binding sites. In bullous pemphigoid, cicatricial pemphigoid and pemphigoid gestationis the antibodies bind to the lamina lucida and are termed anti-lamina lucida antibodies. In epidermolysis bullosa acquisita they bind below the lamina densa and are termed anti-sublamina densa antibodies (see Figure 2.15). Therefore distinguishing between the anti-lamina

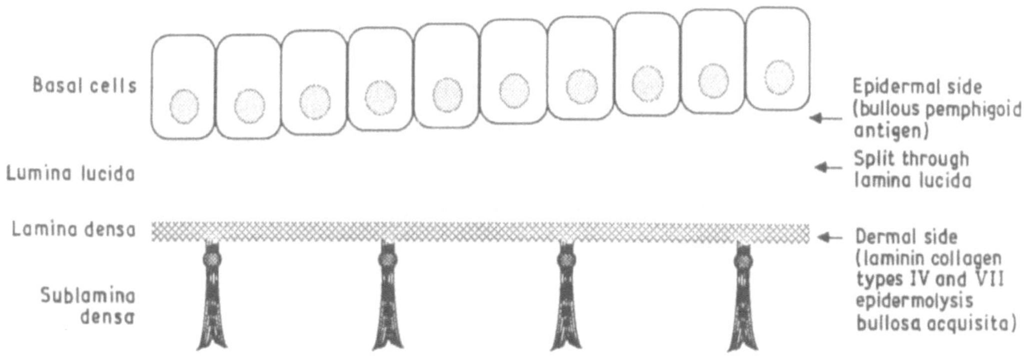

Figure 2.12 Plane of cleavage after 1 M NaCl separation.

lucida antibodies and anti-sublamina densa antibodies is essential for accurate diagnosis, especially in those cases of bullous pemphigoid, cicatricial pemphigoid and epidermolysis bullosa acquisita where diagnostic features considered characteristic of one disease may be present in another. Furthermore, routine determination of the antibody-binding site may provide a better understanding of the clinical, pathological and immuno-ultrastructural correlation in all bullous conditions associated with anti-BMZ antibodies. The split-skin IIF technique provides a simple and

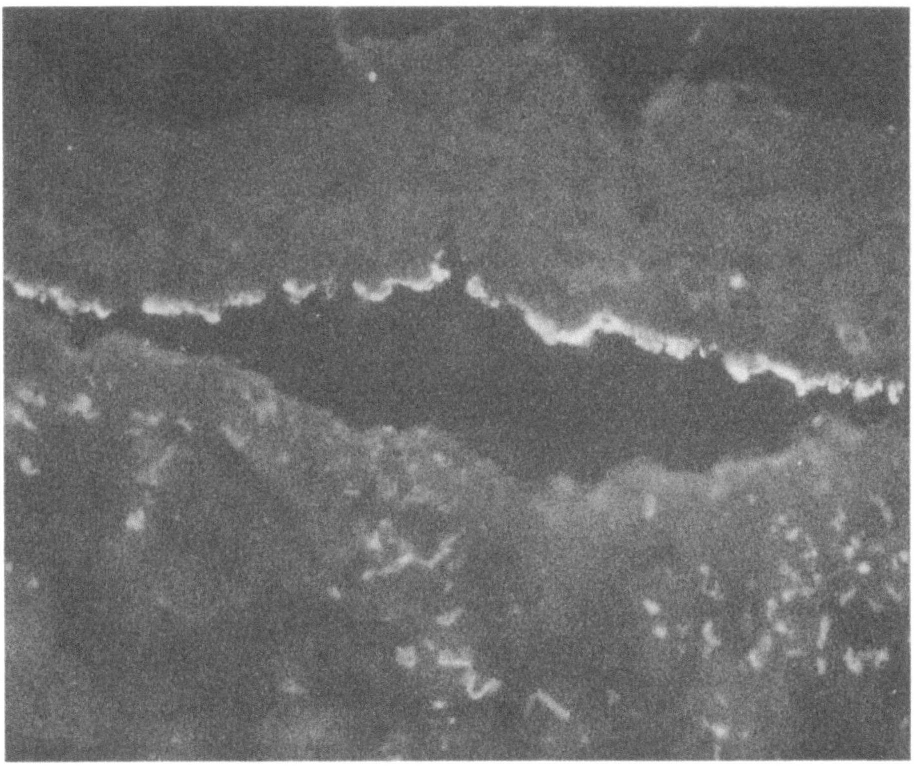

Figure 2.13 IIF showing bullous pemphigoid antibodies binding to the epidermal side of 1 M NaCl-split skin (IgG).

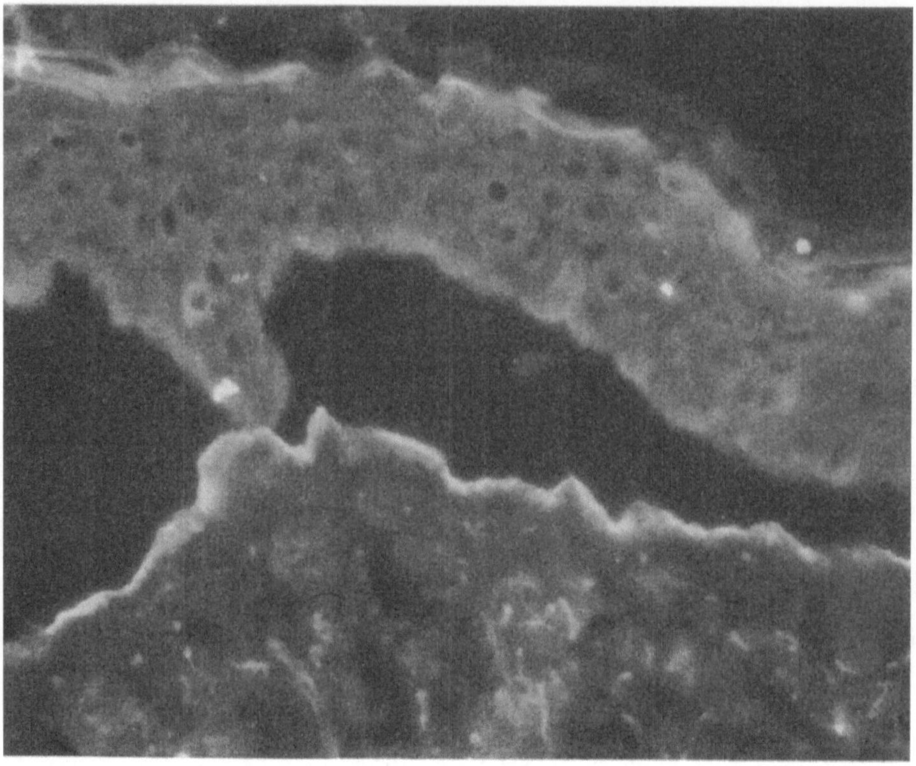

Figure 2.14 IIF showing epidermolysis bullosa acquisita antibodies binding to the base of 1 M NaCl-split skin (IgG).

reliable alternative to IEM for identifying anti-lamina lucida antibodies but will not distinguish low lamina lucida from sublamina densa antibodies [13]. This method relies on splitting normal skin through the lamina lucida whereby the bullous pemphigoid antigen adheres to the epidermal side with components of lamina densa, epidermolysis bullosa acquisita antigen, type IV collagen and type VII collagen on the dermal side (Figures 2.12–2.14). The split skin is then used as a substrate for the indirect immunofluorescence technique. There is also an increase in the sensitivity for detecting anti-BMZ antibodies using split skin as substrate, increasing antibody detection to 95% in bullous pemphigoid and 50% in cicatricial pemphigoid [14]. This may be due to improved exposure of the antigen in the split skin. The separation can be achieved by three different procedures each involving a different mechanism [15].

(a) Skin-separation procedures

Tissue extraction (cold 1 M NaCl) Thin strips of normal skin are incubated with 1 M NaCl solution at 4° C for 72 h with continuous stirring. The NaCl solution is renewed at 24 h and 48 h.

Enzymic (cold trypsinization) Thin strips of normal skin are floated on precooled 0.25% trypsin solution and maintained at 4° C for 18 h. At the end of the incubation the skin strips are washed in fresh PBS and placed with the epidermis upwards on blotting paper. The epidermis is gently dislodged from the dermis with fine forceps. The dislodged epidermis is then placed back on the dermis and cut into 1 mm blocks. These blocks are embedded in OCT compound, snap-frozen and stored at −70° C until required.

Induction of suction blister (mechanical) Sunction blisters are induced in normal adult volunteers using a suction blistering device as described by Kobza-Black *et al.* [16]. As soon as the blister reaches a diameter of 3 mm a punch biopsy of the blister is performed under local anaesthesia. The biopsy is snap-frozen as described before and stored at −70° C until required.

2.2.4 Electron microscopy

Electron microscopy is mandatory in the differential diagnosis of the genetically determined group of mechanobullous skin conditions, namely epidermolysis bullosa. The characteristic feature of epidermolysis bullosa appears to be structural abnormalities at the dermo–epidermal junction area (BMZ). The different forms of epidermolysis bullosa (simplex, junctional and dystrophic) can be distinguished by determining the level of split at the BMZ by electron microscopy (see Chapter 12).

(a) Fixation and processing of specimen for electron microscopy

Generally the basic principles of fixation and preservation applied to light-microscopic studies apply equally well to higher-resolution studies. The use of a primary and secondary fixation sequence is now generally accepted as being a flexible method of fixing specimens for electron microscopy [17]. The primary fixative of choice for a skin specimen is Karnovsky fixative [18], which is a mixture of glutaraldehyde and paraformaldehyde in cacodylate buffer at pH 7.4.

Skin specimens for electron-microscopy studies are cut into thin slices (1 mm × 2 mm) and immersed in Karnovsky fixative for 4 h at 4° C. They are then thoroughly washed in cacodylate buffer containing 0.44 M sucrose overnight at 4° C and postfixed in 1% osmium tetroxide (secondary fixative) for 1 h at room temperature. The skin slices are then dehydrated in graded ethanol, impregnated with epoxy resin (araldite) and embedded in gelatine capsules size 00 which fit the chucks of most ultramicrotomes. Semithin sections (1 μm thick) mounted on a glass slide are either stained with 1% Toluidine Blue for light-microscope examination or unstained sections are viewed with a phase-contrast microscope. This enables suitable areas for ultrathin sectioning to be selected. The ultrathin sections are collected on to grids and stained with uranyl acetate and lead citrate before examination with an electron microscope.

2.2.5 Immunoelectron microscopy (Appendix H)

Immunoelectron-microscopic techniques provide a precise correlation between the clinical and the immunological events in the subepidermal autoimmune blistering diseases. The subepidermal blistering conditions bullous pemphigoid, cicatricial pemphigoid and epidermolysis bullosa acquisita have identical immunofluorescence staining patterns. Immunoelectron-microscopic techniques are used to distinguish accurately between these conditions by demonstrating the exact antibody-binding sites (Figures 2.15–2.17). The application of these techniques has led to important advances in the understanding of the immunopathological mechanisms involved in the acquired blistering diseases.

The conventional immunoelectron-microscopic techniques using free floating sections [19] are not easy to perform, and because of freezing artefacts good morphological results are rarely obtained. This handicap is overcome by using thin slices of tissues freshly cut without freezing. The slices are easy to manipulate and give excellent morphological results [20].

The specimens are cut into thin slices (1 mm thick) either manually or by using a hand microtome [21]. They are then washed, with agitation, in 50 ml of PBS for 1 h at 4° C. Prolonged washing of the fresh slices in a large volume of PBS eliminates the extracellular immunoglobulins that are present in the tissue. If the washing is insufficient these extracellular immunoglobulins react with the anti-Ig antibodies making penetration of the antibodies to the specific binding sites impossible.

The slices are lightly fixed in 2% buffered paraformaldehyde for 1 h at 4° C with agitation. The initial fixation with paraformaldehyde provides good morphological preservation for the subsequent long incubation periods and also

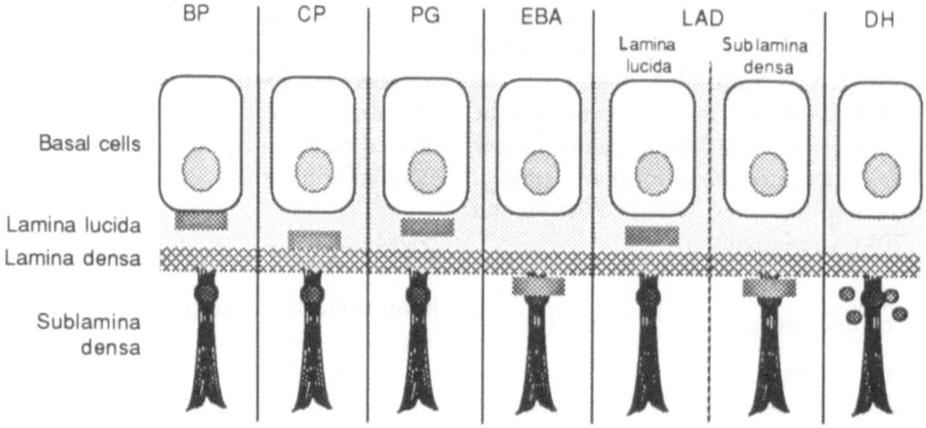

Figure 2.15 Immunoelectron microscopic localization of immunoreactants at the basement membrane zone in blistering disorders. Key: BP, bullous pemphigoid; CP, cicatricial pemphigoid, PG, pemphigoid gestationis; EBA, epidermolysis bullosa acquisita; LAD, linear IgA disease; DH, dermatitis herpetiformis.

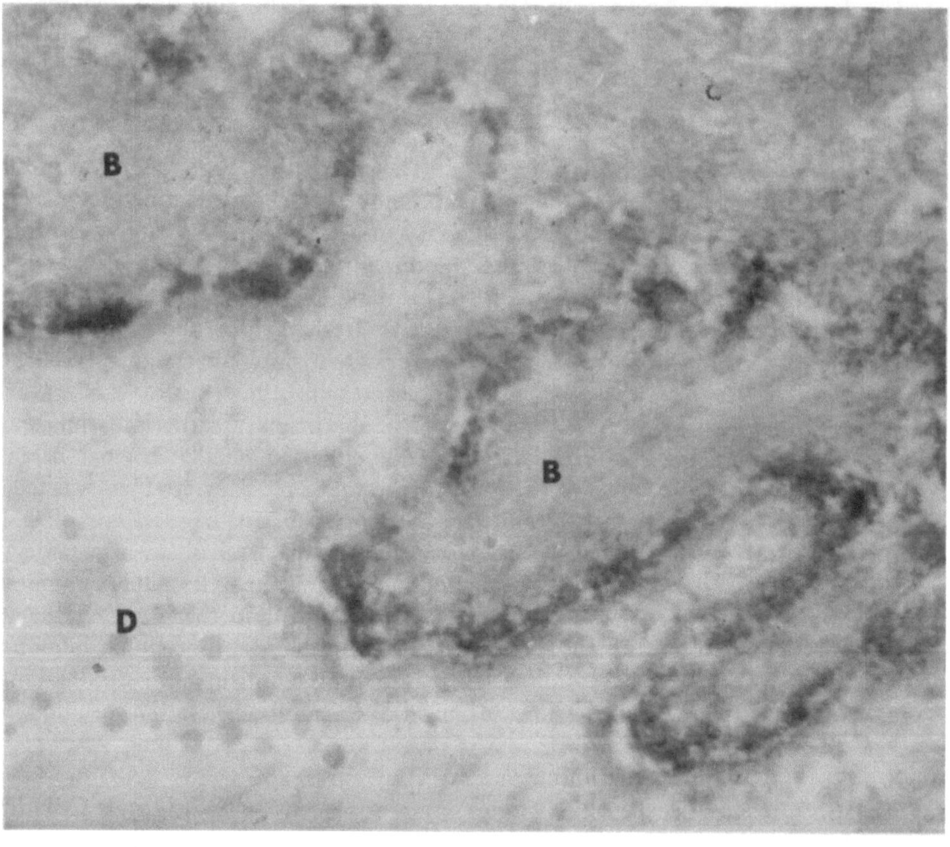

Figure 2.16 Immunoelectron microscopy showing IgG deposits in lamina lucida (bullous pemphigoid). B, Basal cell; D, dermis.

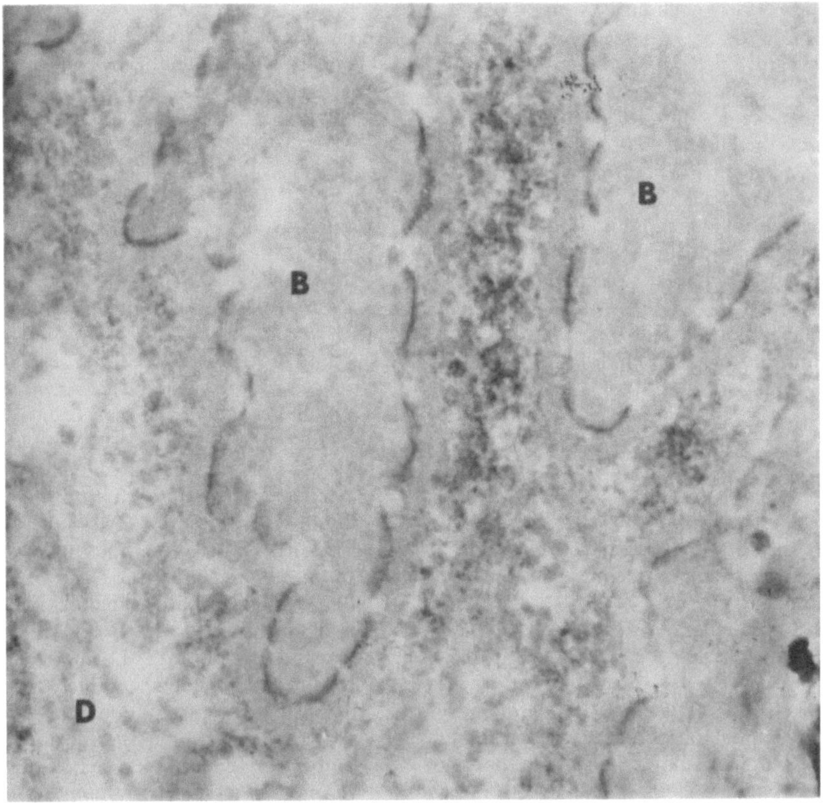

Figure 2.17 Immunoelectron microscopy showing IgG deposits in sublamina densa (epidermolysis bullosa acquisita). B, Basal cell; D, dermis.

preserves the antigenicity of the binding sites. They are then washed in PBS for a further 1 h at 4° C. For the direct reaction the slices are incubated with horseradish peroxidase-labelled antisera [anti-human immunoglobulins] for 18 h at 4° C. For the indirect reaction the slices are incubated with unlabelled primary antibody (patient's serum) for 18 h at 4° C, washed for 1 h at 4° C and incubated again with horseradish peroxide-labelled antisera for a further 18 h at 4° C. All washings and dilutions of primary antibody and antisera are carried out in PBS. The slices are then washed for 30 min (three 10-min changes), postfixed in Karnovsky's fixative for 4 h at 4° C and washed in cacodylate buffer containing 0.44 M sucrose at pH 7.4. The horseradish peroxidase is developed by incubating the slices in Graham/Karnovsky's medium [22] for 1 h in the dark with agitation at room temperature. The slices are finally fixed in osmium tetroxide, impregnated and embedded in epoxy resin. The unstained ultrathin sections are viewed by electron microscope.

2.3 DIAGNOSIS

The main diagnostic histological features and immunopathological findings in the major acquired blistering disorders are summarized in Table 2.1.

REFERENCES

1. Beutner, E.H., Nisengard, R.J. and Kumar, V. (1979) Defined immunofluorescence: basic concepts

and their application to clinical dermatology. In *Immunopathology of the Skin* (eds E.H. Beutner, T.P. Chorzelski and S.F. Bean), John Wiley and Sons, New York, pp. 29–75.

2. Chayen, J., Bitensky, L., Butcher, R. and Poulter, L. (1973) *A Guide to Practical Histochemistry*, John Wiley and Sons, New York, p. 5.
3. Michel, B., Milner, Y. and David, K. (1973) Preservation of tissue-fixed immunoglobulins in skin biopsies of patients with lupus erythematoses and bullous diseases. Preliminary report. *J. Invest. Dermatol.*, **59**, 449–52.
4. Nisengard, R.J., Jablonska, S., Chorzelski, T.P. *et al.* (1978) Immunofluorescence studies. Comparisons of methods of transportation. *Arch. Dermatol.*, **144**, 1329.
5. Skeete, M.V.H. and Black, M.M. (1977) The evaluation of a special liquid fixative for direct immunofluorescence. *Clin. Exp. Dermatol.*, **2**, 49–56.
6. Lever, W.F. and Schaumburg-Lever, G. (1983) *Histopathology of the Skin,* 6th edn, J.B. Lippincott Co., Philadelphia.
7. Pinkus, H. and Mehregan, A.H. (1981) *A Guide to Dermatopathology*, 3rd edn, Appleton-Crofts, New York.
8. Beutner, E.H., Hale, W.L., Nisengard, R.J., Chorzelski, T.P. and Holubar, K. (1973) Defined immunofluorescence in clinical immunopathology. In *Immunopathology of Skin. Labelled Antibody Study* (eds E.H. Beutner, T.P. Chorzelski, S.F. Bean and R.E. Jordon), Dowden, Hutchinson and Ross, Pennsylvania, pp. 197–247.
9. Sobolinski, M.L., Beutner, E.H., Kransky, S., *et al.* (1987) Substrate specificity of anti-epithelial antibodies of pemphigus vulgaris and pemphigus foliaceous sera in immunofluorescence tests on monkey and guinea pig oesophagus sections. *J. Invest. Dermatol.*, **88**, 545–9.
10. Matis, L.W., Anhalt, G.I., Diaz, L.A., *et al.* (1987) Calcium enhances the sensitivity of immunofluorescence for pemphigus antibodies. *J. Invest. Dermatol.*, **89**, 302–4.
11. Goldberg, D.J., Sobolinski, M. and Bystryn, J.C. (1984) Regional variation in the expression of bullous pemphigoid antigen and location of lesions in bullous pemphigoid. *Invest. Dermatol.*, **82**, 326–8.
12. Woodley, D.T., Ernst, T., Roose, M.C., *et al.* (1987) Neonatal foreskin substrate has limitations for the immunofluorescence screening of monoclonal antibodies. *J. Invest. Dermatol.*, **88**, 167–71.
13. Logan, R.A., Bhogal, B., Das, A.K., *et al.* (1987) Localisation of bullous pemphigoid antibody – an indirect immunofluorescence study of 228 cases using a split-skin technique. *Brit. J. Dermatol.*, **117**, 471–8.
14. Kelly, S.E. and Wojnarowska, F. (1988) The use of chemically split tissue in the detection of circulating anti-basement membrane zone antibodies in bullous pemphigoid and cicatricial pemphigoid. *Brit. J. Dermatol.*, **118**, 31–40.
15. Woodley, D., Sounder, D., Talley, M.J., *et al.* (1983) Localisation of basement membrane component after dermal–epidermal junction separation. *J. Invest. Dermatol.*, **81**, 149–53.
16. Kobza-Black, A., Greaves, M.W., Hensby, C.N., *et al.* (1977) A new method for recovery of exudates from normal and inflamed human skin. *Clin. Exp. Dermatol.*, **2**, 199–316.
17. Nunn, R.E. (1970) *Electron Microscopy. Preparation of Biological Specimens*, Butterworths, London.
18. Karnovsky, M.J. (1965) A formaldehyde-glutaraldehyde fixative of high osmolality for use in electron microscopy. *J. Cell Biol.*, **27**, 137A.
19. Albini, B., Holubar, K., Shu, S., *et al.* (1979) Enzymes antibody methods in immunodermatology. In *Immunopathology of The Skin*, 2nd edn (eds E.H. Beutner, T.P. Chorzelski and S.F. Bean), John Wiley and Sons, New York, pp. 93–134.
20. Prost, C., Dubertret, L. and Fosse, M. (1984) A routine immunoelectron microscopic technique for localising an autoantibody on epidermal basement membrane. *Brit. J. Dermatol.*, **110**, 1–7.
21. Dubertret, L., Bertaux, M., Fosse, M., *et al.* (1986) A simple method for correlating observations on skin at the light and electron microscopic levels. *Brit. J. Dermatol.*, **102**, 149–59.
22. Graham, R.C. and Karnovsky, M.J. (1966) The early stages of absorption of injected horseradish peroxidase in the proximal tubules of a mouse kidney. Ultrastructural cytochemistry by a new technique. *J. Histochem. Cytochem.*, **14**, 291.

APPENDICES

Appendix A

Phosphate-buffered saline (PBS) pH 7.4 (Coon's buffer)

Sodium chloride	= 20.25 g
Disodium hydrogen phosphate	= 3.20 g
Sodium dihydrogen phosphate	= 0.39 g
Distilled water	= 2.5 l

Check pH. Adjust if necessary.

Appendix B

Michel's liquid fixative (transport medium)

A. BUFFER

1. 1 M potassium citrate buffer (pH 7.0)	= 2.5 ml
2. 0.1 M magnesium sulphate	= 5.0 ml
3. 0.1 M *N*-ethylmaleimide (Sigma)	= 5.0 ml
4. Distilled water	= 87.5 ml

B. FIXATIVE

1. Buffer A	= 100 ml
2. Ammonium sulphate	= 55 g

Adjust pH to 7.0.

C. POTASSIUM CITRATE BUFFER (pH 7.0)

1. Disodium hydrogen phosphate 14.2 g/ml of distilled water.
2. Citric acid 21.0 g/100 ml of distilled water. To 82.3 ml of disodium hydrogen phosphate solution add citric acid solution (approximately 17.3 ml) drop by drop until the pH of solution is 7.

Appendix C

Buffered glycerol (mounting medium)

Sodium hydrogen carbonate	= 0.072 g
Disodium hydrogen carbonate	= 0.016 g
p-Phenylenediamine (Sigma)	= 10 mg
Glycerol	= 90 ml
Distilled water	= 10 ml

Dissolve *p*-phenylenediamine in distilled water and then add sodium hydrogen carbonate and disodium hydrogen carbonate. Mix well and add glycerol. Adjust pH to between 8.0 and 9.0.

Appendix D

Complement diluting buffer

Barbitone	= 0.56 g
Sodium chloride	= 8.5 g
Magnesium chloride	= 0.17 g
Calcium chloride	= 0.03 g
Barbitone soluble	= 0.19 g
Distilled water	= 1.0 l

This buffer is commercially available as oxoid complement fixation test diluent tablets.

Appendix E

DIF technique (skin biopsy)

1. Cut 4 μm-thick section of snap-frozen biopsies in a cryostat set at −18° C. Five coverslips are needed for each biopsy.
2. Dry section with an electric fan for 10 min.
3. Wash sections in PBS for 10 min.
4. Fan-dry sections for 10 min.
5. Cover sections of each coverslip with one of the following FITC-labelled antisera.
   IgM diluted 1 : 100
   IgG diluted 1 : 200
   IgA diluted 1 : 100
   C3 diluted 1 : 100
   Fibrinogen diluted 1 : 200
   All dilutions are made with PBS. These dilutions are for Dako FITC-labelled antisera.
6. Incubate in a moist chamber at 37° C for 30 min.
7. Wash section in PBS for 30 min (three 10-min changes).
8. Fan-dry sections, mount in buffered glycerol and examine with fluorescence microscope.

Appendix F

IIF technique (patient serum)

1. Cut 4 μm-thick frozen sections of substrate (normal human skin). Two coverslips per serum are required.
2. Fan-dry sections for 10 min.
3. Wash sections in PBS for 10 min.
4. Fan-dry sections for 10 min.
5. Cover sections of each coverslip with one of the following:
   Patient's serum diluted 1 : 10 with PBS.
   Patient's serum diluted 1 : 80 with PBS.
6. Incubate in a moist chamber at 37° C for 30 min.
7. Wash sections in PBS for 30 min (three 10-min changes).
8. Fan-dry sections for 10 min.
9. Cover sections with FITC-labelled anti-(human IgG) diluted 1 : 200 in PBS.

10. Incubate in a moist chamber at 37° C for 30 min.
11. Wash sections in PBS for 30 min (three 10-min changes).
12. Fan-dry sections, mount in buffered glycerol and examine with a fluorescence microscope.

Appendix G

Indirect C3 technique (patient serum)

1. Cut 4 μm-thick frozen sections of normal human skin (substrate). Two coverslips per serum are required.
2. Fan-dry sections for 10 min.
3. Wash sections in PBS for 10 min.
4. Fan-dry sections for 10 min.
5. Cover sections of each coverslip with one of the following:
   Patient's serum diluted 1 : 2 with PBS.
   Patient's serum diluted 1 : 4 with PBS.
6. Incubate in a moist chamber at 37° C for 30 min.
7. Wash sections in PBS for 30 min (three 10-min changes).
8. Fan-dry sections for 10 min.
9. Cover sections with source of complement (normal human serum diluted 1 : 5 with complement diluting buffer).
10. Incubate in a moist chamber at 37° C for 30 min.
11. Wash sections with PBS for 30 min (three 10-min changes).
12. Fan-dry sections for 10 min.
13. Cover sections with anti-human Cs dilute 1 : 100 with PBS and incubate at 37° C for 30 min.
14. Wash sections in PBS for 30 min (three 10-min changes).
15. Fan-dry sections, mount in buffered glycerol and examine with a fluorescence microscope.

Appendix H

Immunoelectron-microscopic technique (IEM)

1. Cut thin slices of fresh tissue with a sharp razor or by hand microtome.
2. Wash slices in 50 ml of PBS for 1 h at 4° C.
3. Fix slices in 2% buffered paraformaldehyde for 1 h at 4° C with agitation.
4. Wash sections in PBS for 1 h at 4° C.
5. Incubate slices with horseradish peroxidase-labelled Ig or complement 3 (C3) diluted 1 : 10 with PBS for 18 h at 4° C.
6. Wash slices in PBS for 1 h at 4° C.
7. Fix slices in Karnovsky fixative for 1 h at 4° C.
8. Wash slices in cacodylate buffer for 30 min.
9. Wash slices in 0.1 M Tris–HCl buffer, pH 7.6, for 30 min.
10. Develop horseradish peroxidase in Graham/Karnovsky medium for 1 h at room temperature with agitation in dark.
11. Wash slices in cacodylate buffer for 15 min.
12. Postfix slices in 1% osmium tetroxide for 4 h.
13. Dehydrate and embed slices in araldite resin.
14. Cut ultrathin sections and examine under electron microscope.

Three

Treatment of the immunological bullous diseases

G. M. Levene

The aim of treatment of most diseases is to prevent them if possible, to use the appropriate amount of topical or systemic therapy to cure or at least to control them, and to manage any adverse effects of therapy. These aims apply equally to the bullous disorders.

3.1 PREVENTION

Since the initiating cause of most bullous disorders is little understood it is not easy to give advice on how to prevent them. The inflammatory bullous disorders such as pemphigus and pemphigoid undoubtedly have genetic and immunological factors in their aetiology but so far no environmental triggers of the conditions have been discovered, apart from certain drugs in the case of pemphigus and pemphigoid. Pemphigus has been associated with administration of penicillamine [1–3], and with the similar sulphydryl drugs thiopronine [4] and captopril [5] as well as with rifampicin [6,7]. So far there is no known marker to indicate why a small proportion of patients taking these drugs develop pemphigus. Penicillamine has also been associated with the development of cicatricial pemphigoid [8], and indomethacin has been shown to exacerbate dermatitis herpetiformis [9].

Radiotherapy can initiate pemphigus [10] and can result in a rather intractable exacerbation at the site of radiation in patients with existing pemphigus (unpublished observations).

Clues as to aetiology might be obtained from the more frequent association of blistering with other diseases; examples that can be mentioned are diabetes with bullous pemphigoid, particularly of the localized type [11], and psoriasis with pemphigoid [12–14]. Photochemotherapy has been implicated in inducing bullous pemphigoid during treatment of psoriasis [15]. Unfortunately such associations may indicate only a propensity to develop autoimmune or other phenomena without helping to explain what triggers the bullous disease.

A dietary factor, such as sensitivity to gluten, has been implicated for certain only in dermatitis herpetiformis (DH) in this group of disorders; the expression of the disease comes only after ingestion of gluten, and a strict gluten-free diet can lead to virtually complete remission. This is of some importance since the chronic small bowel inflammation (coeliac disease) associated with gluten sensitivity can subsequently give rise to small bowel lymphoma. It is possible that keeping to a strict gluten-free diet will prevent the development of such lymphomas. Unfortunately many patients with DH find a gluten-free diet distasteful and will not continue it; these patients require long-term anti-inflammatory drug medication.

There is no good evidence for the role of psychological factors in the development of bullous disorders although the presence of blisters can be very alarming, and the chronicity of pemphigus and its often slow and incomplete response to treatment can make patients very despondent.

3.2 TOPICAL THERAPY IN THE BULLOUS DISORDERS

It has been the custom to emphasize the role of systemic drugs in the treatment of bullous diseases. This has been understandable in that powerful systemic drugs were discovered early and supplanted the rather bland and ineffectual topical agents then in use. However, the development of very potent topical corticosteroids (e.g. clobetasol propionate) has meant that some bullous problems can be treated topically or intralesionally without resort to systemic therapy, or at least rather less systemic therapy need be used. The topical preparation can be supplemented with antibiotic and anti-*Candida* activity, e.g. in Dermovate-NN cream or ointment, which contains neomycin and nystatin in addition to the steroid.

3.2.1 Dermatitis herpetiformis

This is probably best treated with a combination of a gluten-free diet and a sulphone or appropriate sulphonamide drug (Chapter 11). It must be kept in mind that DH with its associated coeliac disease is a systemic disorder with implications for general malaise, malabsorption and the possibility of gut lymphoma. Whilst it is likely that some relief can be obtained with topical therapy, this cannot be recommended other than as a temporary measure whilst waiting for systemic measures to take effect. When starting a trial of oral dapsone one expects a prompt and unequivocal improvement; the interpretation of the response could be blurred if a potent topical steroid is given at the same time.

3.2.2 Linear IgA disease (Chapters 7 and 8)

Linear IgA disease tends to present clinically with lesions similar to both dermatitis herpetiformis and pemphigoid, but small bowel changes are not found. Sulphones and certain sulphonamides alone can produce resolution of this disorder although some patients also require systemic steroids. Topical corticosteroid therapy is worth trying if pruritus is severe and can be particularly helpful for mucosal lesions.

3.2.3 Bullous pemphigoid (Chapter 5)

This can be localized in type and particularly affects the fronts of the shins. In some cases topical therapy with clobetasol proprionate ointment or selective intralesional therapy with triamcinolone acetonide suspension can control this problem. Many of the patients are elderly, and topical therapy can limit the dose of systemic therapy needed. Sometimes classical bullous pemphigoid in elderly patients is of rapid but not abrupt onset. This type of bullous pemphigoid can be treated with a very potent topical corticosteroid associated with minimal systemic steroid.

3.2.4 Cicatricial pemphigoid

Topical steroid is helpful for some patients with cicatricial pemphigoid. A moderately potent or very potent variety is needed, and, particularly when the anogenital area is involved, concomitant therapy with nystatin or clioquinol is desirable. Topical or intralesional therapy is said to be helpful for conjunctival disease in combination with systemic therapy.

3.2.5 Pemphigus

Topical therapy has an important part to play in the control of pemphigus both in the early stages and subsequently. Some patients with mild pemphigus foliaceus can be controlled using only topical therapy for many years and in some cases no other therapy is required. Topical antimicrobial measures help to prevent exacerbation of lesions by infection but care should be taken to choose preparations that are dilute enough not to cause toxicity if absorbed through the broken skin. Neomycin and clioquinol should be used only on small areas of erosion. If there are extensive erosions they can be painted with aqueous 0.5% Gentian Violet solution, alternating with topical steroid. In general, topical antiseptics should be used with caution in view of the possibility of local delay in healing [16] and of absorption.

3.2.6 Oral lesions

Manifestations of bullous disease inside the mouth often cause much discomfort. Topical therapy has a large part to play in helping these lesions. Whereas sucking hydrocortisone hemisuccinate tablets is rarely of value, coating the lesions with triamcinolone in Orabase is helpful. If lesions are present in the vestibule or sulci of the mouth, application of clobetasol propionate ointment topical is an awkward but helpful nocturnal treatment. This ointment can be applied under a denture to appropriate lesions on the hard palate or alveolar margin, achieving the effect of a topical steroid under occlusion. Another method is the use of a soft dental impression carrier bearing fluocinonide gel held inside the mouth for 1h four times daily [17]. A simpler method is to spray the lesions with a potent corticosteroid aerosol of the type used for hay fever (e.g. beclomethasone dipropionate, 250 μg per dose).

Particularly recalcitrant mouth ulcers or erosions can be injected with intralesional triamcinolone, a procedure which is usually well tolerated by the patient and sometimes rapidly effective. Pemphigus lesions on the vermilion of the lips often respond well to potent topical steroid therapy.

3.3 MANAGEMENT OF ACTIVE BULLOUS DISEASE

Inflammatory bullous disorders can be of all grades of severity and the requirements for treatment can likewise vary from no therapy at all to the maximum of the therapeutic armoury. Over the past few years there has been an increasing trend to treat dermatological patients as out-patients rather than as in-patients. This trend has affected the management of bullous disorders. Whilst there has been little problem in managing dermatitis herpetiformis and minor degrees of pemphigus in the clinic it has been customary to admit patients with extensive bullous pemphigoid and those with more severe pemphigus. For patients with large areas of blistering and erosions there will always be need for in-patient facilities if the disease is to be controlled without causing the patient unnecessary distress.

The importance of skilled nursing care for these severely affected patients cannot be overemphasized. A bed with a mattress that evens out pressure is desirable and the patient should lie on a sheet of absorbant non-stick material. A mattress such as that made by Spenco Medical Corporation, of polyester fibre, is a simple one which provides gentle support for eroded areas. If erosions are very severe a sheet of Lyofoam avoids the sticking which is a feature of fabric sheets. In extreme cases a pneumatic mechanical air or water bed, as used for patients with severe burns, may need to be employed but these are not widely available.

Frequent mouthwashes are desirable if there are painful mouth lesions; hexetidine (0.1% solution) (Oraldene) and benzydamine hydrochloride (0.15% solution) (Difflam Oral Rinse) are examples of suitable preparations. Buccal *Candida* infection will need treatment with amphotericin B lozenges, and Vincent's stomatitis, recognized by unpleasant foetor oris, requires metronidazole or systemic penicillin.

3.4 DRUG THERAPY OF BULLOUS DISEASES

When considering drug treatment it is convenient to divide the stages of treatment into three phases; phase 1, initial treatment; phase 2, maintenance treatment; phase 3, withdrawal of treatment.

3.4.1 Phase 1: initial treatment

The aim of treatment is to achieve control as quickly and as safely as possible.

(a) Dermatitis herpetiformis and linear IgA disease

Initial treatment of dermatitis herpetiformis and linear IgA disease is usually by administration of dapsone, perhaps starting with 50 mg daily for 3 days to ensure no ill effects and then increasing to a dose of 100 mg daily. This therapy is usually so prompt and complete in its action that it has been used as a diagnostic test for the disease. This drug is completely contraindicated if the patient has glucose-6-phosphate-dehydrogenase deficiency which would result in acute haemolysis; some negro and various other populations (e.g. Asian and Mediterranean) have a high incidence of this genetic disorder and a blood screening test may be necessary before starting treatment. If dapsone otherwise makes the patient feel unwell or if there is unacceptable anaemia due to haemolysis it may be necessary to change to alternative drugs, these being sulphapyridine at a dose of 0.5–2 g daily or sulphamethoxypyridazine also at 0.5–2 g daily. Linear IgA disease likewise often responds to dapsone, but usually more slowly.

(b) Bullous pemphigoid

Bullous pemphigoid is traditionally treated initially with a moderate dose of systemic prednisolone, usually between 40 and 80 mg daily, the dose being slowly lowered as the condition improves. Azathioprine is often added as a steroid-sparing drug. High doses of prednisolone are not always well tolerated in elderly people and it is desirable to avoid them if possible. One can often successfully treat pemphigoid by using intermittent depot tetracosactrin together with azathioprine and topical steroid therapy [18]. In this technique an injection of depot tetracosactrin (2 mg IM) is given and oral azathioprine (50 mg b.d.*) is started at the same time. Topical clobetasol propionate ointment is applied sparingly to all inflammatory lesions. After 3 or 4 days a second dose of tetracosactrin is given and the azathioprine increased to 50 mg t.d.s†. The depot adrenocorticotropin is then given once or twice weekly for 2–3 weeks until the condition is well controlled. At this stage the azathioprine dose may be sufficiently effective by itself to prevent relapse, but otherwise a relatively small dose of prednisolone, e.g. 10–15 mg daily orally, will be needed as a supplement. Under some circumstances successful treatment can be achieved without admission to hospital, but in others the severity of the initial blistering may indicate the need for admission for a week or two. The use of azathioprine in bullous pemphigoid is well established [19–21].

* Twice daily.
† Three times daily.

Some patients with bullous pemphigoid respond completely to dapsone or the sulphones, particularly when the disease starts below the age of 60 and in whose histology neutrophils predominate over eosinophils [22–25].

Although in most instances bullous pemphigoid comes readily under control there are individual cases who are resistant to systemic steroid therapy, and who are unable to tolerate azathioprine or dapsone. These patients present a considerable problem and, as in pemphigus, cyclophosphamide [26] and methotrexate [11] can rescue the situation. In one French study there was a high mortality when systemic corticosteroids were used either alone or with azathioprine [27]. Recently success in treating pemphigoid has been described using oral tetracycline or erythromycin, and nicotinamide (niacinamide USP) [28], and by oral tetracycline alone [29]. The role of these preparations in pemphigoid as sole or supplementary therapy deserves further evaluation.

(c) Cicatricial pemphigoid

Cicatricial pemphigoid often responds well to dapsone [30] and this is the drug of first choice. Sometimes combined therapy with dapsone and sulphapyridine or sulphamethoxypyridazine is needed. Systemic steroids are not as helpful as one would wish and often an unacceptably high dose is necessary to produce any response.

(d) Pemphigus

Pemphigus is more variable in its mode of onset than the other bullous disorders. It is often helpful for therapeutic purposes to classify pemphigus as 'major' or 'minor' according to the extent and severity of skin lesions and systemic upset [18]. In patients with insidious onset of intermittent minor lesions of pemphigus foliaceus one can debate whether treatment, apart from topical therapy, is required at all. Help will come from the indirect immunofluorescence titre which will give an indication of the activity of the pemphigus. A low titre will justify minimal treatment whereas a high or rising titre will indicate the need for more active intervention. If only a few superficial lesions are present a moderately potent topical steroid can heal the lesions. A bacteriology swab will indicate whether pathogenic staphylococci are present and hence the need for a systemic antistaphylococcal antibiotic such as flucloxacillin.

More active but still 'minor' pemphigus requires systemic therapy, but it is not always necessary to opt for high-dose systemic steroids. Initial treatment with injected gold [31] or with dapsone [32, 33] can produce a good remission, often accelerated by concomitant topical therapy, and these agents can also be used as steroid-sparing therapy either together with moderate-dose alternate-day steroid therapy or given subsequently in the event of incomplete response to steroid alone [34]. Gold is given in a similar regime as that used by rheumatologists for joint disease; after initial screening tests for normality of blood, liver and kidneys a test dose of 10 mg IM of sodium aurothiomalate (Myocrisin) is given. A week later, if all is well, a dose of 25 mg IM is given and subsequently weekly doses of 50 mg IM are administered. Alternatively dapsone tablets are given in doses of 50–200 mg with careful screening of haemoglobin etc., to ensure that there is no leucopenia or undue haemolysis. If it is desired to add a systemic steroid for these relatively 'minor' cases, a dose of 40 mg of prednisolone on alternate days may be all that is required initially, the success of the treatment being monitored by the clinical response and by the fall in immunofluorescent titre. Recently an oral gold preparation (auranofin) has been described to be of value in pemphigus [35]. Other drugs of great value in pemphigus are azathioprine [21, 36] and cyclophosphamide [37, 38].

In patients with pemphigus of clinically 'major' severity, particularly if it is of recent onset or is deteriorating rapidly, the mainstay of treatment is large doses of systemic steroid [39, 40]. Prednisolone is the most usual preparation employed. A morning dose of 150–300 mg of prednisolone is given in association with a steroid-sparing drug such as azathioprine, cyclophosphamide, methotrexate, gold or dapsone. Staphylococcal skin infection or *Candida* mouth infection should be sought and appropriately treated. Systemic therapy is supplemented by potent topical steroid therapy. Many of these patients can now be managed without admission to hospital [39]. It is commonly found that severe pemphigus can be rather slow to improve even with very high prednisolone doses, and new lesions may continue to appear. In such cases it is often necessary to continue high-dose steroid therapy for 5–10 weeks before the disease is controlled since the anti-inflammatory or immunosuppressive steroid-sparing drugs may take several weeks or even months to achieve their maximum effect. The activity of the disease is monitored by weekly indirect immunofluorescent blood tests. If erosions increase or totally fail to heal and the titre does not fall, it may be necessary to increase the dose of systemic steroid to as high as 400 mg daily for some weeks.

As the condition comes under control the systemic steroid dose can be reduced by half, and halved again a week or two later. A falling immunofluorescent titre together with the clinical finding of improvement and lack of relapse will encourage reduction of steroid dose. An alternate-day regime of systemic steroid should be adopted as soon as possible in order to minimize side effects.

Severe pemphigus is a rather rare disease, at least in Europe and the USA, so that detailed comparisons of diverse treatment regimes is by no means easy [41]. It was suggested [18] that bolus therapy of methylprednisolone should be considered for severe pemphigus and this has been used with success [42, 43]; however, in view of the possible hazards of pulse therapy this technique should probably be reserved for younger patients in the initial episode of severe pemphigus.

Cyclophosphamide, as an independently effective and steroid-sparing drug, has been praised on numerous occasions over the years, and it can be most useful [26, 37]. Pasricha [44] has enthusiastically advocated a combination of bolus parenteral dexamethasone with cyclophosphamide and continued low-dose oral cyclophosphamide therapy.

(e) Epidermolysis bullosa acquisita

Acquired epidermolysis bullosa (Chapter 10) has gradually become established as a bullous disease in its own right [45]. The clinical and immunopathological features have been delineated and various treatments have been used. Success has been claimed with dapsone, vitamin E, gold and systemic steroids.

(f) Newer methods of treating bullous diseases

There have been reports of plasmaphaeresis in pemphigus [43, 46, 47] and pemphigoid [48, 49, 49a]. This is a highly specialized and expensive treatment which is not without risk and of transient benefit. It is probably to be considered only in severe pemphigus associated with a very high antibody titre, where plasmapheresis will produce a temporary remission whilst the systemic therapy takes effect.

The organ transplant anti-rejection drug, cyclosporin A, has been used with success in cases of pemphigus and pemphigoid [50, 51]. It is variably effective but not very easy to use in view of the necessity to monitor blood levels of the drug and its tendency to cause renal damage and hypertension. It is probably best reserved as alternative therapy in major pemphigus where conventional treatment is not proving effective.

3.4.2 Phase 2: medium-term treatment

After the disease has been brought under control the next problem is to maintain the patient in remission. There is usually no difficulty with DH and bullous pemphigoid which stay controlled for long periods with a stable drug regime. If a strict gluten-free diet is being used in the former it may be possible to reduce the daily requirement for dapsone or sulphapyridine. Bullous pemphigoid is usually no problem so far as controlling blisters is concerned but some individual patients are troubled by continued pruritus and reactivation of the disease which can be very intractable and does not respond well to systemic steroids, even in quite high maintenance dose. Topical steroid application helps but the problem can often by solved by adding systemic dapsone or a sulphonamide to the existing treatment [52].

As always in this group of diseases, pemphigus presents the greatest challenge to therapeutic endeavour. It is a common problem that patients have survived the acute stage of the illness with the use of large-dose systemic steroids but after the dose has been reduced to low maintenance levels the patient is still having lesions in the mouth, on the face, and sometimes on the skin. Chronic infection can be overlooked, especially *Candida* in the mouth which is cleared rapidly by amphoteracin B lozenges, and *Staphylococcus aureus* infection in skin lesions which responds to flucloxacillin or other appropriate systemic antibiotic. It must be remembered that staphylococcal impetigo can look almost identical to pemphigus both clinically and histologically. Apart from the clinical evidence the blood immunofluorescence titre of pemphigus antibody will help to establish the activity of the disease. Some patients are chronically undertreated in the medium term. This often comes about by attempts to reduce the systemic steroid dose to very low maintenance levels and a reluctance to introduce extra immunosuppressive medication. In this situation it is usually necessary temporarily to increase the dose of prednisolone and to introduce one or more of the steroid-sparing drugs if these are not already being employed. If azathioprine is already being used a possible sequence is gold, dapsone and cyclophosphamide. These drugs usually show a beneficial effect within a few weeks if they are going to work but there is no way of assessing in advance which one or combination will work best.

A suitable regime of injected gold is to give 50 mg weekly until 1 g is given, then 50 mg on alternate weeks until 2 g is given and then 50 mg monthly until a total of 3 g is reached, at which time it can probably be stopped. Complications of gold therapy are relatively common but not usually devastating and it can be stopped if unpleasant side effects appear. Dapsone is given in the same regime as for DH, but it does not always work. Cyclophosphamide is undoubtedly an excellent antipemphigus treatment but caution is needed in view of its possible effects on the bladder (haemorrhagic cystitis) and its tendency to cause gonadal atrophy and consequent male and female infertility, a consideration of importance in young patients.

3.4.3 Phase 3: stopping treatment and late events

If the disease is well controlled by systemic steroid with or without a mixture of other drugs there is no need to be hasty in reducing or stopping these drugs. All of the bullous diseases can relapse after many years of inactivity. The relapse can come after stopping treatment or whilst the patient is still on maintenance therapy. Usually only a modest increase in the treatment is required to control the exacerbation.

It is unwise to reintroduce very-high-dose steroid in patients already on maintenance steroid therapy in view of the great risk of skeletal problems in already weakened bones. Patients can be incapacitated as much by the pain of collapsed dorsal vertebrae or by ischaemic necrosis of the head of the femur as by the original bullous disease.

If the disease is genuinely inactive the therapy can be progressively tapered off over the course of 2 or 3 years. Remarkably some patients claim that a dose of prednisolone of even 1 or 2 mg weekly is needed to keep them free of mouth or skin lesions, and at this level no harm is likely to come to them even if this is continued indefinitely.

With many patients it is possible to cease treatment completely. It is uncertain, however, whether any of these diseases can be regarded as cured or whether they are best regarded as quiescent. Long-term follow up is needed.

REFERENCES

1. Benveniste, M., Crouzet, J., Homberg, J.C., Lessana, M., Camus, J.P. and Hewitt, J. (1985) Pemphigus induits par la D-pénicillamine dans la polyarthrite rhumatoïde. *Nouv. Presse Med.* **4**, 3125–8.
2. Marsden, R.A., Ryan, T.J., Vanhegan, R.I., Walshe, M., Hill, H. and Mowat, A.G. (1976) Pemphigus foliaceus induced by penicillamine. *Brit. Med. J.*, **ii**, 1423–4.
3. Ho, V.C., Stein, H.B., Ongley, R.C. and McLeod, W.A. (1985) Penicillamine induced pemphigus. *J. Rheumatol.*, **12**, 583–6.
4. Trotta, F., Scaramelli, M., Cervi, G. and Virgili, A.R. (1984) Thiopronine-induced pemphigus vulgaris in rheumatoid arthritis. *Scand. J. Rheumatol.*, **13**, 93–5.
5. Parfrey, P.S., Clement, M., Vandenberg, M.J. and Wright, P. (1980) Captopril-induced pemphigus. *Brit. Med. J.*, **281**, 194.
6. Gange, R.W., Rhodes, E.L., Edwards, C.O. and Powell, M.E.A. (1976) Pemphigus induced by rifampicin. *Brit. J. Dermatol.*, **95**, 445–8.
7. Lee, C.W., Lim, J.H. and Kang, H.J. (1984) Pemphigus foleaceus induced by rifampicin. *Brit. J. Dermatol.*, **111**, 619–22.
8. Shuttleworth, D., Graham-Brown, R.A.C., Hutchinson, P.E. and Jolliffe, D.S. (1985) Cicatricial pemphigoid in D-Penicillamine-treated patients with rheumatoid arthritis: a report of three cases. *Clin. Exp. Dermatol.* **10**, 392–7.
9. Griffiths, C.E.M., Leonard, J. and Fry, L. (1985) Dermatitis herpetiformis exacerbated by indomethacin. *Brit. J. Dermatol.*, **112**, 443–5.
10. David, M. and Feuerman, E.J. (1987) Induction of pemphigus by X-ray irradiation. *Clin. Exp. Dermatol.*, **12**, 197–9.
11. Downham, T.F. and Chapel, T.A. (1978) Bullous pemphigoid: therapy in patients with and without diabetes mellitus. *Arch. Dermatol.*, **114**, 1639–42.
12. Koeber, W.A., Price, N.M. and Watson, W. (1978) Coexistent psoriasis and bullous pemphigoid. A report of 6 cases. *Arch. Dermatol.*, **114**, 1643–6.
13. Grunwald, M.H., David, M. and Feuerman, E.J. (1985) Coexistence of psoriasis vulgaris and bullous diseases. *J. Amer. Acad. Dermatol.*, **13**, 224–8.
14. Grattan, C.E.H. (1985) Evidence of an association between bullous pemphigoid and psoriasis. *Brit. J. Dermatol.*, **113**, 281–3.
15. Brun, P. and Baran, R. (1982) Pemphigoïde bulleuse induite par la photochimiotherapie du psoriasis. *Ann. Dermatol. Vénéréol. (Paris).* **109**, 461.
16. Deas, J., Billings, P., Brennan, S., Silver, I. and Leaper, D.J. (1986) The toxicity of commonly used antiseptics on fibroblasts in tissue culture. *Phlebology,* **1**, 205–9.
17. Aufdemorte, T.B., De Villez, R.L. and Parel, S.M. (1985) Modified topical steroid therapy for the treatment of oral mucous membrane pemphigoid. *Oral Surg.*, **59**, 256–60.
18. Levene, G.M. (1982) The treatment of pemphigus and pemphigoid. *Clin. Exp. Dermatol.*, **7**, 643–52.
19. Greaves, M.W., Burton, J.L., Marks, J. and Dawber, R.P.R. (1971) Azathioprine in the treatment of bullous pemphigoid. *Brit. Med. J.*, **i**, 144–5.
20. Burton, J.L. and Greaves, M.W. (1974) Azathioprine for pemphigus and pemphigoid: 4-year follow-up. *Brit. J. Dermatol.*, **92**, 103–9.
21. Aberer, W., Wolff-Schreiner, E.C., Stingl, G. and Wolff, K. (1987) Azathioprine in the treatment of

pemphigus vulgaris: a long-term follow up. *J. Amer. Acad. Dermatol.*, **16**, 527–33.

22. **Piamphongsant, T. and Ausawamongkonpan, S. (1976) Bullous pemphigoid controlled by dapsone.** *Dermatologica*, **152**, 352–7.
23. **Person, J.R. and Rogers, R.S. III** (1977) Bullous **pemphigoid responding to sulfapyridine and the sulphones.** *Arch. Dermatol.*, **113**, 610–15.
24. **Piamphongsant, T.** (1983) Dapsone for the **treatment of bullous pemphigoid.** *Asian Pacific J. Allerg. Immunol.*, **1**, 19–21.
25. **Venning, V., Millard, P.R. and Wojnarowska, F.** (1989) Dapsone as first line treatment for bullous pemphigoid. *Brit. J. Dermatol.*, **120**, 83–92.
26. **Krain, L.S., Landau, J.W. and Newcomer, V.D. (1972) Cyclophosphamide in the treatment of pemphigus vulgaris and bullous pemphigoid.** *Arch. Dermatol.*, **106**, 657–61.
27. **Bernard, P., Venot, J., Rommel, A., Bonnetblanc, J.M. and Texier, L. (1986) Pemphigoïde bulleuse: étude du prognostic à propos de cinquante-sept observations.** *Semin. Hôp. Paris*, **62**, 1229–32.
28. **Berk, M.A. and Lorincz, A.L. (1986) The treatment of bullous pemphigoid with tetracycline and niacinamide: a preliminary report.** *Arch. Dermatol.*, **122**, 670–4.
29. **Thornfeldt, C.R. and Menkes, A.W.** (1987) Bullous **pemphigoid controlled by oral tetracycline.** *J. Amer. Acad. Dermatol.*, **16**, 305–10.
30. **Rogers, R.S.III, Seehafer, J.R. and Perry, H.O. (1982) Treatment of cicatricial (benign mucous membrane) pemphigoid with dapsone.** *J. Amer. Acad. Dermatol.*, **6**, 215–23.
31. **Pennys, N.S., Eaglstein, W.H., Indgin, S. and Frost, P. (1973) Gold sodium thiomalate treatment of pemphigus.** *Arch. Dermatol.*, **108**, 56–60.
32. **Piamphongsant, T. (1979) Treatment of pemphigus with corticosteroids and cyclophosphamide.** *J. Dermatol. (Tokyo)*, **6**, 359.
33. **Basset, N., Guillot, B., Michel, B.,** *et al.* (1987) **Dapsone as initial treatment in superficial pemphigus: report of nine cases.** *Arch. Dermatol.*, **123**, 783–5.
34. **Poulin, Y., Perry, H.O. and Muller, S.A.** (1984) **Pemphigus vulgaris: results of treatment with gold as a steroid-sparing agent in a series of 13 patients.** *J. Amer. Acad. Dermatol.*, **11**, 851–7.
35. **Salomon, D. and Saurat, J-H.** (1986) Oral gold **therapy (Auranofin) in pemphigus** vulgaris. *Dermatologica*, **172**, 310–14.
36. **Roenigk, H.H. and Deodhar, S.** (1973) Pemphigus **treatment with** azathioprine, clinical **and immunological** correlation. *Arch. Dermatol.*, **107**, 353–7.
37. **Fellner, M.G., Katz, J.M. and McCabe, J.B.** (1978) **Successful use of cyclophosphamide** and prednisone for initial treatment of pemphigus vulgaris. *Arch. Dermatol.*, **114**, 889–94.
38. Ahmed, A.R. and Hombal, S. (1987) Use of cyclophosphamide in azathioprine failures in pemphigus. *J. Amer. Acad. Dermatol.*, **17**, 437–42.
39. Lever, W.F. and Schaumberg-Lever, G. (1984) Treatment of pemphigus vulgaris: results obtained in 84 patients between 1961 and 1982. *Arch. Dermatol.*, **120**, 44–7.
40. Smolle, J. (1985) Zur Therapie der Pemphiguskrankheiten. Kritische Ammerkungenanhand von 44 Fallen. *Hautarzt*, **36**, 96–102.
41. Bystryn, J.C. (1984) Adjuvant therapy of pemphigus. *Arch. Dermatol.* **120**, 941–51.
42. Siegel, J. and Eaglstein, W.H. (1984) High dose methylprednisolone in the treatment of bullous pemphigoid. *Arch. Dermatol.*, **120**, 1157–65.
43. Fine, J.-D., Appell, M.L., Green, L.K. and Sams, W.M., Jr (1988) Pemphigus vulgaris. Combined treatment with intravenous corticosteroid, pulse therapy, plasmapheresis and azathioprine. *Arch. Dermatol.*, **124**, 236–9.
44. Pasricha, J.S. (1987) Can pemphigus be cured? *Brit. J. Dermatol.*, **117**, *Suppl.* **32**, 42–3.
45. Gammon, W.R., Briggaman, R.H., Woodley, D.T., Heald, P.W. and Wheeler, C.E. (1984) Epidermolysis bullosa acquisita – a pemphigoid-like disease. *J. Amer. Acad. Dermatol.*, **11**, 820–32.
46. Ruocco, V., Rossi, A., Argenziano, G., Astarita, C., Alviggi, L., Farzati, B. and Papaleo, G. (1977) Pathogenicity of the intercellular antibodies of pemphigus and their periodic removal from the circulation by plasmapheresis. *Br. J. Dermatol.*, **98**, 237–41.
47. Swanson, D.L. and Dahl, M.V. (1981) Pemphigus vulgaris and plasma exchange, clinical and serologic studies. *J. Amer. Acad. Dermatol.*, **4**, 325–8.
48. Roujeau, J-C., Guillaume, J-C., Morel, P. *et al.* (1984) Plasma exchange in bullous pemphigoid. *Lancet*, **ii**, 486–9.
49. Guillaume, J.C., Roujeau, J.C., Touzet, C., Revuz, J. and Touraine, R. (1985) Traitement de la pemphigoïde bulleuse par échanges plasmatiques et prednisolone. *Medicine*, **14**, 1139–42.

49a. Goldberg, N.S., Robinson, J.K., Roenigk, H.H. *et al.* (1985) Plasmapheresis therapy for bullous pemphigoid. *Arch. Dermatol.* **121**, 1484–5.

50. Thivolet, J., Barthelemy, M., Rigot-Muller, G. *et al.* (1985) Effects of cyclosporine on bullous pemphigoid and pemphigus. *Lancet*, **i**, 334–5.
51. Balda, B.R. and Rosenzweig, D. (1986) Cyclosporin A in der Behandlung von Pemphigus foliaceus und Pemphigus erythematosus. *Hautarzt*, **37**, 454–7.
52. Jeffes, E.W.B. and Ahmed, A.R. (1989) Adjuvant treatment of bullous pemphigoid with dapsone. *Clin. Exp. Dermatol.*, **49**, 132–6.

Four

Pemphigus: Pemphigus vulgaris and pemphigus foliaceus

Stephan Müller and John R. Stanley

INTRODUCTION

The term pemphigus stems from the Greek pemphix (blister) [1] and describes a group of chronic blistering skin diseases in which autoantibodies are directed against the cell surface of keratinocytes, resulting in the loss of cohesion between epidermal cells, through a process called acantholysis. Pemphigus is divided into pemphigus vulgaris (PV) with a suprabasal acantholysis and pemphigus foliaceus (PF) with acantholysis in the upper parts of the epidermis. With these definitions in mind, we could classify pemphigus vegetans and pemphigus erythematosus, types of pemphigus with certain unique clinical features, as subtypes of PV and PF, respectively.

4.2 CLINICAL FEATURES

4.2.1 Presentation

Pemphigus has a worldwide distribution with an annual incidence of approximately 0.1–0.5 per 100 000 population [2–5]. The prevalence of PV in patients of Jewish origin is increased, and the annual incidence of pemphigus has been reported to be about 1.6–3.2 cases per 100 000 Jewish population. The disease has a peak incidence of occurrence in patients between the fourth and sixth decade [6–8].

4.2.2 Cutaneous distribution, mucous membrane involvement and morphology of lesions

PV is the most common type of pemphigus and comprises about 80% of patients with pemphigus [6, 7]. In more than 50% of cases the disease begins with oral lesions, which may precede the cutaneous lesions by several months or may be the major, if not only, manifestation in some patients [6–9]. Even though 10–15% of patients present with cutaneous lesions only, the mucous membranes are ultimately involved in almost all cases [4, 6]. Mucous membrane lesions in PV usually are seen as painful erosions. Presumably because of trauma, intact bullae are rarely seen in the mouth. Lesions in the oral cavity are usually eroded, painful and heal slowly with peripheral extension through shedding of the epithelium. These lesions are of different sizes with irregular ill-defined borders. Most frequently buccal and palatine mucosa are involved [10]. Extensive erosions and painful lesions in the mouth may result in decreased food intake which in turn may contribute to hypoproteinaemia and hypoalbuminaemia. Other mucous membranes may be involved and ulcerations of the vulva [11, 12] or the conjunctiva [13] may result in an initial misinterpretation of the diagnosis. Lesions of pharynx, larynx [14], oesophagus [15, 16], urethra, cervix [11, 12] and rectal mucosa [17] have been reported. If mucous membranes other than the oral cavity are involved, the course of the disease may be

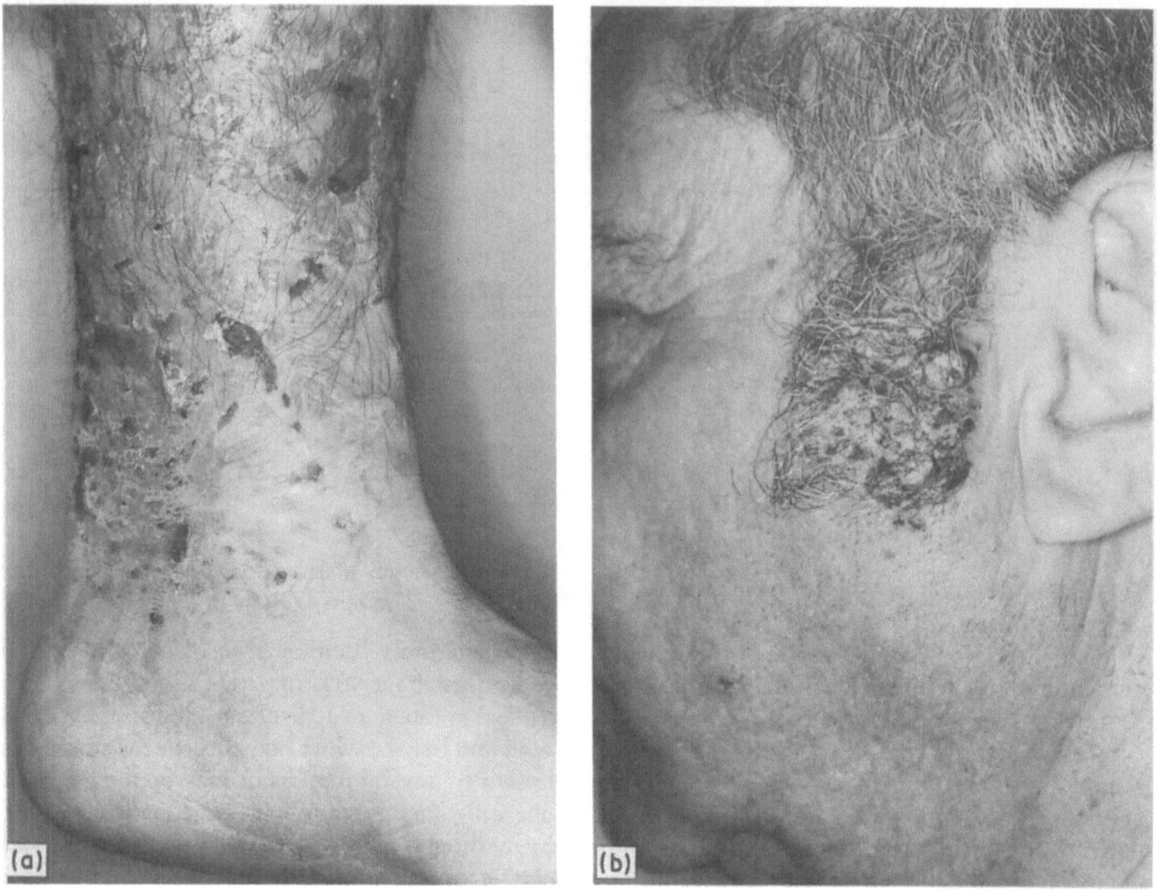

Figure 4.1 Clinical appearance of PV. (a) Patient's ankle shows crusted erosions and flaccid blisters. (b) Patient's sideburn area shows crusted verrucous lesions.

more severe [18]. A more generalized bullous phase occurs in many patients, if untreated, 5 or more months after the onset of oral lesions [19].

Cutaneous lesions in PV can be localized or generalized and usually present primarily as flaccid vesicles or bullae varying in size from less than 1 cm to several cm (Figure 4.1(a)). The scalp, face, axillae and groin are frequent sites of involvement. The content of the lesions is initially clear. The blisters may develop on normal skin or on an erythematous macule or plaque. In a few days the vesicular contents may become turbid, but often the blisters rupture easily and produce painful raw denuded areas. These eroded areas often extend at the edges due to continual peripheral loss of epidermis. Thus, relatively large areas of erosion are the main cutaneous lesions seen in many PV patients. Crusted verrucous lesions may also often develop at sites of ruptured bullae (Figure 4.1(b)) [18, 19].

Pemphigus vegetans, a subtype of PV, has been classically divided into two clinical types, Neumann and Hallopeau [20]. These two differ in their clinical presentation but it is probably accurate to think of PV, pemphigus vegetans Neumann and pemphigus vegetans Hallopeau as a spectrum from most to least severe. In the Neumann type of pemphigus vegetans the denuded areas often develop hypertrophic granulations, so-called vegetations, and in the periphery of extending vegetations pustules may be seen. Older vegetations may become dry, papillomatous and hyperkeratotic. When the disease activity changes to a more severe course the tendency to form vegetations lessens and the clinical picture is dominated by large denuded areas as it is in PV. In the Hallopeau type of pemphigus vegetans pustules are followed rapidly by vegetations with peripheral enlargement. The lesions are mostly found in the intertriginous areas. Older vegetations become firm, verrucous and hyperkeratotic. The course of pemphigus vegetans Hallopeau is said to be more benign than PV and spontaneous remissions are possible. However, some patients go on to develop flaccid bullae and denuded areas and the disease then resembles the Neumann type of pemphigus vegetans. Thus the two types of pemphigus vegetans and PV form a clinical spectrum.

Patients with PF have a very different clinical appearance from patients with PV [20]. PF patients present with scaly and crusted lesions, often in a seborrhoeic distribution on the face and trunk (Figure 4.2(a,b)). The onset of disease is often subtle with a few scattered crusted lesions which come and go, and are frequently mistaken for impetigo. As opposed to the expanding erosions seen in PV, PF lesions are usually sharply demarcated. Along the border of lesions, small vesicles may be present. Because the vesicle is so superficial and fragile, often only the crust and scale that result from a ruptured vesicle are seen. PF lesions can become generalized and the disease can even develop into an erythrodermic exfoliative dermatitis. As opposed to the extensive mucous membrane involvement in PV, mucous membrane lesions in PF are rare. Oral lesions may occur with extensive skin disease, but these are unusual. Other mucous membrane lesions seldom occur. The age of onset in a study of 30 patients varied between 17 and 85 years of age, with a median of 52 years. Occasional occurrence in children has been reported [20].

Pemphigus erythematosus (Senear–Usher Syndrome) [21], a subset of PF, presents clinically with erythematous scaling plaques over the scalp and face. These lesions may resemble lupus erythematosus or seborrhoeic dermatitis. At the same time combinations of bullae, denuded areas and crusted lesions may appear and may resemble psoriasis or impetigo [22]. The disease shows the same histological pattern as PF [20]. However, immunofluorescent studies indicate that, in addition to the epidermal cell surface antibodies found in all PF patients, as discussed below, these patients also have bound immunoglobulins at the dermo–epidermal junction. Some patients also have circulating antinuclear antibodies. Although some of these features may suggest that these patients have lupus erythematosus, frank clinical lupus is not usually seen [22, 23].

Fogo selvagem (wildfire) (FS) or Brazilian PF occurs predominantly in central and southern Brazil. Clinically, histologically and immunohistologically FS and PF share many common features or are identical. However, the epidemiology of FS differs considerably from that of PF. In contrast to the sporadic occurrence of PF, FS occurs in endemic foci. In contrast to PF, FS often affects children, adolescents and young adults, with about one-third of the cases occurring before the age of 20. Familial PF is extremely rare, whereas there have been many cases of familial FS reported [24, 25].

Other unusual aspects of pemphigus include neonatal pemphigus and penicillamine-induced pemphigus. Several cases of neonatal PV are reported in the literature. Transplacental passage of immunoglobulins of the IgG class in women suffering from pemphigus during pregnancy is thought to be the cause [26]. PV developing during pregnancy may be associated with a significant risk of foetal mortality [27]. Newborns not only may have lesions typical for pemphigus but may have typical direct and indirect immunofluorescence patterns as well [28, 29]. However, if the newborn survives the neonatal period, the prognosis is excellent, since the disease subsides as maternal antibody is catabolized. On the other hand, reports on neonatal PF are lacking. Eyre and Stanley recently reported a case of a baby born to a mother with active PF. This newborn had *in vivo* bound epidermal cell surface immunoglobulin, but no clinical disease [30].

In 1969 Degos [31] reported a form of pemphigus that was associated with penicillamine. Since then over 30 cases of penicillamine-associated or penicillamine-induced pemphigus have been

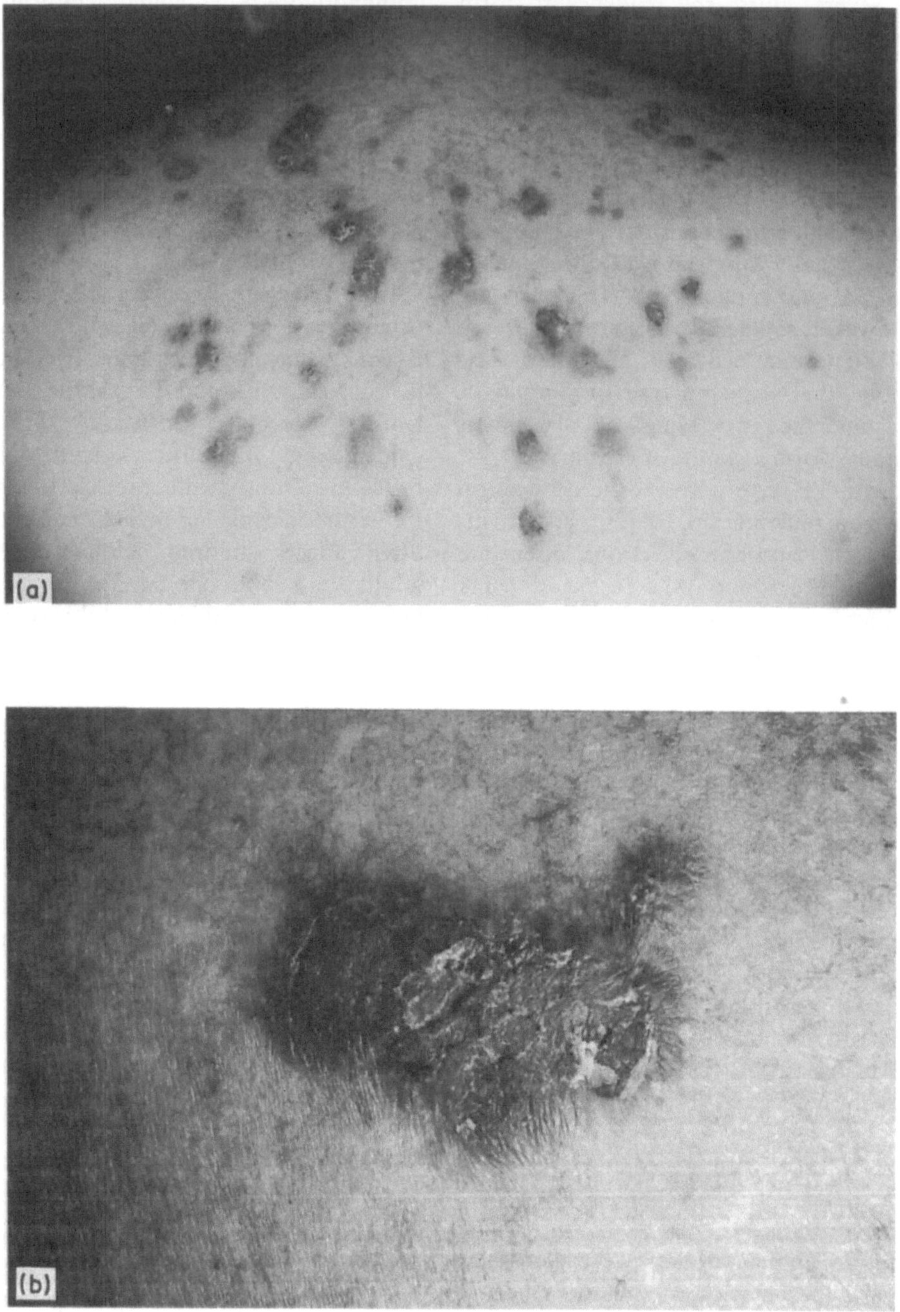

Figure 4.2 Clinical appearance of PF. (a) Patient's back shows scattered well-demarcated crusted scaly lesions. (b) Close-up of a lesion on the patient's back demonstrates the scale and crust.

described [32]. PF is the more common form of pemphigus induced by penicillamine, but PV has also been reported [33], as have other autoimmune diseases such as myasthenia gravis. The appearance and disappearance of the eruption usually is closely related in time to the use of penicillamine. In addition, the limited and localized cutaneous involvement, as well as the rarity of oral lesions, differentiate the penicillamine-associated bullous eruption from the spontaneous forms of pemphigus [32]. However, the issue of whether penicillamine-induced pemphigus is different from spontaneously occurring pemphigus is still uncertain [33]. Although the disease usually remits when the penicillamine is discontinued, cases of persistent pemphigus after penicillamine have been reported. In one report, 7 out of 104 patients who received penicillamine for more than 6 months developed pemphigus [34]. Other medications described to be associated with pemphigus in sporadic reports are captopril [35], penicillin and ampicillin [36, 37], rifampicin [38, 39] and pyrazolon derivatives [40]. Combinations of indomethacin and aspirin [41] and propranolol and mepbromate [42] have also been reported to be associated with pemphigus. The associations of medications other than penicillamine with pemphigus are probably fortuitous.

A number of different diseases have been reported that occur together with pemphigus. The triad of pemphigus with myasthenia gravis and/or thymoma has been reported repeatedly [43–46]. Pemphigus has also been described in connection with mycosis fungoides, other malignancies, cutaneous lupus erythematosus and with bullous pemphigoid, but these associations are probably fortuitous [45, 47–52].

Indirect immunofluorescence studies in patients suffering from severe burns have shown circulating anti-(epithelial cell surface) antibodies in over 50% [53]. These antibodies are termed pemphigus-like antibodies, since no clinical correlate is associated with their presence, and direct immunofluorescence does not reveal antibody bound *in vivo*. The antibodies usually disappear after 2–3 months. These findings are similar to the results of Thivolet and Beyvin [54] and Ablin [55]. The intercellular antibodies contained in these sera are not absorbed by human blood group A and B erythrocytes, confirming that the positive immunofluorescence is not due to naturally occurring haemagglutinins. The relationship of these antibodies to true pemphigus autoantibodies is unclear.

4.3 INVESTIGATIONS

4.3.1 Light microscopy

In PV the early histological changes consist of intercellular oedema and, in the lower epidermis, disappearance of intercellular bridges. The loss of cell cohesion, called acantholysis, leads to the formation of a cleft, and later, to the formation of a bulla in the suprabasal layer of the epidermis (Figure 4.3(a)). The basal cells remain attached to the dermis. Inside the bullae there are rounded acantholytic cells and clusters of epidermal cells (Figure 4.3(a)). During the early phase of blister formation there is usually little inflammation. However, early lesions sometimes show invasion of eosinophils in an epidermis with intercellular oedema, but without acantholysis, a pattern called eosinophilic spongiosis [20, 56, 57].

In PF the acantholysis occurs in the upper portions of the epidermis, usually in the granular layer. Accordingly the cleft can be found in a superficial subcorneal location (Figure 4.3(b)). There is a mild inflammatory infiltrate in the dermis; often eosinophils are present. Frequently neutrophils collect in the subcorneal cleft, with the resulting histology being indistinguishable from impetigo [57]. Eosinophilic spongiosis can also be seen in early lesions of PF.

4.3.2 Electron microscopy

In lesions of PV, early change in the epidermis shows a widening of the intercellular spaces, while the desmosomes are still intact. These desmosomes eventually become separated from the opposing attachment plaques, but the tonofilaments are still adherent at the attachment plaques. With advancing acantholysis the desmosomes gradually disappear altogether. The basal cells are not only separated from the overlying epidermal cells but are

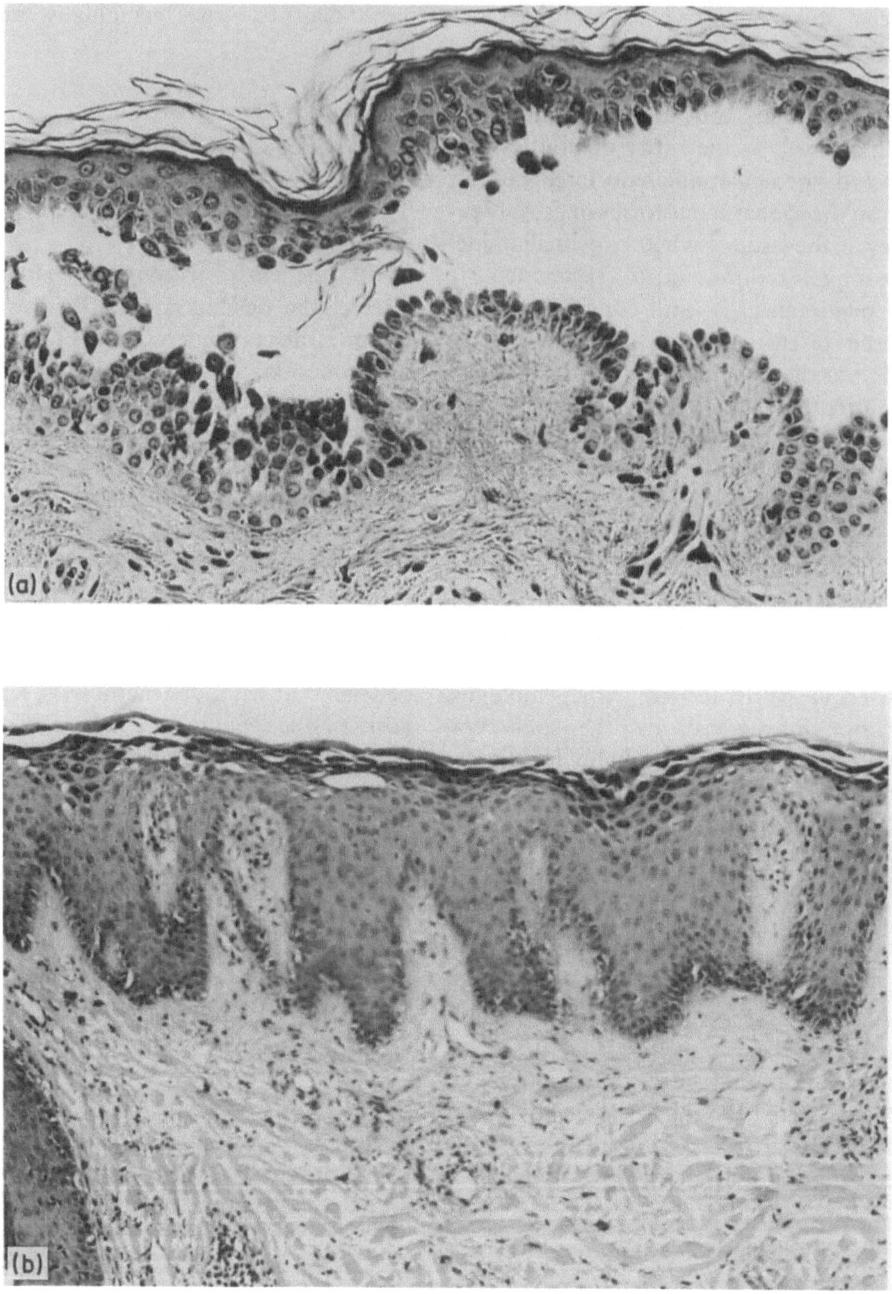

Figure 4.3 Histology of PV and PF. (a) PV lesion demonstrates a suprabasilar blister with acantholysis (× 225). (b) PF lesion shows a subcorneal blister (× 88).

also separated from each other. However, the basal cells stay attached to the basement membrane through their hemidesmosomes [58, 59].

Contrary to the electron-microscopic findings in PV, early change in at least some lesions of PF shows a separation of the tonofilaments from the attachment plaque of their corresponding desmosome. This is followed by a loss of desmosomes leading to acantholysis and by loss of orientation of the tonofilaments, resulting in dyskeratosis [60].

In summary, the desmosomal damage may be more pronounced in PF than in PV. PV lesions show severe alteration of the basal cell layer whereas in PF the ultrastructural changes occur in the higher layers of the epithelium.

4.3.3 Immunofluorescence findings

Beutner and Jordon [61] first demonstrated antibodies to the cell surface of epidermal cells in the sera of patients with PV by indirect immunofluorescence (Figure 4.4(a)). Similar antibodies are present in the sera of patients with PF (Figure 4.4(b)). A correlation of disease activity and indirect immunofluorescence titre has been observed [62, 63], even though exceptions have been reported [64, 65]. In a small percentage of patients with clinically active disease no circulating anti-epithelial cell surface antibodies can be demonstrated with indirect immunofluorescence. In these cases direct immunofluorescence must be employed to demonstrate the antibody already bound to the patient's epidermis, but not circulating in his blood.

Direct immunofluorescence is carried out by incubating frozen sections of lesional or perilesional skin from the patient with a fluorescein-conjugated anti-human IgG. Skin from patients with PV or PF demonstrates a staining of the epidermal cell surface. In addition to IgG, complement deposits can also be detected on the surface of epidermal cells in some patients by direct immunofluorescence. Beutner *et al.* [66] and Jordon *et al.* [67] showed, with direct immunofluorescence studies, that deposition of IgG on the epidermal cell surface occurs in over 90% of patients with PV. Direct immunofluorescence is probably more sensitive than indirect studies [64], and it is now generally accepted that a positive direct or indirect immunofluorescence result is necessary to confirm a diagnosis of pemphigus. Usually a differentiation between PV and PF on the basis of either the direct or indirect immunofluorescence pattern is not possible, even though the staining in PF can sometimes be limited to the upper portions of the epidermis [68, 69].

To localize PV antibody at an ultrastructural level, Wolff and Schreiner [70] performed immunoelectron microscopy on lesional skin from a patient with PV. A peroxidase-conjugated anti-human IgG was used to precipitate an electron-dense product where the patient's autoantibodies were bound in the skin. PV IgG was localized to the keratinocyte cell surfaces and within the extracellular portion of the desmosomes. Acantholytic cells were also coated with a thick layer of the electron-dense reaction product. Similar studies with Brazilian PF skin demonstrated a distribution of the antibody bound *in vivo* similar to that seen in PV [71, 72].

4.3.4 Studies to characterize pemphigus antigen

Several approaches have been used to characterize the pemphigus antigen at the molecular level. In 1977 Wood and Beutner [73] used an immunofluorescence blocking technique to study differences in specificity of antisera to PV and PF antigens. This technique is based on the assumption that if antibodies in two sera have identical specificities, then the binding of antibodies from the first serum will block further antibody binding from the second serum. In particular, a non-fluoresceinated serum sample from each of four patients with PV and two patients with Brazilian PF was tested for the ability to block the other serum samples, that were fluoresceinated, from binding to the frozen section of an epithelial substrate. PV sera blocked other PV sera from binding. Similarly, one Brazilian PF serum blocked the other from binding. In contrast, PV serum did not block Brazilian PF serum or vice versa. These findings suggested that PV and Brazilian PF antigens were distinct. However, there are difficulties in unambiguously interpreting the results of immunofluorescence

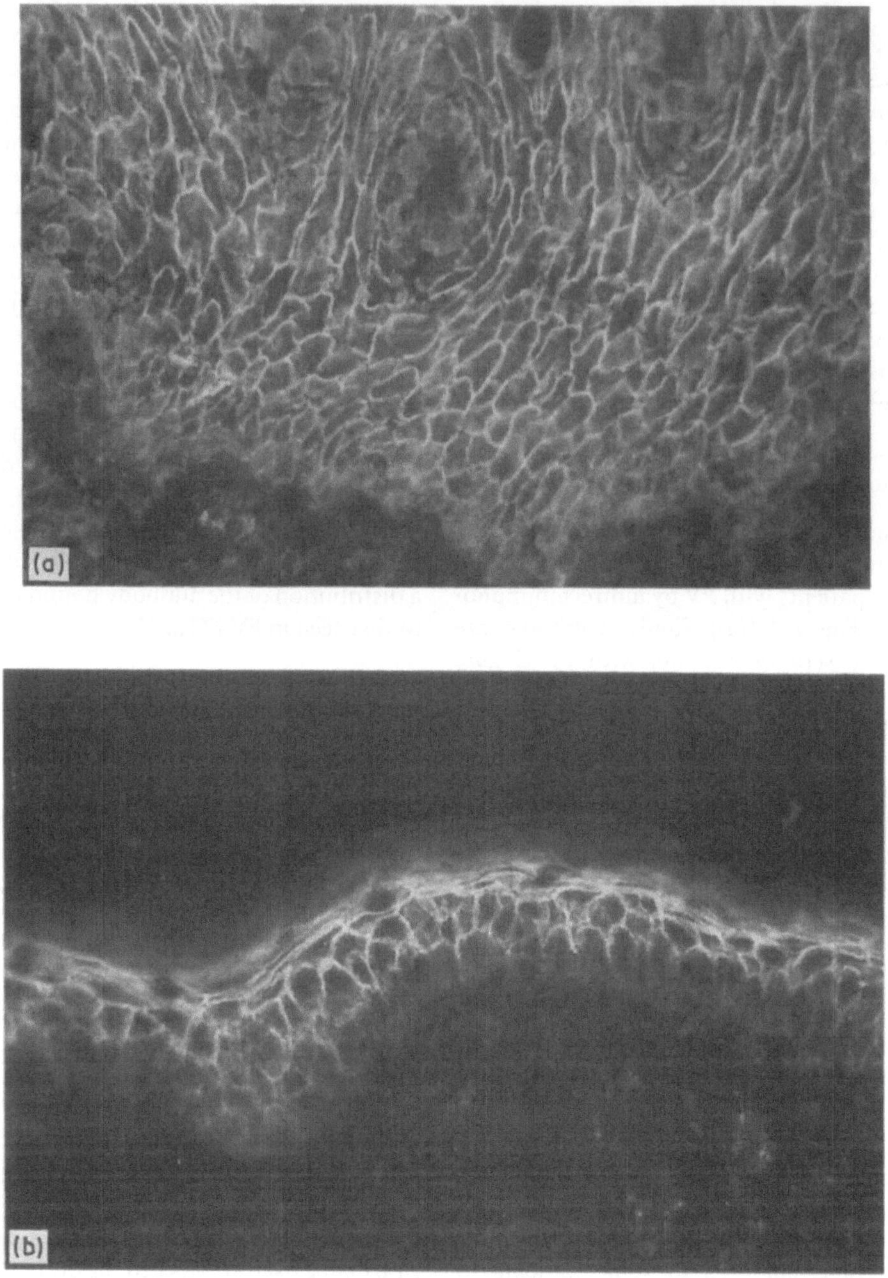

Figure 4.4 Indirect immunofluorescence with pemphigus sera. (a) PV serum on a monkey oesophagus substrate shows cell surface binding (× 350). (b) PF serum on a normal human skin substrate demonstrates cell surface binding (× 350).

blocking studies. One serum may be capable of blocking the binding of a second serum, not because the two sera bound the same antigen or molecule, but because of steric hindrance if one antigen is near another on the cell surface. On the other hand, if two sera bind different epitopes on the same antigen or molecule, then one may not block the binding of another. With these reservations in mind, the above study suggests, but does not absolutely prove, that PV antigens are identical and distinct from Brazilian PF antigens. These conclusions have been confirmed with the use of immunochemical studies (see below).

Similarly, binding of pemphigus antibody to the surface of epidermal cells can be blocked by the plant lectin concanavalin A [74–76]. This led to the interpretation that pemphigus antigen contains carbohydrate linkages (probably α-D-mannose residues), known to be bound by concanavalin A. Again, because of steric hindrance, these results must be interpreted cautiously. Recent studies, however, do confirm that pemphigus antigens are glycoproteins (see below).

Using absorption studies to define pemphigus antigens further, extracts from various tissues were biochemically fractionated and the fractions were incubated with PV sera. A particular fraction was assumed to contain pemphigus antigen if its incubation with pemphigus serum prevented subsequent positive immunofluorescence with this serum. Using these techniques various groups have isolated, from different sources, a diverse array of molecules purported to be pemphigus antigen: a 12-kDa antigen from bovine oesophagus [77], a group of glycoproteins with molecular masses of 50, 25 and 20 kDa from human saliva [78], a 18-kDa glycoprotein with ribonucleic acid from guinea-pig epidermis [79], a 75-kDa glycoprotein from human urine [80], and a 68-kDa protein from human oesophageal mucosa [81]. The relationship of these diverse molecules to the higher-molecular-weight molecules recently defined by the immunochemical studies discussed below is unclear.

Several immunochemical approaches were used to demonstrate directly the biosynthesis of the pemphigus antigen by human and mouse keratinocytes [82]. Extracts of [^{14}C]glucosamine-labelled keratinocytes were used to immunoprecipitate antigen with different sera from pemphigus patients using a protein A immunoprecipitation technique. Sera from five of seven pemphigus patients specifically precipitated a molecule that, when reduced, was 130 kDa. The fact that this molecule was also labelled with ^{14}C-labelled amino acids and with [^{3}H]mannose, but not with $^{35}SO_4$, indicated that the molecule was a glycoprotein and not a sulphated proteoglycan. In 1984 it was shown that the antigen described above reacted only with sera from patients with PV and not with sera from patients with PF [83]. This molecule, the PV antigen, was further characterized by electrophoresis under non-reducing conditions as a glycoprotein of molecular mass 210 kDa with disulphide-linked chains of molecular mass 130 kDa, a highly glycosylated polypeptide, and of 85 kDa (Figure 4.5) [83]. These experiments established that all PV sera tested had antibodies against this same molecule, but that PF sera do not bind the PV antigen. Recent experiments performed by immunoprecipitation of ^{125}I-labelled extracts of normal human epidermis, have demonstrated the same 130-kDa and 85-kDa chains of PV antigen *in vivo* as are synthesized *in vitro* [84].

Several studies have employed immunoblotting procedures to define pemphigus antigens. Using bovine tongue epithelium as substrate, Jones, Yokoo and Goldman [85] isolated a 140-kDa protein that reacted with four PV sera. This is probably a similar molecule to the 130-kDa glycopeptide chain demonstrated by immunoprecipitation of extracts of human keratinocytes. Immunoblots of bovine snout [85] and human epidermis [83], on the other hand, were negative when incubated with PV sera, probably because denatured PV antigen from these sources no longer bound antibody. However, Peterson and Wuepper [86], by concentrating human PV sera, were able to identify a 33-kDa molecule in immunoblots of epidermal cell membrane glycoproteins, affinity purified on a concanavalin A column. How this smaller molecule is related to the larger PV antigen is not known, but it may represent a degradation product of the 130 kDa, 85 kDa complex.

PF antigen has also been identified by immunoblotting. In initial experiments, four

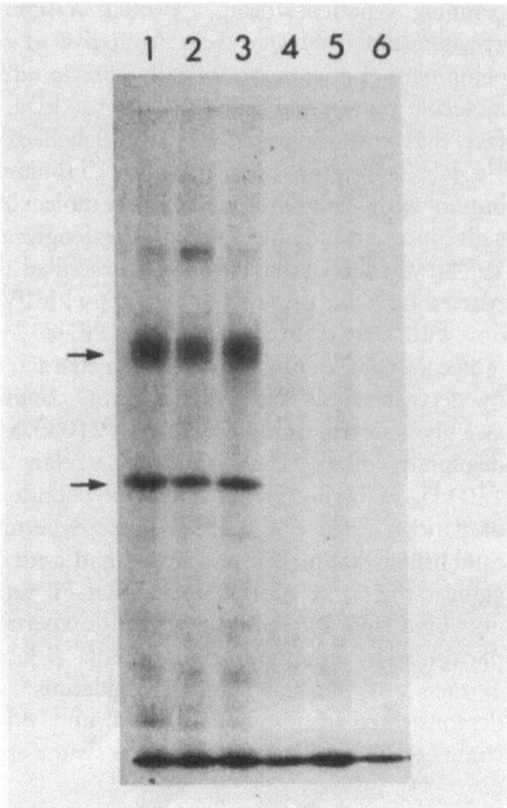

Figure 4.5 Immunoprecipitation of PV antigen from extracts of [^{14}C]amino acid labelled cultured keratinocytes. Lanes 1–3: different PV sera were used to precipitate the PV antigen, polypeptide bands of molecular mass 130 kDa and 85 kDa (arrows). Lanes 4–6: normal human sera were used as controls in the same immunoprecipitation procedure.

of eight PF sera had antibodies that identified a 160-kDa polypeptide in extracts of normal human epidermis [83]. Further studies demonstrated that about one-third of PF patients had antibodies that bound this 160 kDa polypeptide by immunoblotting (Figure 4.6) [87]. In addition, antibodies to desmoglein I, a core desmosomal glycoprotein, identified the same 160-kDa band on immunoblots [88].

Two-dimensional gel electrophoresis confirmed that the 160-kDa PF antigen is identical to desmoglein I. When extracts of normal human epidermis were separated by such two-dimensional gel electrophoresis, then transferred to nitrocellulose for immunoblotting, PF sera and antibodies to desmoglein I identified comigrating polypeptides with molecular masses of approximately 160 kDa and isoelectric points of approximately 5.5 [88]. Similar studies were performed with a monoclonal antibody to desmoglein I which also bound PF antigen (Figure 4.7) [89]. Finally further proof of identify of PF antigens and desmoglein I comes from studies in which antibodies in PF serum were affinity purified by the 160-kDa PF antigen polypeptide. IgG that bound this polypeptide was eluted and then shown to bind specifically to desmoglein I [88]. Thus,these studies demonstrated that about one-third of PF patients have autoantibodies against desmoglein I.

To determine why only one-third of patients with PF could be shown to have antibodies to desmoglein I by immunoblotting, further studies were performed. The hypothesis on which these studies was based is that all PF patients have antibodies to desmoglein I in its native state, but that only a subgroup of sera are capable of binding denatured antigen as seen by immunoblotting. To address this problem, a minimally denaturing extraction procedure was used on normal human epidermis. Extracted proteins were labelled with ^{125}I then subjected to immunoprecipitation with PF sera. All tested PF sera brought down the same complex of polypeptides with molecular masses of 260, 160, 110 and 85 kDa [90]. The 160-kDa polypeptide in this complex was identified as desmoglein I by two-dimensional gel analysis. In addition, antibodies to desmoglein I precipitated the same complex as PF antibodies. Finally it was shown that there is a calcium-sensitive conformational epitope on this complex, so that in the absence of calcium only about one-third of the PF sera still bound the complex. These are the same one-third of sera capable of binding denatured antigen. In summary, then, all PF sera bind a complex of polypeptides that includes desmoglein I, a core desmosomal glycoprotein. Most PF sera bind a calcium-sensitive conformational epitope on this complex. Since Ca^{2+} is important in

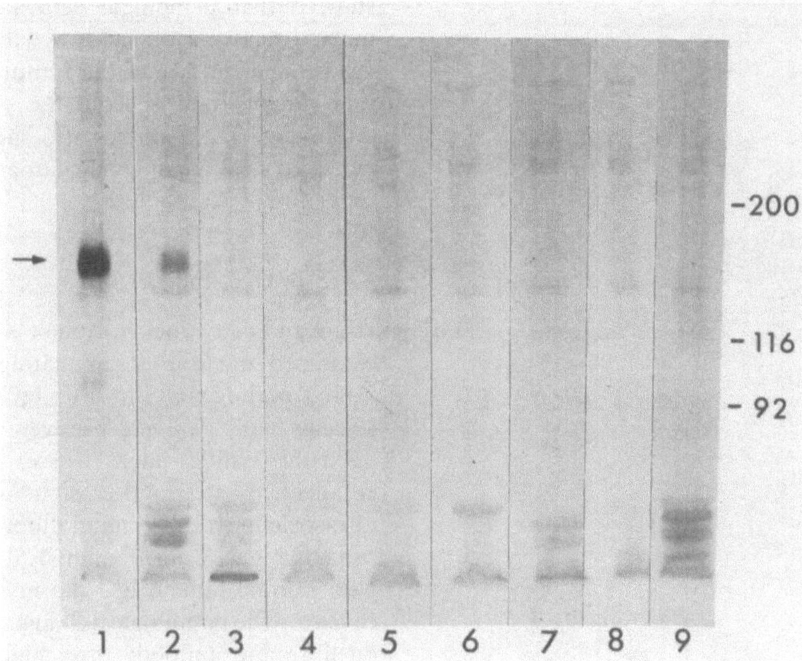

Figure 4.6 Immunoblot of extracts of normal human epidermis demonstrates PF antigen, a 160 kDa polypeptide band (arrow). Lanes 1–6: each lane was stained with a different PF serum. Only two (shown in lanes 1, 2) of the six sera bind the 160-kDa band on this immunoblot. Lanes 7–9: each lane was stained by a different normal human serum, as controls. Numbers at far right indicate migration of known mol. wt standards (mol. wt × 10^{-3}).

desmosome function, these findings suggest that some PF sera might interfere with a Ca^{2+}-sensitive mechanism of desmosome assembly.

Studies with FS sera have demonstrated that the antigen bound by these sera is identical to that bound by sporadic North American PF sera [87, 90].

Several general conclusions regarding pemphigus antigens can be drawn from the findings in the above studies. All PV sera thus far tested have antibodies to a characteristic glycoprotein consisting of polypeptides of 130 and 85 kDa, capable of forming disulphide bonds. PF sera do not bind the PV antigen complex, but contain antibodies against a characteristic complex of polypeptides, consisting of desmoglein I and other, possibly desmosomal, proteins. These findings indicate that PV and PF sera have distinct and unique antigen specificities at a molecular level.

4.4 PATHOPHYSIOLOGY

4.4.1 Organ and cell culture studies

Schiltz and Michel [91] demonstrated that human skin in organ culture developed acantholysis when incubated with pooled sera or purified IgG from patients with pemphigus. The resulting acantholysis was indistinguishable from the typical histological finding in PV. Direct immunofluorescence studies using fluorescein-labelled anti-human IgG showed that pemphigus IgG was detectable on the epidermal cell membrane in these organ cultures. Finally, acantholysis in these experiments could be induced in the absence of complement [92]. These studies were the first to demonstrate that PV autoantibodies are pathogenic and capable of causing acantholysis. Similar studies with PF antibodies have also been performed [93].

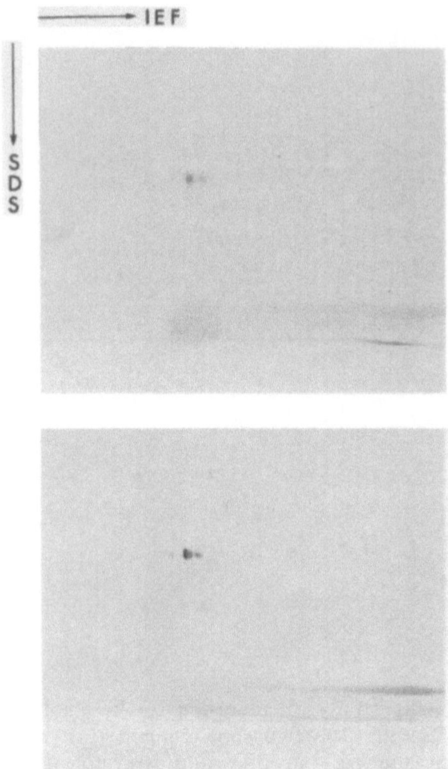

Figure 4.7 Immunoblot of PF antigen (top) and desmoglein I (bottom), a core desmosomal glycoprotein, on extracts of normal human epidermis separated by two dimensional gel electrophoresis (isoelectric focusing, IEF, and SDS-PAGE). Top blot was stained with a PF serum, and the bottom blot was stained with a monoclonal antibody against desmoglein I. PF antigen and desmoglein I comigrate with isoelectric point about 5.5 and mol. wt about 160 000.

When this *in vitro* model was examined by electron microscopy it was seen that the intercellular spaces widened 12 h after incubating pemphigus IgG with cultures of normal human epidermis. After 24–48 h tonofilaments retracted from the cell periphery and desmosomes were lost. At 72 h isolated cells without desmosomes were noticed in the suprabasilar layer; basal cells, however, remained attached to the basement membrane [94].

Farb *et al.* [95] and Diaz and Marcelo [96] showed that pemphigus sera added to primary murine epidermal cell cultures will cause epidermal cell detachment, which the authors consider highly reproducible and specific for pemphigus autoantibodies. These studies also support the pathogenic role of pemphigus autoantibodies in the induction of acantholysis.

4.4.2 In vivo studies

Using an *in vivo* model, Anhalt *et al.* [97, 98] also examined the role of circulating autoantibodies in the pathogenesis of PV. IgG fractions from patients with PV were passively transferred into neonatal Balb/c mice. These mice developed cutaneous blisters and erosions with histological, ultrastructural and immunofluorescence features of pemphigus. Control animals that were injected with normal human IgG did not develop similar changes. The pathological changes were dependent on dose and antibody titre; high-titre sera were most effective. The circulating antibody titre in the mice was correlated to the severity of the disease. Electron microscopy of lesions from these mice revealed a widening of the epidermal intercellular spaces between desmosomes in early lesions, and complete cell–cell detachment, even at desmosomes in older lesions [99]. Using this same *in vivo* model, Roscoe *et al.* [100] demonstrated that PF IgG is also capable of causing acantholysis in the superficial epidermis of neonatal mice.

4.4.3 Mechanism of acantholysis

Pemphigus antibodies may mediate acantholysis by triggering release of proteolytic enzymes from epidermal cells. Using the organ culture system discussed above, Schiltz and coworkers [91, 92] came to the conclusion that when pemphigus IgG autoantibody binds to the epidermal cell surface, cells respond by secreting a factor capable of causing acantholysis. This factor, called pemphigus acantholysis factor (PAF), did not appear in control cultures incubated with normal IgG. PAF was capable of causing suprabasilar acantholysis in organ cultures, identical to that seen with PV serum. PAF was thought to be a proteolytic enzyme, active near neutral pH. These studies suggested that the binding of the pemphigus antibody to the epidermal cell surface resulted in activation, release or synthesis of a non-lysosomal proteolytic enzyme that was involved in the loss of cell adhesion.

There are some recent data to suggest that the PAF proteolytic enzyme is a plasminogen activator. In non-keratinocyte cell systems, Becker *et al.* [101] reported that production of plasminogen activator, a serine proteinase that catalyses the conversion of plasminogen to plasmin, could be activated by incubating cells with antibodies. In addition, the purified anti-cell surface IgG produced a rapid change in morphology of these cells with 2 h. Cells became rounded and detached from the culture dish surface. Keratinocytes incubated with pemphigus anti-cell surface antibodies show a similar effect. Singer *et al.* [102] incubated confluent primary cultures of neonatal human epidermal cells with affinity-purified plasminogen-free IgG from patients with pemphigus. After 24 h a tenfold increase in extracellular plasminogen activator and a fivefold increase in cell-associated plasminogen activator was found with PF IgG. After incubation with PV IgG, the increase in extracellular plasminogen activator was sevenfold and the increase in cell-associated plasminogen activator sixfold. Biochemically and immunologically, two types of human plasminogen activator can be identified: a urokinase type with a molecular weight of 52 000–55 000 and a tissue type with a molecular weight between 60 000 and 74 000 [103]. By SDS-PAGE (SDS polyacrylamide-gel electrophoresis) it was shown that the plasminogen activator activity secreted by cultured human epidermal cells had a molecular weight of 55 000, suggesting it to be a urokinase-type enzyme. The importance of plasminogen activator and plasmin in causing acantholysis was studied in organ cultures. Addition of plasmin inhibitors such as aprotinin and lima bean trypsin inhibitor prevented the development of acantholysis when either PV or PF IgG were added to skin in organ cultures. In addition, both plasminogen and PF IgG were required to cause acantholysis [102].

The stimulation of plasminogen activator could be inhibited by corticosteroids. Dexamethasone at a concentration of 10^{-10}M inhibited extracellular plasminogen activator activity by 60% after incubation of epidermal cells with PF IgG. At 10^{-8}M, dexamethasone inhibition reached 95% [93]. These findings may account for the beneficial effects of corticosteroids on the course of pemphigus.

In summary, these findings indicate that the first step in the pathogenesis of pemphigus is the binding of autoantibody to the surface of human epidermal cells, which may stimulate the production of a plasminogen activator of the urokinase type. Plasminogen would then be converted to plasmin which may be responsible for the loss of cellular adhesion. This pathophysiological scheme is tentative and other proteins, such as complement [104], and/or other mechanisms, including direct effects of IgG on cell adhesion, may also prove to be important.

4.5 TREATMENT

Currently the first-choice therapy for both types of pemphigus is corticosteroids, usually in the form of oral prednisone. The goal of therapy is to control the disease at the lowest possible dose of prednisone. If the disease is severe then daily prednisone at a high dose (60 mg a day or greater) is given to get the disease under control. If the initial disease activity is mild or limited, then lower doses can be tried. Once the disease is under control, the prednisone dose is tapered, if possible, to an alternate-day regimen. The object is to control the disease at the lowest possible alternate-day dose of prednisone [105]. PF is often mild enough to require only topical corticosteroids for control.

If the disease cannot be controlled on a low alternate-day dose of prednisone, then adjuvant therapy is often used to try to lower the dose of prednisone needed. The most effective adjuvant therapy is not known. However, there are three main drugs used – gold, azathioprine and cyclophosphamide [105].

The mechanisms responsible for the effects of gold treatment in pemphigus are not known [106]. It is speculated that gold compounds act *in vivo* by altering the pathways of inflammatory response [107], such as mediator generation and/or the activation of degradative enzymes. Gold might also alter phagocytic cell function, or T lymphocyte function [106]. Dermatological side effects of gold therapy are manifold. In a series of patients studied by Penneys [106] non-specific eczematous reactions are described. Lichen planus-like eruptions, pityriasis rosea-like eruptions, generalized erythroderma and gold cheilitis and stomatitis were observed as well. An acute vasomotor reaction, which may lead to myocardial infarction, has been reported with intramuscular gold, especially the thiomalate preparation [108]. Further complications of gold therapy include anaphylaxis, proteinuria [106, 109], nephrotoxicity, leucopenia and thrombocytopenia, aplastic anaemia [106], intrahepatic cholestasis [110], pulmonary fibrosis [111] and deposition of gold compounds in the cornea and lens leading to chrysiasis [112]. An intramuscular preparation such as aurothioglucose or gold sodium thiomalate is usually administered for pemphigus [113]. Experience with oral gold therapy and pemphigus is limited [114]. In summary, gold therapy may have a corticosteroid-sparing effect and some patients can be controlled on gold medication alone [115]. However, gold, like corticosteroids, can have serious side effects.

The most commonly used adjuvant therapy in pemphigus is the administration of cyclophosphamide or azathioprine [116–119]. Usually one of these drugs is given together with corticosteroids, but after a latent period of between 4 and 8 weeks it may be sufficient, especially in mild forms of pemphigus, to control disease activity. In patients with more active disease, these immunosuppressive drugs may provide a corticosteroid-sparing effect [8, 118]. Since no controlled studies are available on the efficacy of these drugs and since spontaneous remissions may occur even in untreated pemphigus, especially in PF, the evaluation of case reports is difficult. The belief that immunosuppressive drugs do, indeed, have a corticosteroid-sparing effect is based on individual observations [105]. Serious side effects of these drugs include toxic effects on bone marrow and liver. Cyclophosphamide can also induce sterility in men and women as well as haemorrhagic cystitis [105]. The long-term administration of immunosuppressives may be associated with a higher risk of developing malignant neoplasias [120, 121].

In severe uncontrollable pemphigus other therapeutic approaches have also been tried. Plasmaphaeresis is a procedure that decreases the level of circulating antibodies, including pemphigus anti-epithelial cell surface antibodies. Since the antibody level rebounds due to the feedback regulation of antibody synthesis [122] it is necessary to combine this therapy with immunosuppressive drugs such as cyclophosphamide [123]. Following repeated plasmaphaeresis, a gradual decline in antibody levels associated with a concurrent improvement in clinical symptoms has been reported [105, 124, 125]. Another alternative is the so-called corticosteroid pulse therapy. High doses of methylprednisolone are administered once a day for 5 days. Patients must be in electrolyte balance prior to the initiation of pulse therapy and carefully monitored during therapy. Sudden death resulting from electrolyte shifts may occur [126].

Finally, in a recent report nine patients with PF were treated with dapsone. The authors reported improvement in the five patients who had low or negative levels of circulating anti-epithelial cell surface antibodies [127].

4.6 PROGNOSIS AND THERAPY

In the precorticosteroid era PV was usually a fatal disease. Most patients died within 5 years of the onset of the disease [20, 126]. On the other hand prognosis was better in patients with PF. Except for occasional acute cases with generalized involvement, PF follows, in the majority of patients, a very chronic course, that may extend over many years with rare acute exacerbations [20]. One reason for the difference in prognosis between PV and PF is probably the difference in the level of the epidermis at which blister formation occurs. In PF only the very superficial epidermis is lost, whereas in PV the entire epidermis, with the exception of the basal layer, is gone.

The advent of corticosteroid therapy dramatically improved the prognosis of pemphigus. Subsequent to the widespread use of corticosteroids, the mortality rate has drastically dropped from 73% reported between 1941 and 1950 to less than 30% soon after the introduction of corticosteroids and, recently, is down to probably less than 10% [5, 7, 128].

With current therapy most of the fatal outcomes are due to infections, secondary to a combination of difficult-to-control disease with persistent skin erosions and immunosuppression from therapy [129–131].

REFERENCES

1. *Steadman's Medical Dictionary* (1982) Williams and Wilkins, Baltimore, MD, 24th edn, p. 487.
2. Lynch, P., Gallego, R.E. and Saied, N.K. (1976) Pemphigus – a review. *Ariz. Med.*, **33**, 1030–7.
3. Simon, D.G., Krutchkoff, D., Kaslow, R.A. and Zarbo, R. (1980) Pemphigus in Hartford county, Connecticut, from 1972 to 1977. *Arch. Dermatol.*, **116**, 1035–7.
4. Pisanti, S., Sharav, Y., Kaufman, E. and Posner, L.N. (1974) Pemphigus vulgaris; incidence in Jews of different ethnic groups, according to age, sex and initial lesion. *Oral Surg.*, **38**, 382–7.
5. Hietanen, J. and Salo, O.P. (1982) Pemphigus: An epidermiological study of patients treated in Finnish hospitals between 1969 and 1978. *Acta Dermatovener.*, **62**, 491–6.
6. Rosenberg, F.R., Sanders, S. and Nelson, C.T. (1976) Pemphigus. A 20-year review of 107 patients treated with corticosteroids. *Arch. Dermatol.*, **112**, 962–70.
7. Krain, L.S. (1974) Pemphigus-epidemiologic and survival characteristics of 59 patients, 1959–1973. *Arch. Dermatol.*, **110**, 862–5.
8. Ryan, J.G. (1971) Pemphigus. A 20 year survey of experience with 70 cases. *Arch. Dermatol.*, **104**, 14–20.
9. Beutner, E.H. and Chorzelski, T.P. (1976) Studies on etiologic factors in pemphigus. *J. Cutan. Path.*, **3**, 67–74.
10. Zegarelli, D.J. and Zegarelli, E.V. (1977) Intraoral pemphigus vulgaris. *Oral Surg.*, **44**, 384–93.
11. Mikhail, G.R., Drukker, B.H. and Chow, C. (1967) Pemphigus vulgaris involving the cervix uteri. *Arch. Dermatol.*, **95**, 496–8.
12. Sagher, F., Bercovici, B. and Romem, R. (1974) Nikolsky sign on cervix uteri in pemphigus. *Brit. J. Dermatol.*, **90**, 407–11.
13. Bean, S.F., Holubar, K. and Gillett, R.B. (1975) Pemphigus involving the eyes. *Arch. Dermatol.*, **111**, 1484–6.
14. Block, L.J., Caldarelli, D.D., Holinger, P.H. and Pearson, R.W. (1977) Pemphigus of the air and food passage. *Ann. Otol. Rhinol. Laryngol.*, **86**, 584–7.
15. Raque, C.J., Stein, K.M. and Samitz, M.H. (1970) Pemphigus vulgaris involving the esophagus. *Arch. Dermatol.*, **102**, 371–3.
16. Wood, D.R., Patterson, J.B. and Orlando, R.C. (1982) Pemphigus vulgaris of the esophagus. *Ann. Intern. Med.*, **96**, 189–91.
17. Epstein, J.H., Feigen, G.M. and Epstein, N.N. (1958) Pemphigus vulgaris with lesions of the rectal mucosa. *Arch. Dermatol.*, **78**, 36–8.
18. Ahmed, A.R. (1983) Pemphigus vulgaris: clinical features. *Dermatol. Clin.*, **1**, 171–7.
19. Pye, R.J. (1986) Bullous eruptions. In *Textbook of Dermatology*, 4th edn (eds A., Rook, D.S. Wilkinson, F.J.G. Ebling, R.H. Champion and J.L. Burton), Blackwell Scientific Publications, Oxford, pp. 1619–63.
20. Lever, W.F. (1965) *Pemphigus and Pemphigoid*, Charles C. Thomas, Springfield, IL.
21. Senear, F.E. and Usher, B. (1926) An unusual type of pemphigus combining features of lupus erythematosus. *Arch. Dermatol. Syphil.*, **13**, 761–81.
22. Perry, H.O. (1987) Pemphigus erythematodes (pemphigus erythematosus, Senear-Usher Syndrome). In *Clinical Dermatology*, 14th edn (ed. J.D. Demis), Harper & Row, Cambridge, pp. 6–10, 1–3.
23. American, M.L. and Ahmed, A.R. (1985) Pemphigus erythematosus. *Int. J. Dermatol.*, **24**, 16–25.
24. Castro, R.M. and Proenca, N.G. (1982) Ähnlichkeiten und Unterschiede zwischen brasilianischem "Fogo selvagem" und Pemphigus foliaceus Cazenave. *Hautarzt*, **33**, 574–7.
25. Castro, R.M., Roscoe, J.T. and Sampaio, S.A.P. (1983) Brazilian pemphigus foliaceus. *Clin. Dermatol.*, **1**, 22–41.
26. Storer, J.S., Galen, W.K., Nesbitt, L.T. and DeLeo, V.A. (1982) Neonatal pemphigus vulgaris. *J. Amer. Acad. Dermatol.*, **6**, 929–32.
27. Ross, M.G., Kane, B., Frieder, R., *et al.* (1986) Pemphigus in pregnancy: a reevaluation of fetal risk. *Amer. J. Obstet. Gynecol.*, **155**, 30–3.
28. Merlob, P., Metzker, A., Hazaz, B., *et al.* (1986) Neonatal pemphigus vulgaris. *Pediatrics*, **78**, 1102–5.
29. Green, D. and Maize, J.C. (1982) Maternal pemphigus vulgaris with *in vivo* bound antibodies in the stillborn fetus. *J. Amer. Acad. Dermatol.*, **7**, 388–92.
30. Eyre, R.W. and Stanley, J.R. (1988) Maternal pemphigus foliaceus with cell surface antibody bound in neonatal epidermis. *Arch. Dermatol.*, **124**, 25–7.

31. Degos, R., Touraine, R., Belaich, S. and Revuz, J. (1969) Pemphigus chez un malade traite par penicillamine pour maladie de Wilson. *Bull. Soc. Fr. Dermatol. Syphiligr.*, **76**, 751–3.
32. Troy, J.L., Silvers, D.N., Grossman, M.E. and Jaffe, I.A. (1981) Penicillamine-associated pemphigus: is it really pemphigus? *J. Amer. Acad. Dermatol.*, **4**, 547–55.
33. Hashimoto, K., Singer, K. and Lazarus, G.S. (1984) Penicillamine-induced pemphigus. *Arch. Dermatol.*, **120**, 762–4.
34. Marsden, R.A., Ryan, T.J., Van Hegan, R.I., *et al.* (1976) Pemphigus foliaceus induced by penicillamine. *Brit. Med. J.*, **4**, 1423.
35. Parfrey, P.S., Clement, M., Vandenburg, M.J. and Wright, P. (1980) Captopril-induced pemphigus. *Brit. Med. J.*, **281**, 194.
36. Fellner, M.J. and Mark, A.S. (1980) Penicilline- and ampicillin-induced pemphigus vulgaris. *Int. J. Dermatol.*, **7**, 392–3.
37. Ruocco, V., Rossi, A., Pisani, M., *et al.* (1979) An abortive form of pemphigus vulgaris probably induced by penicillin. *Dermatologica*, **159**, 266–73.
38. Gange, W., Rhodes, E.L., Edwards, C.O. and Powell, M.E.A. (1976) Pemphigus induced by rifampicin. *Brit. J. Dermatol.*, **95**, 445–8.
39. Lee, C.W., Lim, J.H. and Kang, H.J. (1984) Pemphigus foliaceus induced by rifampicin. *Brit. J. Dermatol.*, **111**, 619–22.
40. Chorzelski, T.P., Jablonska, S. and Blaszczyk, M. (1966) Autoantibodies in pemphigus. *Acta Dermatol. Venerol.*, **46**, 26.
41. DeMento, F.J. and Grover, R.W. (1973) Acantholytic herpetiform dermatitis. *Arch. Dermatol.*, **107**, 883–7.
42. Goddard, W., Lambert, D., Gavanou, J. and Chapius, J.L. (1980) Pemphigus inquit après treatment par l'association propranolol-mepbromate. *Ann. Dermatol. Venerol.*, **107**, 1213–16.
43. Maize, J.C., Dobson, R.I. and Provost, T.T. (1975) Pemphigus and myasthenia gravis. *Arch. Dermatol.*, **111**, 1134–9.
44. Peck, S.M. and Osserman, K.E. (1969) Studies in bullous diseases: Treatment of pemphigus vulgaris with methotrexate, two patients (one with concurrent myasthenia gravis). *J. Mt. Sinai Hosp. NY*, **36**, 71–6.
45. Cruz, P.D., Coldiron, B.M. and Sontheimer, R.D. (1987) Concurrent features of cutaneous lupus erythematosus and pemphigus erythematosus following myasthenia gravis and thymoma. *J. Amer. Acad. Dermatol.*, **16**, 472–80.
46. Tagami, H., Imamura, S., Noguchi, S. and Nishitani, H. (1976) Coexistence of peculiar pemphigus, myasthenia gravis and malignant thymoma. *Dermatologica*, **152**, 181–90.
47. Krain, L.S. and Bierman, S.M. (1974) Pemphigus vulgaris and internal malignancy. *Cancer*, **33**, 1091–9.
48. Krain, L.S. (1974) The association of pemphigus with thymoma or malignancy: a critical review. *Brit. J. Dermatol.*, **90**, 397–405.
49. Sarnoff, D.S. and DeFeo, C.P. (1985) Coexistence of pemphigus foliaceus and mycosis fungoides. *Arch. Dermatol.*, **121**, 669–72.
50. Naysmith, A. and Hancock, B.W. (1976) Hodgkin's disease and pemphigus. *Brit. J. Dermatol.*, **94**, 695–6.
51. McKee, P.H., McClelland, M. and Sandford, J.C. (1978) Co-existence of pemphigus, anti-skeletal muscle antibody and a retroperitoneal paraganglioma. *Brit. J. Dermatol.*, **99**, 441–5.
52. Chorzelski, T.P., Maciejowski, E., Jablonska, S., *et al.* (1974) Coexistence of pemphigus and bullous pemphigoid. *Arch. Dermatol.*, **109**, 849–53.
53. Quismorio, F.P., Bland, S.L. and Friou, G.J. (1971) Autoimmunity in thermal injury: occurrence of rheumatoid factors, antinuclear antibodies and antiepithelial antibodies. *Clin. Exp. Immunol.*, **8**, 701–11.
54. Thivolet, J. and Beyvin, A.J. (1968) Recherche par immunofluorescence d'autoanticorps serique vis-à-vis des constituants de l'epiderme chez les brules. *Experimentia* **24**, 945–6.
55. Ablin, R.J., Milgrom, F., Kano, K., Rapaport, F.T. and Beutner, E.H. (1969) Pemphigus-like antibodies in patients with skin burns. *Vox Sang.* **16**, 73–5.
56. Lever, W.F. (1983) *Histopathology of the Skin*, 6th edn, J.B. Lippincott, Philadelphia, pp. 104–13.
57. Ackerman, B.A. (1978) *Histologic Diagnosis of Inflammatory Skin Diseases*, Lea and Feabiger, Philadelphia, pp. 525–32.
58. Hashimoto, K. and Lever, W.F. (1967) An electron microscopic study on pemphigus vulgaris of the mouth and the skin with special reference to the intercellular cement. *J. Invest. Dermatol.*, **48**, 540–52.
59. Lever, W.F. (1979) Pemphigus and pemphigoid. A review of the advances made since 1964. *J. Amer. Acad. Dermatol.*, **1**, 2–31.
60. Wilgram, G.F., Caulfield, J.B. and Madgic, E.B. (1964) An electron microscopic study of acantholysis and dyskeratosis in pemphigus foliaceus. *J. Invest. Dermatol.*, **43**, 287–99.
61. Beutner, E.H. and Jordon, R.E. (1964) Demonstration of skin antibodies in sera of pemphigus vulgaris patients by indirect immunofluorescence staining. *Proc. Soc. Exp. Biol. Med.*, **117**, 505–10.
62. Sams, W.M. and Jordan, R.E. (1971) Correlation of pemphigoid and pemphigus antibody titres with activity of disease. *Brit. J. Dermatol.*, **84**, 7–13.
63. O'Loughlin, S., Goldman, G.C. and Provost, T.T.

(1978) Fate of pemphigus antibody following successful therapy. *Arch. Dermatol.*, **114**, 1769–72.
64. Judd, K.P. and Lever, W.F. (1979) Correlation of antibodies in skin and serum with disease severity in pemphigus. *Arch. Dermatol.*, **115**, 428–32.
65. Fitzpatrick, R.E. and Newcomer, V.D. (1980) The correlation of disease activity and antibody titers in pemphigus. *Arch. Dermatol.*, **116**, 285–90.
66. Beutner, E.H., Lever, W.F., Witebsky, E., *et al.* (1965) Autoantibodies in pemphigus vulgaris. *J. Amer. Med. Assoc.*, **192**, 98–104.
67. Jordon, R.E., Triftshauser, C.T. and Schroeter, A.L. (1971) Direct immunofluorescent studies of pemphigus and bullous pemphigoid. *Arch. Dermatol.*, **103**, 486–91.
68. Bystryn, J.C., Abel, E. and DeFeo, C. (1974) Pemphigus foliaceus. Subcorenal intercellular antibodies of unique specificity. *Arch. Dermatol.*, **110**, 857–61.
69. Bystryn, J.C. and Rodriguez, J. (1978) Absence of intercellular antigens in the deep layers of the epidermis in pemphigus foliaceus. *J. Clin. Invest.*, **61**, 339–48.
70. Wolff, K. and Schreiner, E. (1971) Ultrastructural localization of pemphigus autoantibodies within the epidermis. *Nature (London)*, **229**, 59–61.
71. Konrad, K., Stingl, G. and Holubar, K. (1977) Ultrastructural localization of *in vivo* bound immunoglobulin in epidermis of Brazilian pemphigus foliaceus (fogo selvagem). *Brit. J. Dermatol.*, **96**, 449–51.
72. Sotto, M.N., Shimizu, S.H., Costa, J.M. and De Brito, T. (1980) South American pemphigus foliaceus: electron microscopy and immunoelectron localization of bound immunoglobulin in the skin and oral mucosa. *Brit. J. Dermatol.*, **102**, 521–7.
73. Wood, G.W. and Beutner, E.H. (1977) Blocking-immunofluorescence studies on the specificity of pemphigus autoantibodies. *Clin. Immunol. Immunopathol.*, 7, 168–75.
74. Hashimoto, K., King, L.E., Yamanishi, Y., *et al.* (1974) Identification of the substance binding pemphigus antibody and concanavalin A in the skin. *J. Invest. Dermatol.*, **52**, 423–35.
75. Van Lis, J.M.J. and Kalsbeek, G.L. (1975) The interaction of concanavalin A and the surface coat of stratified squamous epithelium. *Brit. J. Dermatol.*, **92**, 27–35.
76. Nishikawa, T., Harada, T., Hatano, H., *et al.* (1975) Epidermal intercellular binding of concanavalin A and pemphigus antibody. *Acta Dermatovenerol.*, **55**, 309–11.
77. Ablin, R.J., Bronson, P. and Beutner, E.H. (1969) Immunochemical characterization of epithelial antigen(s) reactive with pemphigus-like antibodies of rabbit and human pemphigus autoantibodies. *J. Hyg. Epidemiol. Microbiol. Immunol.*, **13**, 321–9.
78. Diaz, L.A., Patel, H. and Calvanico, N.J. (1980) Isolation of pemphigus antigen from human saliva. *J. Immunol.*, **124**, 760–5.
79. Miyagawa, S., Hojo, T., Ishii, H., *et al.* (1977) Isolation and characterization of soluble epidermal antigens reactive with pemphigus antibodies. *Acta Dermatovenerol.*, **57**, 7–13.
80. Murahata, R.I. and Ahmed, A.R. (1983) Partial purification and characterization of pemphigus-like antigens in urine. *Arch. Dermatol. Res.*, **275**, 118–23.
81. Shu, S.Y. and Beutner, E.H. (1973) Isolation and characterization of antigens reactive with pemphigus antibodies. *J. Invest. Dermatol.*, **61**, 270–6.
82. Stanley, J.R., Yaar, M., Hawley-Nelson, P. and Katz, S.I. (1982) Pemphigus antibodies identify a cell surface glycoprotein synthesized by human and mouse keratinocytes. *J. Clin. Invest.*, **70**, 281–8.
83. Stanley, J.R., Koulu, L. and Thivolet, C. (1984) Distinction between epidermal antigens binding pemphigus vulgaris and pemphigus foliaceus autoantibodies. *J. Clin. Invest.*, **74**, 313–20.
84. Eyre, R.W. and Stanley, J.R. (1987) Characterization of pemphigus vulgaris antigen extracted from normal human epidermis and comparison with pemphigus foliaceus antigen. *J. Clin. Invest.*, **81**, 807–12.
85. Jones, J.C.R., Yokoo, K.M. and Goldman, R.D. (1986) Further analysis of pemphigus autoantibodies and their use in studies on the heterogeneity, structure, and function of desmosomes. *J. Cell Biol.*, **102**, 1109–17.
86. Peterson, L.L. and Wuepper, K.D. (1984) Isolation and purification of a pemphigus vulgaris antigen from human epidermis. *J. Clin. Invest.*, **73**, 1113–20.
87. Stanley, J.R., Klaus-Kovtun, V. and Sampaio, S.A.P. (1986) Antigenic specificity of fogo selvagem autoantibodies is similar to North American pemphigus foliaceus and distinct from pemphigus vulgaris autoantibodies. *J. Invest. Dermatol.*, **87**, 197–201.
88. Koula, L., Kusumi, A., Steinberg, M.S., Klaus-Kovtun, V. and Stanley, J.R. (1984) Human autoantibodies against a desmosomal core protein in pemphigus foliaceus. *J. Exp. Med.*, **160**, 1509–18.
89. Stanley, J.R., Koulu, L., Klaus-Kovtun, V. and Steinberg, M.S. (1986) A monoclonal antibody to the desmosomal glycoprotein desmoglein I binds the same polypeptide as human autoantibodies in pemphigus foliaceus. *J. Immunol.*, **136**, 1227–30.
90. Eyre, R.W. and Stanley, J.R. (1987) Human autoantibodies against a desmosomal protein complex with a calcium-sensitive epitope are

characteristic of pemphigus foliaceus patients. *J. Exp. Med.*, **165**, 1719–24.
91. Schiltz, J.R. and Michel, B. (1976) Production of epidermal acantholysis in normal human skin *in vitro* by the IgG fraction from pemphigus serum. *J. Invest. Dermatol.*, **67**, 254–60.
92. Schiltz, J.R., Michel, B. and Papay, R. (1978) Pemphigus antibody interaction with human epidermal cells in culture. *J. Clin. Invest.*, **62**, 778–88.
93. Hashimoto, K., Shafran, K.M., Webber, P.S., *et al.* (1983) Anti-cell surface pemphigus auto-antibody stimulates plasminogen activator activity of human epidermal cells: a mechanism for the loss of epidermal cohesion and blister formation. *J. Exp. Med.*, **157**, 259–72.
94. Hu, C.H., Michel, B. and Schiltz, J.R. (1978) Epidermal acantholysis induced *in vitro* by pemphigus autoantibody. *Amer. J. Pathol.*, **90**, 345–62.
95. Farb, R.M., Dykes, R. and Lazarus, G.S. (1978) Anti-epidermal-cell-surface pemphigus antibody detaches viable epidermal cells from culture plates by activation of proteinase. *Proc. Natl. Acad. Sci. Usa*, **75**, 459–63.
96. Diaz, L.A. and Marcelo, C.L. (1978) Pemphigoid and pemphigus antigens in cultured epidermal cells. *Brit. J. Dermatol.*, **98**, 631–7.
97. Anhalt, G.J., Labib, R.S., Voorhees, J.J., *et al.* (1982) Induction of pemphigus in neonatal mice by passive transfer of IgG from patients with the disease. *New Engl. J. Med.*, **306**, 1189–96.
98. Anhalt, G.J., Till, G.O., Diaz, L.A., *et al.* (1986) Defining the role of complement in experimental pemphigus vulgaris in mice. *J. Immunol.*, **137**, 2835–40.
99. Takahashi, Y., Patel, H.P., Labib, R.S., *et al.* (1985) Experimentally induced pemphigus vulgaris in neonatal BALB/c mice: a time-course study of clinical, immunologic, ultrastructural, and cytochemical changes. *J. Invest. Dermatol.*, **84**, 41–6.
100. Roscoe, J.T., Diaz, L., Sampaio, S.A.P., *et al.* (1985) Brazilian pemphigus foliaceus auto-antibodies are pathogenic to BALB/c mice by passive transfer. *J. Invest. Dermatol.*, **85**, 538–41.
101. Becker, D., Ossowski, L. and Reich, E. (1981) Induction of plasminogen activator synthesis by antibodies. *J. Exp. Med.*, **154**, 385–96.
102. Singer, K.H., Hashimoto, K., Jensen, P.J., *et al.* (1985) Pathogenesis of autoimmunity in pemphigus. *Annu. Rev. Immunol.*, **3**, 87–108.
103. Wilson, E.L., Becker, M.L.B., Hoal, E.G. and Dowdle, E.B. (1980) Molecular species of plasminogen activator secreted by normal and neoplastic human cells. *Cancer Res.*, **40**, 933–8.
104. Kawana, S., Geoghegan, W.D. and Jordan, R.E. (1985) Complement fixation by pemphigus antibody. II. Complement enhanced detachment of epidermal cells. *Clin. Exp. Immunol.*, **61**, 517–25.
105. Bystryn, J.C. (1984) Adjuvant therapy of pemphigus. *Arch. Dermatol.*, **120**, 941–51.
106. Penneys, N.S. (1979) Gold therapy: dermatologic uses and toxicities. *J. Amer. Acad. Dermatol.*, **1**, 315–20.
107. Penneys, N.S., Ziboh, V., Gottlieb, N.L. and Katz, S. (1974) Inhibition of prostaglandin synthesis and human epidermal enzymes by aurothiomalate *in vitro*: possible actions of gold in pemphigus. *J. Invest. Dermatol.*, **63**, 356–61.
108. Gottlieb, N.L. and Brown, H.E. (1977) Acute myocardial infarction following gold sodium thiomalate induced vasomotor (nitritoid) reaction. *Arthr. Rheum.*, **20**, 1026–8.
109. Gibbons, R.B. (1979) Complications of chrysotherapy. A review of recent studies. *Arch. Intern. Med.*, **139**, 343–6.
110. Favreau, M., Tannenbaum, H. and Lough, J. (1977) Hepatic toxicity associated with gold therapy. *Ann. Intern. Med.*, **87**, 717–19.
111. Winterbauer, R.H., Wilske, K.R. and Wheelis, R.F. (1976) Diffuse pulmonary injury associated with gold treatment. *New Engl. J. Med.*, **294**, 919–21.
112. Hashimoto, A., Maeda, Y., Ito, H., *et al.* (1972) Corneal chrysiasis: a clinical study in rheumatoid arthritis patients receiving gold therapy. *Arthr. Rheum.*, **15**, 309–12.
113. Poulin, Y., Perry, H.O. and Muller, S.A. (1984) Pemphigus vulgaris: results of treatment with gold as a steroid sparing agent in a series of thirteen patients. *J. Amer. Acad. Dermatol.*, **11**, 851–7.
114. Salomon, D. and Saurat, J.H. (1986) Oral gold therapy (Auranofin) in pemphigus vulgaris. *Dermatologica*, **172**, 310–14.
115. Penneys, N.S., Eaglstein, W.H. and Frost, P. (1976) Management of pemphigus with gold compounds. *Arch. Dermatol.*, **112**, 185–7.
116. Roenigk, H.H. and Deodhar, S. (1973) Pemphigus treatment with azathioprine. *Arch. Dermatol.*, **107**, 353–7.
117. Aberer, W., Wolff-Schreiner, E.C., Stingl, G. and Wolff, K. (1987) Azathioprine in the treatment of pemphigus vulgaris. *J. Amer. Acad. Dermatol.*, **16**, 527–33.
118. Lever, W.F. and Schaumburg-Lever, G. (1977) Immunosuppressants and prednisone in pemphigus vulgaris. Therapeutic results obtained in 63 patients between 1961 and 1975. *Arch. Dermatol.*, **113**, 1236–41.
119. Fellner, M.J., Katz, J.M. and McCabe, J.B. (1978) Successful use of cyclophosphamide and prednisone for initial treatment of pemphigus vulgaris. *Arch. Dermatol.*, **114**, 889–94.
120. Penn, I. (1979) Tumor incidence in human allograft recipients. *Transpl. Proc.*, **11**, 1047–51.

121. Notes and News (1982) Anti-cancer drugs causing cancer. *Lancet*, i, 234.
122. Bystryn, J.C., Graf, M.W. and Uhr, J.W. (1970) Regulation of antibody formation by serum antibody. II. Removal of specific antibody by means of exchange transfusion. *J. Exp. Med.*, **132**, 1279–87.
123. Roujeau, J.C., Andre, C., Fabre, M.J., *et al.* (1983) Plasma exchange in pemphigus. Uncontrolled study in ten patients. *Arch. Dermatol.*, **119**, 215–21.
124. Swanson, D.L. and Dahl, M.V. (1981) Pemphigus vulgaris and plasma exchange: clinical and serologic studies. *J. Amer. Acad. Dermatol.*, **4**, 325–8.
125. Roujeau, J.C., Kalis, B., Lauret, P., *et al.* (1982) Plasma exchange in corticosteroid-resistant pemphigus. *Brit. J. Dermatol.*, **106**, 103–4.
126. Singer, K.H., Hashimoto, K. and Lazarus, G.S. (1983) Pathophysiology of pemphigus. *Dermatol. Clin.*, **1**, 179–86.
127. Basset, N., Guillot, B., Michel, B., *et al.* (1987) Dapsone as initial treatment in superficial pemphigus. *Arch. Dermatol.*, **123**, 783–5.
128. Savin, J.A. (1981) Some factors affecting prognosis in pemphigus vulgaris and pemphigoid. *Brit. J. Dermatol.*, **104**, 415–20.
129. Ahmed, A.R. and Moy, R. (1982) Death in pemphigus. *J. Amer. Acad. Dermatol.*, 7, 221–8.
130. Lynch, P.J., Rather, E.P. and Rutala, P.J. (1978) Pemphigus and coccidioidomycosis. *Cutis*, **22**, 581–3.
131. Tomecki, K.J. and Provost, T.T. (1979) Pemphigus vulgaris and herpes simplex. *NY State J. Med.*, **11**, 1760–2.

Five

Bullous pemphigoid

Lynne H. Morrison, Luis A. Diaz
and Grant J. Anhalt

5.1 INTRODUCTION

Bullous pemphigoid (BP) is an acquired blistering disease of the elderly with a substantially lower mortality than pemphigus vulgaris (PV). It is characterized histologically by subepidermal bullae and immunopathologically by *in vivo* deposition of autoantibodies and complement components along the epidermal basement membrane zone (BMZ). The majority of these patients also have circulating autoantibodies directed against the BMZ of stratified squamous epithelium. Because of these characteristics, BP is felt to be an autoimmune disease in which the cutaneous lesions may result as a consequence of these anti-BMZ antibodies.

Lever [1], in 1953, was the first to recognize that BP was a distinct bullous disease by its clinical and histological features. He chose to call the disease bullous pemphigoid because it was clinically similar to pemphigus vulgaris, but histologically lacked acantholysis. In 1967, Jordon [2] described the typical immunopathological characteristics of BP, which have been amply confirmed and are now considered important criteria in establishing the diagnosis of BP.

BP is considered to be part of the pemphigoid spectrum of diseases which also includes herpes gestationis, cicatricial pemphigoid and localized scarring pemphigoid (Brunsting–Perry). These diseases share clinical, histological and immunopathological similarities, but their exact relationship to one another remains to be determined.

5.2 CLINICAL FEATURES

5.2.1 Presentation

The true incidence of BP is not known, but it is thought to be twice as common as pemphigus vulgaris [3] and its incidence in Great Britain was estimated at 1 per 100 000 per year in 1985 [4].

Bullous pemphigoid occurs most frequently in the elderly with the vast majority of patients being over 60 years old at the time the eruption begins [3]. Rarely, it may occur in infancy or childhood and the clinical features of the few reported cases are similar to those seen in adults [5]. The age of onset in childhood BP varies, with the youngest patient being 3 months old [6].

In general, men and women are equally affected, but one series suggests that over the age of 70, men are more frequently affected than women [7]. No racial or geographic predilection is recognized in BP and, in contrast to PV, there is no increased incidence in the Jewish population [8]. Additionally, there is no known specific HLA association [9, 10].

5.2.2 Cutaneous distribution

The distribution of lesions in BP is most often generalized, but in 15–30% of patients the bullae may be localized [11, 12]. Although the distribution is usually widespread, sites of predilection include the lower abdomen, inner thighs, groin, axillae and flexural aspects of the arms and legs

[13]. This distribution may correlate with recent immunofluorescent (IF) studies which demonstrate the greatest amounts of antigen(s) reacting with BP sera in axillae, groin and low back, and lowest amounts on the face and scalp [14]. These data suggest that the areas commonly involved with bullous lesions correspond to the skin sites with highest expression of BP antigen.

In a minority of cases, BP may also present as a localized blistering eruption confined to one area of the body, most often the lower extremities [12]. The blisters are non-scarring, a feature that helps separate localized BP from localized cicatricial pemphigoid of Brunsting–Perry. This form of the disease most often occurs in middle aged to elderly women, and may remain localized or may progress to generalized disease.

5.2.3 Mucosal lesions

Mucosal lesions occur less often and with less severity than in PV and are usually restricted to the mouth [3] but may also involve the pharynx, nose and rarely the eyes and oesophagus [14a]. They are rarely the initial presenting feature [8, 13]. The incidence of oral lesions in BP varies from 8 to 58% among four reported series [14a, 15–17]. Oral lesions consist of small bullae which often remain intact, but if they rupture, heal rapidly without scarring. Involvement of the vermilion border of the lips is rare [13]. Other mucous membranes reported to be involved include the oesophagus, vagina and anus [18].

5.2.4 Morphology of lesions

The most characteristic clinical feature of BP is the presence of large tense bullae which arise on either an erythematous base or on normal skin [3, 13] (Figure 5.1). Grouping may be present, but is not a constant feature. Because the blisters arise subepidermally, the roof often has enough integrity to remain intact, accounting for their tense nature. The blisters may be filled with clear fluid or may be haemorrhagic, and when they rupture, leave denuded areas which may become covered with crust or debris. These erosions do not tend to spread peripherally, as may happen in PV, and generally heal well without scarring. The Nikolsky sign (extension of a blister with lateral pressure) is typically negative in BP. In addition to tense blisters, patients may also have erythematous macules, papules and urticarial plaques which may have a serpiginous configuration and may have superimposed bullae. In many patients, such urticarial plaques and papules, and less often an eczematous dermatitis, can precede the appearance of bullae by weeks to months [3, 8, 19].

The degree of pruritis in BP varies from non-existent to intense. About one-third of patients have pruritis severe enough to require systemic antihistamines [8, 16]. A few have prolonged pruritis preceding the onset of BP [20].

There are, in addition to the classical presentation of BP, several clinical variants. Vesicular pemphigoid is characterized by small tense vesicles, which may be grouped, giving the clinical impression of atypical dermatitis herpetiformis (DH) [12, 21–22]. Direct IF (DIF) studies in these patients show linear deposition of IgG and C3 along the BMZ, suggesting that these are cases of vesicular BP, not DH. The term polymorphic pemphigoid has been used by Honeyman *et al.* [23] to describe a group of patients who had small pruritic papules, vesicles and blisters on the trunk and extremities, without evidence of jejunal atrophy. DIF in most patients showed linear deposition of IgG and C3 along the BMZ, but others showed only IgA at the BMZ. The former group of patients probably has vesicular pemphigoid, while the latter group probably represents patients with linear IgA disease.

Pemphigoid vegetans is a rare variant of BP, reported in only three patients to date [24–26]. All three presented with purulent vegetating plaques in the groin and axillae, similar in appearance to pemphigus vegetans. Two of the patients also had inflammatory bowel disease. DIF was consistent with BP in all cases.

Another uncommon variant is pemphigoid nodularis, characterized by scattered hyperkeratotic nodules and plaques on which bullae may arise [12, 27–28]. These patients have chronic lesions which have often been recalcitrant to therapy. Clinically and histologically, they are similar to prurigo nodules, but direct and indirect IF (IIF) shows findings consistent with BP.

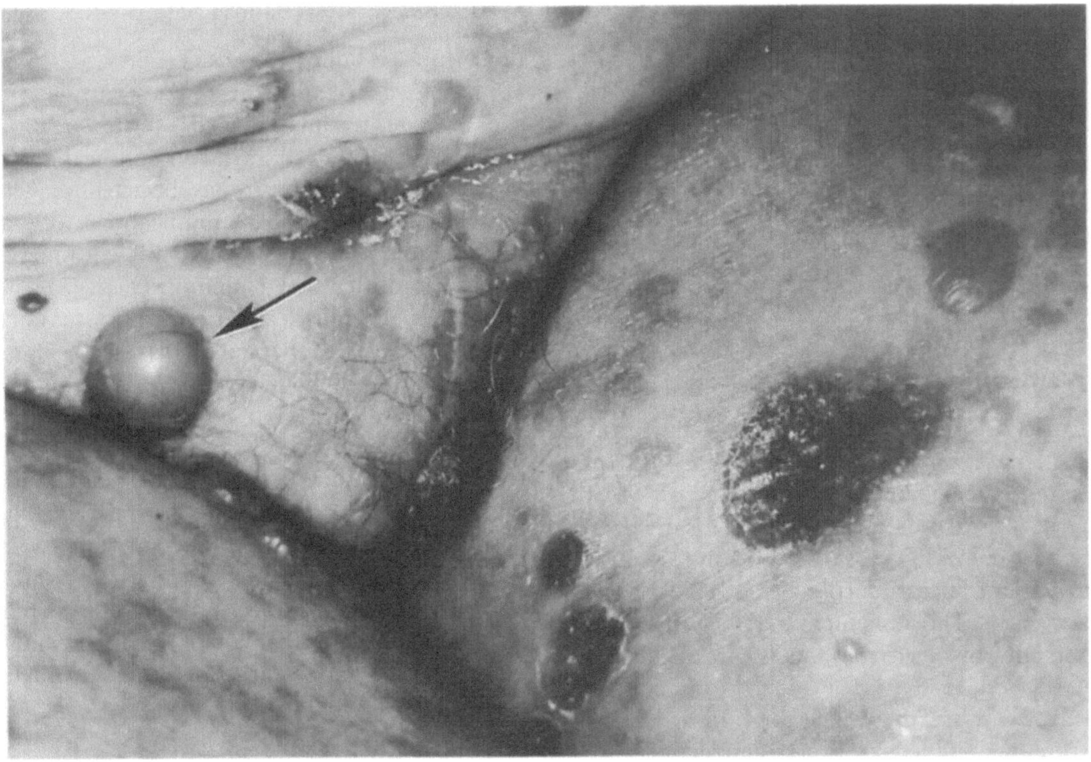

Figure 5.1 Clinical photograph showing tense bulla (arrow) and crusted erosions.

5.3 DIFFERENTIAL DIAGNOSIS

During the early urticarial or eczematous phase of BP the diagnosis may be difficult to make without immunopathological studies. When bullae appear, the diagnosis is generally more evident. However, several other bullous and vesicular diseases must be considered in the differential diagnosis, including herpes gestationis, cicatricial pemphigoid, epidermolysis bullosa acquisita, dermatitis herpetiformis, linear IgA disease, bullous lupus erythematosus and bullous drug eruptions.

5.3.1 Herpes gestationis

Herpes gestationis (HG) (see Chapter 7) is a rare subepidermal bullous disease of pregnancy and the post-partum period. HG characteristically presents during the second trimester with urticarial papules and plaques around the umbilicus, with subsequent development of both vesicles and bullae [29]. The lesions are intensely pruritic, and will spread to involve the trunk and often, the palms and soles, but usually spare the oral mucosa. Exacerbation of the disease typically occurs shortly after delivery, but patients most often go into remission within several weeks after delivery. In some cases recurrent flare ups are seen with the use of oral contraceptives and menses.

The histological findings are generally indistinguishable from BP and DIF shows linear deposition of C3 along the BMZ and, in about 30% of cases, weak deposition of IgG [29]. IIF is negative in most cases, but indirect complement fixation IF shows the presence of the 'HG factor' in the great majority of cases, which is a circulating IgG with avid complement-binding ability [30].

The relationship between BP and HG is currently unresolved. Although they share clinical, histological and immunopathological similarities, there are differences that suggest that they may be distinct entities. Unique features of HG include: (1) its association with pregnancy, (2) exacerbation by oestrogens or progesterone, (3) the characteristic avidity with which the autoantibody binds complement, and (4) the presence of basal cell necrosis seen with electron microscopy [31].

5.3.2 Cicatricial pemphigoid

Cicatricial pemphigoid (CP) (see Chapter 6), or benign mucous membrane pemphigoid, is a chronic scarring subepidermal bullous disease of the elderly, primarily affecting the mucosal surfaces. The oral mucosa is most often involved, with the gingiva and buccal mucosa being typical sites of onset [32]. The conjunctiva is the next most commonly involved site and is affected in most cases [17, 32–34]. The ocular inflammation resolves with scarring which can lead to trichiasis, entropion, symblepharon and destruction of the inferior fornix. These in turn may result in blindness due to corneal ulceration or vascularization. Nasal, pharyngeal, vaginal and, rarely, oesophageal lesions also occur.

Skin lesions occur in 24% of CP patients [35]. The lesions may be either scattered tense bullae which heal without scarring or one to several areas of recurrent bullae on an erythematous base that resolve with atrophic scars, usually found on the head and neck. A variant of CP, Brunsting–Perry pemphigoid, presents with scarring bullae, usually found on the face and scalp, in the absence of mucosal lesions [19, 33].

Routine histology shows a subepidermal blister, generally with fewer eosinophils than seen in BP. DIF is similar to that seen in BP. Less than 20% of CP patients have circulating anti-BMZ antibodies detectable with IIF [36], in contrast to BP, in which 70% are seropositive [2, 16]. Indirect immunoelectron-microscopic studies have suggested that the deposition of immune reactants in CP is at a lower level in the lamina lucida than those seen in BP, suggesting that these may be two distinct diseases [36].

5.3.3 Epidermolysis bullosa acquisita

Epidermolysis bullosa acquisita (EBA) (see Chapter 10) is a disease of adult onset, classically described as having trauma-induced blisters, usually occurring on extensor surfaces, and healing with milia and scars [37]. It has been subsequently recognized that EBA can mimic other vesiculobullous diseases, especially BP, leading to diagnostic difficulties. Gammon *et al.* [38] have found that a BP-like clinical presentation may occur in up to 50% of EBA patients. This disease has been associated with diabetes mellitus and inflammatory bowel disease and is often relatively resistant to steroid therapy. Neither histopathology nor routine DIF studies will necessarily differentiate EBA from BP, since similar linear deposition of IgG occurs in both diseases [38]. Definitive separation can be accomplished by direct or indirect immunoelectron microscopy. In EBA, the immune deposits are seen either in the lamina densa or in the immediate sublamina densa area, while in BP, they reside in the lamina lucida [39].

5.3.4 Dermatitis herpetiformis

Dermatitis herpetiformis (see Chapter 11) most often presents in young adults with intensely pruritic papules and vesicles, in a highly characteristic distribution over extensor surfaces. More than 80% of DH patients have an associated gluten-sensitive enteropathy, and also have an increased prevalence of HLA-B8 and DR3 haplotype [40]. DH may be confused with vesicular pemphigoid, but the latter usually lacks the classic DH distribution [12, 22]. The two may be further distinguished by DIF, which in DH usually shows granular deposits of IgA in the papillary tips, and by IIF, which shows circulating IgA in only 2% of patients with granular IgA deposits on DIF [41].

5.3.5 Linear IgA disease

The term linear IgA disease (LAD) (see Chapter 8) encompasses a clinically heterogeneous group of patients with vesiculobullous disease whose IF studies show linear BMZ deposits consisting mainly of IgA with or without complement components. Patients with linear IgA deposits include those with clinical features of chronic bullous disease of childhood (Chapter 9), those with mixed clinical features of DH and BP, and some patients resembling classic DH [6, 40, 42]. These latter patients have also been referred to as linear DH. LAD patients differ from classic DH by the much lower incidence of jejunal enteropathy, a less complete response to sulphones, and no increase in the incidence of HLA-B8 histocompatibility antigen in adult patients [40, 43]. LAD patients differ from those with classic BP by the relatively younger age group affected, the presence of linear IgA rather than IgG at the BMZ by DIF, and a lower incidence of anti-BMZ antibodies, with these antibodies being of the IgA rather than IgG isotype [42]. Immunoelectron microscopy has shown deposition of IgA in both the lamina lucida and the subbasal lamina, suggesting that two immunological variants may exist [40]. Although these patients are immunohistologically distinct from both typical DH and BP, their precise relationship to the latter diseases remains unclear.

5.3.6 Bullous systemic lupus erythematosus

Bullous systemic lupus erythematosus (BSLE) (Chapter 18), an uncommon cutaneous manifestation of systemic lupus, may also mimic BP. The following criteria have been suggested for the diagnosis of bullous SLE: (1) diagnosis of SLE based on American Rheumatism Association (ARA) criteria, (2) presence of vesicles or bullae on either sun- or non-sun-exposed skin, (3) histopathology showing a subepidermal vesicle with a predominantly neutrophilic infiltrate, (4) negative IIF for anti-BMZ antibodies and (5) DIF showing granular or linear deposition of IgG and/or IgM and often IgA at the BMZ [44]. Since many of these features may be shared with authentic BP, definitive diagnosis of bullous lupus depends on immunoelectron microscopy studies, which shows the immune deposits present beneath the lamina densa, a feature not seen in BP [45] (see below).

5.3.7 Bullous drug eruptions

Finally, bullous drug eruptions (Chapter 17) may resemble BP clinically. Immunofluorescent studies can help differentiate these cases from those in which drugs may have induced BP lesions. Drugs that have been associated with onset of BP lesions include furosemide [46], sulphasalazine [47], phenoxymethylpenicillin [48] and topical 5-fluorouracil [49].

5.4 INVESTIGATIONS

5.4.1 Histopathology

Histological findings in BP can vary depending on the type of lesion biopsied. The most characteristic histological finding in a biopsy from a bulla is a subepidermal blister with a mixed dermal inflammatory infiltrate consisting of numerous eosinophils, mononuclear cells and some neutrophils [50] (Figure 5.2(a)). The degree of dermal infiltrate depends on whether the bulla selected for biopsy arose on inflamed or normal skin, with the former showing a denser dermal infiltrate than the latter [51]. Rarely, the neutrophil is the predominant inflammatory cell type. The blister cavity typically contains fibrin, eosinophils and neutrophils, and the surrounding epidermis may show eosinophilic spongiosis and basal cell vacuolization.

Biopsy of an urticarial lesion typically shows the eosinophil-rich infiltrate, basal cell vacuolization and papillary oedema, without a subepidermal blister. Pemphigoid vegetans and nodularis have epidermal hyperplasia and hyperkeratosis in addition to the histological changes of classic BP [25, 27, 50].

A biopsy for histopathology is best taken from an early bulla, since regeneration of the epidermis on the blister floor, which begins in about 2 days, can give the false impression of an intraepidermal blister in older lesions [51].

The histological differential diagnosis includes CP and HG which may be impossible to differentiate from BP [51]. In rare cases where neutrophils predominate in the infiltrate, DH, LAD and BSLE should also be considered.

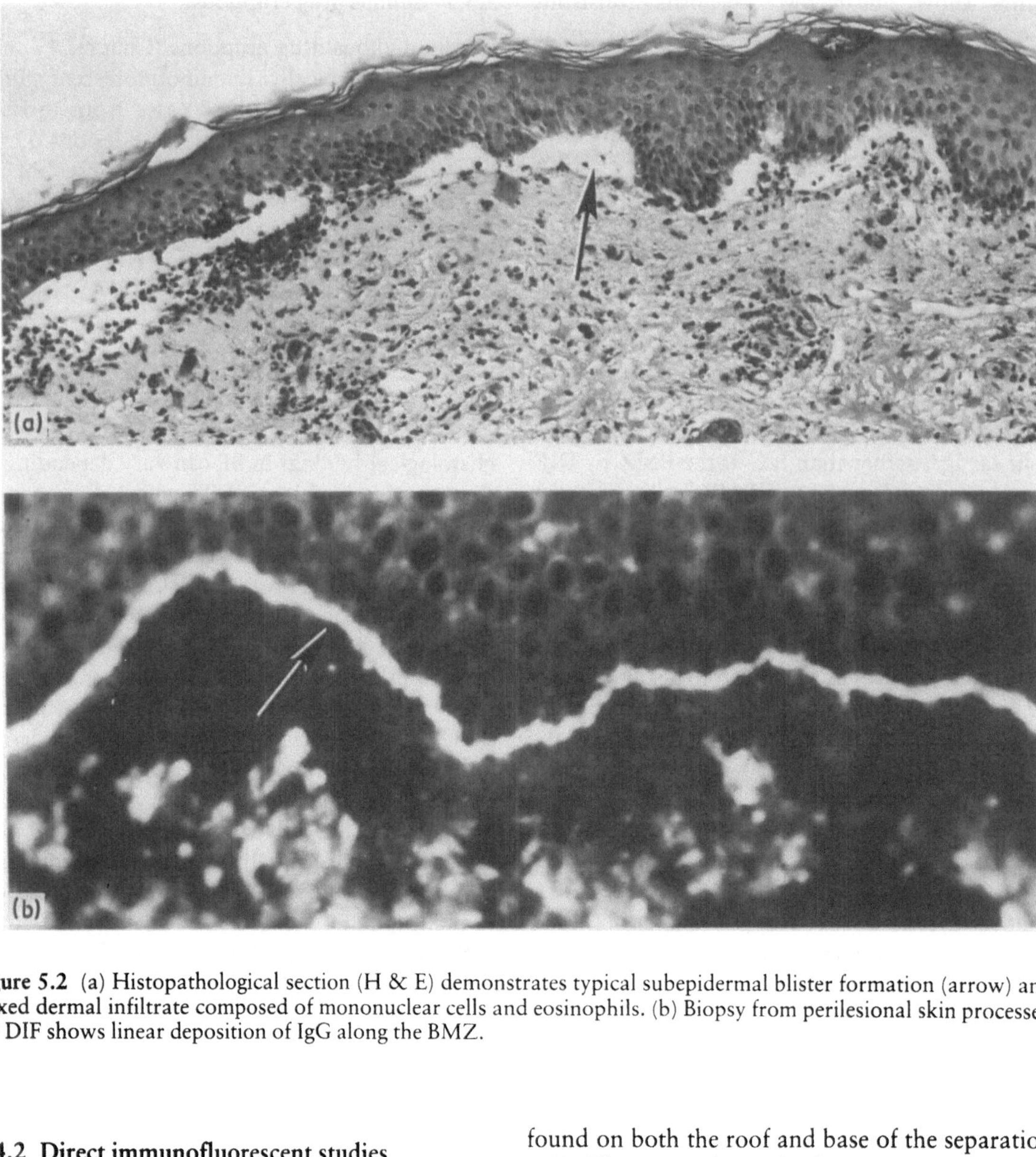

Figure 5.2 (a) Histopathological section (H & E) demonstrates typical subepidermal blister formation (arrow) and mixed dermal infiltrate composed of mononuclear cells and eosinophils. (b) Biopsy from perilesional skin processed for DIF shows linear deposition of IgG along the BMZ.

5.4.2 Direct immunofluorescent studies

In BP, biopsies for DIF reflect *in vivo* deposition of anti-BMZ antibodies and complement. A typical positive result from perilesional skin shows immune deposits present in a continuous fine linear pattern along the BMZ (Figure 5.2(b)). This pattern may appear granular in some areas due to oblique tissue sectioning. In biopsies with dermo–epidermal separation, the immune deposits may be absent entirely, seen only on the blister roof, or found on both the roof and base of the separation [53]. The optimal site for biopsy is on clinically normal skin, within 2 cm of a lesion since biopsies from either clinically involved areas or from skin too distant from a lesion can give false negative results [53]. Positive results may also be obtained from clinically uninvolved oral mucosa and bulbar conjuctiva [14a].

The immune deposits in BP characteristically consist of IgG and complement [17, 52–54]. Approximately 90% of patients demonstrate IgG deposition, while C3 is detected more often, in nearly 100% of patients [16, 53]. Occasionally, C3 is the only immune deposit detected at the BMZ. Other classes of immunoglobulins are seen less frequently, usually in combination with IgG. IgM is the second most frequently detected immunoglobulin, followed by IgA. IgE and IgD have both been found, but in a minority of patients [16–17, 53, 54].

Linear deposits of IgG and C3 along the BMZ are typical of, but not specific for, BP. These findings can also appear in CP, HG, EBA and BSLE. The latter two diseases may be differentiated by immunoelectron microscopy [53].

5.4.3 Indirect immunofluorescent studies

IIF in BP is used to detect the presence of anti-BMZ autoantibodies in patient sera [52].

Approximately 70% of patients with active BP have circulating anti-BMZ antibodies detectable by routine IIF methods [2, 16–17, 53]. These antibodies produce a linear pattern at the BMZ resembling what is seen on DIF. The vast majority are of the IgG class, but circulating IgA and IgE anti-BMZ antibodies have also been detected [12, 55, 56]. In general, these titres correlate poorly with disease activity [16]. They are, however, most often absent when the disease is in remission and detectable when BP is active [16, 53].

Several authors have reported the presence of circulating antibodies which were not detected by routine IIF. Herrmann detected circulating anti-BMZ antibodies in the sera of four seronegative BP patients only after dissociating circulating immune complexes [57]. In addition, patients with high anti-nuclear antibody titres may have false negative IIF results unless the substrate is pretreated to extract nuclear antigen [58]. In a few patients, the titre of circulating BP antibody may be so low as to be undetectable by routine IIF, but its presence is implied by the detection of complement in indirect complement fixation IF [59]. In all studies, substrate selection should be noted, since the results may vary on substrates from different sources [60, 61] and may be enhanced by the use of chemically split tissue [61a].

Circulating anti-BMZ antibodies exist not only in BP, but also in EBA, and less frequently in HG and CP [53]. EBA antibodies can be differentiated either by immunoelectron microscopy or by IIF on skin which has been split through the lamina lucida with 1 M NaCl. EBA antibodies will bind only to the base of the separation, whereas BP antibodies bind to the roof, or to both the roof and base [61a, 62, 62a].

Rarely, circulating anti-BMZ IgG has been found in cases of psoriasis, leg ulcers and in burn patients [63]. This finding is uncommon and not considered a characteristic feature of these diseases.

5.4.4 Other laboratory studies

Few associated laboratory abnormalities have been reported in patients with BP. In 70% there was an elevated serum IgE level [64] and peripheral blood eosinophilia has been noted in 50% [65].

5.5 ASSOCIATED DISEASES

BP has been reported in association with a variety of diseases, including systemic lupus erythematosus (SLE), diabetes mellitus (DM), psoriasis, lichen planus (LP) and rheumatoid arthritis (RA). The validity of these associations may be altered by the fact that case reports and studies prior to 1967 were based on clinical and histological data without the benefit of IF confirmation. Thus, these early studies may have included patients with a number of vesiculobullous diseases other than BP.

5.5.1 Systemic lupus erythematosus

Early reports on patients with vesiculobullous eruptions and SLE indicated that these patients had coexisting SLE and BP, although generally there were questions concerning complete diagnosis of one of the two diseases [45, 66, 67]. Subsequently, patients with clearly established SLE by ARA criteria and vesiculobullous eruptions have been more carefully studied [44, 45, 68, 69]. These patients were often young black females with active SLE who developed subepidermal vesicles or bullae, either on an erythematous base or on normal skin. Their histopathology showed subepidermal bullae with a predominantly neutrophilic infiltrate, similar to DH. Their DIF revealed linear or granular deposition of IgG, IgM and/or IgA and less often C3 along the BMZ while IIF was negative in most cases. Most importantly, immunoelectron microscopy showed that the immune reactants are deposited beneath the lamina densa as seen in lupus, rather than in the lamina lucida, as seen in BP [45]. Hence, these patients probably do not have coexisting BP and SLE; rather they represent a bullous form of SLE which mimics BP both clinically and as assessed by DIF.

Gammon *et al.* [70] have recently reported three patients with bullous lupus erythematosus who have circulating autoantibodies against the BMZ. These antibodies have several features of the EBA autoantibody, including *in vitro* binding to the dermal side of an artifactually induced dermo–epidermal separation, and recognition of a 290- and 145-kDa dermal protein. These data suggest that cases of bullous lupus erythematosus with circulating anti-BMZ antibodies may represent co-occurrence of SLE and EBA or may be a distinct subset of bullous lupus erythematosus.

5.5.2 Diabetes mellitus

Chuang *et al.* [71] evaluated the frequency of primary DM in patients with BP in a retrospective case-controlled study. He identified 30 patients with histologically and immunopathologically diagnosed BP, and chose as controls patients whose names appeared before and after each case of BP from their histopathology record book. They found that 20% of BP patients had DM prior to the use of systemic steroids compared to only 2.5% of the control population. Because the controls had a lower average age, they also compared the frequency of DM in BP patients to a subgroup of controls over 50, and still found a significantly higher prevalence of DM among BP patients.

5.5.3 Psoriasis

Several reports describe the coexistence of psoriasis and BP. In most cases, BP was apparently precipitated by psoriatic therapy, including psoralen and ultraviolet A (PUVA), ultraviolet light and tar, and ultraviolet light and anthralin [72–75]. Grattan, however, has reported an increased incidence of psoriasis in BP patients unrelated to therapy [4]. In a retrospective case-controlled study, he reviewed 62 cases of BP, most confirmed by immunopathology, and 62 control cases with leg ulcers. He found that psoriasis occurred in 11% of BP patients, but in no controls. Although this is higher than the general prevalence of 0.25–2%, further studies are required to confirm this association.

5.5.4 Rheumatoid arthritis

A number of patients with long-standing rheumatoid arthritis (RA) have been reported to develop BP [72–79]. In 1980 Callen reviewed 10 cases of RA and BP from the literature and noted that in most the diagnosis of BP was well documented, but the diagnosis of RA did not always meet the ARA criteria [77]. However, he suggested that the relationship may be more than coincidental, citing a study by Salo and Rasanen [80], who found that 12% of 94 BP patients had RA and hypothesized that the two diseases may share a similar pathogenesis.

5.5.5 Lichen planus

Lichen planus pemphigoides (LPP) has been described many times in the literature [81–84]. It is usually characterized by a typical outbreak of lichen planus followed by a bullous eruption occurring on the LP lesions and on normal skin. It is currently unclear whether these patients have coexisting LP and BP or represent a distinct entity. A complete description of these patients is not available in all cases, but most show histological changes of LP in their papular lesions and histological and DIF findings consistent with BP in bullous or peribullous skin [82–85]. The majority also have circulating autoantibodies directed against the BMZ. Immunoelectron microscopy has demonstrated immune deposits in the lamina lucida of perilesional skin, similar to BP. However, in blister cavities, they are located on the floor rather than on the roof as expected in BP [82]. An immunoprecipitation study has not reproduced the findings reported in BP [86], again suggesting that these antibodies are not reacting with the BP antigen [82]. It has been hypothesized that destruction of the BMZ in LP could lead to unmasking of a previously hidden antigen(s) which may result in autoantibody production, causing a bullous disease similar to BP [81].

5.5.6 Malignancy

BP has been reported in association with malignancies of the lymphoreticular system, skin, lung, breast, pancreas, kidney, gastrointestinal and genitourinary tract [87]. No consistent correlations exist with the type of malignancy, the clinical course, or time of onset of the two diseases. The significance of this association is somewhat controversial but most large series have concluded that there is no increased incidence of malignancy in BP patients compared to age- and sex-matched controls [79, 87, 88].

Stone and Schroeter reviewed the records of 73 patients with BP, most of whom were diagnosed by immunofluorescent studies [87]. These were compared with 73 patients with psoriasis and 73 with contact dermatitis, matched for age, sex and calendar year of diagnosis to determine the incidence of malignancy within a 5-year period before or after the diagnosis of BP. Their data demonstrated that malignancy occurred no more often in patients with BP, than in the two control groups. Similarly, Ahmed *et al.* [88] found a 3% incidence of malignancy in 33 patients with BP compared to 4.2% in an age-matched population. Paslin [89] reviewed 19 cases of BP between 1960 and 1972, 18 of whom were evaluated for malignancy and nine of whom had autopsies performed. Only one patient was found to have a malignancy, a 5% incidence. Savin [79] as well, in reviewing the events leading to death in BP patients, noted no increased incidence of malignancy.

In contrast, Chorzelski *et al.* [90] found malignant disease in 12 of 110 BP patients which, according to the Poisson equation, is significantly higher than expected in an age- and sex-matched group of the Polish population. These authors recommended a careful evaluation for malignancy in BP patients.

Several authors [17, 91] have reported that a subset of BP patients who are seronegative by IIF have a higher frequency of malignancy than those who are seropositive. The frequency of malignancy in this seronegative group has not been evaluated in a controlled study.

5.6 PATHOGENESIS AND RECENT ADVANCES

BP is probably an autoimmune disease mediated by autoantibodies directed against an antigen in the BMZ of stratified squamous epithelia. Evidence that supports this concept includes the presence of circulating anti-BMZ antibodies, deposition of these antibodies at the site of clinical lesion formation [53], the association with other autoimmune diseases [92], and *in vitro* [93] and *in vivo* [94] models using BP antibody to reproduce features of the spontaneously occurring disease.

5.6.1 The BP antigen(s)

The BP antigen(s) is a normal constituent of the BMZ of stratified squamous epithelia in all vertebrates [95] and is also found in the BMZ of the gall-bladder, urethra, bladder and bronchi [96]. It is defined by its interaction with autoantibodies present in the sera of patients with BP. The antigen(s) is synthesized by epidermal basal cells [97] and has been produced by keratinocytes in culture [86, 98].

The localization of the BP antigen has been studied previously by both IF and immunoelectron microscopic techniques. Using standard IIF methods, it has been established that BP antibodies bind to an antigen in the BMZ. Direct and indirect immunoelectron microscopy using immunoperoxidase techniques have shown that BP antibodies are deposited within the lamina lucida of the BMZ, implying that the antigen is located there as well [99–101].

Recent observations in our laboratory on both intact epidermis and basal cell suspensions show that, contrary to previous assumptions, the majority of the BP antigen is located intracellularly in association with hemidesmosomes, and only a small portion is found extracellularly in the lamina lucida [102]. These observations have now been confirmed by several other investigators [103, 104].

Mutasim *et al.* [102] have shown that viable murine epidermal sheets, separated below the basal lamina, incubated with BP sera, then cryosectioned and treated with FITC-conjugated anti-human IgG show no linear BMZ fluorescence. When epidermal sheets were first pretreated with agents to permeabilize the cell membrane, then incubated with BP sera, cryosectioned and treated with FITC-conjugated anti-human IgG, they then revealed linear fluorescence along the BMZ. Epidermal sheets processed by standard IIF, in which the epidermis is first sectioned (exposing intracellular antigens), then treated with BP serum and FITC-labelled anti-human IgG, show typical continuous linear fluorescent staining along the BMZ. Control sections incubated with normal human sera did not show any fluorescence regardless of treatment sequence. Since antibodies do not cross membranes of viable cells, these observations suggest that the BP antigen in epidermal sheets is intracellular.

Similar results have been demonstrated using suspensions of epidermal basal cells [102]. If a suspension of trypsinized basal cells is prepared from fresh viable epidermis, about 10–15% of the cells are non-viable. If this cell suspension is incubated with BP serum and then FITC-labelled anti-human IgG, only the non-viable basal cells (10–15%) will show positive fluorescence, which is limited to one pole of the cell. When these epidermal cell suspensions are permeabilized prior to IIF, essentially all basal cells show the polar fluorescence (Figure 5.3(a)).

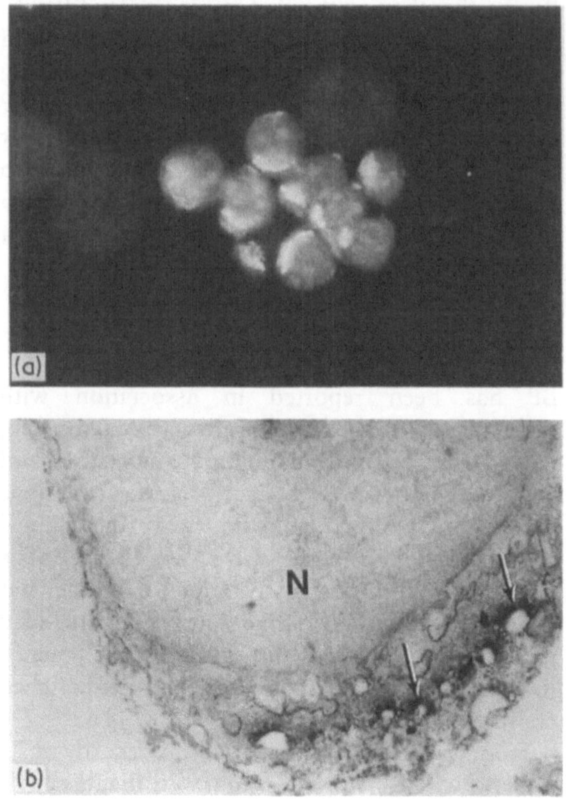

Figure 5.3 (a) Murine basal cells which have been separated by trypsinization, then permeabilized prior to incubation with BP sera and FITC-labelled anti-human IgG, showing polar fluorescence presumably corresponding to the dermal pole of the cell. (b) Immunoelectron photomicrograph of these trypsinized cells which have been incubated with BP sera and peroxidase-labelled anti-human IgG. Near one end of the cell are multiple vesicles, with the immunoreactants located on their cytoplasmic side (arrows). These vesicles represent internalized hemidesmosomes. N = nucleus.

Using similar methods, we have also studied the ultrastructural localization of the BP antigen. In murine epidermal sheets permeabilized prior to BP sera and peroxidase conjugate exposure, 100% of the basal cells demonstrated regularly spaced intracellular dense clumps on the dermal pole of the cell membrane. These sites of deposition corresponded to basal cell hemidesmosomes. No immunoreactants were seen in the desmosomes. Similar experiments on non-permeabilized epidermal sheets demonstrated no deposition of immunoreactants in the majority of basal cells. In the few basal cells that were non-viable, immunoreactants were seen deposited intracellularly in sites corresponding to the location of hemidesmosomes (Figure 5.4). There was faint deposition of immunoreactants in the lamina lucida. Permeabilized trypsin-dissociated basal cells exposed to BP sera and peroxidase conjugate

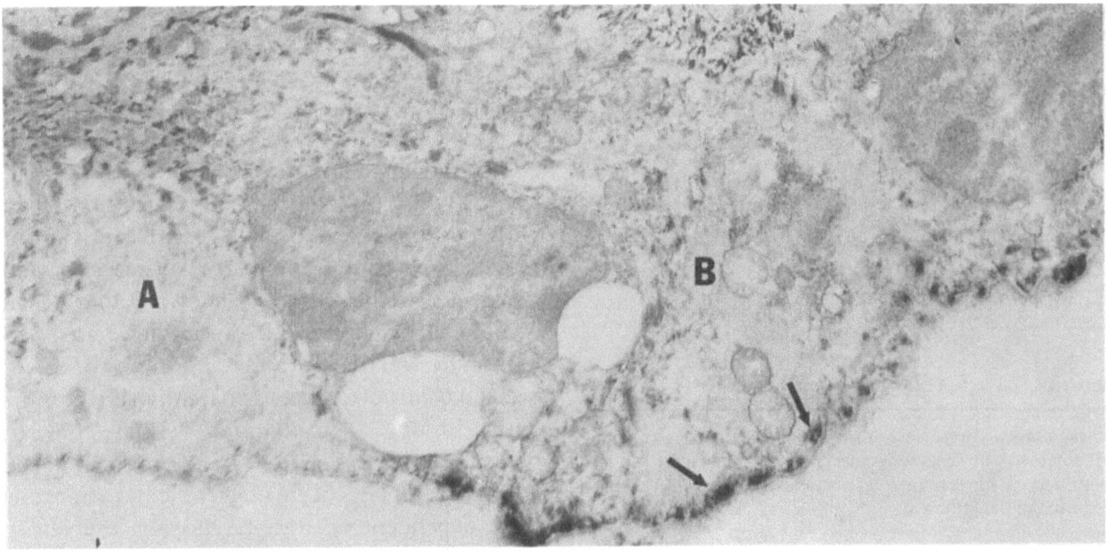

Figure 5.4 Immunoelectron photomicrograph of a murine epidermal sheet which has been incubated with BP sera and peroxidase-labelled anti- human IgG . Two adjacent basal cells are shown; the cell on the left (A) is viable and no immune deposition is seen. The cell on the right (B) is non-viable and BP autoantibodies have been able to cross the permeabilized membrane and deposit intracellularly in areas corresponding to hemidesmosomes (arrows).

showed clumps of immunoreactants only in the cytoplasm on the outer surface of intracellular vesicles (Figure 5.3(b)). This location corresponds to a recognized ultrastructural site of internalized hemidesmosomes in trypsinized basal cells [105].

The deposition of immunoreactants predominantly at sites of hemidesmosomes in both epidermal sheets and in dissociated basal cells implies that the major part of BP antigen lies in the tonofilament-attachment plaque complex. Studies performed on human skin using dissociated basal cells and intact epidermis from suction blisters have given similar results.

These findings do not discount previous work suggesting that BP antigen resides in the lamina lucida [99–101]. The immunoelectron microscopy studies that demonstrated this finding reflected *in vivo* deposition of antibody in perilesional skin or were done under conditions in which the basal cell membranes may not have been permeable, and therefore only extracellular antigen would be detectable.

There is increasing evidence for the heterogeneity of BP antigens. In 1977 Diaz *et al.* [106] identified a 20-kDa saline-soluble protein extracted from the epidermis of sodium thiocyanate (NaSCN)-split human skin, which was able to adsorb BP antibodies from serum as shown by IIF methods. Stanley *et al.* [86] immunoprecipitated a protein from cultured human epidermal cells which was soluble in non-ionic detergent and from spontaneously transformed mouse epidermal cells which was soluble in buffered saline using BP sera. The protein, which consisted of disulphide-linked chains of approximately 220 kDa, was immunoprecipitated by nine different BP sera, suggesting that there is a single BP antigen. This antigen was different from fibronectin and laminin, two other components of the BMZ with similar molecular weights. Subsequently, using immunoblotting, Stanley *et al.* [107] demonstrated a 220–240-kDa non-disulphide-linked BP antigen extracted with sodium dodecyl sulphate (SDS) from suction-blister-derived human epidermis.

Finally, Labib, from our laboratory, has analysed 28 BP sera and 24 control sera by immunoblotting

Table 5.1 Frequency of detection of protein bands with immunoblotting using BP and control sera

Protein bands	*Bullous pemphigoid* (n = 28)	*Cicatricial pemphigoid* (n = 4)	*Normals and other controls** (n = 24)
240 kDa	12 (43)†	1	0
200 kDa	7 (25)		0
180 kDa	8 (29)	0	0
97 kDa	2 (7)	0	0
77 kDa	2 (7)	0	0
No bands	3 (11)	3	24

* These controls were sera from patients with systemic lupus erythematosus, mycosis fungoides, psoriasis or eczema.
† Number of BP sera giving positive reactions. Percentages are shown in parentheses.

to characterize the BP antigen extracted from human epidermis in SDS [108]. The majority of BP sera recognized both a 240-kDa and a 180-kDa epidermal protein. However, a total of five bands of 240 kDa, 200 kDa, 180 kDa, 97 kDa and 77 kDa were recognized by BP sera (Table 5.1). Although one control serum from a CP patient recognized a 240-kDa band, none of the other controls detected any of these bands. This suggests that there may be a variety of autoantibodies in BP serum as defined by the antigens with which they react. The relationship between the various antigens described by different investigators and to the antigens demonstrated in the hemidesmosomes and lamina lucida by immunoelectron microscopy is currently unclear.

The function of the BP antigen has not been determined, but several possible roles have been suggested. Wound-healing experiments [109, 110] have suggested that the BP antigen may be important in cell substrate attachment during early epidermal migration. In addition, since it is selectively absent from the BMZ of basal cell carcinoma, it may have a role in directing normal keratinocyte differentiation [111].

5.6.2 The BP autoantibodies

Although it is not established unequivocally, there is considerable evidence suggesting that BP autoantibodies are pathogenic. Gammon *et al.* [93] have described an *in vitro* model for BP, referred to as a leucocyte attachment (LA) assay, which has been useful in evaluating the functional properties of BP antibodies and their interaction with complement and inflammatory cells. Using indirect LA, in which normal human skin is first treated with BP sera, then incubated with fresh normal human sera as a complement source and viable leucocytes, they have shown that when complement-binding BP antibodies are used, leucocytes will migrate and attach to the BMZ. The attached leucocytes were apparently activated and, with prolonged incubation, dermal epidermal separation occurred, similarly to that seen in early lesions of BP. Leucocyte migration and attachment were dependent on the presence of complement-fixing BP antibodies, complement and viable leucocytes.

Using direct LA, in which biopsies from BP patients are incubated with complement and leucocytes, they have also shown that there is a greater degree of leucocyte attachment in lesional skin compared to perilesional skin, although there was no difference in the intensity of IgG or C3 deposition in these two sites [112]. This suggests that immune complexes in lesional skin from BP patients have greater complement-activating capacity than do those from adjacent normal skin.

This model provides functional evidence that BP antigen–antibody complexes can activate complement, produce chemotactic activity, and recruit activated leucocytes to the BMZ and it suggests that all three entities play a role in mediating the inflammatory events in BP.

Further evidence that BP antibodies are pathogenic has been obtained by *in vivo* passive transfer studies. Anhalt *et al.* [94] have demonstrated that purified IgG from BP patients injected into the corneal stroma of rabbits produced corneal inflammatory lesions, with visible blisters. Histologically, the lesions showed subepithelial blister formation with polymorphonuclear cells along the BMZ, and DIF demonstrated linear depostion of human IgG and rabbit C3 along the BMZ. The intensity of the inflammation correlated with the complement fixation titres of the IgG, supporting a role for complement in mediating BP lesion production. It was not possible to produce similar changes by intradermal injection into rabbit skin.

Naito *et al.* [113] have reported the development of dermal–epidermal separation and dermal inflammation in guinea-pigs at the site of intradermally injected, concentrated sera and IgG fractions from BP patients. Gammon *et al.* have not been able to reproduce these findings [114].

Since the above models all suggest that complement is an important mediator of the inflammatory response, it would be expected that BP antibodies, should be capable of fixing complement, but this is not true in all cases. Although essentially all tissue-bound antibodies fix complement *in vivo*, as evidenced by DIF [53], many but not all circulating antibodies are capable of fixing complement [115, 116]. Sams and Schur [117] have suggested that complement-activating antibodies are primarily of the IgG3 subclass, and may play the major role in lesion formation. However, Bird *et al.* [118], using monoclonal antibodies to the four subclasses of IgG, have shown that IgG4, which is not capable of fixing complement, is the predominant subclass found both in sera and deposited in tissue of BP patients. The reason for this discrepancy is unclear, but since IgG4 may have homocytotropic properties for mast cells [119], it may play a role in mast cell degranulation and provide an additional mechanism for mediating inflammation.

5.6.3 The complement system

Several lines of evidence support the role of complement in the pathogenesis of BP, including the regular detection of C3 with DIF studies [53], the ability of most circulating anti-BMZ antibodies to fix complement *in vitro* [116], and immunoelectron-microscopic studies showing C3 deposition at the site of blister formation (lamina lucida) [120]. Levels of total haemolytic complement and of individual complement components have been found to be reduced in blister fluid compared to sera of BP patients, suggesting local activation of the complement cascade [121]. Additionally, *in vivo* and *in vitro* models for BP have, in general, required the presence of complement-fixing antibodies and/or complement to produce positive results [93, 94].

Components of both the classic and alternative pathways have been detected both in skin lesions and fixed *in vitro* by serum anti-BMZ antibodies, including C1q, C4, C3, C5, C5–9, factor B, B1H globulin and properdin [122]. These findings most likely reflect the activation of the classic pathway with amplification through the alternative pathway [52].

Using a monoclonal antibody to a neoantigen on C9, Dahl *et al.* [123] have demonstrated the presence of the membrane attack complex (MAC) at the BMZ in biopsies from BP patients. The detection of this complex in some lesions with a paucity of inflammatory cells suggested a direct cytopathic role for complement in production of BP lesions.

5.6.4 The inflammatory cellular events

The role of inflammatory cells in BP has been studied by several investigators. Wintroub *et al.* [124] studied the histological abnormalities seen at various clinical stages of BP lesions, and found a functional and morphological role for mast cells in production of BP lesions. Histological examination of clinically normal perilesional skin, which showed deposition of C3 by DIF, revealed an increased number of mast cells in the papillary dermis. Biopsies from early erythematous macules showed mast cell hypogranulation, and an inflammatory infiltrate consisting of only mononuclear cells. More advanced lesions demonstrated progressive hypogranulation of mast cells and an influx of eosinophils. The suggestion that mast cell degranulation induces influx of eosinophils is supported by the finding of an eosinophilic chemotactic factor (ECF-A) in blister fluid, with biochemical properties similar to the type derived from mast cells [56, 124]. Elevated levels of histamine in blister fluid further support a role for mast cell activation in the pathogenesis of BP [125].

Ultrastructural studies have shown that once eosinophils accumulate near the BMZ, they release their granules, which contain proteolytic enzymes, and a cytotoxic agent, eosinophilic major basic protein (MBP) [126]. Deposition of eosinophil-derived enzymes has been demonstrated on the epidermal basement membrane in perilesional skin and on the floor of blisters from BP patients [127], supporting the proposal that proteolytic enzymes of eosinophils play a role in the early stages of blister formation.

5.6.5 Proposed hypothesis for the immunopathological events in BP

Current evidence has prompted the following hypothesis for subepidermal blister formation in BP [122, 128]. The initial event is presumed to be the alteration of the BP antigen in some way, causing stimulation of B cells/plasma cells which produce various classes of anti-BMZ antibodies, with the IgG class predominating. These autoantibodies attach to the BP antigen(s), probably in the lamina lucida, and activate the complement cascade, which generates the anaphylatoxins C3a and C5a. Mast cells degranulate, in response to the anaphylatoxins and possibly in response to IgG4, release ECF-A, neutrophilic chemotactic factor, histamine and proteolytic enzymes. Eosinophils and neutrophils are recruited, both by mast cell factors and by C5a, and adhere to the BMZ by virtue of their Fc and C3b receptors, where they release tissue-destructive enzymes. Injury to the BMZ may be mediated by these enzymes, producing dermo–epidermal separation.

5.7 TREATMENT

Generalized BP requires systemic therapy, using agents similar to those effective in PV, but in lower doses and for shorter periods of time. The majority of patients with localized BP have responded well to therapy with topical steroids alone without recurrences of their disease [12, 16]. Systemic corticosteroids are the mainstay of therapy in generalized BP; the most widely used preparation is prednisone. Most large series show that the majority of patients with generalized disease were controlled with 40–80 mg daily of prednisone [16, 17, 130, 131] and only rarely was it necessary to exceed 80 mg daily. The severity of disease, age of the patient and presence of underlying diseases, especially diabetes mellitus, tuberculosis and hypertension, must be considered in determining the dose of corticosteroids. Mild disease, which has been arbitrarily defined as presence of 20 lesions or less [130], usually responds to lower doses of prednisone than does moderate (20–40 lesions) or severe (greater than 60 lesions) disease. Healing of existing lesions and cessation of new blister formation reflects a response to therapy. Once the disease is under control, the prednisone dose should be tapered slowly and eventually changed to an alternate-day regimen to minimize the steroid side effects.

Long-term therapy with corticosteroids can produce a number of well-known complications including hypertension, diabetes mellitus, gastrointestinal bleeding, osteoporosis, cataracts and increased susceptibility to bacterial, fungal and viral infections [132]. These potential adverse effects must be considered and appropriate parameters monitored during therapy.

A minority of patients may not respond to, or may require a high maintenance dose of, corticosteroids. These patients may benefit from the addition of an immunosuppressive agent. The most frequently used agents are azathioprine and cyclophosphamide. Greaves and Ahmed have both found that use of azathioprine in combination with prednisone has allowed a significant reduction or discontinuation of corticosteroid therapy, and Ahmed additionally noted a decrease in the total duration of therapy [16, 133, 134]. Important adverse effects of azathioprine which require monitoring include bone marrow suppression and cholestasis; it additionally may confer an increased risk of long-term development of malignancy [135]. Experience with cyclophosphamide is more limited, but it has also been shown to have steroid-sparing effects [136]. The more serious adverse effects include bone marrow suppression, haemorrhagic cystitis, sterility and possible carcinogenic potential [137]. Methotrexate has also been used in a limited number of patients with success [11].

Person and Rogers reported good response to dapsone or sulphapyridine in six of 41 BP patients [138]. Interestingly, those who improved had a predominance of neutrophils on their biopsy. Rook and Waddington [139] have also been able to control BP patients with sulphone therapy. Although these are not drugs of first choice in BP, they may be useful in management of patients in whom corticosteroids are contraindicated or not tolerated. Corticosteroid pulse therapy, in which patients are given 1 g of methylprednisolone intravenously for 3 consecutive days, has recently been reported to be successful in initial control of patients with severe BP [140]. However, since there is only limited experience with its use in BP patients, it is currently considered an experimental mode of therapy. Plasmaphaeresis has also been used with success in treating patients with BP [141, 142]. This procedure, which acts presumably by removing pathogenic antibodies, is costly, time consuming and has only temporary beneficial effects, so is generally reserved for cases of BP in which routine therapy has proven unsuitable. Finally, cyclosporin, an immunosuppressive agent originally used to prevent graft rejection, has proven beneficial in the treatment of two BP patients [143]. Further studies are needed to determine the role of this agent in the treatment of BP.

5.8 PROGNOSIS

In most patients with generalized BP, the disease is self-limited, lasting anywhere from months to years [13]. The course of treated disease varies probably due to heterogeneous clinical presentation and differing therapeutic regimens, but in general, the majority of treated patients go into remission within 3–6 years without need for further therapy [8, 16, 17]. Remissions and exacerbations, usually occurring over a period of months, are not uncommon and recurrent disease may be less severe than the initial episode [13, 17]. Recurrences are rare in localized non-scarring BP [16]. In contrast to PV, the mortality rate is low, even without treatment [8, 13]. However, BP is still a potentially fatal disease, with a mortality rate of 10–20% in treated patients [8]. Savin has found that the risk of death in BP increases with the age of onset of disease and that death in BP most often occurs within the first 12 weeks of starting treatment [129]. It is uncommon for bullous lesions themselves to be the direct cause of death, but side effects of treatment, general debilitation of severe illness, and underlying associated illness in the elderly may contribute to the demise of BP patients [129].

ACKNOWLEDGEMENT

This work was supported in part by US Public Health Service Grants RO1-AM32599, RO1-AM32081, RO1-AM32490, KO4-ARO1686, R23-AM32079 and T32-AM07324 from the National Institutes of Health.

REFERENCES

1. Lever, W.F. (1953) Pemphigus. *Medicine,* **32**, 1–123.
2. Jordon, R.E., Beutner, E.H., Witebsky, E., *et al.* (1967) Basement zone antibodies in bullous pemphigoid. *J. Amer. Med. Assoc.*, **200**, 751–8.
3. Rook, A., Wilkinson, D.S. and Ebling, F.J.G. (eds) (1979) *Textbook of Dermatology*, Blackwell Scientific Publications, Oxford, pp. 1462–5.
4. Grattan, C.E.H. (1985) Evidence of an association between bullous pemphigoid and psoriasis. *Brit. J. Dermatol.*, **113**, 281–3.
5. Bean, S.F. (1987) in *Clinics in Dermatology: Bullous Pemphigoid*, Vol. 5 (ed. A.R. Ahmed), J.B. Lippincott, Philadelphia, pp. 13–17.
6. Marsden, R.A., McKee, P.H., Bhogal, B., *et al.* (1980) A study of benign chronic bullous dermatosis of childhood and comparison with dermatitis herpetiformis and bullous pemphigoid occurring in childhood. *Clin. Exp. Dermatol.*, **5**, 159–72.
7. Lim, C.C., MacDonald, R.H. and Rook, A.J. (1968) Pemphigoid eruptions in the elderly. *Trans. St. Johns Hosp. Dermatol. Soc. Lond.*, **54**, 148–51.
8. Ahmed, A.R. and Newcomer, V.D. (1987) in *Clinics in Dermatology: Bullous Pemphigoid* (ed. A.R. Ahmed), J.B. Lippincott, Philadelphia, pp. 6–12.
9. Ahmed, A.R., Cohen, E., Blumenson, L.E. and Provost, T.T. (1977) HLA in Bullous Pemphigoid. *Arch. Dermatol.*, **113**, 1121.
10. Ahmed, A.R., Konqui, A., Park, M.S., Tiwari, J.L. and Terasaki, P.I. (1984) DR antigens in bullous pemphigoid. *Arch. Dermatol.*, **120**, 795.

11. Downham, T.F. and Chapel, T.A. (1978) Bullous pemphigoid therapy in patients with and without diabetes mellitus. *Arch. Dermatol.*, **114**, 1639–42.
12. Provost, T.T., Maiz, J.C., Ahmed, A.R., Strauss, J.S. and Dobson, R.L. (1979) Unusual subepidermal bullous diseases With immunologic features of bullous pemphigoid. *Arch. Dermatol.*, **115**, 156–60.
13. Jordon, R.E. (1987) in *Dermatology in General Medicine* (eds T.B. Fitzpatrick, A.Z. Eisen, K. Wolff, I.M. Freedberg and K.F. Austen), McGraw-Hill, New York, pp. 580–6.
14. Sison-Fonacier, L. and Bystryn, J.C. (1986) Regional variations in antigenic properties of skin. A possible cause for disease-specific distribution of skin lesions. *J. Exp. Med.*, **164**, 2125–30.
14a. Venning, V.A., Frith, P.A., Bron, A.J., Millard, P.R. and Wojnarowska, F. (1988) Mucosal involvement in bullous and cicatricial pemphigoid. A clinical and immunopathological study. *Brit. J. Dermatol.*, **118**, 7–15.
15. Lever, W.F. (1965) *Pemphigus and Pemphigoid*, Charles C. Thomas, Springfield, IL, p. 222.
16. Ahmed, A.R., Maize, J.C. and Provost, T.T. (1977) Bullous pemphigoid. Clinical and immunologic follow-up after successful therapy. *Arch. Dermatol.*, **113**, 1043–6.
17. Person, J.R. and Rogers, R.S. (1977) Bullous and cicatricial pemphigoid. Clinical, histopathologic, and immunopathologic correlations. *Mayo Clin. Proc.*, **52**, 54–66.
18. Perry, H.O. (1967) Skin disease with mucocutaneous involvement. *Oral Surg.*, **24**, 800.
19. Korman, N. (1987) Bullous pemphigoid. *J. Amer. Acad. Dermatol.*, **16**, 907–24.
20. Bingham, E.A., Burrow, D. and Sanford, J.C. (1984) Prolonged pruritus and bullous pemphigoid. *Clin. Exp. Dermatol.*, **9**, 564–70.
21. Gruber, G.G., Owen, L.G. and Callen, J.P. (1980) Vesicular pemphigoid. *Amer. Acad. Dermatol.*, **3**, 619–22.
22. Bean, S.F., Michel, B., Furey, N., Thorne, E.G. and Meltzer, L. (1976) Vesicular pemphigoid. *Arch. Dermatol.*, **112**, 1402–4.
23. Honeyman, J.F., Honeyman, A.R., De la Parra, M.A., Pinto, A. and Eguiguren, G.J. (1979) Polymorphic pemphigoid. *Arch. Dermatol.*, **115**, 423–7.
24. Al-Najjar, A., Reilly, G.D. and Bleehen, S.S. (1984) Pemphigoid vegetans: A case report. *Acta Dermatol. Venereol.*, **64**, 450–2.
25. Winkelmann, R.K. and Daniel Su, W.P. (1979) Pemphigoid vegetans. *Arch. Dermatol.*, **115**, 446–8.
26. Kuokkanen, K. and Helin, H. (1981) Pemphigoid vegetans. Report of a case. *Arch. Dermatol.*, **117**, 56.
27. Yung, C.W., Soltani, K. and Lorincz, A.L. (1981) Pemphigoid nodularis. *Amer. Acad. Dermatol.*, **5**, 54–60.
28. Massa, C. and Connolly, S.M. (1982) Bullous pemphigoid with features of prurigo nodularis. *Arch. Dermatol.*, **118**, 937–9.
29. Shornick, J.K., Banger, J.L., Freeman, R.G., *et al.* (1983) Herpes gestationis: clinical and histologic features of 28 cases. *J. Amer. Acad. Dermatol.*, **8**, 214–24.
30. Katz, S.I., Hertz, K.C. and Yaoita, H. (1976) Herpes gestationis: immunopathology and characterization of the HG factor. *J. Clin. Invest.*, **57**, 1434–41.
31. Katz, S.I. and Provost, T.T. (1987) in *Dermatology in General Medicine.* (eds T.B. Fitzpatrick, A.Z. Eisen, K. Wolff, I.M. Freedberg and K.F. Austen), McGraw Hill, New York, pp. 586–9.
32. Hardy, K.M., Perry, H.O., Pingree, G.C., Kirby, T.J. and Minn, R. (1971) Benign mucous membrane pemphigoid. *Arch. Dermatol.*, **104**, 467–73.
33. Lever, W.F. (1979) Pemphigus and pemphigoid. *Amer. Acad. Dermatol.*, **1**, 1–32.
34. Shklar, G. and McCarthy, P.L. (1971) Oral lesions of mucous membrane pemphigoid. A study of 85 cases. *Arch. Otolaryngol.*, **93**, 354–64.
35. Liu, H.N., Daniel Su, W.P. and Rogers, R.S. (1986) Clinical variants of pemphigoid. *Int. J. Dermatol.*, 17–27.
36. Fine, J.D., Neises, G.R. and Katz, S.I. (1984) Immunofluorescence and immunoelectron microscopic studies in cicatricial pemphigoid. *J. Invest. Dermatol.*, **82**, 39–43.
37. Roenigk, H., Ryan, J.G. and Bergfeld, W.F. (1971) Epidermolysis bullosa acquisita. *Arch. Dermatol.*, **103**, 1–10.
38. Gammon, W.R., Briggaman, R.A., Woodley, D.T., Heald, P.W. and Wheeler, C.E. (1984) Epidermolysis bullosa acquisita – a pemphigoid-like disease. *J. Amer. Acad. Dermatol.*, **11**, 820–32.
39. Briggaman, R.A., Gammon, W.R. and Woodley, D.T. (1985) Epidermolysis bullosa acquisita of the immunopathological type (dermolytic pemphigoid). *J. Invest. Dermatol.*, **85**, 79s–84s.
40. Lawley, T.J., Strober, W., Yaoita, H. and Katz, S.I. (1980) Small intestinal biopsies and HLA types in dermatitis herpetiformis patients with granular and linear IgA skin deposits. *J. Invest. Dermatol.*, **74**, 9–12.
41. Yaoita, H. and Katz, S.I. (1977) Circulating IgA antibasement membrane zone antibodies in dermatitis herpetiformis. *J. Invest. Dermatol.*, **69**, 558–60.
42. Chorzelski, T.P., Jablonska, S., Beutner, E.H., *et al.* (1987) in *Immunopathology of the Skin* (eds E.H. Beutner, T.P. Chorzelski and V. Kumar), John Wiley and Sons, New York, pp. 407–20.

43. Leonard, J.N., Haffenden, G.P., Ring, NP., *et al.* (1982) Linear IgA disease in adults. *Brit. J. Dermatol.*, **107**, 301–16.
44. Camisa, C. and Sharma, H.M. (1983) Vesiculobullous systemic lupus erythematosus. Report of two cases and a review of the literature. *J. Amer. Acad. Dermatol.*, **9**, 924–32.
45. Olansky, A.J., Briggaman, R.A., Gammon, W.R., Kelly, T.F. and Sams, W.M. (1982) Bullous systemic lupus erythematosus. *J. Amer. Acad. Dermatol.*, **7**, 511–20.
46. Fellner, M.J. and Katz, J.M. (1976) Occurrence of bullous pemphigoid after furosemide therapy. *Arch. Dermatol.*, **112**, 75–7.
47. Bean, S.F., Good, R.A. and Windhorst, D.B. (1970) Bullous pemphigoid in an 11-year-old boy. *Arch. Dermatol.*, **102**, 205–8.
48. Fincher, D.F., Dupree, E., Tex, G. and Bean, S.F. (1971) Bullous pemphigoid in childhood. Immunofluorescent studies. *Arch. Dermatol.*, **103**, 88–90.
49. Bart, B.J. and Bean, S.F. (1970) Bullous pemphigoid following the topical use of fluorouracil. *Arch. Dermatol.*, **102**, 457–9.
50. Flotte, T.J. (1987) in *Clinics in Dermatology: Bullous Pemphigoid* (ed. A.R. Ahmed), J.B. Lippincott, Philadelphia, pp. 71–80.
51. Lever, W.F. and Schaumburg-Lever, G. (1983) *Histopathology of the Skin*, J.B. Lippincott, Philadelphia, pp. 113–17.
52. Imber, M.J., Murphy, G.F. and Jordon, R.E. (1987) in *Clinics in Dermatology: Bullous Pemphigoid* (ed. A.R. Ahmed), J.B. Lippincott, Philadelphia, pp. 81–92.
53. Gammon, W.R. (1987) in *Immunopathology of the Skin* (eds E.H. Beutner, T.P. Chorzelski and V. Kumar), John Wiley and Sons, New York, pp. 323–36.
54. Jordon, R.E. (1975) Complement activation in bullous skin diseases. *J. Invest. Dermatol.*, **65**, 162–9.
55. Nieboer, C. and van Leeuwen, J.E. (1980) IgE in the serum and on mast cells in bullous pemphigoid. *Arch. Dermatol.*, **116**, 555–6.
56. Baba, T., Sonozaki, H., Seki, K., *et al.* (1976) An eosinophil chemotactic factor present in blister fluids of bullous pemphigoid patients. *J. Immunol.*, **116**, 112–16.
57. Herrmann, K., Lohrisch, I., Bohme, H.J. and Haustein, U.F. (1978) Detection of antibodies after immune complex splitting in serum of patients with bullous pemphigoid and systemic lupus erythematosus. *Brit. J. Dermatol.*, **99**, 635–40.
58. Danno, K., Okamoto, H., Miyauchi, H. and Imamura, S. (1982) Bullous pemphigoid and antinuclear antibodies. Unmasking of basement membrane fluorescence in sodium chloride-treated substrates. *Arch. Dermatol.*, **118**, 37–9.
59. Millns, J.L., Meurer, M. and Jordon, R.E. (1979) The complement system in bullous pemphigoid. VI. C3 fixing activity in the absence of detectable antibody. *Clin. Immunol. Immunopathol.*, **13**, 475.
60. Chorzelski, T.P. and Beutner, E.H. (1972) Factors contributing to occasional failures in the laboratory diagnosis of bullous pemphigoid by indirect immunofluorescence. *Brit. J. Dermatol.*, **86**, 111–17.
61. Zhu, X.J. and Bystryn, J.C. (1983) Heterogeneity of pemphigoid antigens. *J. Invest. Dermatol.*, **80**, 16–20.
61a. Kelly, S.E. and Wojnarowska, F. (1988) The use of chemically split tissue in the deletion of circulating anti-basement zone antibodies in bullous pemphigoid. *Brit. J. Dermatol.*, **118**, 31–40.
62. Gammon, W.R., Briggaman, R.A., Inman, A.O., *et al.* (1984) Differentiating anti-lamina lucida and anti-sublamina densa anti-BMZ antibodies by indirect immunofluorescence on 1.0 M sodium chloride-separated skin. *J. Invest. Dermatol.*, **82**, 139–44.
62a. Logan, R.A., Bhogal, B., Das, A.K., McKee, P.M. and Black, M.M. (1987) Localization of bullous pemphigoid antibody – an indirect study of 228 cases using a split-skin technique. *Brit. J. Dermatol.*, **117**, 471–8.
63. Ullman, S., Halberg, P. and Nielsen, R. (1975) Anti-basement membrane antibodies in sera from patients without bullous pemphigoid. *Acta Dermatovenereol.*, **55**, 305–8.
64. Arbesman, C.E., Eypych, J.I., Reisman, R.E., *et al.*, (1974) IgE levels in sera of patients with pemphigus or bullous pemphigoid. *Arch. Dermatol.*, **110**, 378–81.
65. Sushkell, L.L. and Jordon, R.E. (1983) Bullous pemphigoid: a cause of peripheral blood eosinophilia. *J. Amer. Acad. Dermatol.*, **8**, 648–51.
66. Jordon, R.E., Muller, S.A., Minn, R., Hale, W.L. and Beutner, E.H. (1969) Bullous pemphigoid associated with systemic lupus erythematosus. *Arch. Dermatol.*, **99**, 17–25.
67. Stoll, D.M. and King, Jr. L.E. (1984) Association of bullous pemphigoid with systemic lupus erythematosus. *Arch. Dermatol.*, **120**, 362–6.
68. Pedro, S.D., Tex, L. and Dahl, M.V. (1973) Direct immunofluorescence of bullous systemic lupus erythematosus. *Arch. Dermatol.*, **107**, 118–20.
69. Gammon, W.R. and Lewis, D.M. (1986) Bullous eruption of system lupus erythematosus. *Curr. Concepts Skin Disorders*, **7**, 5–9.
70. Gammon, W.R., Woodley, D.T., Dole, K.C. and Briggaman, R.A. (1985) Evidence that anti-basement membrane zone antibodies in bullous eruption of systemic lupus erythematosus recognize epidermolysis bullosa acquisita autoantigen. *J. Invest. Dermatol.*, **84**, 472–6.

71. Chuang, T.Y., Korkij, W., Soltani, K., Clayman, J. and Cook, J. (1984) Increased frequency of diabetes mellitus in patients with bullous pemphigoid: A case-control study. *J. Amer. Acad. Dermatol.*, **11**, 1099–102.
72. Koerber, W.A., Price, N.M. and Watson, W. (1978) Coexistent psoriasis and bullous pemphigoid. *Arch. Dermatol.*, **114**, 1643–6.
73. Person, J.R. and Rogers, R.S. (1976) Bullous pemphigoid and psoriasis: does subclinical bullous pemphigoid exist? *Brit. J. Dermatol.*, **95**, 535–40.
74. Robinson, J.K., Baughman, R.D. and Provost, T.T. (1978) Bullous pemphigoid induced by PUVA therapy. Is this the aetiology of the acral bullae produced during PUVA treatment? *Brit. J. Dermatol.*, **99**, 709–13.
75. Cram, D.L. and Fukuyama, K. (1972) Immunohistochemistry of ultraviolet-induced pemphigus and pemphigoid lesions. *Arch. Dermatol.*, **106**, 819–24.
77. Callen, J.P. (1980) Internal disorders associated with bullous disease of the skin. *Amer. Acad. Dermatol.*, **3**, 107–19.
78. Giannini, J.M., Callen, J.P. and Gruber, G.G. (1981) Bullous pemphigoid and rheumatoid arthritis. *Amer. Acad. Dermatol.*, **4**, 695–7.
79. Savin, J.A. (1979) The events leading to the death of patients with pemphigus and pemphigoid. *Brit. J. Dermatol.*, **101**, 521–6.
80. Salo, O.P. and Rasanen, J.S. (1972) Pemphigoid and rheumatoid arthritis. *Ann. Clin. Res.*, **4**, 173–7.
81. Chorzelski, T.P., Jablonska, S., Beutner, E.H., *et al.* (1987) in *Immunopathology of the Skin* (eds E.H. Beutner, T.P. Chorzelski and V. Kumar), John Wiley and Sons, New York, pp. 337–54.
82. Lang, P.G. and Maize, J.C. (1983) Coexisting lichen planus and bullous pemphigoid or lichen planus pemphigoides? *J. Amer. Acad. Dermatol.*, **9**, 133–40.
83. Mora, R.G., Nesbitt, L.T. and Brantley, J.B. (1983) Lichen planus pemphigoides: Clinical and immunofluorescent findings in four cases. *J. Amer. Acad. Dermatol.*, **8**, 331–6.
84. Prost, C., Tesserand, F., Laroche, L. *et al.* (1985) Lichen planus pemphigoides: an immuno-electron microscopic study. *Brit. J. Dermatol.*, **113**, 31–6.
85. Stingl, G. and Holubar, K. (1975) Coexistence of lichen planus and bullous pemphigoid. An immunopathological study. *Brit. J. Dermatol.*, **93**, 313–20.
86. Stanley, J.R., Hawley-Nelson, P., Yuspa, S.H., *et al.* (1981) Characterization of bullous pemphigoid antigen: a unique basement membrane protein of stratified squamous epithelia. *Cell.*, **24**, 897–903.
87. Stone, S.P. and Schroeter, A.L. (1975) Bullous pemphigoid and associated malignant neoplasms. *Arch. Dermatol.*, **111**, 991–4.
88. Ahmed, A.R., Chu, T.M. and Provost, T.T. (1977) Bullous pemphigoid. Clinical and serologic evaluation for associated malignant neoplasms. *Arch. Dermatol.*, **113**, 969.
89. Paslin, D.A. (1973) Bullous pemphigoid and hypernephroma: a critical review of the association of bullous pemphigoid and malignancy. *Oral Glucocorticoids*, **14**, 554–5.
90. Chorzelski, T.P., Jablonska, S., Maciejowska, E., *et al.* (1978) Coexistence of malignancies with bullous pemphigoid. *Arch. Dermatol.*, **114**, 964.
91. Hodge, L., Marsden, R.A., Black, M.M., *et al.* (1981) Bullous pemphigoid: the frequency of mucosal involvement and concurrent malignancy related to indirect immunofluorescence findings. *Brit. J. Dermatol.*, **105**, 65–9.
92. Dahl, M.V. (1987) in *Clinics in Dermatology: Bullous Pemphigoid* (ed. A.R. Ahmed), J.B. Lippincott, Philadelphia, pp. 64–70.
93. Gammon, W.R., Merritt, C.C., Lewis, D.M., *et al.* (1982) An *in vitro* model of immune complex-mediated basement membrane zone separation caused by pemphigoid antibodies, leukocytes, and complement. *J. Invest. Dermatol.*, **78**, 285–90.
94. Anhalt, G.J., Bahn, C.F., Labib, R.S. *et al.* (1981) *J. Clin. Invest.*, **68**, 1097–101.
95. Diaz, L.A., Weiss, H.J., Calvanico, N.J., *et al.* (1978) Phylogenetic studies with pemphigus and pemphigoid antibodies. *Acta Dermatol. Venereol.*, **58**, 537–40.
96. Beutner, E.H., Jordon, R.E. and Chorzelski, T.P. (1968) The immunopathology of pemphigus and bullous pemphigoid. *J. Invest. Dermatol.*, **51**, 63–80.
97. Woodley, D., Didierjean, L., Regnier, M. *et al.* (1980) Bullous pemphigoid antigen synthesized *in vitro* by human epidermal cells. *J. Invest. Dermatol.*, **75**, 148–51.
98. Stanley, J.R., Hawley-Nelson, P., Poirier, M., *et al.* (1980) Detection of pemphigoid antigen, pemphigus antigen, and keratin filaments by indirect immunofluorescence in cultured human epidermal cells. *J. Invest. Dermatol.*, **75**, 183–6.
99. Holubar, K., Wolff, K., Konrad, K. and Beutner, E.H. (1975) Ultrastructural localization of immunoglobulins in bullous pemphigoid skin. *J. Invest. Dermatol.*, **64**, 220–7.
100. Schaumburg-Lever, G., Rule, A., Schmidt-Ullrich, B. and Lever, W.F. (1975) Ultrastructural localization of *in vivo* bound immunoglobulins in bullous pemphigoid – a preliminary report. *J. Invest. Dermatol.*, **64**, 47–9.
101. Pehamberger, H., Gschnait, F., Konrad, K., *et al.* (1980) Bullous pemphigoid, herpes gestationis and linear dermatitis herpetiformis: circulating anti-basement membrane zone. *J. Invest. Dermatol.*, **74**, 105–8.

102. Mutasim, D.F., Takahashi, Y., Labib, R.S., *et al.* (1985) A pool of bullous pemphigoid antigen(s) is intracellular and associated with the basal cell cytoskeleton–hemidesmosome complex. *J. Invest. Dermatol.*, **84**, 47–53.
103. Regnier, M., Vaigot, P., Michel, S. and Prunieras, M. (1985) Localization of bullous pemphigoid antigen (BPA) in isolated human keratinocytes. *J. Invest. Dermatol.*, **85**, 187–90.
104. Westgate, G.E., Weaver, A.C. and Couchman, J.R. (1985) Bullous pemphigoid antigen localization suggests an intracellular association with hemidesmosomes. *J. Invest. Dermatol.*, **84**, 218–24.
105. Takahashi, Y., Mutasim, D.F., Patel, H.P., *et al.* (1985) The use of human pemphigoid autoantibodies to study the fate of epidermal basal cell hemidesmosomes after trypsin dissociation. *J. Invest. Dermatol.*, **85**, 309–13.
106. Diaz, L.A., Calvanio, N.J., Tomasi, T.B. and Jordon, R.E. (1977) Bullous pemphigoid antigen: isolation from normal human skin. *J. Immunol.*, **118**, 455–60.
107. Stanley, J.R., Woodley, D.T. and Katz, S.I. (1984) Identification and partial characterization of pemphigoid antigen extracted from normal human skin. *J. Invest. Dermatol.*, **82**, 108–111.
108. Labib, R.S., Anhalt, G.J., Patel, H.P., *et al.* (1986) Molecular heterogeneity of the bullous pemphigoid antigens as detected by immunoblotting. *J. Immunol.*, **136**, 1231–5.
109. Stanley, J.R., Alvarez, O.M., Bere, E.W., *et al.* (1981) Detection of basement membrane zone antigens during epidermal wound healing in pigs. *J. Invest. Dermatol.*, **77**, 240–3.
110. Hintner, H., Fritsch, P.O., Foidart, J.M., *et al.* (1980) Expression of basement membrane zone antigens at the dermoepibolic junction in organ cultures of human skin. *J. Invest. Dermatol.*, **74**, 200–4.
111. Stanley, J.R., Beckwith, J.B., Fuller, R.P., *et al.* (1982) A specific antigenic defect of the basement membrane is found in basal cell carcinoma but not in other epidermal tumors. *Cancer*, **50**, 1486–90.
112. Gammon, W.R., Merritt, C.C., Lewis, D.M., *et al.* (1982) Functional evidence for complement-activating immune complexes in the skin of patients with bullous pemphigoid. *J. Invest. Dermatol.*, **78**, 52–7.
113. Naito, K., Morioka, S., Ikeda, S. and Ogawa, H. (1984) Experimental bullous pemphigoid in guinea pigs: the role of pemphigoid antibodies, complement, and migrating cells. *J. Invest. Dermatol.*, **82**, 227–30.
114. Gammon, R.W. and Briggaman, R.A. (1987) Absence of specific changes in guinea pig skin treated with bullous pemphigoid antibodies. *Clin. Res.*, **35**, 388A.
115. Jordon, R.E., Nordby, J.M. and Milstein, H. (1975) The complement system in bullous pemphigoid. III. Fixation of C1q and C4 by pemphigoid antibody. *J. Lab. Clin. Med.*, **86**, 733–40.
116. Jordon, R.E., Sams, W.M. and Beutner, E.H. (1969) Complement immunofluorescent staining in bullous pemphigoid. *J. Lab. Clin. Med.*, **74**, 548–56.
117. Sams, W.M. and Schur, P.H. (1973) Studies of the antibodies in pemphigoid and pemphigus. *J. Lab. Clin. Med.*, **82**, 249–254.
118. Bird, P., Friedmann, P.S., Ling, N., *et al.* (1986) Subclass distribution of IgG autoantibodies in bullous pemphigoid. *J. Invest. Dermatol.*, **86**, 21–5.
119. Nakagawa, T. and DeWeck, A.L. (1983) Membrane receptors for the IgG4 subclass on human basophils and mast cells. *Clin. Rev. Allergy*, **1**, 197–206.
120. Schmidt-Ullrich, B., Rule, A., Schaumburg-Lever, G. and Leblanc, C. (1975) Ultrastructural localization of *in vivo*-bound complement in bullous pemphigoid. *J. Invest. Dermatol.*, **65**, 217–19.
121. Jordon, R.E., Day, N.K., Sams, W.M. and Good, R.A. (1973) The complement system in bullous pemphigoid. I. Complement and component levels in sera and blister fluids. *J. Clin. Invest.*, **52**, 1207–14.
122. Jordon, R.E., Kawana, S. and Fritz, K.A. (1985) Immunopathologic mechanisms in pemphigus and bullous pemphigoid. *J. Invest. Dermatol.*, **85**, 72s–8s.
123. Dahl, M.V., Falk, R.J., Carpenter, R. and Michael, A.F. (1984) Deposition of the membrane attack complex of complement in bullous pemphigoid. *J. Invest. Dermatol.*, **82**, 132–5.
124. Wintroub, B.U., Mihm, M.C., Goetzl, E.J., *et al.* (1978) Morphologic and functional evidence for release of mast-cell products in bullous pemphigoid. *New England J. Med.*, **298**, 417–21.
125. Katayama, I., Doi, T. and Nishioka, K. (1984) High histamine level in the blister fluid of bullous pemphigoid. *Arch. Dermatol. Res.*, **276**, 126–7.
126. Dvorak, A.M., Mihm, M.C., Osage, J.E., *et al.* (1982) Bullous pemphigoid, an ultrastructural study of the inflammatory response: eosinophil, basophil and mast cell granule changes in multiple biopsies from one patient. *J. Invest. Dermatol.*, **78**, 91–101.
127. Dubertret, L., Bertaux, B., Fosse, M. and Touraine, R. (1980) Cellular events leading to blister formation in bullous pemphigoid. *Brit. J. Dermatol.*, **104**, 615–24.
128. Sams, W.M. and Gammon, W.R. (1982) Mechanism of lesion production in pemphigus and pemphigoid. *J. Amer. Acad. Dermatol.*, **6**, 431–49.

129. Savin, J.A. (1987) in *Clinics in Dermatology: Bullous Pemphigoid* (ed. A.R. Ahmed), J.B. Lippincott, Philadelphia, pp. 52–9.
130. Ahmed, A.R. and Rogers, R.S. (1987) in *Clinics in Dermatology: Bullous Pemphigoid* (ed. A.R. Ahmed), J.B. Lippincott, Philadelphia, pp. 146–54.
131. Church, R. (1960) Pemphigoid treated with corticosteroids. *Brit. J. Dermatol.*, 72, 431–41.
132. Gallant, C. and Kenny, P. (1986) Oral glucocorticoids and their complications. *J. Amer. Acad. Dermatol.*, **14**, 161–75.
133. Greaves, M.W., Burton, J.L., Marks, J. and Dawber, R.P.R. (1971) Azathioprine in treatment of bullous pemphigoid. *Brit. Med. J.*, **1**, 144–5.
134. Burton, J.L. and Greaves, M.W. (1974) Azathioprine for pemphigus and pemphigoid – a 4 year follow-up. *Brit. J. Dermatol.*, **91**, 103–9.
135. Ahmed, A.R. and Moy, R. (1981) Azathioprine. *Int. J. Dermatol.*, 20, 461–9.
136. Krain, L.S., Landau, J.W. and Newcomer, V.D. (1972) Cyclophosphamide in the treatment of pemphigus vulgaris and bullous pemphigoid. *Arch. Dermatol.*, **106**, 657–61.
137. Ahmed, A.R. and Hombal, S.M. (1984) Cyclophosphamide review of relevant pharmacology and clinical uses. *J. Amer. Acad. Dermatol.*, **6**, 1115–26.
138. Person, J.R. and Rogers, III, R.S. (1977) Bullous pemphigoid responding to sulfapyridine and the sulfones. *Arch. Dermatol.*, **113**, 610–15.
139. Rook, A. and Waddington, E. (1953) Pemphigus and pemphigoid. *Brit. J. Dermatol.*, **65**, 425–31.
140. Siegel, J. and Eaglstein, W.H. (1984) High-dose methylprednisolone in the treatment of bullous pemphigoid. *Arch. Dermatol.*, **120**, 1157–65.
141. Goldberg, N.S., Robinson, J.K., Roenigk, Jr., H.H., *et al.* (1985) Plasmapheresis therapy for bullous pemphigoid. *Arch. Dermatol.*, **121**, 1484–5.
142. Roujeau, J.C., Morel, P., Dalle, E., *et al.* (1984) Plasma exchange in bullous pemphigoid. *Lancet*, **ii**, 486–9.
143. Thivolet, J., Barthelemy, H., Rigot-Muller, G. and Bendelac, A. (1985) Effects of cyclosporin on bullous pemphigoid and pemphigus. *Lancet*, **i**, 334–5.

Six
Cicatricial pemphigoid

Jo-David Fine

6.1 INTRODUCTION

Cicatricial pemphigoid is a chronic blistering disorder which primarily involves mucous membranes; lesions characteristically heal with scarring. Depending on the tissues involved, this disease has been referred to by a variety of names including ocular pemphigoid, chronic cicatricial conjunctivitis, essential shrinkage of the conjunctivae, oral pemphigoid and benign mucous membrane pemphigoid. In addition, it is occasionally incorrectly referred to as pemphigus conjunctivae or ocular pemphigus, despite the presence of subepithelial rather than intraepithelial blister formation in cicatricial pemphigoid.

6.2 CLINICAL FEATURES

6.2.1 Presentation

The actual frequency of cicatricial pemphigoid is unknown, although it appears to be seen less commonly than either bullous pemphigoid or pemphigus vulgaris. Cicatricial pemphigoid is a disease primarily of middle-aged and elderly patients, although it has been observed in all age groups including children; the mean age of onset is 66 years [7, 8]. There is a 1.5 : 1 female-to-male ratio in this disease [7]. There does not appear to be any racial or geographic predilection.

6.2.2 Cutaneous distribution

Skin involvement is infrequent (10–25%) in cicatricial pemphigoid [5, 9, 10]. When it does occur, there are usually a paucity of lesions, and they most often arise on the face, neck and scalp, similar to the Brunsting–Perry variant of bullous pemphigoid. However, lesions may also appear on other body parts, including genitalia (glans penis, foreskin, scrotum, labia), umbilicus, extremities and shoulders. In some patients, skin lesions are asymptomatic; in others, pruritus or a painful burning sensation of the skin may be noted.

6.2.3 Mucous membrane involvement

Cicatricial pemphigoid is primarily a disease of mucous membranes. The actual frequency of involvement of specific tissues varies among different series, reflecting biases in patient referrals. For example, the incidence of oral involvement is greater in patients reported in the oral surgical than in the ophthalmological literature. It is clear, however, that oral cavity and ocular lesions are very common, being seen in nearly 100% and 61–80% of patients, respectively, in some series [6, 7, 9–11]. In addition, ocular involvement, when present, is usually (up to 87%) bilateral [9]. Other mucosal surfaces that may be involved in cicatricial pemphigoid, in order of prevalence, include the pharynx (43%), nasal mucosa (38%), larynx (30%), genital mucosal surfaces (such as the urethral meatus, labia, foreskin, vagina) (up to 20–35%), rectum (11%) and oesophagus (7%) [9].

Within the oral cavity, the most common sites of involvement by cicatricial pemphigoid include the gingivae (64%), buccal mucosa (58%), palate (26%), alveolar ridge (16%), tongue (15%) and lower lip (7%) [7]. In contrast, oral lesions are uncommon in patients with bullous pemphigoid, and, when present, tend to arise with different frequencies frrom those reported for cicatricial pemphigoid. For example, lesions occur on the gingivae in only 16% and do not arise on the alveolar ridge. Furthermore, whereas the incidence of buccal mucosal involvement is similar (52%), the frequencies of involvement of the palate (40%), tongue (24%) and lower lip (20%) are higher in bullous than in cicatricial pemphigoid (7).

6.2.4 Morphology of lesions

(a) Cutaneous

When skin lesions arise in cicatricial pemphigoid, they appear as tense clear fluid-filled vesicles and bullae, indistinguishable from those observed in bullous pemphigoid. Approximately one-third of the latter are reported to heal subsequently with scarring [12].

(b) Oral cavity

The most common presentation within the oral cavity in cicatricial pemphigoid, observed in 64% of patients, is desquamative gingivitis [7]. The latter is a descriptive term which refers to a spectrum of gingival inflammation, ranging from mild cases with asymptomatic focal erythema along the gumline to more severe forms characterized by more diffuse and painful erythema, induration, erosions and scarring of the gingivae, occasionally accompanied by the presence of intact vesicles (Figure 6.1). Whereas cicatricial pemphigoid is the underlying cause of most cases of desquamative gingivitis, it should be recognized that the latter may also infrequently result from several otherwise unrelated conditions including lichen planus, pemphigus vulgaris, chronic intraoral irritation, chronic periodontal infection and the menopause [13]. When buccal mucosa or palate is involved by cicatricial pemphigoid, lesions are characterized by erythema, erosions and, if chronic, by scar formation (Figure 6.2).

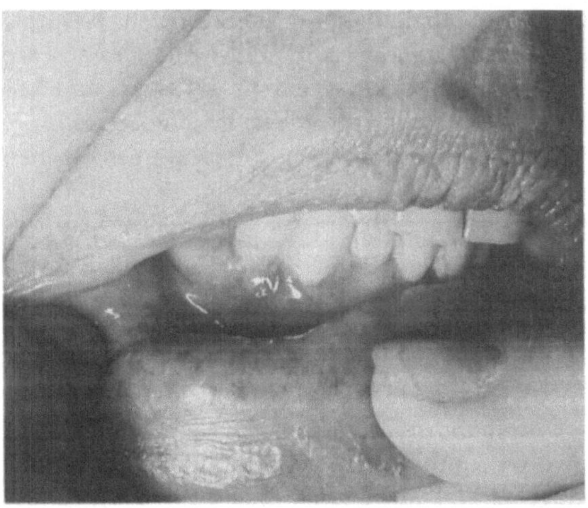

Figure 6.1 Early desquamative gingivitis, characterized by focal erythema, oedema and erosions along the gumline.

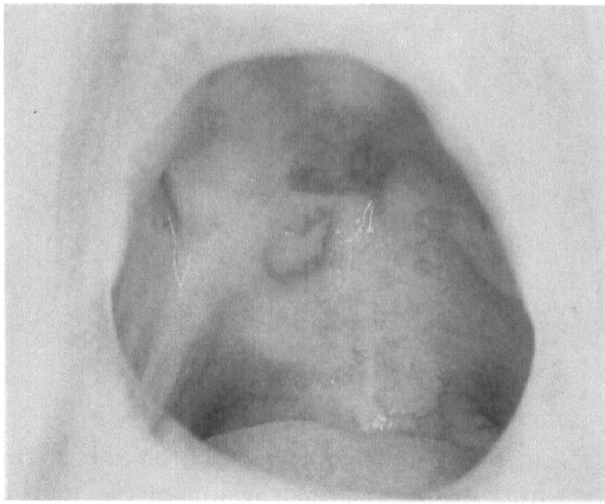

Figure 6.2 Erythema and erosions along the hard palate of a patient with cicatricial pemphigoid.

Milder oral lesions may be asymptomatic; with more extensive involvement, patients may experience either spontaneous pain, particularly in gingival tissues, or pain upon eating.

(c) Ocular

The earliest and least specific ocular finding is chronic conjunctivitis [9, 14]. If ocular involvement is progressive, conjunctival vesicles or bullae may develop. Significant oedema of the eyelids may

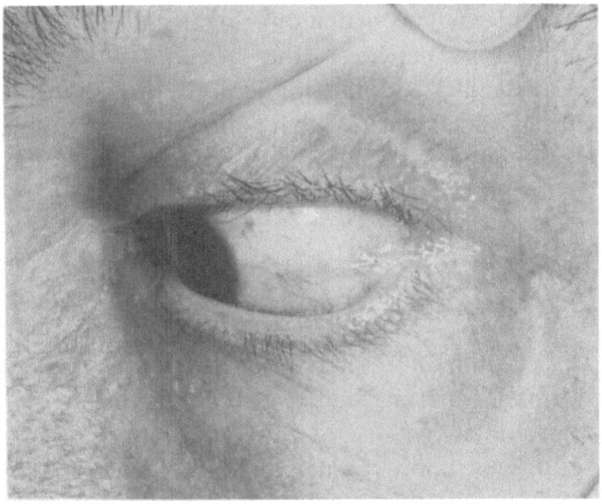

Figure 6.3 Symblepharon formation along the lateral conjunctival surface.

occur, even early in the course of the disease. As the latter heal, scarring occurs, characterized by either focal white subepithelial fibrotic striae or by fibrous tracts connecting the bulbar and palpebral conjunctive (referred to as ankyloblepharons). If symblepharon formation is extensive, then conjuctivae (referred to as ankyloblepharons). If symblepharon formation is extensive, then entropions may develop, leading if untreated to superficial punctate keratopathy, dry eye, inversion of lashes (trichiasis), corneal neovascularization, corneal ulceration and eventually to blindness. Ocular symptoms include burning and dryness.

(d) Nasopharynx

Involvement of the nasopharynx leads to nasal mucosal erosions, crusting, discharge and epistaxis; when disease activity is severe, nasal obstruction may occur due to progressive scar formation and nasopharyngeal stenosis. Upper throat involvement may be associated with painful erosions or vesiculation.

(e) Tracheolarynx

Tracheolaryngeal involvement is rare. When present, however, vocal cord injury may lead to intermittent hoarseness or aphonia. Laryngeal stenosis may lead to progressive bronchitic symptoms, including dyspnoea and sputum production, and, if severe, rarely may necessitate tracheostomy [14].

(f) Oesophagus

The oesophagus may be affected by this disease. Signs of oesophageal involvement include mucosal erosions, blister formation and scarring (leading to stenosis); symptoms include dysphagia and phagodynia.

(g) Rectum

Involvement of the rectum may be associated with intermittent bleeding or pain with defaecation [14].

(h) Genitourinary tract

Genitourinary tract involvement may be associated with recurrent erosions, blisters and scar formation. Pain may be experienced with urination or intercourse. If disease activity is more severe, urethral stenosis may develop, necessitating dilatation [14].

6.3 GENETICS

Cicatricial pemphigoid is an acquired disorder. One study suggests an increased incidence of the HLA allele B12 in such patients, although this has not been as yet confirmed by other investigators [15].

6.4 DIFFERENTIAL DIAGNOSIS

There is virtually no differential diagnosis in patients with long-standing disease when more characteristic ocular and oral lesions are present in the absence of more than an occasional skin lesion, with the possible exception of rare patients with epidermolysis bullosa acquisita. Unfortunately, the differential diagnosis becomes more extensive in the presence of incomplete expression of the disease. For example, several otherwise different disease processes may present as desquamative gingivitis, as previously discussed. However, the presence of more characteristic accompanying skin findings (i.e. violaceous papules with Wickham striae in lichen planus) usually permit ready diagnosis. Similarly, whereas conjunctivitis and ocular scarring are non-specific, the presence of conjunctival vesiculation suggests the diagnosis of cicatricial pemphigoid.

6.5 INVESTIGATIONS

6.5.1 Routine histology

Light microscopy of oral lesions reveals a subepithelial blister or cleft formation, accompanied by a mixed mononuclear inflammatory cell infiltrate comprised of lymphocytes and plasma cells, within the lamina propria [16]. Histological examination of an intact skin lesion reveals subepidermal vesiculation (Figure 6.4). In the author's experience, the blister cavity and perivascular regions contain eosinophils in a pattern identical to that observed in bullous pemphigoid, although others have suggested that neutrophils may predominate [17, 18].

6.5.2 Direct immunofluorescence

Direct immunofluorescence of perilesional or normal-appearing buccal mucosa is positive in approximately 80% of patients for the presence of one or more tissue-bound immunoreactants (immunoglobulins, complement, fibrin) in a thin linear homogeneous pattern along the epithelial–connective tissue basement membrane zone (Figure 6.5(a)) [19–23]. Similar findings are noted in perilesional conjunctiva (Figure 6.5(b)) or skin Positive findings also have been noted from some patients when obtained from normal-appearing buccal mucosa in the absence of any detectable oral mucosal involvement. Furthermore, although least

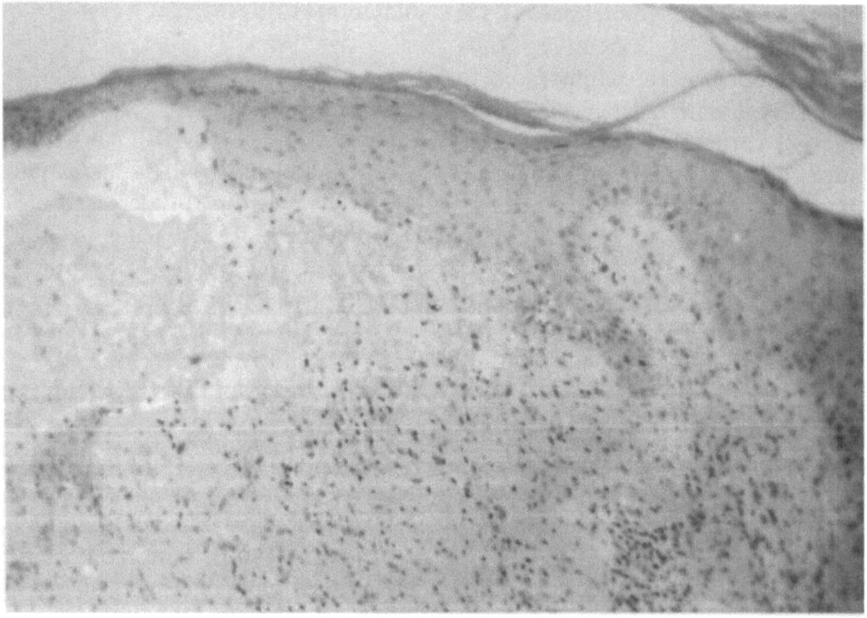

Figure 6.4 Light microscopy of an intact blister arising on the skin of a patient with cicatricial pemphigoid Subepidermal separation and eosinophilic infiltration are present (× 35).

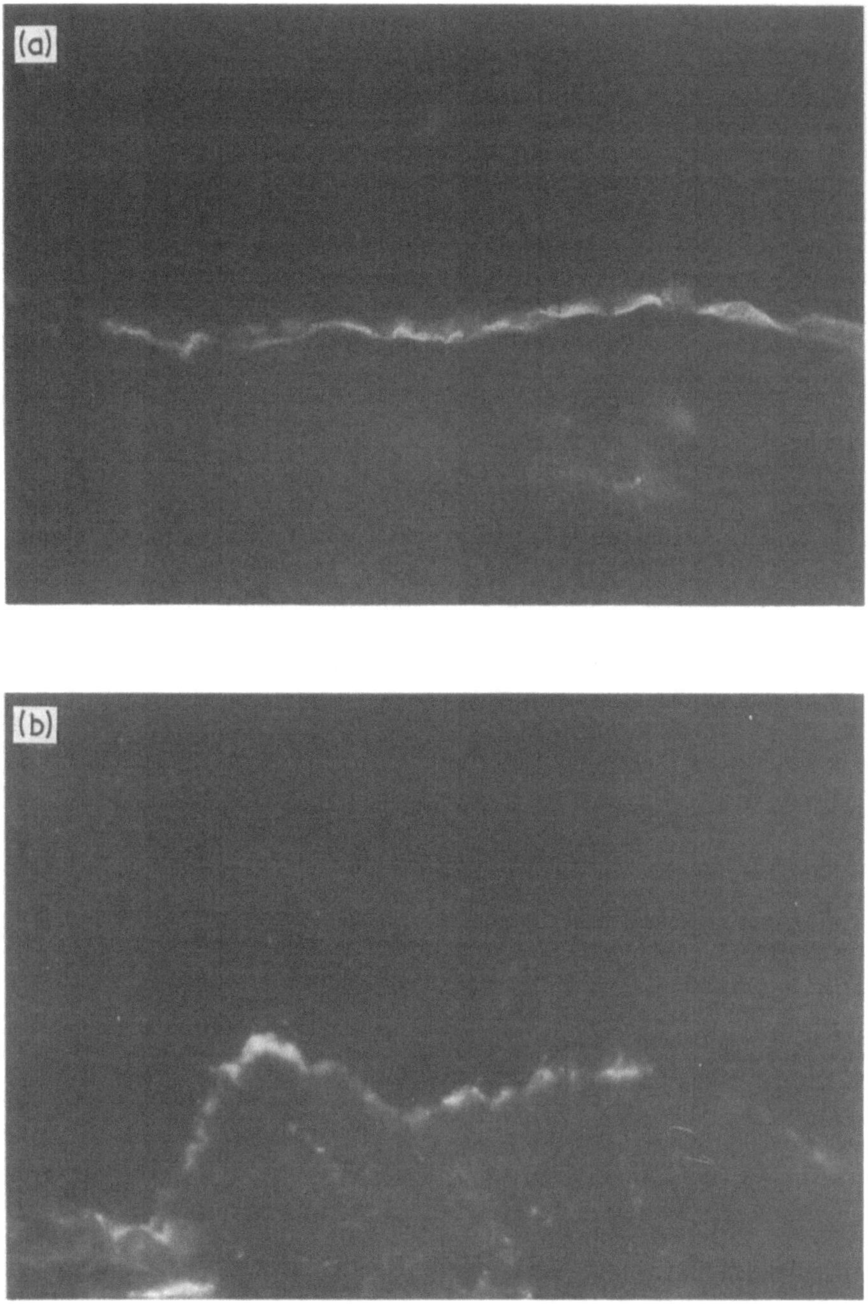

Figure 6.5 Direct immunofluorescence of buccal mucosa (A) and scleral conjunctiva (B) from a patient with cicatricial pemphigoid, demonstrating tissue-bound immunoreactants along the basement membrane zone separating epithelium (above) from connective tissue (below). (A, × 239; B, × 187).

commonly seen, direct immunofluorescence has been shown to be positive in approximately 20% of patients when specimens are obtained from normal-appearing deltoid skin, even in the absence of any detectable skin involvement [23].

The most frequently detectable immunoreactants are IgG and C3; less commonly, IgA, IgM, and/or fibrin may be noted. Although some specimens contain only IgG and/or C3, in the author's experience the presence of at least three tissue-bound immunoreactants appears to favour the diagnoses of cicatricial pemphigoid and epidermolysis bullosa acquisita rather than bullous pemphigoid. Furthermore, when blister formation is present in a specimen from a patient with cicatricial pemphigoid, immunoreactants are either absent within the blister itself (presumably due to enzymic digestion) or are usually present solely on the dermal side of the cleft; in contrast, bound immunoreactants are present along the epidermal roof of the blister in bullous pemphigoid. Finally, considerable differences in the number and/or intensity of different bound immunoreactants may be noted in direct immunofluorescence findings when multiple tissues (i.e. skin, buccal mucosa, conjunctiva) are simultaneously examined from the same individual.

6.5.3 *Indirect immunofluorescence*

Circulating anti-basement membrane autoantibodies are detectable in approximately 10–36% of cicatricial pemphigoid patients when conventional substrates (monkey oesophagus, normal human skin) are employed [20, 21, 23]. The titres of such autoantibodies do not appear to correlate with the extent of disease activity. When present, these autoantibodies are almost invariably of the IgG class (although IgA class autoantibodies have been reported) and are detectable in very low titres (i.e. 1 : 2 – 1 : 10). In those sera negative by routine indirect immunofluorescence technique, complement fixation assays (analogous to herpes gestationis) also have proven negative [23]. Other investigators have suggested that the use of normal oral mucosa as tissue substrate yields a much higher frequency of positive indirect immunofluorescence results, presumably due to preferential expression of the basement membrane antigen(s) identified by such autoantibodies [21]. Unfortunately, these results have not been confirmed by others [23].

6.5.4 *Electron microscopy*

Electron microscopy of lesional tissue confirms lamina lucida cleavage in cicatricial pemphigoid [16]. Although in advanced lesions the basement membrane appears partially or largely destroyed, these findings do not adequately explain the characteristic scarring in this disease since similar findings also have been noted in lesions from patients with bullous pemphigoid.

6.5.5 *Immunoelectron microscopy*

Direct immunoelectron microscopic studies of perilesional skin, conjunctiva and oral mucosa have demonstrated that the tissue-bound immunoreactants in cicatricial pemphigoid are present within the lamina lucida (Figure 6.6), the same ultrastructural location of immunoreactants

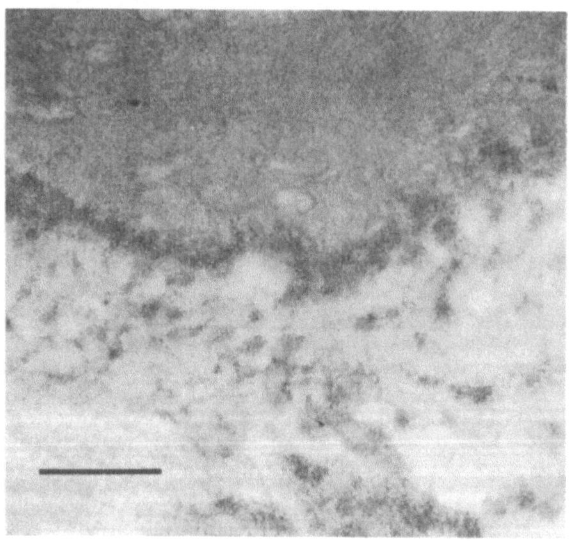

Figure 6.6 Immunoelectron micrograph of buccal mucosa of a patient with cicatricial pemphigoid, demonstrating tissue-bound IgG within the lamina lucida. (Bar = 0.5 μm). (Reproduced from ref. [23] with permission of the publisher.)

in several other autoimmune skin diseases, including bullous pemphigoid and herpes gestationis [23–25]. In addition, in one patient in which a perilesional specimen revealed early cleft formation, tissue-bound immunoreactants were detectable along the base of the lamina lucida cleft, consistent with direct immunofluorescence findings (unpublished work).

6.6 SYSTEMIC MANIFESTATIONS AND ASSOCIATED DISEASES

There are no known associations in cicatricial pemphigoid patients with other systemic diseases.

6.7 PATHOGENESIS AND RECENT ADVANCES

At the present time, very little is known about the pathogenesis of cicatricial pemphigoid, in part because of the small number of patients available for study, the technical difficulties associated with elution of tissue-bound autoantibodies from necessarily small biopsy specimens, the rarity of detectable circulating anti-basement membrane autoantibodies in this patient population, and the lack of organ culture or animal models for this disease.

Despite these disclaimers, several issues should be addressed. First, it is assumed that the observation of tissue-bound immunoreactants along the epithelial–connective tissue basement membrane zone in the majority of patients implies an antibody-mediated autoimmune basis for the disease. This does not, however, explain the 20% of patients with identical clinical findings who lack positive direct immunofluorescence, presuming that they indeed have the same disease process. Further studies are warrented to determine whether such negative immunofluorescence findings simply reflect our inability to detect minute amounts of bound immunoreactants by conventional immunohistochemical techniques or whether identical blister formation and scarring can actually develop in the absence of such a humoral immune response. Second, the striking predilection for mucosal involvement and scar formation in this disease, compared to bullous pemphigoid, has suggested to some that cicatricial pemphigoid is indeed an entity distinct from bullous pemphigoid, despite the fact that both have tissue-bound immunoreactants and blister formation at the level of the lamina lucida. Proof of the latter hypothesis awaits demonstration that the tissue-bound autoantibodies present in most patients with cicatricial pemphigoid recognize a different antigen from those recently characterized in bullous pemphigoid.

Several lines of investigation indirectly suggest that different lamina lucida antigens are recognized in cicatricial and bullous pemphigoid. First, when mechanical suction blisters are performed on bullous pemphigoid skin, tissue-bound immunoreactants are detectable along the epidermal roof of the lamina lucida-separated skin, consistent with recent work demonstrating close association of bullous pemphigoid antigens with the basal keratinocyte plasma membrane in the region of the hemidesmosomes [26, 27]. In contrast, when identical studies were performed on two cicatricial pemphigoid patients, tissue-bound immunoreactants were detected on the dermal side of the blister; subsequent counterstaining with bullous pemphigoid autoantibodies confirmed their binding to the epidermal roofs of the same skin specimens [23]. Similar spatial differences in the two groups of antigens have been noted when lesional or perilesional specimens have been examined in both patient populations by direct immunofluorescence and direct immunoelectron microscopy, as previously discussed.

Second, in a recent study, the human organ specificities of anti-basement membrane autoantibodies from two patients with cicatricial pemphigoid were compared to those from patients with bullous pemphigoid and epidermolysis bullosa acquisita [28]. Whereas all three groups of autoantibodies bound consistently to basement membrane in some organs (skin, buccal mucosa, tongue, oesophagus, anal canal), expression in some other mucosal tissues (urethra, ureter, vagina) was noted primarily with antibodies from patients with cicatricial pemphigoid and epidermolysis bullosa acquisita, suggesting a possible explanation for the predilection for mucosal involvement in these two conditions.

Third, when these same autoantibodies were applied to normal human skin previously separated at the level of the lamina lucida with 1 M NaCl solution, differences were noted in the location of the antigens defined by each group of antibodies [28]. Each bullous pemphigoid antiserum uniformily bound to the epidermal portion of the tissue preparation, consistent with recently published data demonstrating localization of the bullous pemphigoid antigens to the region of the basal keratinocyte hemidesmosomes. Epidermolysis bullosa acquisita antisera bound almost exclusively to the dermal portion, consistent with the localization of its antigen to the lamina densa. One of two cicatricial pemphigoid antisera bound to the epidermal portion in a manner indistinguishable from that observed in the case of bullous pemphigoid. The second cicatricial pemphigoid antiserum, however, bound solely to the dermal portion of NaCl-split skin, consistent with previously discussed findings by direct immunofluorescence and direct immunoelectron microscopy in mechanical suction blisters and lesional tissue, respectively, obtained from some patients with cicatricial pemphigoid.

Fourth, using the same three groups of autoantibodies, distinctive differences have been observed in the ability of each group of autoantibodies to bind to skin specimens from patients with each of the three inherited forms of epidermolysis bullosa, again suggesting the likelihood that different basement membrane antigens are recognized by these antibodies [29].

In general, attempts at immunoprecipitation of basement membrane antigens with cicatricial pemphigoid autoantibodies from extracts known to contain bullous pemphigoid antigens have proven unsuccessful. One interpretation of such negative data is that these autoantibodies do not recognize the same antigens and that cicatricial pemphigoid antigens are either not present in these extracts or are present in such minute quantities as to preclude their detection by this technique. Alternatively, these findings may simply reflect the technical limitation of immunoprecipitation when autoantibodies in such low concentration as those found in cicatricial pemphigoid sera are employed for such a procedure. Recently a single antiserum from a patient purported to have cicatricial pemphigoid has been shown to recognize a protein band with the same molecular weight as that observed with some but not all bullous pemphigoid antisera [30]. Since competitive blocking studies were not performed, it is unknown whether these findings represent co-recognition of the same protein or simply recognition of different proteins having similar molecular weights. Furthermore, insufficient clinical and immunopathological data were given to substantiate that this latter antiserum was indeed from a patient with cicatricial pemphigoid rather than a variant of bullous pemphigoid (i.e. Brunsting–Perry; other). Clearly additional studies are warranted with medium-to-high-titre anti-basement membrane autoantibodies from patients with well-documented cicatricial pemphigoid before it can be concluded that these autoantibodies recognize the same antigens as those in bullous pemphigoid, and therefore, that this disease is simply a phenotypic variant of bullous pemphigoid.

6.8 TREATMENT

6.8.1 Local

When oral manifestations are localized and mild or asymptomatic, simple topical therapy usually suffices. Such measures may include the use of topical anaesthetics, local corticosteroids (topical; intralesional), frequent mouth rinses and meticulous dental care [5, 31]. In addition, some patients benefit from split-thickness grafting to localized non-healing areas [32].

In a similar manner, some ophthalmologists prefer to treat mild ocular disease conservatively with corticosteroids, administered either topically as drops or intralesionally. Furthermore, some patients with more advanced disease benefit from surgical interventions including surgical lysis of fibrous scar tracts, removal of eyelashes from eyelids inverted by entropion formation, and in selected cases, by placement of mucous membrane grafts on to damaged external ocular tissue.

6.8.2 Systemic

(a) Immunosuppressants

The standard therapy for patients with moderate to severe disease activity, especially when ocular or laryngeal structures are involved, is prednisone [33, 34]. This drug is usually initiated at a dosage of 60–80 mg/day as a single daily dose. Compared to some other blistering diseases, including bullous pemphigoid, the response to prednisone in cicatricial pemphigoid is often slow and partial, necessitating the addition of one or more other drugs both to enhance clinical response and subsequently allow reduction of the corticosteroid dosage. The two most commonly used immunosuppressant agents in this disease are azathioprine and cyclophosphamide [35, 36]. Other immunosuppressant agents, such as methotrexate, cyclosporin A and chlorambucil, found to be useful in selected patients with bullous pemphigoid, are as yet unproven in cicatricial pemphigoid.

(b) Dapsone

A few years ago dapsone was reported to be of benefit in patients with cicatricial pemphigoid, with 11 of 24 patients achieving complete remission [37]. On the basis of this finding, additional clinical trials with long-term follow up are warranted to determine the role of dapsone, either alone or in combination with prednisone and/or other immunosuppressant agents, in the treatment of this disease. In addition, it is still to be determined whether use of this drug should be confined to patients with primarily oral involvement or whether it can be appropriately used early in the management of patients with rapidly progressive ocular disease.

6.9 PROGNOSIS AND SEQUELAE

The course of cicatricial pemphigoid is highly variable. Some patients with localized oral involvement remain stable for years or decades in the absence of more aggressive systemic therapy. Some other patients, however, may develop rapidly progressive ocular involvement which eventuates in blindness despite treatment with two or more immunosuppressant agents. Similarly, rare patients may eventually undergo tracheostomy due to unresponsive disease activity within the tracheolaryngeal tree, while others may initially present with active ocular involvement and then go into indefinite spontaneous remission of disease within the eyes while still continuing to develop blisters and erosions within other mucous membranes or skin.

REFERENCES

1. Thost, A. (1911) Der chronische schleim haut Pemphigus der oberen Luftwege. *Arch. Laryng. Rhinol.*, **25**, 459–78.
2. McCarthy, P.L. and Shklar, G. (1980) *Diseases of the Oral Mucosa*, Lea & Febiger, Philadelphia.
3. Lever, W. (1953) Pemphigus. *Medicine*, **32**, 1–123.
4. Church, R.E. and Sneedon, L.B. (1956) Ocular pemphigus with generalized bullous eruption. *Brit. J. Dermatol.* **68**, 128–32.
5. Foster, M.E. and Nally, F.F. (1977) Benign mucous membrane pemphigoid (cicatricial pemphigoid): a reconsideration. *Oral. Surg.*, **44**, 697–705.
6. Nisengard, R.J. and Neiders, M. (1981) Desquamative lesions of the gingiva. *J. Periodontol.*, **52**, 500–10.
7. Laskaris, G., Sklavounou, A. and Stratigos, J. (1982) Bullous pemphigoid, cicatricial pemphigoid, and pemphigus vulgaris: a comparative clinical survey of 278 cases. *Oral Surg.*, **54**, 656–62.
8. Rosenbaum, M.M., Esterly, N.B., Greenwald, M.J., *et al.* (1984) Cicatricial pemphigoid in a 6-year old child: report of a case and review of the literature. *Pediat. Dermatol.*, **2**, 13–22.
9. Hardy, K.M., Perry, H.O., Pingree, G.C., *et al.* (1971) Benign mucous membrane pemphigoid. *Arch. Dermatol.*, **104**, 467–75.
10. Shklar, G. and McCarthy, P. (1971) Oral lesions of mucous membrane pemphigoid. *Arch. Otolaryngol.*, **93**, 354–64.
11. Lever, W. (1965) *Pemphigus and Pemphigoid.* Charles C. Thomas, Springfield, IL.
12. Lever, W.F. (1944) Pemphigus conjunctivae with scarring of the skin. *Arch. Dermatol.*, **49**, 113–17.
13. Rogers, R.S. III, Sheridan, R.J. and Jordan, R.E. (1976) Desquamative gingivitis: clinical, histopathologic, and immunopathologic investigations. *Oral Surg.*, **42**, 316–27.
14. Marx, R.E. and Sanders, D.W. (1980) Cicatricial pemphigoid (benign mucous membrane pemphigoid). *J. Oral Surg.*, **38**, 834–40.

15. Mondino, B.J., Brown, S.I. and Rabin, B.S. (1979) HLA antigens in ocular cicatricial pemphigoid. *Arch. Ophthalmol.*, 97, 479.
16. Shafer, W.G., Hine, M.K. and Levy, B.M. (1983) *A Textbook of Oral Pathology*, W.E. Saunders Co., Philadelphia.
17. Lever, W.F. and Schaumburg-Lever, G. (1983) *Histopathology of the Skin* (6th edn), J.B. Lippincott Co., Philadelphia.
18. Ackerman, A.B. (1978) *Histologic Diagnosis of Inflammatory Skin Diseases – A Method by Pattern Analysis.* Lea & Febiger, Philadelphia.
19. Bean, S.F., Waisman, M., Michel, B. *et al.* (1972) Cicatricial pemphigoid. Immunofluorescent studies. *Arch. Dermatol.*, **106**, 195–9.
20. Nisengard, R.J., Jablonska, S., Beutner, E.H., *et al.* (1975) Diagnostic importance of immunofluorescence in oral bullous diseases and lupus erythematosus. *Oral Surg.*, **40**, 365–75.
21. Laskaris, G. and Angelopoulos, A. (1981) Cicatricial pemphigoid: direct and indirect immunofluorescent studies. *Oral Surg.*, **51**, 48–54.
22. Daniels, T.E. and Quadra-White, C. (1981) Direct immunofluorescence in oral mucosal disease: a diagnostic analysis of 130 cases. *Oral Surg.*, **51**, 38–47.
23. Fine, J.-D., Neises, G.R. and Katz, S.I. (1984) Immunofluorescence and immunoelectron microscopic studies in cicatricial pemphigoid. *J. Invest. Dermatol.*, **82**, 39–43.
24. Honigsmann, H., Stingl, G., Holubar, K., *et al.* (1976) Anto-antibodies and immune complexes in immune dermatoses. Mapping of fine structural binding sites (abstr.). *J. Invest. Dermatol.*, **66**, 263.
25. Neiboer, C., Boorsma, D.M. and Woerdeman, M.J. (1983) Immunoelectron microscopic findings in cicatricial pemphigoid: their significance in relation to epidermolysis bullosa acquisita. *Brit. J. Dermatol.*, **106**, 419–22.
26. Mutasim, D.F., Takahashi, Y., Labib, R.S., *et al.* (1985) A pool of bullous pemphigoid antigen(s) is intracellular and associated with basal cell cytoskeleton–hemidesmosome complex. *J. Invest. Dermatol.*, **84**, 47–53.
27. Westgate, G.E., Weaver, A.C. and Couchman, J.R. (1985) Bullous pemphigoid antigen localization suggests an intracellular association with hemidesmosomes. *J. Invest. Dermatol.*, **84**, 218–24.
28. Fine, J.-D. (1985) Cicatricial pemphigoid, bullous pemphigoid, and epidermolysis bullosa acquisita antigens: differences in organ and species specificities and localization in chemically-separated human skin of three basement membrane antigens. *Collagen Related Res.*, **5**, 369–77.
29. Fine, J.-D. (1985) Epidermolysis bullosa: variability of expression of cicatricial pemphigoid, bullous pemphigoid, and epidermolysis bullosa acquisita antigens in clinically uninvolved skin. *J. Invest. Dermatol.*, **85**, 47–9.
30. Labib, R.S., Anhalt, G.J., Patel, H.P., *et al.* (1986) Molecular heterogeneity of the bullous pemphigoid antigens as detected by immunoblotting. *J. Immunol.*, **136**, 1231–5.
31. Aufdemorte, T.B., De Villez, R.L. and Parel, S.M. (1985) Modified topical steroid therapy for the treatment of oral mucous membrane pemphigoid, *Oral Surg.* **59**, 256–60.
32. O'Hara, D.B., Herzig, E., Goldberg, M.H. *et al.* (1980) Split-thickness skin graft for treatment of benign mucous membrane pemphigoid. *Oral Surg.*, **49**, 487–90.
33. Person, J.R. and Rogers, R.S. III. (1977) Bullous and cicatricial pemphigoid: clinical, histopathologic, and immunopathologic correlations. *Mayo Clin. Proc.*, **52**, 54–66.
34. Herron, B.E. (1975) Immunologic aspects of cicatricial pemphigoid. *Amer. J. Ophthalmol.*, **79**, 271–8.
35. Dave, V.K. and Vickers, C.F.H. (1974) Azathioprine in treatment of mucocutaneous pemphigoid. *Brit. J. Dermatol.*, **90**, 183–6.
36. Brody, H.J. and Perozzi, D.J. (1977) Benign mucous membrane pemphigoid. *Arch. Dermatol.*, **113**, 1598–9.
37. Rogers, R.S. III, Seehafer, J.R. and Perry, H.O. (1982) Treatment of cicatricial (benign mucous membrane) pemphigoid with dapsone. *J. Amer. Acad. Dermatol.*, **6**, 215–23.

Seven
Herpes gestationis

Robert Charles-Holmes and
Martin M. Black

7.1 INTRODUCTION

Herpes gestationis (HG) is a rare bullous dermatosis which develops in association with either pregnancy or the trophoblastic tumours, hydatidiform mole and choriocarcinoma. There is a considerable clinical and pathological overlap between HG and the pemphigoid group of disorders. In view of this the disorder is now frequently termed pemphigoid gestationis [1, 2].

7.2 CLINICAL FEATURES

7.2.1 Presentation

By definition HG is a disorder of women of child-bearing age. Its frequency has been variably estimated at 1 in 3000 [3] and 1 in 60 000 pregnancies [4]. No information is available with regard to its geographical distribution. Most reported cases have been in caucasians; however, Shornick *et al.* recently reported HG in two black patients [5]. They suggested that on the basis of HLA genetic variations between different racial groups one might expect the frequency of HG in blacks to be one-third that in caucasians.

The onset of HG may vary from the ninth week of gestation to 1 week postpartum with an average onset at 21 weeks gestation [6]. In 75% of patients the severity of HG increases immediately post-partum [6]. The duration of the eruption after birth is variable. Recently patients have been described with clinical activity persisting for more than 10 years [7, 8]. However, in the majority of cases the bullous lesions resolve within 2 months of delivery and the urticarial lesions within a year [6]. In subsequent episodes the eruption tends to begin earlier in pregnancy.

7.2.2 Cutaneous distribution

The eruption usually begins on the abdomen with a predilection for the periumbilical region (Figure 7.1). The next most common sites of presentation are the palms and soles. At the height of the eruption it has a widespread distribution [6, 9].

7.2.3 Mucous membrane involvement

The oral and vaginal mucous membranes may be involved in HG. However, this is uncommon, occurring in no more than 20% of cases [9]. There have been no reports of involvement of the ocular mucous membranes.

7.2.4 Morphology

The initial lesions consist of urticarial papules, plaques, target lesions and annular wheals. An interval of a month may elapse before the development of the bullous lesions [6]. Despite the fact that HG is an exceedingly pruritic eruption many of the vesicles survive excoriation to become larger tense blisters. The bullae are usually filled with straw-coloured fluid, although some may be haemorrhagic. The bullae develop within the areas of urtication. When annular urticated lesions are

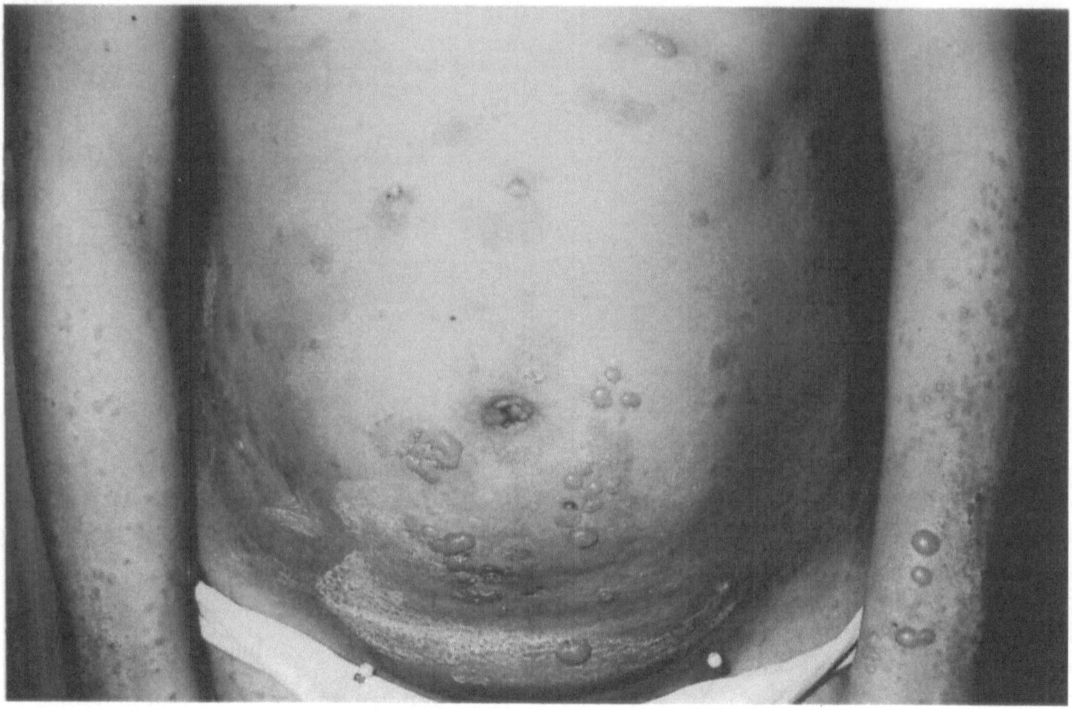

Figure 7.1 Herpes gestationis: urticated papular and bullous lesions on the abdomen and arms during a postpartum flare.

present this may result in blisters arranged in a ringed configuration. Recently pustular lesions have also been described [10].

7.3 GENETICS

Mothers with HG frequently enquire whether there is any risk of their daughters developing HG when they, in turn, become pregnant. As yet no familial cases have been described. However, HLA studies have shown that there is a strong genetic component in determining predisposition to HG. Patients with HG have a significant increase in A1, B8 and DR3 [11, 12]. These antigens occur in linkage disequilibrium and it seems likely that the association with DR3 is the most important aetiologically. It has been suggested that DR antigens are themselves in linkage disequilibrium with immune response determinants. An increased frequency of DR3 has been identified in various immunologically mediated diseases including dermatitis herpetiformis, coeliac disease, Sjögren's syndrome, Addison's disease, Graves' disease, myasthenia gravis and systemic lupus erythematosus [13]. It is possible that DR3 confers a non-specific increase in immune responsiveness.

The most significant HLA association with HG is the possession of both DR3 and DR4 [11, 12]. DR4 has been associated with insulin-dependent diabetes, rheumatoid arthritis and hydralazine-induced systemic lupus erythematosus [13]. It may well be that DR4 confers a similar susceptibility to immunological disease as does DR3, making individuals with both antigens particularly at risk.

7.4 DIFFERENTIAL DIAGNOSIS

The most frequent problem in the differential diagnosis of HG is distinguishing it from the much more common pregnancy dermatosis, polymorphic eruption of pregnancy (PEP). Synonyms for this disorder are pruritic urticarial papules and plaques of pregnancy, toxaemic rash of pregnancy and late-onset prurigo of pregnancy [14]. As has been mentioned, in HG the eruption may be present for a month or more before bullous lesions develop and it is during this time that there may be problems in differentiating HG from PEP. Two clinical features may be helpful at this stage. The first is the site of the onset of the eruption. Lesions beginning in the periumbilical area would suggest a diagnosis of HG. The periumbilical skin is often relatively spared in PEP. The second feature is the presence of florid striae distensae. These are found in 81% of the cases of PEP, but occur in only 3% of cases of HG [6]. A summary of the clinical differences between HG and PEP is given in Table 7.1.

The histopathology of vesicular lesions may help in the differentiation of HG and PEP. The vesicles in HG are usually subepidermal, whereas they are intraepidermal in PEP. However, two cases of PEP have been described in which the histopathology demonstrated subepidermal vesicles [15]. Fortunately immunofluorescence studies do enable HG and PEP to be confidently differentiated. Direct immunofluorescence of perilesional skin consistently demonstrates C3 deposition at the basement membrane zone in HG, whereas the findings are consistently negative in PEP [6].

Table 7.1 Differentiation of HG and PEP

	HG	*PEP*
Incidence	1 : 60 000 pregnancies	1 : 240 pregnancies
Primigravida	30%	76%
Onset (mean gestation)	21 weeks	35 weeks
Duration of urticarial lesions postpartum (mean)	60 weeks	1 week
Morphology		
Urticarial papules	100%	100%
Vesicles	95%	44%
Target lesions	95%	19%
Bullae	95%	0%
Striae	3%	81%
Periumbilical lesions	87%	12%

Data from Holmes *et al.* [6].

7.5 INVESTIGATIONS

7.5.1 Histopathology and ultrastructure

The histopathology of the early urticarial lesions demonstrates epidermal and papillary dermal oedema with occasional foci of eosinophilic spongiosis. In the dermis there is a perivascular infiltrate composed of lymphocytes, histiocytes and frequently eosinophils. The bullous lesions are subepidermal and they invariably contain numerous eosinophils [16–18]. Focal areas of basal cell necrosis have also been described [17, 19].

Ultrastructural studies of HG have demonstrated degenerative changes in epidermal cells leading to cellular necrosis which is particularly prominent in the basal layer [16, 20]. Studies of the normal skin in HG have shown that even here some of the basal cells demonstrate degeneration of their plasma membrane adjacent to the basement membrane [21]. Blister formation occurs within the lamina lucida between necrotic epidermal cells and the lamina densa [19, 21, 22]. These findings are in contrast to bullous pemphigoid where the blister formation appears to arise within the lamina lucida with intact basal cells [21].

7.5.2 Immunopathology

Immunofluorescence studies demonstrate that in all cases of HG there is deposition of C3 at the basement membrane zone of skin and usually one can demonstrate a C3 binding factor in the serum [6]. The frequency of positive direct and indirect immunofluorescence findings for C3 and IgG are shown in Table 7.2.

7.6 AETIOLOGY

There have been considerable advances recently in our understanding of the aetiology of HG. It occurs

Table 7.2 Immunofluorescence findings in HG

Direct	C3	100%
	IgG	27%
Indirect	C3	91%
	IgG	21%

Data from Holmes *et al.* [6].

only in association with pregnancy, hydatidiform mole and choriocarcinoma [23–26]. One feature in common with pregnancy and these trophoblastic tumours is that the patient's immune system is exposed to trophoblastic antigens. Therefore it was suggested that HG could develop as a result of an immune response to trophoblastic antigens and that this immune response could cross-react with and damage antigens at the basement membrane zone of skin [12]. Since this hypothesis was proposed, various clinical and laboratory evidence has accumulated in its support. Ortonne *et al.* demonstrated that there were, indeed, antigenic determinants shared by both trophoblastic tissue and skin [27]. Kelly *et al.* have shown that the complement-binding factor (HG factor) binds to epidermal basal keratinocytes and to amnion of placenta and umbilical cord after 22 weeks gestation [28] (Figure 7.2). This cross-reactivity is not surprising as skin and amnion are both derived from the ectodermal germ layer during embryogenesis [28]. Borthwick and Stirrat have studied the placentae of women with HG and confirmed evidence of an immune attack [29, 30]. They studied seven patients with HG. Immunohistological studies of their placentae showed abnormal expression of Class II MHC antigens. The area affected in all of the placentae

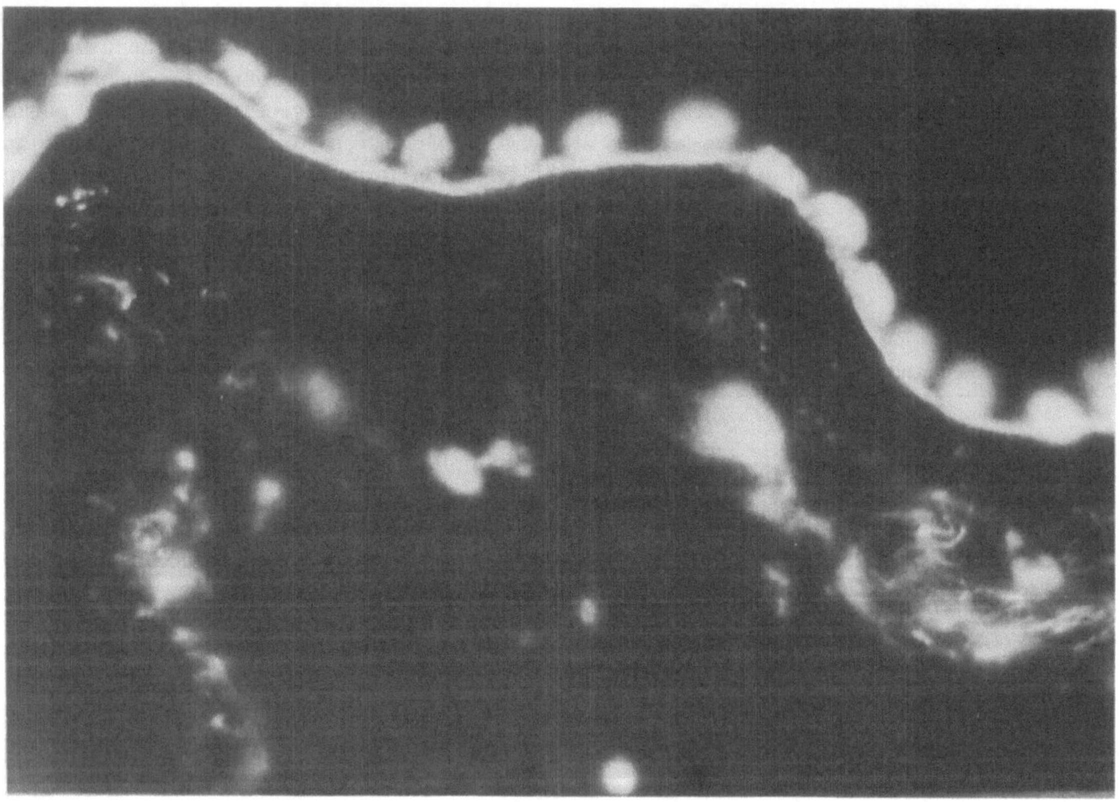

Figure 7.2 Binding of herpes gestationis serum to amnion placentae.

was the chorionic villi adjacent to the maternal decidua. It is possible that the Class II MHC antigens present in the villous stroma of the placentae may be involved in antigen presentation to the maternal immune system leading to an autoimmune attack on the placenta. A similar role for aberrant Class II MHC expression has been proposed in the induction of autoimmune disease of other organs [31, 32]. In accord with the laboratory evidence of an immune attack on the placenta there is clinical evidence of impaired placental function in HG [33]. Finally a most unusual case has been reported which appears to encapsulate and confirm all of the preceding speculations about the aetiology of HG [34]. The patient was an 80-year-old man who received multiple intramuscular injections of placental extracts as a rejuvenating treatment and subsequently developed a pemphigoid-like bullous eruption.

Having established a possible mechanism for the induction of HG which is potentially applicable to all pregnancies, we need to consider why the disorder is, in fact, so uncommon. It would seem that for the immune response to occur certain further factors need to be contributed by both the patient and her consort. The HLA association of HG with the haplotype A1, B8, DR3 and the pairing of DR3 and DR4 has already been discussed. These HLA findings are associated with increased immune responsiveness. Therefore, perhaps for HG to occur one needs a patient with an inherent tendency to autoimmune disease. The suggestion that the consort is important in determining whether HG will develop stems from cases in which the eruption has only developed when women have changed their sexual partner [12]. In normal pregnancy 50% of the foetal and trophoblastic tissues are derived from the consort and 100% in hydatidiform mole [35]. Perhaps there are inheritable minor variations in membrane antigens and it requires exposure to particular trophoblastic antigens, only derived from certain consorts, to initiate the sequence that results in HG. Investigation of the fathers in affected pregnancies has so far been limited to HLA antigen studies. Shornick *et al.* found a slight increase in the frequency of HLA DR2 in the consorts [36], but in a further study the frequency of HLA antigens was normal [12]. Several studies have noted an increased frequency of HLA antibodies in patients with HG directed against their husbands' HLA antigens [12, 36–38]. However, these antibodies may be of no importance aetiologically, but may simply reflect the high immune responsiveness of the patients [39].

7.7 PATHOGENESIS

Our understanding of the pathogenesis of HG has increased considerably since the first immunopathological studies by Provost and Tomasi in 1973 [40]. They demonstrated deposition of C3, C5 and Properdin along the basement membrane zone (BMZ) of lesional skin in HG. They were unable to demonstrate any immunoglobulins of the G, M or A classes. Sera were examined by an indirect immunofluorescence (IIF) technique employing normal human skin as a substrate, and this revealed a factor in the serum that was capable of binding C3 to the BMZ of skin. This was termed the HG factor. Serial serum samples were studied in one patient and these showed disappearance of the HG factor from the serum at 5 months postpartum concomitant with resolution of the skin eruption. Provost and Tomasi felt that the HG factor was probably not an immunoglobulin (Ig) as it was thermolabile and they had been unable to demonstrate immunoglobulin at the BMZ by DIF. They concluded that as Properdin, C3 and C5 were present along the BMZ, in the absence of immunoglobulin or C1q, activation of complement in HG was occurring via the alternative pathway. However, subsequent investigations into the character of the HG factor and its pathological significance have shown that it is, in fact, an immunoglobulin of the G class [41, 42]. Chromatography and sucrose gradient ultracentrifugation was used to separate the IgG fraction of serum and it was within this fraction that the HG factor was demonstrated. Immunoabsorption of HG patients' sera with anti-human IgG removed the HG factor, and the HG factor could be destroyed by papain digestion. Although Provost and Tomasi [40] had reported that the HG factor was thermolabile and therefore unlikely to be an IgG, both Katz, Hertz and Yaoita [42] and Jordon *et al.* [41] found it to be thermostable at 56–60 °C. In addition, both reports noted cases in which immunofluorescence studies were positive for IgG as well as C3, as had previously been described by Bushkell, Jordon and Goltz. [43]. A further study by Carruthers and Ewins [44] employing chromatography and immunoabsorption confirmed that the HG factor was indeed an IgG. They also demonstrated that, in common with the IgG subclasses IgG_1, IgG_2 and IgG_4, it bound to staphylococcal protein A. As the subclasses that bind complement avidly are IgG_1 and IgG_3 they proposed that the HG factor probably belonged to the IgG_1 subclass. Immunofluorescence studies using monoclonal antibodies to the IgG subclasses have confirmed that complement fixation in HG is dependent on an immunoglobulin of IgG_1 subclass [45].

In addition to defining the character of the HG factor the studies of Jordon *et al.* [41], Katz, Hertz and Yaoita [42] and Carruthers and Ewins [44] also examined the pathway of complement activation in HG. Provost and Tomasi [40] had concluded from their studies that complement activation in HG occurred via the alternative pathway. However, the following year Bushkell, Jordon and Goltz [43] described a patient with IgG, C1q, C3 and Properdin deposition at the BMZ and therefore evidence of classical, as well as alternative, pathway activation. The question as to whether complement is activated primarily by the classical or alternative pathway in HG was clarified by the results of IIF experiments using serum deficient in specific complement components as the source of complement. Jordon *et al.* [41] performed IIF studies with HG sera employing C2-deficient human serum as the source of complement. This resulted in failure to demonstrate C3 at the BMZ, whereas C3 deposition had been noted with normal human serum as the complement source. As C2 is a component of the classical pathway alone, Jordon *et al.* [41] concluded that complement activation in HG is primarily via the classical pathway. Similar evidence for classical pathway activation was obtained by Katz, Hertz and Yaoita [42] using C4-deficient guinea-pig serum as the complement source. Carruthers and Ewins [44] subsequently confirmed these findings. While these studies showed that complement activation in HG is primarily via the classical pathway DIF may also demonstrate deposition of the alternative pathway components, Properdin and factor B, at the BMZ [40–43]. The most likely explanation for involvement of these alternative pathway components is activation of the C3 amplification loop by C3b generated via the classical pathway. A case of HG has been described in which C3 nephritic factor (C3NF) was demonstrated in the patient's serum [46]. This is an IgG autoantibody to alternative pathway C3 convertase (C3b Bb) which prolongs the half-life of this convertase and therefore enhances the alternative pathway [47]. The presence of C3NF could be the explanation for significant alternative pathway activation in other patients with HG.

While conclusive evidence has been accumulated that the HG factor is an IgG and that activation of complement is primarily by the classical pathway, one has to acknowledge that in most cases of HG it is not possible to demonstrate IgG with standard immunofluorescence. Holubar, Konrad and Stingl [48] proposed that the reason for this was that conventional immunofluorescence methods were simply not sensitive enough. They supported this suggestion by reporting a patient with negative DIF for IgG in whom deposition of IgG along the BMZ could be demonstrated by immunoelectron microscopy (IEM). The IEM technique used was a peroxidase–antiperoxidase multistep method which had been likely, on theoretical considerations, to be more sensitive than standard immunofluorescence [49]. Jurecka *et al.* have used this technique in a further three active cases of HG and shown IgG deposition on the BMZ in all cases [50].

There have been conflicting findings with regard to the localization of immunoreactants in HG. Honigsmann *et al.* [51] and Harrington and Bleehen [22] reported that the fine structural localization of the deposits in HG was in the lamina lucida localized around hemidesmosomes and therefore identical to that seen in bullous pemphigoid (BP). However, in contrast to this, Yaoita, Gullino and Katz [21] found that the pattern of immunoglobulin deposition in the lamina lucida was uniform and therefore slightly different from that seen in bullous pemphigoid. Immunofluorescence blocking experiments have also produced conflicting results. Jordon *et al.* [41] found that BMZ fluorescence with fluorescein isothiocyanate-labelled BP antibody could be almost completely blocked with HG serum, suggesting that the antibodies might be directed against a common antigen, whereas Carruthers and Ewins [44] performed a series of similar experiments and were unable to confirm these findings. They suggested that the explanation for this might be that in both BP and HG there are a number of autoantibodies directed at different, though closely related, sites in the BMZ. In support of this hypothesis $F(ab^1)_2$ prepared from pooled BP sera did, indeed, block BMZ fluorescence for C3 with five out of seven HG sera. Therefore immunopathological evidence suggests that, while HG has a pathogenesis that is very similar to BP, it is probably a distinct disorder.

Although the pathogenic role of the HG factor has been questioned [52], there is clinical evidence that strongly supports its role in the pathogenesis of HG. Firstly, neonatal HG has been described, with positive DIF in the infant, in which it has been claimed that passive placental transfer of the HG factor to the neonate was responsible for its clinical involvement [53–55]. Secondly, support for the pathogenicity of the HG factor has been derived from the observation that plasmapheresis in patients with HG has led to clinical improvement. Carruthers and Ewins [44] described a single case in which rapid resolution of lesions was noted on two separate occasions following plasma exchange. A further case of HG that responded well to plasmapheresis was reported by van de Wiel *et al.* [56].

7.8 SYSTEMIC MANIFESTATIONS AND ASSOCIATED DISEASES

HG has been described in association with Graves' disease [57]. In view of the strong association between HG and the HLA haplotype A1, B8, DR3 one would expect an increased frequency of autoimmune associations.

7.9 TREATMENT

HG usually responds very well to treatment with systemic corticosteroids. We have found that in most patients the eruption comes under good control on prednisolone 40 mg daily. One can then reduce the dose to the minimum which will control the disease and subsequently titrate the dose against disease severity. Many patients experience a brisk flare in the severity of their eruption immediately postpartum [6] and this will necessitate a temporary increase in their steroid treatment. Fortunately the administration of systemic corticosteroids in the second and third trimesters does not appear to confer any appreciable risk to the foetus [33, 58]. Not all patients, however, do require systemic steroid treatment. In mild episodes, treatment with a topical corticosteroid may be sufficient. In patients in whom corticosteroids are contra-indicated, treatment with plasmapheresis should be considered. This has been used successfully in HG during pregnancy [56] and also in cases persisting postpartum [44]. Further treatments that have been recommended in HG include the sulphonamides [59] and pyridoxine [60]. In our experience both these treatments have been disappointing.

Recently a case was reported in which severe HG went into remission when the patient was prescribed ritodrine to prevent premature labour [61]. This is a beta-adrenergic drug with pre-dominantly a beta-2-receptor agonist action. In premature labour it is used to reduce uterine contractility. If this drug does have an inhibitory effect on HG, the mechanism whereby it produces this effect remains unclear.

7.10 PROGNOSIS

7.10.1 Maternal prognosis

In the majority of patients the bullous lesions resolve within 2 months postpartum and the urticarial lesions within 1 year of delivery. However, two cases have been reported recently in which the eruption persisted for more than 10 years postpartum [7, 8]. Once a patient has developed HG it almost invariably recurs in subsequent pregnancies. Occasionally subsequent pregnancies are unaffected and this has been associated with either changed paternity or if the mother and foetus are fully compatible at the DR locus [12]. Recurrence in later pregnancies is usually more severe and tends to develop earlier in pregnancy with each succeeding episode.

Recurrence of HG is not only limited to pregnancy but may also occur if the patient is prescribed an oral contraceptive [62–66]. The activity of HG persisting postpartum not infrequently varies throughout the menstrual cycle. Exacerbations usually occur premenstrually, but may also coincide with ovulation in the mid-cycle [12]. The recurrence of HG with oral contraceptives and menstruation probably represents hormonal modulation of the disease activity rather than any more fundamental role in the aetiology of HG. In some autoimmune disorders it appears that the HLA type of the patient may serve as a guide to the prognosis. For example, in autoimmune thyrotoxicosis, patients that are HLA-DR3 have a worse prognosis [67]. We did consider that this might be the case in HG [52], but our own further personal experience has not borne this out. As yet there are no published studies comparing the disease severity of HG in HLA-DR3 positive and negative patients.

7.10.2 Foetal prognosis

There has been some divergence of opinion with regard to the foetal prognosis in HG. This matter has recently been clarified by a study of 50 affected pregnancies [33]. This showed a significant increase in small-for-dates babies suggesting that there may be impaired placental function in HG. It did not appear to be possible to predict from the

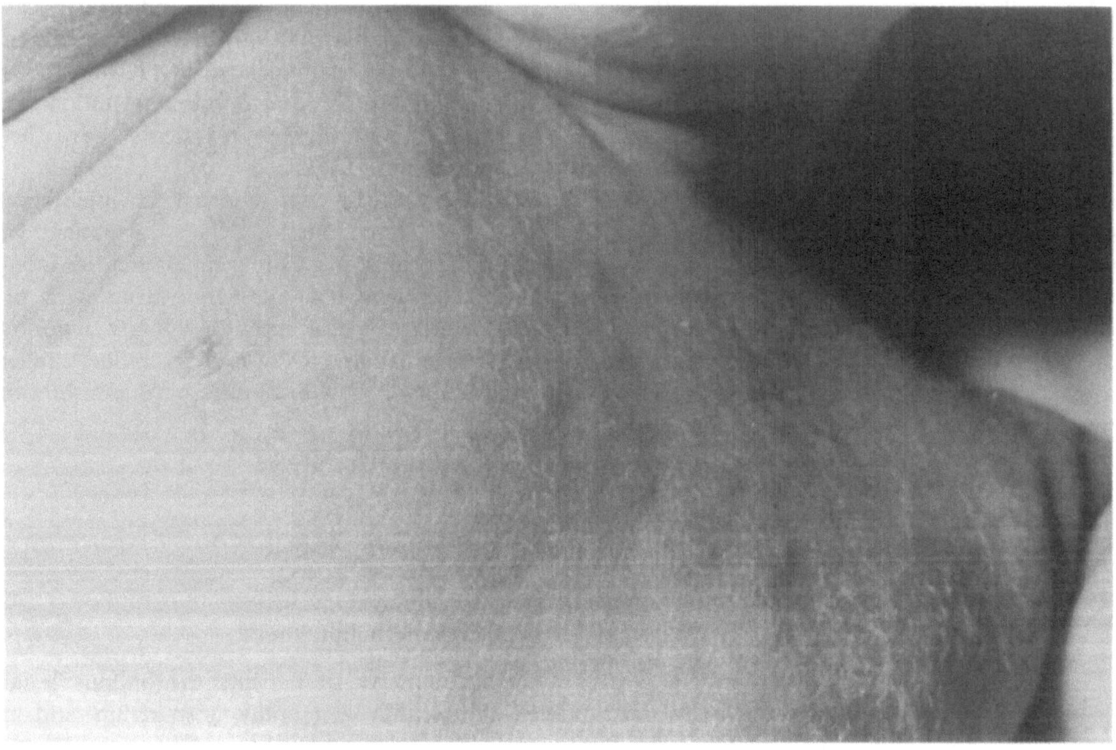

Figure 7.3 Blistering in a neonate born to a patient with herpes gestationis.

severity of HG which pregnancies were particularly at risk for the delivery of small-for-dates infants. Despite the increase in infant risk, the mortality and morbidity which could actually be ascribed to HG in the cases were small. In the 50 infants there were four infant deaths and no stillbirths. Of the four infant deaths it seems more likely that three were unrelated to HG.

Infants with bullous lesions resembling HG have occasionally been reported (Figure 7.3). This has been attributed to passive transfer of the mother's anti-basement membrane zone antibody across the placenta [54, 55].

REFERENCES

1. Holmes, R.C. and Black, M.M. (1983) The specific dermatoses of pregnancy. *J. Amer. Acad. Dermatol.*, **8**, 405–12.
2. Rook, A., Wilkinson, D.S., Ebling, F.J.G., Champion, R.H. and Burton, J.L. (1986) *Textbook of Dermatology*, 4th edn, Blackwell Scientific Publications, Oxford.
3. Russell, B. and Thorne, N.A. (1957) Herpes gestationis. *Brit. J. Dermatol.*, **96**, 563–8.
4. Kolodny, R.C. (1969) Herpes gestationis. A new assessment of incidence, diagnosis and fetal prognosis. *Amer. J. Obstet. Gynecol.*, **104**, 39–45.
5. Shornick, J.K., Meek, T.J., Nesbitt, L.T. and Gilliam, J.N. (1984) Herpes gestationis in blacks. *Arch. Dermatol.*, **120**, 511–13.
6. Holmes, R.C., Black, M.M., Dann, J., *et al.* (1982) A comparative study of toxic erythema of pregnancy and herpes gestationis. *Brit. J. Dermatol.*, **106**, 499–510.
7. Fine, J.D. and Omura, E.F. (1985) Herpes gestationis. Persistent disease activity 11 years post partum. *Arch. Dermatol.*, **121**, 924–6.
8. Holmes, R.C., Black, M.M. and Williamson, D.M. (1986) Herpes gestationis persisting for 12 years post partum. *Arch. Dermatol.*, **122**, 375.
9. Shornick, J.K., Bangert, J.L., Freeman, R.G. and Gilliam, J.N. (1983) Herpes gestationis: clinical and histological features of twenty-eight cases. *J. Amer. Acad. Dermatol.*, **8**, 214–24.
10. Bercovitch, L., Bogaars, H.A. and Murray, D.O. (1983) Pustular herpes gestationis. *Arch. Dermatol.*, **119**, 91–3.
11. Shornick, J.K., Stastny, P. and Gilliam, J.N. (1981) High frequency of histocompatibility antigens HLA-DR3 and DR4 in herpes gestationis. *Clin. Invest.*, **68**, 553–5.
12. Holmes, R.C., Black, M.M., Jurecka, W., *et al.* (1983) Clues to the aetiology and pathogenesis of herpes gestationis. *Brit. J. Dermatol.*, **109**, 131–9.
13. Svejgaard, A., Morling, N., Platz, P., *et al.* (1981) HLA and disease associations with special reference to mechanism. *Transplant. Proc.*, **13**, 913–17.
14. Holmes, R.C. and Black, M.M. (1982) The specific dermatoses of pregnancy: A reappraisal with special emphasis on a proposed simplified clinical classification. *Clin. Exp. Dermatol.*, 7, 65–73.
15. Holmes, R.C., McGibbon, D.H. and Black, M.M. (1984) Polymorphic eruption of pregnancy with subepidermal vesicles. *J. R. Soc. Med.*, 77, 22–3.
16. Schaumburg-Lever, G., Saffolc, O.E., Orfanos, C.E. *et al.* (1973) Herpes gestationis: histology and ultrastructure. *Arch. Dermatol.*, **107**, 888–92.
17. Hertz, K.C., Katz, S.I., Maize, J., *et al.* (1976) Herpes gestationis: A clinicopathologic study. *Arch. Dermatol.*, **112**, 1543–8.
18. Holmes, R.C., Jurecka, W. and Black, M.M. (1983) A comparative histopathological study of polymorphic eruption of pregnancy and herpes gestationis. *Clin. Exp. Dermatol.*, **8**, 523–9.
19. Kint, A., Goerts, M.L., Vanneste, B. and De Cuyper, C. (1980) Herpes gestationis. Etude histologique et ultrastructurale. *Ann. Dermatol. Venereol.*, **107**, 113–42.
20. Pierard, J., Thiery, M. and Kint, A. (1969) Histologie et ultrastructure de l'herpes gestationis. *Arch. Belges Dermatol. Syphil.*, **25**, 321–35.
21. Yaoita, H., Guillino, M. and Katz, S.I. (1976) Herpes gestationis. Ultrastructure and ultrastructural localisation of *in vivo* bound complement. *J. Invest. Dermatol.*, **66**, 383–8.
22. Harrington, C.I. and Bleehen, S.S. (1979) Herpes gestationis: Immunopathological and ultrastructural studies. *Brit. J. Dermatol.*, **100**, 389–99.
23. Dupont, C. (1974) Herpes gestationis with hydatidiform mole. *Trans. St. John's Hosp. Dermatol. Soc.*, **60**, 103.
24. Tindall, J.G., Rea, T.H., Shulman, I., *et al.* (1981) Herpes gestationis in association with hydatidiform mole. *Arch. Dermatol.*, **117**, 510–12.
25. Tillman, W.G. (1950) Herpes gestationis with hydatidiform mole and chorion epithelioma. *Brit. Med. J.*, **1**, 1471.
26. Slazinski, L. and Degfu, S. (1982) Herpes gestationis associated with choriocarcinoma. *Arch. Dermatol.*, **118**, 426–8.
27. Ortonne, J.P., Hsi, B.L., Verrando, P., *et al.* (1987) Herpes gestationis in association with hydatidiform epithelial basement membrane. *Brit. J. Dermatol.*, **117**, 147–54.
28. Kelly, S.E., Bhogal, B., Wojnarowska, F. and Black, M.M. (1988) Expression of a pemphigoid gestationis related antigen by human placenta. *Brit. J. Dermatol.*, **118**, 605–13.

29. Borthwick, G.M., Sunderland, C.A., Holmes, R.C., Black, M.M. and Stirrat, G.M. (1984) Abnormal expression of HLA-DR antigen in the placenta of a patient with pemphigoid gestationis. *J. Reprod. Immunol.*, **6**, 393–6.
30. Borthwick, G.M., Holmes, R.C. and Stirrat, G.M. (1988) Abnormal expression of Class II MHC antigens in placentae from patients with pemphigoid gestationis: analysis of Class II MHC sub-region product expression. *Placenta*, **9**, 81–4.
31. Bottazo, G.F., Pujal-Borrell, R., Hanafusa, T. and Feldmann, M. (1983) Hypothesis: role of aberrant HLA-DR expression and antigen presentation to induction of endocrine autoimmunity. *Lancet*, ii, 1115–18.
32. Hanafusa, T., Pujol-Borrell, R., Chiovata, R., Russell, R.C.G., Doniach, D. and Bottazo, G.F. (1983) Aberrant expression of HLA-DR antigen on thyrocytes in Graves' disease: relevance for autoimmunity. *Lancet*, ii, 1111–15.
33. Holmes, R.C. and Black, M.M. (1984) The foetal prognosis in pemphigoid gestationis (herpes gestationis). *Brit. J. Dermatol.*, **110**, 67–72.
34. Fournier, C., Didierjean, L., Carraux, P., Salomon, D., Merot, Y. and Saurat, J.H. (1986) Placental-pemphigoid: a bullous pemphigoid-like dermatosis after injections of placental extracts in a man. Detection of antibodies to cutaneo-placental antigens. *J. Invest. Dermatol.*, **87**, 140.
35. Kajii, T. and Ohama, K. (1977) Androgenic origin of hydatidiform mole. *Nature (London)*, **268**, 663–4.
36. Shornick, J.H., Stastny, P. and Gilliam, J.N. (1983) Paternal histocompatibility (HLA) antigens and maternal anti-HLA antibodies in herpes gestationis. *J. Invest. Dermatol.*, **81**, 407–9.
37. Reunala, T., Karvonen, J., Tiilikainen, A., *et al.* (1977) Herpes gestationis: A high titre of anti-HLA-B8 antibody in the mother and pemphigoid-like immunohistological findings in the mother and the child. *Brit. J. Dermatol.*, **96**, 563–8.
38. Eberst, E., Tongio, M.M., Eberst, B., *et al.* (1981) Herpes gestationis and anti-HLA immunisation. *Brit. J. Dermatol.*, **104**, 553–9.
39. Holmes, R.C., Black, M.M. and James, D.C.O. (1984) HLA-DR and herpes gestationis. *J. Invest. Dermatol.*, **83**, 78–9.
40. Provost, T.T. and Tomasi, T.B. (1973) Evidence of complement activation via the alternative pathway in skin diseases: I. Herpes gestationis, systemic lupus erythematosus and bullous pemphigoid. *J. Clin. Invest.*, **52**, 1779–87.
41. Jordon, R.E., Heine, K.G., Tappeiner, G., *et al.* (1976) The immunopathology of herpes gestationis. Immunofluorescence studies and characterisation of "HG factor". *J. Clin. Invest.*, **57**, 1426–33.
42. Katz, S.I., Hertz, K.C. and Yaoita, H. (1976) Herpes gestationis. Immunopathology and characterisation of the HG factor. *J. Clin. Invest.*, **57**, 1434–41.
43. Bushkell, L.L., Jordon, R.E. and Goltz, R.W. (1974) Herpes gestationis: New immunologic findings. *Arch. Dermatol.*, **110**, 65–9.
44. Carruthers, J.A. and Ewins, A.R. (1978) Herpes gestationis: Studies on the binding characteristics, activity and pathogenic significance of the complement-fixing factor. *Clin. Exp. Immunol.*, **31**, 38–44.
45. Kelly, S., Cerio, R., Bhogal, B.S., and Black, M.M. (1989) The distribution of IgG subclasses in pemphigoid gestationis: PG factor is an IgG_1 autoantibody. *J. Invest. Dermatol.*, **92**, 695–8.
46. Grimwood, R., Arroyave, C.M., Weston, W.L.L. and Aeling, J.L. (1980) Herpes gestationis associated with the C3 nephritic factor. *Arch. Dermatol.*, **116**, 1045–7.
47. Daha, M.R., Austen, K.F. and Fearon, D.T. (1978) Heterogeneity, polypeptide chain composition and antigenic reactivity of C3 nephritic factor. *J. Immunol.*, **120**, 1389–94.
48. Holubar, K., Konrad, K. and Stingl, G. (1977) Detection by immunoelectron microscopy of immunoglobulin G deposits in skin of immunofluorescence negative herpes gestationis. *Brit. J. Dermatol.*, **96**, 569–71.
49. Holubar, K., Wolff, K., Konrad, K. and Beutner, E.H. (1975) Ultrastructural localisation of immunoglobulins in bullous pemphigoid skin. Employment of a new peroxidase–antiperoxidase multistep method. *J. Invest. Dermatol.*, **64**, 220–7.
50. Jurecka, W., Holmes, R.C., Black, M.M., *et al.* (1983) An immunoelectrol microscopy study of the relationship between herpes gestationis and polymorphic eruption of pregnancy. *Brit. J. Dermatol.*, **108**, 147–51.
51. Honigsmann, H., Stingl, G., Holubar, K., *et al.* (1976) Herpes gestationis: Fine structural pattern of immunoglobulin deposits in the skin *in vivo*. *J. Invest. Dermatol.*, **66**, 389–92.
52. Holmes, R.C. and Black, M.M. (1983) Herpes gestationis. *Dermatology Clinics, 1, Symposium on Blistering Diseases*, 195–203.
53. Rimbaud, P., Jean, R., Bonnet, H., Meynadier, J., Rieu, D. and Guilhou, J. (1971) Herpes gestationis. Eruption bulleuse chez le nouveau-né. *Bull. Soc. Fr. Dermatol. Syphil.*, **78**, 419–25.
54. Katz, A., Minta, J.O., Toole, J.W.P., *et al.* (1977) Immunopathologic study of herpes gestationis in mother and child. *Arch. Dermatol.*, **113**, 1069–72.
55. Chorzelski, T.P., Jablonska, S., Beutner, E.H., *et al.* (1976) Herpes gestationis with identical lesions in the newborn. *Arch. Dermatol.*, **112**, 1129–31.
56. Van de Wiel, A., Hart, H., Flinterman, J., *et al.* (1980) Plasma exchange in herpes gestationis. *Brit. Med. J.*, **281**, 1041–2.
57. Holmes, R.C. and Black, M.M. (1980) Herpes gestationis: A possible association with autoimmune

thyrotoxicosis (Graves' disease). *J. Amer. Acad. Dermatol.*, 3, 474–7.
58. Schatz, M., Patterson, R., Zeitz, S., *et al.* (1975) Corticosteroid therapy for the pregnant asthmatic patient. *J. Amer. Med. Assoc.*, **233**, 804–7.
59. Downing, J.G. and Jillson, O.F. (1949) Herpes gestationis. *New Engl. J. Med.*, **241**, 906.
60. Fosnaugh, R.P., Bryan, H.G. and Orders, R.L. (1961) Pyridoxine in the treatment of herpes gestationis. *Arch. Dermatol.*, **84**, 90–5.
61. Macdonald, K.J.S. and Raffle, E.J. (1984) Ritodrine therapy associated with remission of pemphigoid gestationis. *Brit. J. Dermatol.*, **111**, 630.
62. Lynch, F.W., and Albrecht, R.J. (1966) Hormonal factors in herpes gestationis. *Arch. Dermatol.*, **93**, 446–7.
63. Mitchell, C.M. (1966) Herpes gestationis and the "pill". *Brit. Med. J.*, **ii**, 1324.
64. Dupont, C. (1968) Herpes gestationis and the "pill". *Brit. Med. J.*, **ii**, 699.
65. Gordon, G. (1967) Herpes gestationis and the "pill". *Brit. Med. J.*, **i**, 51–2.
66. Morgan, J.K. (1968) Herpes gestationis influenced by an oral contraceptive. *Brit. J. Dermatol.*, **80**, 456–8.
67. McGregor, A.M., Rees Smith, B., Petersen, M.M., *et al.* (1980) Prediction of relapse in hyperthyroid Graves' disease. *Lancet*, **i**, 1101–3.

Eight
Linear IgA disease of adults

Fenella Wojnarowska

8.1 INTRODUCTION

Linear IgA disease of adults (LAD) is defined as a dapsone-responsive subepidermal bullous disease commencing after puberty in which linear IgA deposits are found at the basement membrane zone (BMZ). There may in addition be an associated circulating IgA anti-BMZ antibody.

LAD has progressed in a little over a decade from being regarded as a variant of dermatitis herpetiformis [1–4] or bullous pemphigoid [5–8] to its recognition as a distinct blistering disease. Chorzelski and Jablonska [9, 10] first considered LAD to be a distinct clinical and immunopathological entity in 1975 and this is now widely accepted [11–16]. Its precise relationship to chronic bullous disease of childhood (CBDC) (Chapter 9), of which it seems likely to be the adult counterpart [16], and to cicatricial pemphigoid (CP) (Chapter 6), bullous pemphigoid (BP) (Chapter 5) and epidermolysis bullosa acquisita (EBA) (Chapter 10) has still to be defined.

8.2 CLINICAL FEATURES

8.2.1 Presentation

LAD may present throughout adult life (Figure 8.1). However, some patients are in the 20–40 age group, younger than BP patients, even though the peak incidence is after 60 years of age [2, 10, 12, 13, 15, 16]. There is a slight female preponderance in this disease (Figure 8.2) [5, 6, 10, 12, 14, 15, 16], although this was not observed in all series [2, 13, 14]. This disease is rare and less common

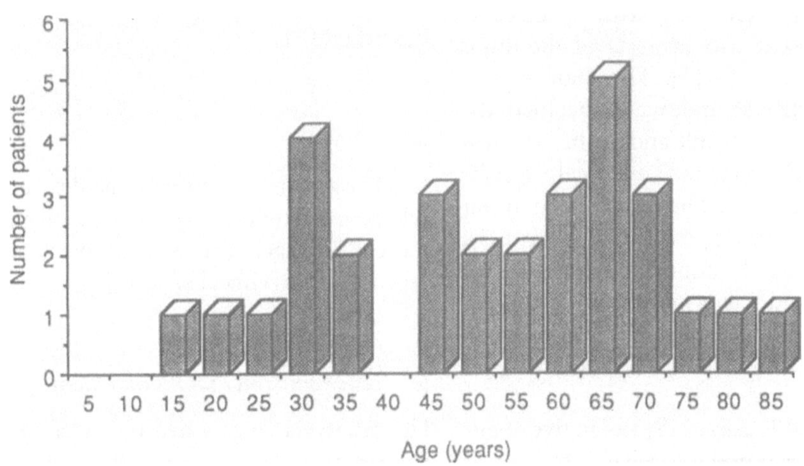

Figure 8.1 Age of onset of linear IgA disease.

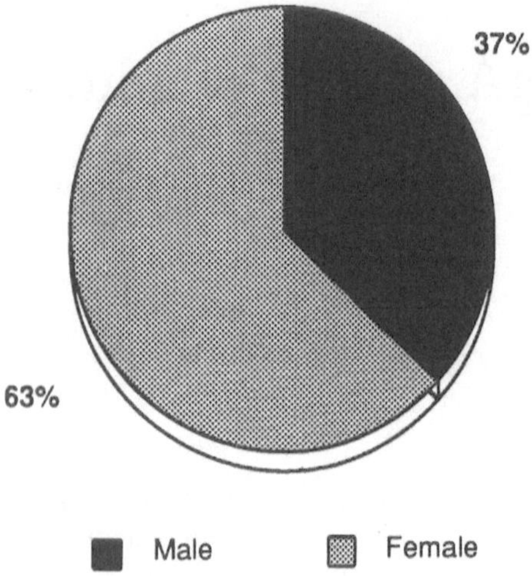

Figure 8.2 Male:female ratio in LAD.

in the West than either BP or dermatitis herpetiformis (DH) and the approximate incidence in Southern England (Oxford Region) is 1 in 250 000 per year. Most cases have been reported from Europe and the USA, however, it is more common than DH in Japan [17] and has been reported from Thailand [18] and occurs in people from the Indian subcontinent (three of 31 patients in our series).

8.2.2 Cutaneous distribution

The distribution is very variable. A minority of patients have an eruption with a DH-like distribution on the extensor aspects of the limbs and buttocks [12, 13, 19–21]. The majority are described as being BP-like and, when specified, the commonest sites are the trunk and limbs, and less commonly the hands, feet, face and scalp can be involved [6, 7, 18, 21–27]. The distribution in our series (30 patients) was the trunk (Figure 8.3), sometimes with localized plaques, and limbs in over 95% (Figure 8.4), and hands and feet in 25%. The face was involved in 40% and the perineum in 30%, which differs from CBDC [28] (see Chapter 9).

The disease may be localized [8] and in five of our cases the disease was initially localized to areas of cutaneous trauma, e.g. a burn or under a plaster cast.

8.2.3 Mucosal involvement

Involvement of mucosa is common, and may be asymptomatic, but is often a troublesome feature of LAD. In a few patients it is so prominent as to make it difficult to distinguish such patients from those with cicatricial pemphigoid [16, 21, 29] (see Chapter 6).

(a) Oral cavity

Oral involvement is common and affects up to 50% of patients [6, 13, 16, 21, 26, 27, 29–32]. There are blisters and erosions (Figure 8.5) which may be asymptomatic or painful enough to prevent eating. In a few patients painful localized erosions persist for years. We have seen one patient with desquamative gingivitis which cleared with the dapsone therapy of her LAD.

(b) Nasopharynx and larynx

Nasopharyngeal involvement with erosions and purpuric lesions have been described [21]. Some 20% of our patients described bleeding and crusting of the nose [16].

(c) Oesophagus

A single case of oesophageal involvement has been described [21].

(d) Larynx

LAD patients describe episodes of hoarseness which may reflect laryngeal involvement. In one patient laryngeal involvement was complicated by episodes of laryngeal stridor [21].

(e) Tracheobronchial involvement

Haemoptysis and wheezing accompanying skin exacerbations have been described in one case, in which bronchoscopy showed vesicles and erosions, and the trachea was distorted and scarred [21].

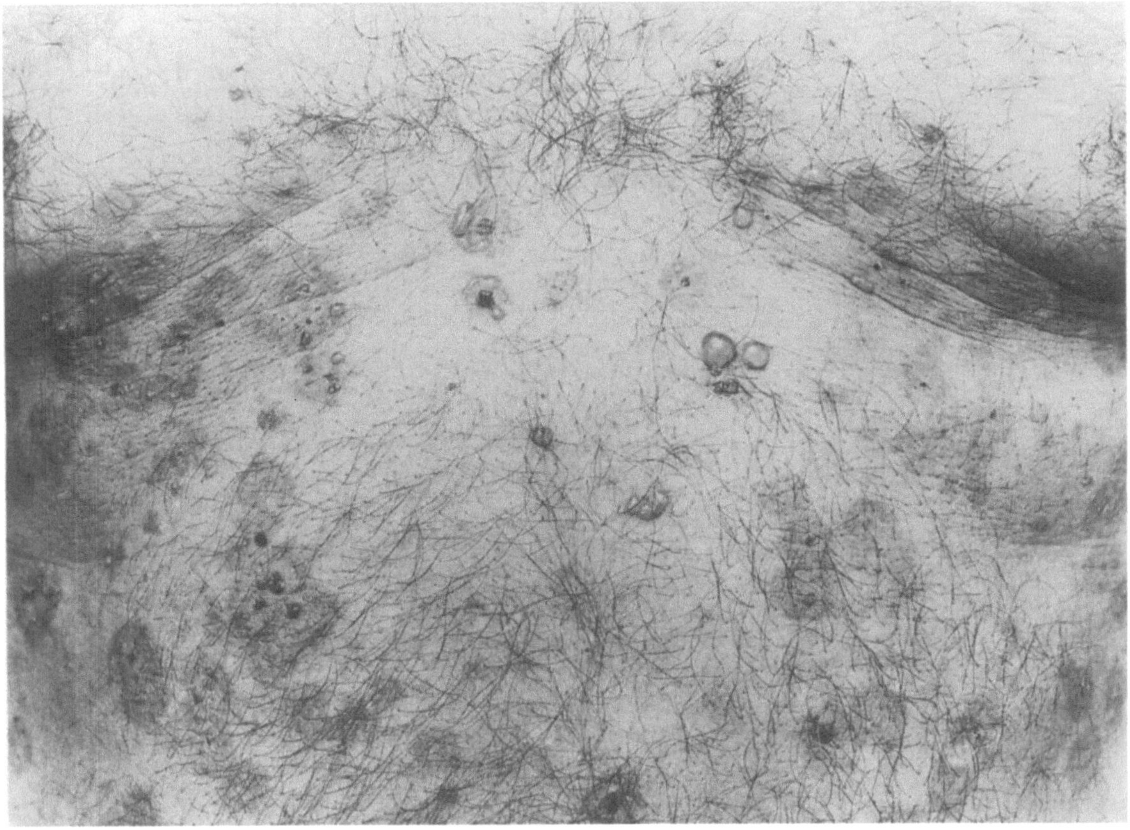

Figure 8.3 LAD: involvement of the trunk with vesicles and urticated lesions.

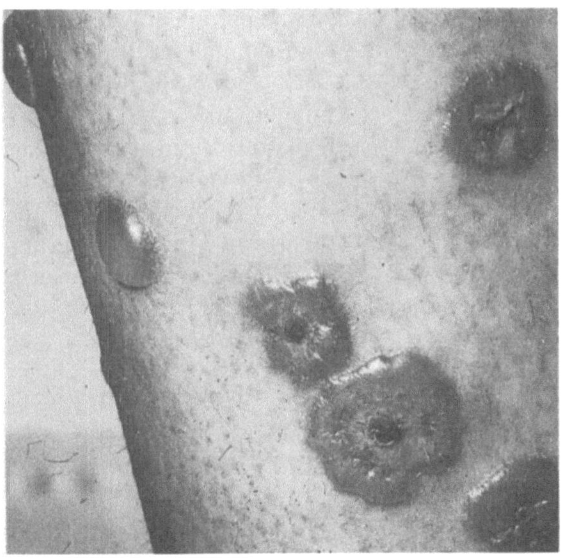

Figure 8.4 LAD: annular lesions and bullae on the thigh.

(f) Anorectal

Haemorrhagic anorectal inflammation has been described in a single case [21].

(g) Genitalia

Involvement of the external genitalia, both vulva and penis, has been described [13, 16, 27, 30] and one patient had sterile dysuria suggesting true mucosal involvement.

(h) Ocular lesions

The eyes are involved in 50% or more of patients [16, 21, 29, 31, 33]. The patients may be asymptomatic or complain of grittiness, dryness and pain; there may be associated eyelid lesions. There may be conjunctivitis, symblepharon

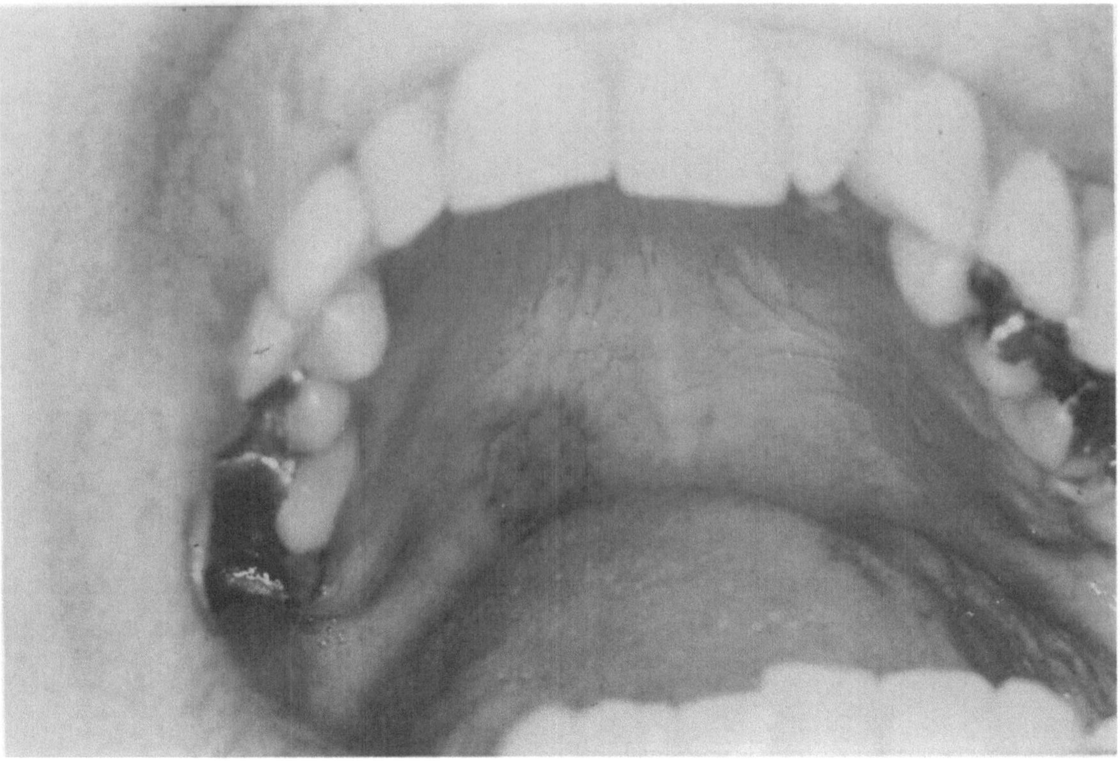

Figure 8.5 LAD: erosion on the palate.

formation (Figure 8.6), cicatrizing conjunctivitis, entropion and trichiasis. Asymptomatic patients have been reported to develop scarring [16, 31]. Eye symptoms should be taken seriously, and ophthalmic examination carried out in all patients. There have as yet been no reports of blindness occurring in adults with LAD, although this has been described in a child with the disease [34].

8.2.4 Morphology of lesions

The lesions are variable not only from patient to patient but also in the same patient at different times, and particularly when modified by treatment. Pruritus may precede the onset of blistering but does not occur in all patients [23, 32]. The initial appearance often suggests a diagnosis of 'atypical' DH, BP or erythema multiforme.

The lesions comprise papulovesicles often arranged in groups or plaques similar to DH [6, 9, 10, 12, 13, 15, 16, 19, 23, 25, 30]. Urticated lesions are common, particularly in partially treated cases, or those going into remission. Vesicles and large bullae (Figures 8.3 and 8.4), which may be haemorrhagic, are common and arise either on normal skin or erythematous or urticated areas [6, 12, 13, 15, 16, 23]. The most characteristic lesion of LAD is the annular, polycyclic or gyrate lesion with a peripheral urticated ring of blistering (Figure 8.4) [15, 16, 30, 32]. The presence of such annular lesions is a pointer to LAD.

8.3 GENETICS

No familial cases of LAD have been reported. There is a raised incidence of HLA-B8 25–60% [4, 12–14, 16] which is, however, lower than in CBDC or DH (see Chapters 9 and 11) suggesting that HLA-B8 may predispose to the development of

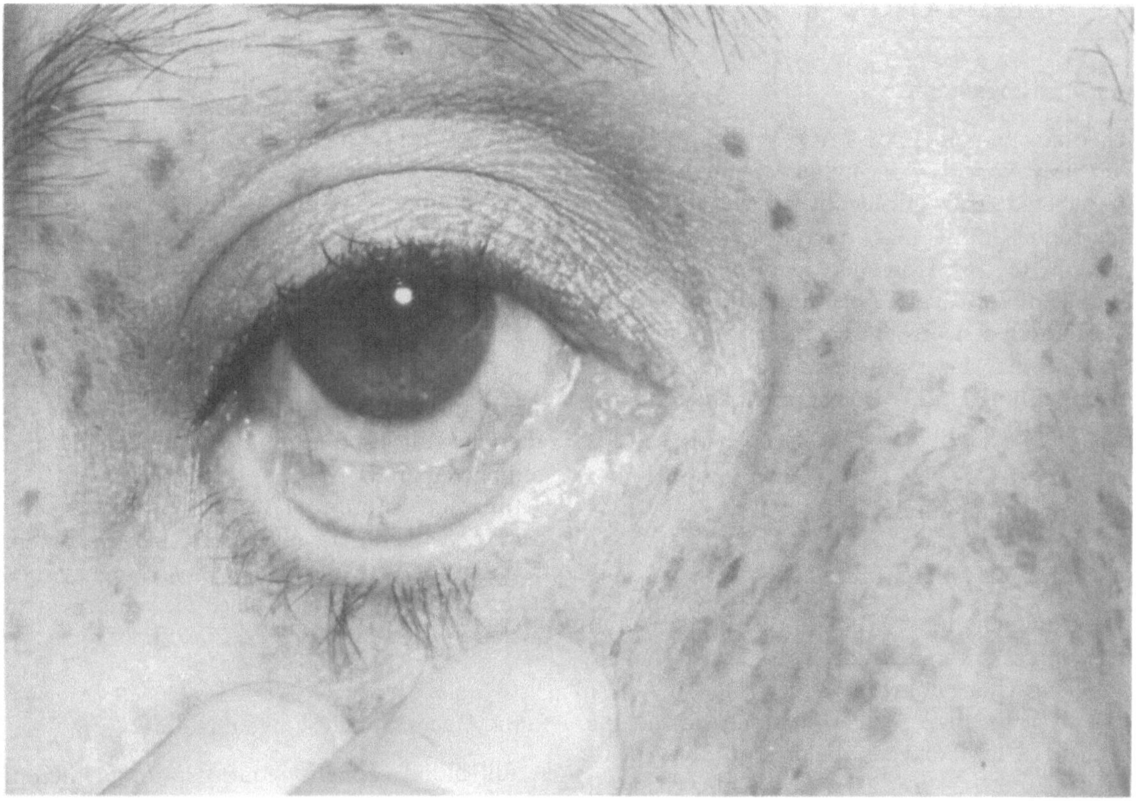

Figure 8.6 LAD: symblepharon in a patient whose disease began in childhood.

adult LAD but is not essential. HLA-B12 which is associated with ocular cicatricial pemphigoid [35] is not increased [13, 16].

8.4 DIFFERENTIAL DIAGNOSIS

Many LAD patients are not clinically diagnosed, are puzzling and often described as 'atypical' forms of other diseases, such as erythema multiforme, DH and BP. The commonest diseases causing confusion are listed below:

1. Erythema multiforme (Chapter 17) is distinguished by its acral distribution and target lesions, even though the combination of annular lesions with hand, foot and mucosal involvement in LAD may cause misdiagnosis. The histopathology and negative immunofluorescence establish the diagnosis.
2. Dermatitis herpetiformis (Chapter 11) is distinguished by the characteristic grouped papulovesicles on the extensor surfaces of the elbows and knees and the presence of granular IgA deposits in the dermal papillae and presence of gluten-sensitive enteropathy. However, many LAD patients were previously regarded as having DH.
3. Bullous pemphigoid (Chapter 5) may be indistinguishable from LAD clinically and histopathologically, but the presence of annular and mucosal lesions points toward a diagnosis of LAD; the diagnosis is confirmed by the response to dapsone and the immunofluorescent pattern.

8.5 INVESTIGATIONS

8.5.1 Histopathology

The histopathology of LAD is not diagnostic. An early vesicular or bullous lesion will show a subepidermal blister with eosinophils or neutrophils, or papillary microabscesses as in DH [12, 13, 15, 36]. However, the histology is closer to that of DH than BP in the majority of cases. The pattern of neutrophils at the dermo–epidermal junction has been suggested to be helpful in distinguishing LAD from DH [37] but this technique is not in routine use.

8.5.2 Immunofluorescence

(a) Direct immunofluorescence

Direct immunofluorescence can be performed on perilesional or clinically uninvolved skin from any site. The major finding is IgA deposited in a linear pattern at the BMZ. Other immunoreactants, i.e. IgG, C3 or IgM, may also be present [2, 6–10, 12, 15, 16, 20, 22–24, 26, 27]. A case with a change in class of immunoreactant from IgG to IgA has been described [38].

Oral mucosa may show linear deposition of IgA at the BMZ [33]. However, linear BMZ IgA is not found in conjunctiva, although other immunoglobulins may be seen [33].

(b) Indirect immunofluorescence

Intact skin. Indirect immunofluorescence may show circulating IgA anti-BMZ antibody, although this occurs in less than 30% of cases [6, 12, 15, 16, 19, 23, 27, 39]. The titres are usually low (1 : 4 – 1 : 64) and both animal oesophagus or normal human skin may be used as substrate. Although there is no consensus as to which is the best substrate, our recent study suggests normal human conjunctiva may be the most sensitive [33].

Split skin. Linear IgA-anti-BMZ circulating antibody binds to the epidermal side of normal skin or oral mucosa which has been artificially cleaved through the lamina lucida with 1 M NaCl (Chapter 2) [33, 40]. The presence of a circulating IgG anti-BMZ antibody excludes the diagnosis of LAD and would be a feature of bullous pemphigoid or epidermolysis bullosa acquisita.

8.5.3 Immunoelectron microscopy

Direct immunoelectron microscopy has shown IgA deposits in both the lamina lucida [4, 20, 22, 38, 41, 42] and sublamina densa which may be associated with anchoring fibrils [4, 19, 26, 27, 41]. In three cases IgA deposits were found both in the lamina lucida and sublamina densa [25, 30] and in one case altered with time from a lamina lucida to a combined pattern [30].

Indirect immunoelectron microscopy has demonstrated the site of the antigen by the binding of the antibody to normal skin. Five cases have been reported, four of which place the antigen in the sublamina densa region [19, 27, 39].

8.5.4 Haematological investigations

A full blood count is required prior to therapy, and, if the patient is of Asian, Mediterranean or Afro-Caribbean origin, glucose-6-phosphate dehydrogenase deficiency should be excluded prior to therapy with dapsone or sulphonamides as deficiency of this enzyme will increase the incidence of drug-induced haemolysis.

8.6 SYSTEMIC MANIFESTATIONS, ASSOCIATED DISEASES AND DRUG ASSOCIATIONS

8.6.1 Systemic manifestations

It is very rare for LAD to have any systemic manifestations other than those arising from mucosal involvement, e.g. difficulties with eating.

8.6.2 Associated diseases

A number of diseases have been described in association with LAD but it is uncertain whether this finding is of biological significance [14].

(a) Gastrointestinal disease

Gluten-sensitive enteropathy (GSE). This was extensively investigated because LAD was considered a variant of DH. Some patients with LAD do have GSE (defined by abnormal jejunal morphology or raised intraepithelial lymphocyte counts) [4, 9, 10, 12, 16, 27]; however, the incidence is low (4–30%). It has been suggested that GSE is specifically associated with sublamina densa deposition of IgA [41] but this has not been confirmed [27]. Anti-gliadin antibodies were not detected in one series [12] but in another study titres of IgA but not IgG anti-gliadin antibodies were elevated compared to controls [43]. Anti-endomysial antibodies have not been detected [44] and anti-reticulin antibodies are absent [12]. There is certainly not the close association between GSE and LAD as is observed in DH (see Chapter 11).

Other gastrointestinal diseases. Ulcerative colitis and gastric hypochlorhydria have been described in association with LAD [13].

(b) Autoimmune diseases

There are two reports of systemic lupus erythematosus (SLE) in association with LAD [2, 18] and bullous LE may be associated with linear IgA deposition (see Chapter 9 and 18).

Thyrotoxicosis has been reported [9] and of our 30 LAD patients one is hypothyroid and two have vitiligo. An autoimmune haemolytic anaemia combined with a labile erythrocyte sedimentation rate (ESR) has been reported [23]. About 50% of patients may have autoantibodies [12].

(c) Other diseases

Rheumatoid arthritis has been reported in a LAD patient [2] and we have seen two patients who have polymyalgia rheumatica. Immune nephritis has been reported in a single case [32].

(d) Malignancy

There are reports in the literature of both carcinomas and lymphomas in association with LAD. Five patients with LAD and lymphoma have been reported [13, 16, 45–47], and in our series one patient developed LAD during therapy for lymphoma and another developed myeloma after remission of LAD [16]. Polycythaemia rubra vera has been documented in a single case [13]. Carcinoma of breast, bladder and oesophagus, basal cell and eccrine carcinoma are described; three tumours were examined for evidence of deposition of IgA and were negative [8, 13, 45, 48, 49]. We have one patient who presented with LAD and a renal carcinoma simultaneously, and one with an adenocarcinoma uterus preceding her LAD.

8.6.3 Drug associations

There are two reports in the literature of LAD being induced by the non-steroidal anti-inflammatory drug (NSAID) diclonophenac sodium [50, 51]; 12% of our patients had taken NSAIDs prior to the onset of the eruption, and 13% had recently received antibiotics [16]. Provocation by lithium has also been described [52].

8.7 PATHOGENESIS AND RECENT ADVANCES

LAD is characterized by deposition of an IgA antibody at the BMZ. This antibody has recently been shown to be pathogenic [53]. The nature of the antigen is unknown, and current studies are concerned with its ultrastructural localization and identity. The relationship of LAD to CBDC (Chapter 9) remains unclear. They were previously regarded as being totally separate [12, 28] but recently the clinical similarities have been emphasized [16]. LAD has been regarded as IgA pemphigoid [5–8]. Its occurrence with systemic lupus erythematosus [2, 18] and the demonstration of IgA deposition below the lamina densa [4, 12, 19, 26, 27] suggest that LAD might in some cases be the IgA counterpart of epidermolysis bullosa acquisita (EBA) (see Chapter 10).

8.7.1 The antigen

(a) Ultrastructural localization

The ultrastructural localization of the LAD antigen has been studied using both immunofluorescence and immunoelectron microscopic techniques.

Immunoelectron microscopy has demonstrated a lamina lucida site for the antigen in a single case [39] and sublamina densa position in four cases [19, 27, 39]. Similar results showing a sublamina densa antigen have been obtained with CBDC [27].

Immunofluoroscence using normal skin artificially blistered through the lamina lucida by suction or by 1 M NaCl has given different results. Using the suction blister, sera from three patients with LAD have been studied and in all cases the antigen has been demonstrated on the dermal side of the blister suggesting the antigen is in the low lamina lucida or below the lamina densa. Two of these sera also demonstrated an epidermal, i.e. lamina lucida, component of the antigen [54]. Similar binding was observed in CBDC [54]. Using NaCl-split skin or mucosa, in all cases the antigen was demonstrated on the epidermal side of both normal skin and normal oral mucosa (Figure 8.7), suggesting that there is a lamina lucida component of the antigen [33, 40]. The same has been found in CBDC [33, 40, 55]. The paradox in these results is that both a lamina lucida and a sublamina densa site have been demonstrated for the antigen. It may well be that the antigen is predominantly intracellular as has been shown for BP [56, 57] and this pool is exposed by prolonged incubation with 1 M NaCl [33]. The extracellular antigen may be incorporated into the lamina densa or sublamina

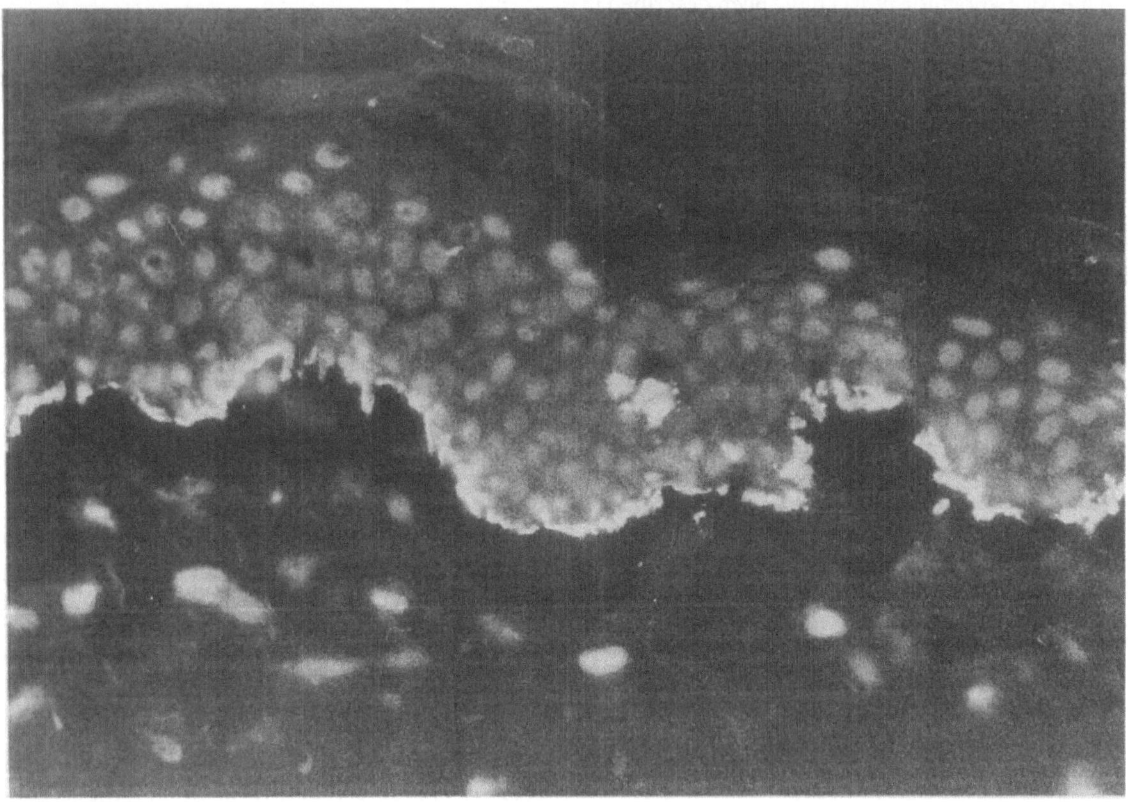

Figure 8.7 Epidermal binding of LAD anti-BMZ antibody to roof of artificially cleaved (1 M NaCl) skin (× 40).

densa, and these epitopes are demonstrated both by immunoelectron microscopy and in suction blisters.

(b) Tissue distribution of the antigen

The antigen has been demonstrated in normal human skin, oral mucosa, conjunctiva, oesophagus, bronchus and vagina [21, 33, 58]. It is therefore present in all stratified squamous epithelia, but absent from neoplastic human bladder [48, 58] and also from normal pig and rodent bladder [58]. Human placenta contains the antigen in the amnion BMZ [58]. It is absent from other epithelial and non-epithelial tissues. The antigen is also present in primates and other mammalian species [58].

(c) Immunoblotting

The LAD antibody does not cross-react with BP [38] and preliminary immunoblotting studies have identified an antigen present in dermal extracts and differing from the BP and EBA antigens [59].

(d) Relationship to chronic bullous disease of childhood

There are marked clinical similarities between CBDC and adult LAD [14, 16] and they share a common immunopathology (see Chapter 9). The ultrastructural localization of the antigen(s) in CBDC and adult LAD is identical using both immunoelectron microscopy and split-skin methods [27, 40, 54] as is the tissue distribution [58]. Preliminary immunoblotting studies suggest that in some patients with CBDC and LAD the BMZ antibody is directed against the same antigen [59].

(e) Relationship to bullous pemphigoid and epidermolysis bullosa acquisita

It is most unlikely that the antigen in LAD is the BP antigen (Chapter 5), because the antigen in many cases has been shown to be below the lamina densa [19, 27, 39]. Suction blister studies have shown a dermal component [54] and the LAD antigen is absent from bladder in which the BP antigen is easily demonstrated [58, 60]. Preliminary immunoblotting studies support this difference [38, 59].

The immunoelectron microscope studies on the LAD antigen suggested that in some patients it might be identical to the EBA antigen (Chapter 10); however, the demonstration of an epidermal-associated epitope with split-skin studies [40, 54] and the differences in species expression [58] suggest that the EBA and LAD antigens are not identical, and immunoblotting has confirmed this [59].

8.7.2 The antibody

Studies on the antibody have comprised its *in vitro* deposition, both as regards relationship to the lesions and also the ultrastructural site of deposition, the nature of the antibodies, the pathogenic role of the antibody and the reason for these patients mounting an IgA response.

(a) Deposition of the antibody in vivo

IgA deposition at the BMZ can be demonstrated in perilesional and clinically uninvolved skin. There is no variation between three sites (forearm, buttock and extensor thigh) (unpublished observations). There is deposition in clinically uninvolved oral mucosa. However, despite the frequent clinical ocular involvement, linear IgA at the BMZ has not been demonstrated in bulbar conjunctiva, even though other immunoreactants present in skin or oral mucosa were retained [33]. This implies either that antibody deposition may not be essential for clinical disease or that there is a specific conjunctival mechanism for clearing IgA.

(b) Ultrastructural site of antibody deposition

Immunoelectron microscopy has demonstrated the antibody in the lamina lucida [4, 14, 20, 22, 38, 41, 42] combined with the sublamina densa [25, 30] and also below the lamina densa [4, 14, 19, 26, 27, 41] (Figure 8.8). Suction blisters have demonstrated antibody on both the epidermal and dermal sides of the split [54], implying lamina lucida and possible sublamina densa deposition.

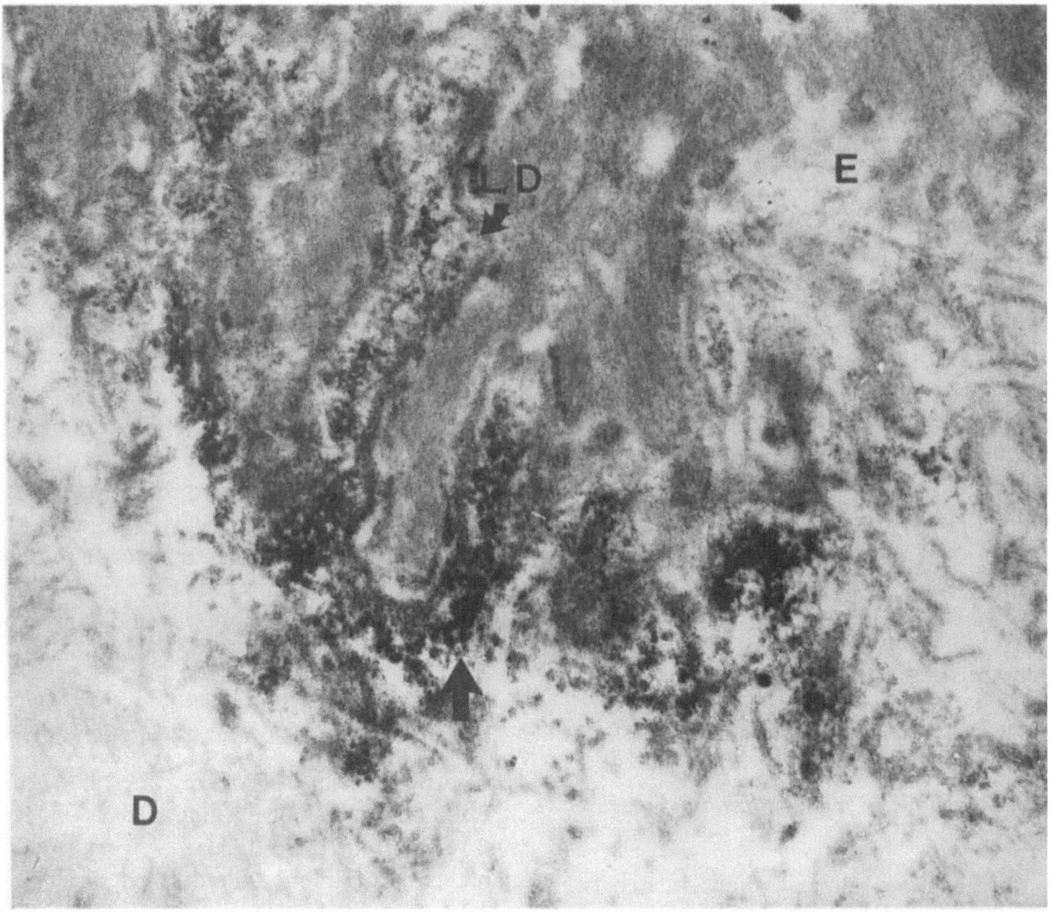

Figure 8.8 Direct immunoelectron microscopy showing antibody deposition in sublamina densa. E, epidermis; D, dermis; LD, lamina densa; the arrow points to the immunoreactants (× 20 000).

(c) The nature of the antibody

There are two subclasses of IgA, IgA_1 and IgA_2, of which IgA_1 is the dominant subclass in serum and IgA_2 in mucosa. In addition, IgA that has been secreted by mucosal tissue is dimeric and contains J chains and this is not usually demonstrated in LAD unless IgM is also present [61]. This implies that the antibody may not originate from mucosa-associated lymphoid tissue, and contrasts with DH in which J chain is present in the skin [62]. The IgA deposited in skin in LAD is almost always IgA_1 (11/12) [63] and (4/4) [63a], again suggesting that the IgA originates in most cases from blood or bone marrow lymphocytes.

(d) The pathogenicity of the antibody

An *in vitro* model using normal human skin cultured in the presence of IgA anti-BMZ antibody has demonstrated the ability of the antibody to bind to the BMZ and to induce dermo–epidermal separation.Complement was not required for the separation which was, however, prevented by proteinase inhibitors [53].

(e) IgA secretion

LAD patients may preferentially mount an IgA response as they have relatively higher titres of IgA anti-gliadin antibodies than IgG antibodies [43].

However, we have not been able to demonstrate increased IgA production by peripheral blood lymphocytes [64].

8.7.3 Other factors

There is evidence that the neutrophils in patients with LAD show enhanced production of oxygen radicals, and this can be transferred to normal neutrophils by LAD serum [65]. This may relate to the induction of blisters, as the presence of IgA deposits does not result in blistering unless the inflammatory cascade is initiated for which proteinases but not complement are necessary [53].

Dapsone is an inhibitor of active oxygens generated by neutrophils [66] and this may relate to its beneficial effects in LAD.

8.8 TREATMENT

The majority of patients with LAD respond to dapsone or sulphonamides, e.g. sulphapyridine and sulphamethoxypyridazine [2, 4–9, 12, 13, 15, 16, 19, 22, 25, 27]. Response is rapid within 48 h [12]. It may be impossible to achieve sufficient doses of these drugs to obtain full control, and prednisone in doses up to 40 mg daily may be necessary to achieve control in a minority of patients [5, 6, 9, 12, 13, 15, 16, 20, 21, 23, 24, 26, 27]. Prednisone alone has been successful in a few cases [5, 7, 10, 12], but has also been unsuccessful despite combination with azathioprine or cyclophosphamide [18, 32, 67]. Azathioprine with dapsone was helpful in one patient [13]. A gluten-free diet is not of benefit [68].

8.8.1 Dapsone

The average dose of dapsone to control the eruption is 100 mg daily [12] but doses as high as 300 or 500 mg daily may be required [12, 22]. The main problems with dapsone are haemolytic anaemia which is universal, but can be precipitous in glucose-6-phosphate dehydrogenase-deficient patients and methaemoglobinaemia. This combination can result in angina, cardiac failure and even myocardial infarction. Dapsone must be used with caution in elderly patients, starting with 50 mg daily, or an alternative drug should be used (see Chapter 11). The dose is increased every 2–3 weeks until control is achieved or side effects become intolerable, and then every few months the patient attempts to reduce the dose. Neutropenia is rare. A full blood count should be performed every 2 weeks in the first 2 months of treatment and, when on a stable dose, every 1–2 months. Many patients feel unwell and complain of lassitude and headache on dapsone, which resolves on transfer to another drug.

We have used dapsone in two patients who have previously had cutaneous reactions to sulphonamides or a history of such without a recurrence of the eruption.

8.8.2 Sulphonamides

The most widely used sulphonamides are sulphamethoxypyridazine and sulphapyridine. Sulphamethoxypyridazine is used at doses of 500 mg – 1.5 g daily, and is our second-line treatment. Sulphapyridine (0.5 – 3 g daily) has been used, but often makes patients feel unwell. Neutropenia or agranulocytosis and severe cutaneous reactions (toxic epidermal necrolysis and erythema multiforme) (Chapter 17) are the potential hazards of sulphonamide therapy. Frequent full blood counts, particularly during the first few months of therapy, are mandatory. Reduction of dosage to control the eruption should be attempted every few months.

The combination of dapsone and sulphamethoxypyridazine has been useful in some of our patients who could not be controlled on either drug alone.

8.8.3 Prednisone

Prednisone in high doses (30–120 mg) may suppress the eruption but is usually used in doses of 5–30 mg daily in addition to dapsone or sulphonamides to achieve complete control.

8.8.4 Colchicine

There is a single report of successful treatment with colchicine (1.5 mg daily) [67].

8.8.5 Topical therapy

Topical therapy with potent (betamethasone valerate, 0.1% etc.) or very potent (clobetasol propionate, 0.05%) steroids may be helpful in suppressing a minor eruption and thus obviating the need for increased dosage of systemic therapy. Topical steroids may be very useful in alleviating mucosal symptoms, conjunctivitis and also oral erosions (see Chapter 3) which often do not respond as well as the skin to systemic therapy.

8.9 PROGNOSIS AND SEQUELAE

8.9.1 Prognosis

The early literature is rather gloomy about the prognosis of LAD with only four papers mentioning remission, i.e. absence of lesions off all treatment, and giving a remission rate of 10–15% [12, 13, 48, 68]. However, our own experience and that of Chorzelski *et al.* are somewhat different with remission rates of 30% [69] and 48% [16]. We have now followed 30 patients for a number of years and the current remission rate is 60%, most of those remitting within 2 years and losing their immune deposits from the skin. In some patients there are no cutaneous lesions but the mucous membranes have continued to be active.

8.9.2 Sequelae

The long-term sequelae concern the mucous membranes. Mucous membrane involvement can be severe and persistent [16, 21, 31]. There have been no reports of blindness due to ocular involvement, unlike cases beginning in childhood [34], but until the disease has been studied for longer it is too early to exclude that possibility and at present ophthalmic monitoring is advised.

8.9.3 Malignancy

The other cause for concern is the number of cases associated with lymphoma and carcinoma. It is not known if this is a chance occurrence or whether it reflects a genetic predisposition to both LAD and lymphoma, a common cause, or cross-reaction between skin and tumour.

REFERENCES

1. Seah, P.P. and Fry, L. (1975) Immunoglobulins in the skin in dermatitis herpetiformis and their relevance in diagnosis. *Brit. J. Dermatol.*, **92**, 157–66.
2. Davies, M.G., Marks, R. and Nuki, G. (1978) Dermatitis herpetiformis a skin manifestation of a generalized disturbance in immunity. *Q.J. Med.*, **186**, 221–48.
3. Katz, S.I. and Strober, W. (1978) The pathogenesis of dermatitis herpetiformis. *J. Invest. Dermatol.*, **70**, 63–75.
4. Lawley, T.J., Strober, W., Yaoita, H. and Katz, S.I. (1980) Small intestinal biopsies and HLA types in dermatitis herpetiformis patients with granular and linear IgA skin deposits. *J. Invest. Dermatol.*, **74**, 9–12.
5. Provost, T.T., Maize, J.C., Razzak Ahmed, A., *et al.* (1979) Unusual subepidermal bullous diseases with immunologic features of bullous pemphigoid. *Arch. Dermatol.*, **115**, 156–60.
6. Honeyman, J.F., Robles Honeyman, A., De la Parra, M.A., *et al.* (1979) Polymorphic pemphigoid. *Arch. Dermatol.*, **115**, 423–7.
7. Van Joost, Th., Faber, W.R., Westerhof, W. and de Mari, F. (1979) Linear dermo–epidermal IgA deposition in bullous pemphigoid. *Acta Dermatovenereol. (Stockholm)*, **59**, 463–5.
8. Russell Jones, R. and Goolamali, S.K. (1980) IgA bullous pemphigoid: a distinct blistering disorder. *Brit. J. Dermatol.*, **102**, 719–25.
9. Chorzelski, T.P. and Jablonska, S. (1975) Diagnostic significance of the immunofluorescent pattern in dermatitis herpetiformis. *Int. J. Dermatol.*, **14**, 429–36.
10. Jablonska, S., Chorzelski, T.P. Beutner, E.H., *et al.* (1976) Dermatitis herpetiformis and bullous pemphigoid. *Arch. Dermatol.*, **112**, 45–8.
11. Wojnarowska, F. (1980) Linear IgA dapsone responsive bullous dermatosis. *J. R. Soc. Med.*, **73**, 371–3.
12. Leonard, J.N., Haffenden, G.P., Ring, N.P., *et al.* (1982) Linear IgA disease in adults. *Brit. J. Dermatol.*, **107**, 301–16.
13. Mobacken, H., Kastrup, W., Ljunghall, K., *et al.* (1983) Linear IgA dermatosis: a study of ten adult patients. *Acta Dermatovenereol. (Stockholm)*, **63**, 123–8.
14. Meurer, M., Schmoeckel, C. and Braun-Falco, O. (1984) Dermatitis herpetiformis Duhring mit lineären Ablagerungen von IgA (lineäre IgA-Dermatose). *Hautarzt*, **35**, 230–9.

15. Wilson, B.D., Beutner, E.H., Kumar, V., *et al.* (1986) Linear IgA bullous dermatosis: an immunologically defined disease. *Int. J. Dermatol.*, **24**, 564–74.
16. Wojnarowska, F., Marsden, R.A., Bhogal, B. and Black, M.M. (1988) Chronic bullous disease of childhood, childhood cicatricial pemphigoid and linear IgA disease of adults, a comparative study demonstrating clinical and immunopathological overlap. *J. Amer. Acad. Dermatol.*, **19**, 792–805.
17. Hashimoto, K., Miki, Y., Nishioka, K., *et al.* (1980) HLA antigens in dermatitis herpetiformis among Japanese. *J. Dermatol.*, **7**, 289–91.
18. Thaipisuttikul, Y., Piamphongsant, T. and Suwanwela, N. (1983) Coexistence of linear IgA dermatitis herpetiformis and systemic lupus erythematosus. *J. Dermatol.*, **10**, 161–6.
19. Pehamberger, H., Konrad, K. and Holubar, K. (1977) Circulating IgA anti-basement membrane antibodies in linear dermatitis herpetiformis (Duhring): immunofluorescence and immunoelectronmicroscopic studies. *J. Invest. Dermatol.*, **9**, 490–3.
20. Dabrowski, J., Chorzelski, T.P., Jablonska, S., *et al.* (1978) The ultrastructural localization of IgA in skin of a patient with mixed form of dermatitis herpetiformis and bullous pemphigoid. *J. Invest. Dermatol.*, **70**, 76–9.
21. Verhelst, G., Demedts, M., Verschakelen, J. *et al.* (1987) Adult linear IgA bullous dermatosis with bronchial involvement. *Brit. J. Dermatol.*, **116**, 587–90.
22. Yaoita, H., Hertz, K.C. and Katz, S.I. (1976) Dermatitis herpetiformis: immunoelectron-microscopic and ultrastructural studies of a patient with linear deposition of IgA. *J. Invest. Dermatol.*, **67**, 691–5.
23. Dahle, J.S., Tjora, S., Daae, L.N.W. and Wereide, K. (1979) Mixed bullous disease with labile erythrocyte sedimentation rate. *Acta Dermatovenereol. (Stockholm)*, **59**, 531–3.
24. Falk, E.S. and Rekvig, O.P. (1980) Mixed form of dermatitis herpetiformis and bullous pemphigoid. *Acta Dermatovenereol. (Stockholm)*, **60**, 229–34.
25. Yamasaki, Y., Hashimoto, T. and Nishikawa, T. (1982) Dermatitis herpetiformis with linear IgA deposition: ultrastructural localization of *in vivo* bound IgA. *Acta Dermatovenereol. (Stockholm)*, **62**, 401–5.
26. Tanita, Y., Masu, S., Kato, T. and Tagami, H. (1986) Linear IgA bullous dermatosis clinically simulating pemphigus vulgaris. *Arch. Dermatol.*, **122**, 246–8.
27. Bhogal, B., Wojnarowska, F., Marsden, R.A., *et al.* (1987) Linear IgA bullous dermatosis of adults and children: an immunoelectron microscopic study. *Brit. J. Dermatol.*, **117**, 289–96.
28. Marsden, R.A., McKee, P.H., Bhogal, B., *et al.* (1980) A study of benign chronic bullous dermatosis of childhood and comparison with dermatitis herpetiformis and bullous pemphigoid occurring in childhood. *Clin. Exp. Dermatol.*, **5**, 159–72.
29. Kumar, V., Rogozinski, T., Yarbrough, C., *et al.* (1980) A case of cicatricial pemphigoid or cicatricial linear IgA bullous dermatosis. *J. Amer. Acad. Dermatol..*, **2**, 327–31.
30. Dabrowski, J., Chorzelski, T., Jablonska, S., *et al.* (1979) Immunoelectron microscopic studies in IgA linear dermatosis. *Arch. Dermatol. Res.*, **265**, 389–98.
31. Leonard, J.N., Wright, P., Williams, D.M., *et al.* (1984) The relationship between linear IgA disease and benign mucous membrane pemphigoid. *Brit. J. Dermatol.*, **110**, 307–14.
32. Van Joost, T., Muntendam, J., Heule, F., *et al.* (1986) Subepidermal bullous autoimmune disease associated with immune nephritis. *J. Amer. Acad. Dermatol.*, **14**, 214–20.
33. Kelly, S.F., Frith, P.A., Millard, P.R., *et al.* (1988) A clinicopathological study of mucosal involvement in linear IgA disease. *Brit. J. Dermatol.*, **119**, 161–70.
34. Wojnarowska, F., Marsden, R.A., Bhogal, B. and Black, M.M. (1984) Childhood cicatricial pemphigoid with linear IgA deposits. *Clin. Exp. Dermatol.*, **9**, 407–15.
35. Mondino, B.J., Brown, S.I. and Rabin, B.S. (1978) HLA antigens in ocular cicatricial pemphigoid. *Brit. J. Ophthalmol.*, **62**, 265–7.
36. Blenkinsopp, W.K., Haffenden, G.P., Fry, L. and Leonard, J.N. (1983) Histology of linear IgA disease, dermatitis herpetiformis, and bullous pemphigoid. *Amer. J. Dermatopathol.*, **5**, 547–54.
37. Smith, S.B., Harrist, T.J., Murphy, G.F., *et al.* (1984) Linear IgA bullous dermatosis *v* dermatitis herpetiformis: quantitative measurements of dermoepidermal alterations. *Arch. Dermatol.*, **120**, 324–8.
38. Petersen, M.J., Gammon, W.R. and Briggaman, R.A. (1986) A case of linear IgA disease presenting initially with IgG immune deposits. *J. Amer. Acad. Dermatol.*, **14**, 1014–19.
39. Yaoita, H. and Katz, S.I. (1977) Circulating IgA anti-basement membrane zone antibodies in dermatitis herpetiformis. *J. Invest. Dermatol.*, **69**, 558–60.
40. Wojnarowska, F., Pothupitiya, G.M., Bhogal, B.S., *et al.* (1987) in *Immunodermatology* (ed. R. Caputo), CIC Edizioni Internazionali, Roma, pp. 237–40.
41. Haffenden, G.P., Ring, N.P., Leonard, J.N. and Fry, L. (1983) Immuno electron microscopical studies in patients with linear IgA deposits. *J. Invest. Dermatol.*, **80**, 363 (abstract).
42. Prost, C., Dubertret, L., Fosse, M., *et al.* (1984) A routine immunoelectron microscopic technique for localizing an auto-antibody on epidermal basement membrane. *Brit. J. Dermatol.*, **110**, 1–7.

43. Ciclitira, P.J., Ellis, H.J., Venning, V.A., *et al.* (1986) Circulating antibodies to gliadin subfractions in dermatitis herpetiformis and linear IgA dermatosis of adults and children. *Clin. Exp. Dermatol.*, **11**, 502–9.
44. Beutner, E.H., Chorzelski, T.P., Kumar, V., *et al.* (1986) Sensitivity and specificity of Iga-class antiendomysial antibodies for dermatitis herpetiformis and findings relevant to their pathogenic significance. *J. Amer. Acad. Dermatol.*, **15**, 464–73.
45. Leonard, J.N., Tucker, W.F.G., Fry, J.S., *et al.* (1983) Increased incidence of malignancy in dermatitis herpetiformis. *Brit. Med. J.*, *286*, 16–18.
46. Vignon, D., Guillaume, J.C., Revuz, J. and Touraine, R. (1982) Association maladie de Hodgkin et dermatose à IgA linéaire. *La Nouv. Presse Méd.*, **11**, 603–4 (lettre).
47. Kienzler, J.-L., Blanc, D., Laurent, R. and Agache, P. (1983) Dermatose bulleuse a IgA linéaire et maladie de Hodgkin. *Ann. Dermatol. Venereol. (Paris)*, **110**, 727–8.
48. Sekula, S.A., Tschen, J.A., Bean, S.F. and Wolf, J.E. (1986) Linear IgA bullous disease in a patient with transitional cell carcinoma of the bladder. *Cutis.*, **38**, 354–62.
49. Green, S.T. and Natarajan, S. (1987) Linear IgA disease and oesophageal carcinoma. *J. R. Soc. Med.*, **80**, 48.
50. Gabrielsen, T.Ø. Stærfelt, F. and Thune, P.O. (1981) Drug-induced bullous dermatosis with linear IgA deposits along the basement membrane. *Acta Dermatovenereol. (Stockholm)*, **61**, 439–41.
51. Valsecchi, R., Tornaghi, A., Serra, M. and Cainelli, T. (1951) Dermatosi bollosa da farmaco a IgA lineari. *Giorn. It. Dermatol. Venereol.*, **117**, 221–3.
52. McWhirter, J.D., Hashimoto, K., Fayne, S. and Ito, K. (1987) Linear IgA bullous dermatosis related to lithium carbonate. *Arch. Dermatol.*, **123**, 1120–2.
53. Akahoshi, Y., Kanda, G., Anan, S. and Yoshida, H. (1987) Dermoepidermal blister formation by linear IgA dermatosis sera in normal human skin in organ culture. *J. Dermatol.*, **14**, 352–8.
54. Aboobaker, J., Bhogal, B., Wojnarowska, F. *et al.* (1987) The localization of the binding site of circulating IgA antibodies in linear IgA disease of adults, chronic bullous disease of childhood and childhood cicatricial pemphigoid. *Brit. J. Dermatol.*, **116**, 293–302.
55. Roberts, L.J. and Sontheimer, R.D. (1987) Chronic bullous dermatosis of childhood: immunopathologic studies. *Paediatr. Dermatol.*, **4**, 6–10.
56. Mutasim, D.F., Takahashi, Y., Labib, R.S., *et al.* (1985) A pool of bullous pemphigoid antigen(s) is intracellular and associated with the basal cell cytoskeleton-hemidesmosome complex. *J. Invest. Dermatol.*, **84**, 47–53.
57. Westgate, G.E., Weaver, A.C. and Couchman, J.R. (1985) Bullous pemphigoid antigen localization suggests an intracellular association with hemidesmosomes. *J. Invest. Dermatol.*, **84**, 218–24.
58. Pothupitiya, G.M., Wojnarowska, F., Bhogal, B.S. and Black, M.M. (1988) Distribution of the antigen in adult linear IgA disease and chronic bullous dermatosis of childhood suggests that it is a single and unique antigen. *Brit. J. Dermatol.*, **118**, 175–82.
59. Wojnarowska, F., Whitehead, P., Bhogal, B., *et al.* (1988) Characterisation of the antigen in chronic bullous dermatosis of childhood and adult linear IgA disease. *Brit. J. Dermatol.*, **118**, 268 (abstract).
60. Diaz, L.A., Weiss, H.J. and Calvanico, N.J. (1978) Phylogenetic studies with pemphigus and pemphigoid antibodies. *Acta Dermatovenereol. (Stockholm)*, 58, 535–9.
61. Leonard, J.N., Haffenden, G.P., Unsworth, D.J., *et al.* (1984) Evidence that the IgA in patients with linear IgA disease is qualitatively different from that of patients with dermatitis herpetiformis. *Brit. J. Dermatol.*, **110**, 315–21.
62. Unsworth, D.J., Leonard, J.N., Payne, A.W., *et al.* (1982) IgA in dermatitis herpetiformis skin is dimeric. *Lancet*, **i**, Feb. 478–80.
63. Hall, R.P. and Lawley, T.J. (1985) Characterization of circulating and cutaneous IgA immune complexes in patients with dermatitis herpetiformis. *J. Immunol.*, 135, 1760–5.
63a. Wojnarowska, F., Delacroix, D. and Gengoux, P. (1988) Cutaneous IgA subclasses in dermatitis herpetiformis and linear IgA disease. *J. Cutan. Pathol.*, **15**, 272–8.
64. Wojnarowska, F. and Perl, S. (1989) Normal IgA production by peripheral blood lymphocytes in dermatitis herpetiformis and linear IgA dermatosis. *Arch. Dermatol. Res.*, **280**, 494–6.
65. Niwa, Y., Sakane, T., Shingu, M., *et al.* (1985) Neutrophil-generated active oxygens in linear IgA bullous dermatosis. *Arch. Dermatol.*, **121**, 73–8.
66. Miyachi, Y. and Niwa, Y. (1982) Effects of potassium iodide, colchicine and dapsone on the generation of polymorphonuclear leukocyte-derived oxygen intermediates. *Brit. J. Dermatol.*, **107**, 209–14.
67. Aram, H. (1984) Linear IgA bullous dermatosis: successful treatment with colchicine. *Arch. Dermatol.*, **120**, 960–1.
68. Leonard, J.N., Griffiths, C.E.M., Powles, A.V., *et al.* (1987) Experience with a gluten free diet in the treatment of linear IgA disease. *Acta Dermatol. Venereol. (Stockholm)*, **67**, 145–8.
69. Chorzelski, T.P., Jablonska, S., Beutner, E.H. and Wilson, B.D. (1987) in *Immunopathology of the Skin*, 3rd edn (eds E.H. Beutner, T.P. Chorzelski and V. Kumar), John Wiley & Sons, New York, pp. 407–20.

Nine

Linear IgA disease of childhood (chronic bullous disease of childhood)

R.A. Marsden

9.1 INTRODUCTION

Linear IgA disease of childhood (LADC) (synonyms juvenile dermatitis herpetiformis, juvenile pemphigoid, chronic bullous disease/dermatosis of childhood) is an acquired blistering disorder of childhood characterized by the presence of a linear band of IgA at the dermo–epidermal junction.

In 1873 Tilbury Fox [1] described a child of 11 years with widespread pruritic small blisters consistent with dermatitis herpetiformis. There followed several reports of similar cases during the late 19th century [2] until 1901 when Bowen described a series of 15 children with a non-itchy eruption consisting of large blisters mainly involving the face and genitalia [3, 4]. This is now considered to be the first report of LAD in childhood but in those early days such cases were thought to represent a variant of dermatitis herpetiformis (DH) unique to children. However, descriptions of DH in childhood/LADC in early literature probably included children with bullous pemphigoid, pemphigus, impetigo and erythema multiforme, and as a result many case reports are difficult to interpret. In 1961, Kim and Winkelmann were the first to separate LADC from DH on clinical grounds [5], and in 1970 the term benign chronic bullous dermatosis of childhood was devised in order to emphasize the self-limiting course of the disease [6]. With the advent of immunofluorescence techniques it became evident that most children with this clinical entity had a linear band of IgA at the dermo–epidermal junction [7]. A minority, however, appeared to have linear deposits of IgG and C3 and thus a disease which was clinically and immunopathologically indistinguishable from bullous pemphigoid [8–10]. LADC is now regarded as a distinctive clinical disorder separate from DH and bullous pemphigoid. Recent findings suggest that LADC and linear IgA dermatosis of adults are different expressions of the same disease [11, 12].

9.2 CLINICAL FEATURES

9.2.1 Presentation and incidence

The onset of the disease is usually below the age of 5 years. In a series of 29 cases known to the author in which blistering began before puberty, 19 were aged 5 or less at the onset of their disease. In the same series 18 patients were female and 11 male. Others have found the disease to be more common in males [5]. LADC has been described in Europe, USA, Jamaica [13], Singapore [14], Malaysia [15], Japan [16], Thailand [17], Zimbabwe [18] and among South African blacks and Sri Lankhans [19]. Personal communications suggest that it is relatively common in India and Kenya.

9.2.2 Precipitating factors

Bowen [4] described the disorder occurring after vaccination. Preceding illnesses such as upper respiratory tract infections or antibiotic ingestion

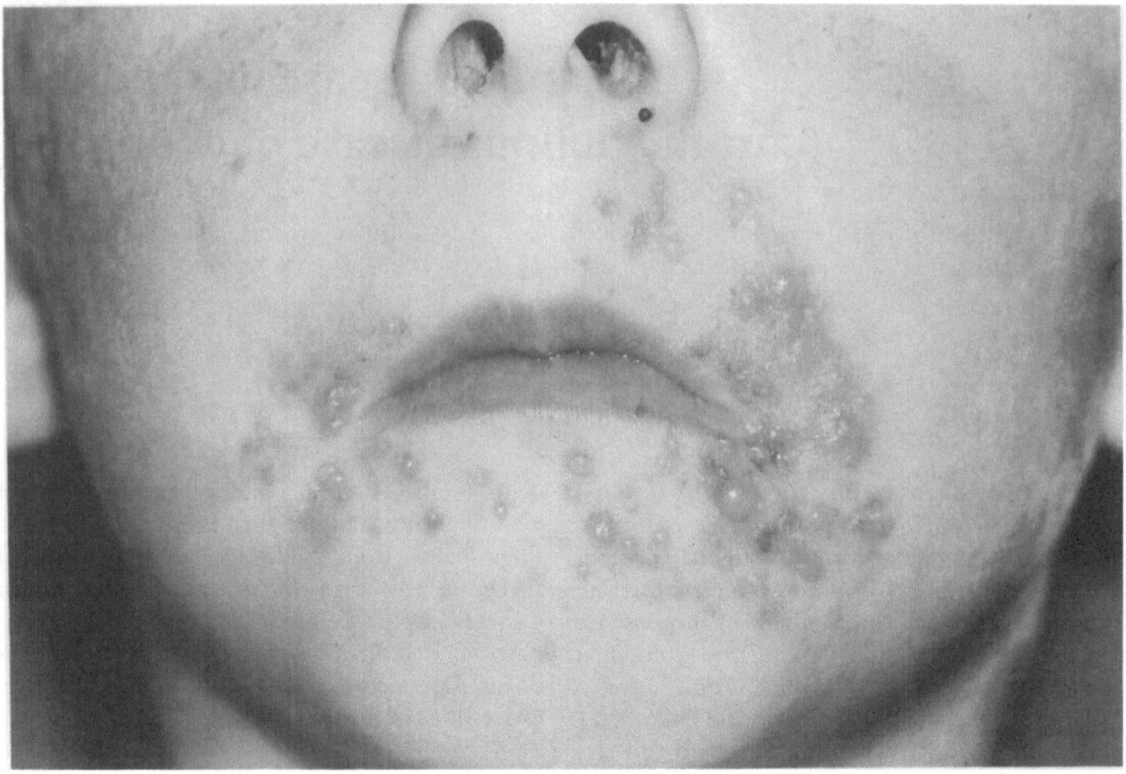

Figure 9.1 Perioral vesicles.

have also been reported [20]. In our own series, 11 out of 29 patients experienced a prodromal illness within 1–2 weeks of the onset of blistering (upper respiratory tract infection, 7; urinary tract infection, 1; measles, 1; typhoid, 1; gastroenteritis, 1) and all were treated with antibiotics mostly of the penicillin group [12]. Two patients have recently been described, one a child the other an adult, with LAD precipitated by a sore throat and fever. In both cases the eruption was accompanied by severe arthralgia [21].

9.2.3 Distribution and morphology of the lesions

Typically the onset is abrupt, with blisters appearing on or near the genitalia or around the mouth (Figures 9.1 and 9.2). In most cases the eruption gradually becomes more extensive and may involve the scalp, eyelids, ears, limbs and the rest of the trunk. In older children, i.e. those aged 7 or more, the eruption may begin on any part of the body and may even spare the pelvic and perioral regions so that in these cases the clinical picture is indistinguishable from that of bullous pemphigoid (Figure 9.3). Pruritus when present is not as intense as that of DH or as painful as that experienced in children with bullous pemphigoid. The bullae, which are sometimes haemorrhagic (Figure 9.4) and may be over a centimetre in diameter, usually arise on normal-looking skin in contrast to the background of urticated erythema seen in many children with bullous pemphigoid. Healing may result in hyperpigmentation but not scarring. New crops of lesions continue to appear spontaneously for several months or years but relapses are not usually as severe as the initial attack. As patients grow older and the disease becomes quiescent, the lesions become predominantly papular or vesicular

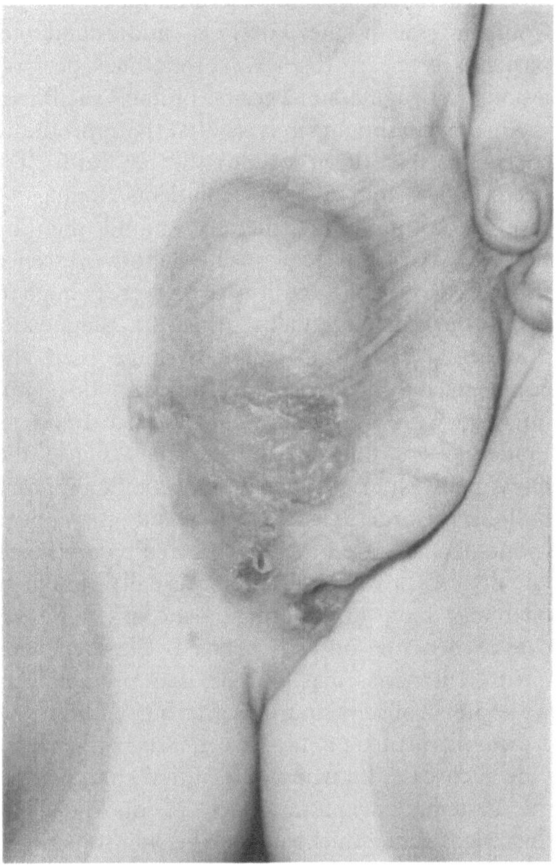

Figure 9.2 Classical scrotal vesicles.

so that the clinical appearance is more like that of DH. 'Jewel-like' clustering of blisters, i.e. fresh vesicles arising around the margin of an old or healing blister, seen in most, but not all, patients during the early stages of the illness, cannot be regarded as diagnostic as it may occur in bullous pemphigoid [10].

9.2.4 Mucous membrane involvement

Mucous membrane involvement is perhaps more common than hitherto suspected. Mouth ulcers and blisters were reported by up to 16 of 29 (55%) patients, and two of these experienced bouts of hoarseness, possibly due to laryngeal involvement. Ocular symptoms such as redness, discomfort and grittiness were described by 14 out of 19 patients (48%) and conjunctival scarring occurred in six out of 29 (21%) patients [12]. One patient developed entropion severe enough to necessitate surgical correction [22] and another became blind at the age of 12 due to corneal damage [23]. The patient illustrated in Figure 8.6 with symblepharon formation first developed her eruption in childhood and then ocular symptoms in adult life. Ocular involvement appears to be more common in those with long-standing disease and it may be relevant that the majority of patients with eye lesions (75%) were HLA-B8-negative [11]. The four patients with severe mucous membrane involvement reported by Wojnarowska *et al.* [23] are now thought to have LADC [12].

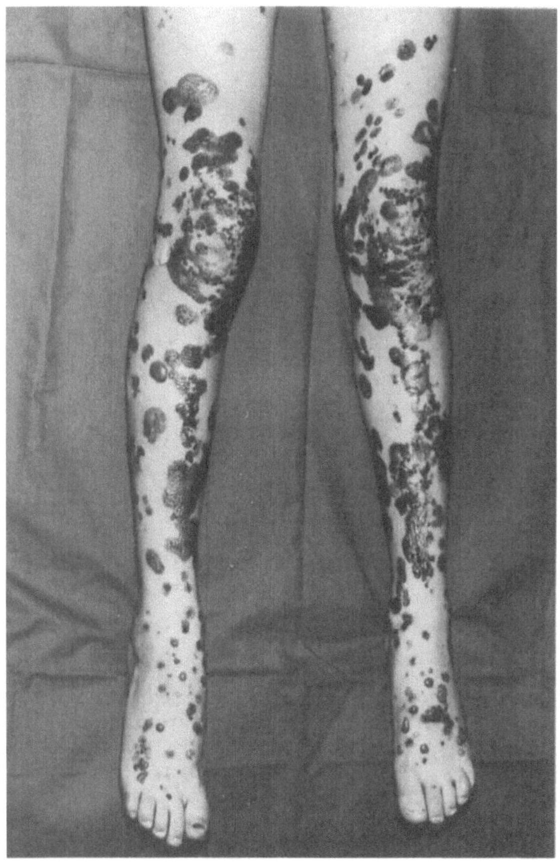

Figure 9.3 This illustrates the extensive nature of the eruption in an older child (age 10). The degree of haemorrhage is most unusual.

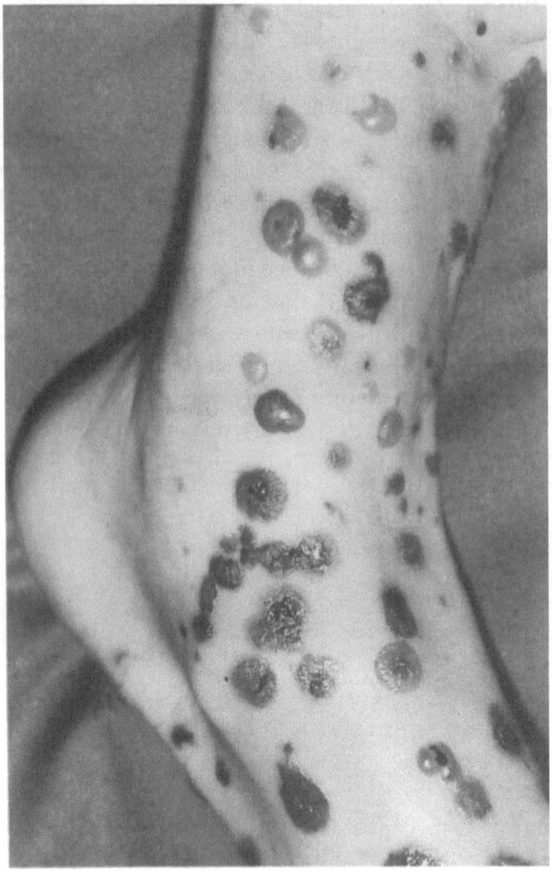

Figure 9.4 Many blisters, some haemorrhagic, arising on a background of normal looking skin. Same patient as in Figure 9.3.

9.3 GENETICS

There are no reports of LADC occurring in families. In 1980 Marsden *et al.* reported a 100% incidence of HLA-B8 in LADC [10] (15 patients were examined). Since then the series has been enlarged and the incidence of HLA-B8 is now 64%, still much higher than in the general population (20–30%) [12].

9.4 DIFFERENTIAL DIAGNOSIS

Patients with LADC are often referred to the dermatologist with a diagnosis of chronic chicken pox, recurrent herpes simplex or bullous impetigo. Confusion with the latter is understandable, particularly in early cases with pronounced perioral lesions. When in doubt a course of flucloxacillin or erythromycin should be given, after the appropriate specimens have been sent to the laboratory for bacteriology and virology. Patients failing to respond to antibiotic therapy should then be biopsied. Where adequate immunofluorescence facilities do not exist or the case is severe enough to justify urgent treatment, then a diagnostic/therapeutic trial of sulphapyridine can be commenced immediately as the drug does not interfere with the immunofluorescence findings. Epidermolysis bullosa simplex, particularly the Dowling Meara type, may mimic an inflammatory bullous disorder, as blisters tend to appear spontaneously, are often surrounded by erythema and do not scar. The condition is usually present at birth but there may be diagnostic difficulties in cases where the onset is delayed. Children with diffuse cutaneous mastocytosis may present with widespread blisters and urticaria but without the typical pigmented papules of urticaria pigmentosa. One such case, known to the author, had neither the systemic symptoms, such as diarrhoea or flushing, nor the thickening of the skin sometimes seen in this disorder, but a biopsy of a blister revealed dermal oedema and an inflammatory infiltrate containing large numbers of mast cells.

As stated above LADC and bullous pemphigoid in children cannot be reliably distinguished from each other on clinical or histological grounds. Direct immunofluorescence or immunoperoxidase techniques are essential. Clinicians without access to such facilities need not despair, however, as both diseases are treated in exactly the same way.

The author has seen several cases of LADC where the initial direct immunofluorescence result was negative and a second biopsy was required to establish the diagnosis. In one patient with the classic pelvic eruption of LADC, two biopsies failed to show IgA but fortunately indirect immunofluorescence showed a circulating IgA antibody. Because of this a third skin biopsy was not deemed necessary. The eruption responded to treatment and eventually went into remission.

9.5 INVESTIGATIONS

9.5.1 Histology

Blisters are subepidermal and in many cases, particularly when the biopsied lesion is more than 24 h old, the findings are relatively non-specific being similar to those seen in the advanced lesions of dermatitis herpetiformis or bullous pemphigoid. However, in the majority of early lesions the findings are best described as DH-like with effacement of dermal papillae in the floor of the blister and an infiltrate containing a large proportion of neutrophils. Papillary neutrophil micro-abscesses may be seen adjacent to the blister [10, 24]. In a minority of cases, however, the infiltrate contains numerous eosinophils and there is festooning of dermal papillae at the base of the blister in a manner reminiscent of bullous pemphigoid. Eosinophilic spongiosis has been described [10]. The histological features in LADC are entirely unpredictable and if one has to decide between a biopsy for histology and a biopsy for immunofluorescence then one should always choose the latter.

9.5.2 Immunopathology

The diagnosis of LADC depends upon the finding of a linear band of IgA at the dermo–epidermal junction. Bands of IgG, IgM or C3 may also be seen upon direct immunofluorescence but these are usually weaker and are often transient. The IgA band itself eventually disappears when the disease is in remission but may be detectable for up to 4 years after the rash has subsided [10]. Treatment appears to have no effect on the direct immunofluorescence findings. Linear IgA deposits have been demonstrated in the mouth but not in the conjunctiva [25]. A 3–4 mm punch biopsy of uninvolved skin is quite adequate for routine diagnostic purposes. Specimens can be obtained from the buttock swiftly and with relative ease. Indeed most children find that the procedure is less traumatic than venepuncture.

A circulating IgA anti-basement membrane zone antibody has been reported in up to 80% of patients with active disease using human skin and rabbit oesophagus substrates [10, 12]. However, titres are often low, i.e. in the 1 : 2 to 1 : 40 range. The use of NaCl-split human skin and human conjunctiva may enhance the detection of circulating antibodies [25]. Both direct and indirect immunoelectron microscopic studies have shown that the IgA antibody is predominantly located beneath the basal lamina in the superficial papillary dermis [26]. However, as in linear IgA disease of adults, there is some controversy regarding the exact binding site, and lamina lucida deposition has been described [16]. Furthermore, indirect immunofluorescence studies using suction blisters, in which the skin is separated through the lamina lucida, have shown that IgA antibody is found in the roof of the blister as well as in the base, thus suggesting that the antigen is present in both the lamina lucida and sublamina region [27]. Similar results have been reported using skin separated chemically using 1 M NaCl [28] which show lamina lucida binding.

9.6 SYSTEMATIC MANIFESTATIONS AND ASSOCIATED DISEASES

There is no firm evidence to suggest that LADC is associated with coeliac disease in spite of a small number of case reports describing such a relationship [13, 29–33]. In the larger series of patients reported to date, jejunal biopsies have been normal, though moderately elevated intraepithelial lymphocyte counts have been found in a few patients. Anti-reticulin and IgA and IgG anti-gliadin antibody titres are within the normal range [9, 10, 12]. If a patient is suspected of having true coeliac disease, rather than transient gluten enteropathy, then a minimum of three jejunal biopsies must be carried out to establish the diagnosis beyond doubt. The first should be taken while the patient is on a normal diet, the second to show recovery of the jejunal mucosa after a gluten-free diet and the third to demonstrate deterioration in response to gluten challenge [34].

9.7 PATHOGENESIS AND RECENT ADVANCES

Pothupitiya *et al.* [35] have shown that the distribution of the LAD antigen in both adults and children is identical. Preliminary immunoblotting studies have been carried out using serum from children and adults with linear IgA dermatosis against keratinocytes and dermal extracts. Both sera reacted against the latter. Not only do these findings suggest that the antigen is dermal in location, they also show that the antigen is identical in both diseases [36]. This is discussed more fully in Chapter 8.

9.8 TREATMENT

Sulphapyridine is still the treatment of choice [37, 38]. An effective dose is 1–2 g daily irrespective of the age or weight of the patient, increasing to 2–3 g daily if there has been no significant improvement within 7 days. When the disease is under control, i.e. when the skin is clear, then the dose can be reduced gradually, sometimes to as little as 0.25 g on alternate days. The dose required to maintain freedom from blisters is entirely unpredictable and may vary from month to month in some patients. The drug is well tolerated by children but if side effects occur, such as allergic rashes, nausea or vomiting, then dapsone (100 mg daily) or sulphamethoxypyridazine (up to 1.5 g daily) can be substituted (bearing in mind that cross-sensitivity occurs between sulphapyridine and sulphamethoxypyridazine). If prednisolone is given, either by itself or as a supplement to sulphapyridine or dapsone, then initial doses in the region of 30 mg daily may be required even in babies and small children. Not all patients respond to sulphapyridine but the author believes that disappointing results can be avoided by giving a sufficiently high dose at the onset of treatment. Clinicians who have difficulty in obtaining supplies of sulphapyridine should contact the manufacturer May and Baker directly.

9.9 PROGNOSIS AND SEQUELAE

LADC is thought of as a benign self-limiting disease invariably resolving before puberty [10, 37]. Unfortunately more recent findings suggest that this is not the case [11, 12, 39]. Half of the patients in our series are in remission, after illnesses persisting for 6 months – 10 years (mean 3.46 years). However, of the 11 patients known to have active disease, seven have had their disease for over 5 years, one for as long as 33 years. Four patients are now well beyond the age of puberty, their current ages being 17, 21, 23 and 39 years; 82% of the patients in remission have HLA-B8 in contrast to only 40% of those with continuing disease [11]. It is possible therefore that the presence or absence of HLA-B8 (and presumably DR3) influences the duration of the disease and possibly even the risk of ocular involvement.

REFERENCES

1. Fox, T. (1873) in *Skin Diseases*, Renshaw, London, pp. 217–22.
2. Alexander, J.O.D. (1975) in *Dermatitis Herpetiformis*, W.B. Saunders Co., London, pp. 31–42.
3. Bowen, J.T. (1901) Five cases of bullous dermatitis (DH) in children following vaccination. *Brit. J. Dermatol.*, **8**, 392–4.
4. Bowen, J.T. (1905) Dermatitis herpetiformis in children. *J. Cutan. Dis.*, **23**, 79–85.
5. Kim, R. and Winkelmann, R.K. (1961) Dermatitis herpetiformis in children. *Arch. Dermatol.*, **83**, 895–902.
6. Jordan, R.E., Bean, S.F., Triftshauser, C.T. and Winkelmann, R.K. (1970) Childhood bullous dermatitis herpetiformis. *Arch. Dermatol.*, **101**, 629–34.
7. Marsden, R.A., Skeete, M.V.H. and Black, M.M. (1979) The chronic acquired bullous diseases of childhood. *Clin. Exp. Dermatol.*, **4**, 227–40.
8. Bean, S.F., Jordan, R.E., Winkelmann, R.K. and Good, R.A. (1971) Chronic non-hereditary blistering diseases in children. *Amer. J. Dis. Childh.*, **122**, 137–41.
9. Chorzelski, T.P. and Jablonska, S. (1979) Linear IgA dermatosis of childhood (chronic bullous diseases of childhood). *Brit. J. Dermatol.*, **101**, 535–42.
10. Marsden, R.A., McKee, P.H., Bhogal, B., *et al.* (1980) A study of benign chronic bullous dermatosis

of childhood and comparison with dermatitis herpetiformis and bullous pemphigoid occurring in childhood. *Clin. Exp. Dermatol.*, 5, 159–72.
11. Marsden, R.A., Wojnarowska, F., McKee, P.H. and Black, M.M. (1988) Chronic bullous disease of *Advances in Diagnosis and Treatment* (eds R. Happle and E. Grosshans), Springer-Verlag, Berlin, pp. 75–81.
12. Wojnarowska, F., Marsden, R.A., Bhogal, B. and Black, M.M. (1989) Chronic bullous disease of childhood, childhood cicatricial pemphigoid and linear IgA disease of adults, a comparative study demonstrating clinical and immunological overlap. *J. Amer. Dermatol.*, 9, 792–805.
13. Warner, J., Brooks, S.E.H., James, W.P.T. and Louisy, S. (1972) Juvenile dermatitis herpetiformis in Jamaica: Clinical and gastrointestinal features. *Brit. J. Dermatol.*, **86**, 226–37.
14. Ratnam, K.V., Lee, C.T. and Tan, T. (1986) Chronic bullous dermatosis of childhood in Singapore. *Int. J. Dermatol.*, **25**, 34–7.
15. Adam, B.A. and Rajagopalan, K. (1979) Immunofluorescence in chronic bullous dermatosis of childhood. *Austr. J. Dermatol.*, **20**, 46–8.
16. Horiguchi, Y., Toda, K.I., Okamoto, H. and Imamura, S. (1986) Immunoelectron-microscopic observations in a case of linear IgA bullous dermatosis of childhood. *J. Amer. Acad. Dermatol.*, **14**, 593–9.
17. Piamphongsant, T., Sirimachan, S. and Himmunknan, P. (1986) Juvenile blistering diseases: the problems of diagnosis and treatment. *Asian-Pacific J. Allergy Immunol.*, **4**, 133–7.
18. Wright, S. and Nkrumah, F.K. (1984) Chronic bullous dermatosis of childhood. *Cent. Afr. J. Med.*, **30**, 165–9.
19. Reid, C., Wojnarowska, F., Pothupitiya, G., *et al.* (1988) Chronic bullous disease of childhood around the world. *Brit. J. Dermatol.*, **119**, Suppl. 33, 41.
20. Berlin, C. (1952) Dermatitis herpetiformis in children. *Brit. J. Dermatol.*, **64**, 281–90.
21. Leigh, G., Marsden, R.A. and Wojnarowska, F. (1988) Linear IgA dermatosis with severe arthralgia. *Brit. J. Dermatol.*, **119**, 789–92.
22. Marsden, R.A. and Greaves, M.W. (1982) Atypical bullous dermatosis of childhood with entropion. *J.R. Soc. Med.*, **75**, 39–41.
23. Wojnarowska, F., Marsden, R.A., Bhogal, B. and Black, M.M. (1984) Childhood cicatricial pemphigoid with linear IgA deposits. *Clin. Exp. Dermatol.*, 9, 407–15.
24. Ackerman, A.B. (1978) Bullous diseases of childhood. In *Histologic Diagnosis of Inflammatory Skin Disease*, Lea and Febiger, Philadelphia, pp. 628–9.
25. Kelly, S.E., Frith, P.A., Millard, P.R., *et al.* (1988) A clinicopathological study of mucosal involvement in linear IgA disease. *Brit. J. Dermatol.*, **119**, 161–70.
26. Bhogal, B., Wojnarowska, F., Marsden, R.A., *et al.* (1987) Linear IgA bullous dermatosis of adults and children. An immunoelectronmicroscopic study. *Brit. J. Dermatol.*, **117**, 289–96.
27. Aboobaker, J., Bhogal, B., Wojnarowska, F., *et al.* (1987) The localisation of circulating IgA antibodies in linear IgA disease, chronic bullous disease of childhood and childhood cicatricial pemphigoid using suction blisters as substrate. *Brit. J. Dermatol.*, **116**, 293–303.
28. Wojnarowska, F., Pothupitiya, G.M., Bhogal, B., *et al.* (1987) in *Immunodermatology* (ed. R. Caputo), CIC Edizioni Internazionali, Rome, pp. 237–9.
29. Meenan, F.O.C. and Cahalane, S.F. (1969) Bullous pemphigoid of childhood and coeliac disease. *Brit. J. Dermatol.*, **81**, 777–9.
30. Del Forno, C., Giannetti, A. and Orecchia, G. (1979) Chronic bullous dermatosis of childhood. *Acta Dermatovenereol. (Stockholm)*, **59**, 178–80.
31. Brandrup, F. and Schmidt, H. (1981) Benign chronic bullous dermatosis associated with coeliac disease. *Clin. Exp. Dermatol.*, **6**, 569–70.
32. Marsden, R.A. (1981) Benign chronic bullous dermatosis of childhood associated with coeliac disease – a reply. *Clin. Exp. Dermatol.*, **6**, 570–1.
33. Meurer, M., Kuhnle, U. and Bertele-Harms, R. (1984) Dermatosis herpetiformis Duhring with coeliac disease and growth retardation: Rapid and complete remission with gluten-free diet. *Clinical Case Report, First Congress of the European Society for Pediatric Dermatology*, Munster, 4–7 October, 1984.
34. Meeuwisse, G.W. (1970) Diagnostic criteria in coeliac disease. *Acta Paediatr. Scand.*, **59**, 461–3.
35. Pothupitiya, G.M., Wojnarowska, F., Bhogal, B.S. and Black, M.M. (1988) Distribution of the antigen in adult linear IgA disease and chronic bullous dermatosis of childhood suggests that it is a single and unique antigen. *Brit. J. Dermatol.*, **118**, 175–82.
36. Wojnarowska, F., Whitehead, P., Bhogal, B., *et al.* (1988) Characterisation of the antigen in chronic bullous dermatosis of childhood and adult linear IgA disease. *Brit. J. Dermatol.*, **118**, 268.
37. Grant, P.W. (1968) Juvenile dermatitis herpetiformis. *Trans. St. John's Hosp. Dermatol. Soc.*, **54**, 128–36.
38. Marsden, R.A. (1982) The treatment of benign chronic bullous dermatosis of childhood and bullous pemphigoid beginning in childhood. *Clin. Exp. Dermatol.*, 7, 653–63.
39. Burge, S., Wojnarowska, F. and Marsden, A. (1989) Chronic bullous dermatosis of childhood persisting into adulthood. *Pediatric Dermatol.*, 5, 246–9.

Ten

Epidermolysis bullosa acquisita

Robert A. Briggaman, W. Ray Gammon and David T. Woodley

10.1 INTRODUCTION

At the turn of the century, patients were recognized with a blistering disorder that resembled hereditary epidermolysis bullosa, but differed by an adult onset and an absence of a family history of epidermolysis bullosa [1–3]. The term, acquired epidermolysis bullosa (EBA), was coined to categorize this group [1,3]. In order to tighten the diagnosis, Roenigk *et al.* [4], in 1971 proposed the following clinical criteria for the disease: (1) trauma-induced bullae over the hands, feet, elbows and knees, atrophic scars, milia and nail dystrophy; (2) adult onset; (3) absence of a family history of epidermolysis bullosa; and (4) exclusion of all other bullous diseases. From its inception, acquired epidermolysis bullosa has represented an operational categorization. Through the years, concepts concerning these patients have gradually evolved. Specific diseases that might have been included in EBA as defined above were removed following their recognition. Examples of this include bullous amyloidosis (Chapter 20) [5], various porphyrias (Chapter 19), various drug-induced bullous disorders (Chapter 17) including those associated with penicillamine and doxorubicin [6], and the pseudoporphyrias which refer to both the photo-induced drug eruptions caused by nalidixic acid, propanolol, furosemide and tetracycline [7] and a bullous eruption associated with chronic dialysis [8] (Chapter 21). During the 1970s, patients that manifested a subepidermal blistering disorder clinically consistent with EBA were reported with immunological features similar to bullous pemphigoid [9–16]. These included linear deposition of IgG and complement components at the epidermo–dermal junction and a circulating IgG anti-basement membrane zone (BMZ) antibody in some patients. Immunoelectron microscopic studies showed that the immune deposits were below the lamina densa and distinguished these patients from other subepidermal blistering diseases [17, 18]. Revised diagnostic criteria were then proposed incorporating these new immunological features [19]. Problems of nosology were still not solved. Some patients were recognized who presented with an inflammatory blistering disease, rather than the mechanobullous non-inflammatory presentation described above, even though they met the other criteria [20–23]. In addition, occasional patients continue to be seen with trauma-induced blisters, scarring, adult onset, lack of a family history of EB and in whom all of the blistering diseases can be excluded including all those enumerated above. Specifically, these patients lack any immunopathological findings [24–26]. Some, but not all, of these patients resemble pseudoporphyria but a specific drug cannot be documented and porphyria can be excluded by appropriate biochemical determinations. A degree of diagnostic confusion has crept back into the use of the term EBA. A case can be made for retaining the designation EBA as a generic term and separating out the immunopathological type as a new distinctive disease entity that might be appropriately termed 'dermolytic pemphigoid'. This has been proposed previously [23]. Another possible solution might be to use the term EBA for the immunopathological form exclusively and lump the above patients in the pseudoporphyria category [26]. The solution to this relatively minor problem is not yet at hand. In any event, a new and distinctive disease entity has been recognized under the designation EBA of the immunopathological type (dermolytic pemphigoid) and has the following criteria: (1) a chronic bullous disease, (2) subepidermal blister, (3) linear deposits of IgG at the BMZ and (4) IgG deposits in the upper dermis beneath the lamina densa recognized by immunoelectron microscopy. The remainder of the present chapter will concentrate on this entity.

10.2 CLINICAL FEATURES

10.2.1 Presentation

Epidermolysis bullosa acquisita is relatively uncommon, although its true incidence is unknown. A rough estimate indicates that its frequency is about one-tenth that of bullous pemphigoid [20, 21]. EBA has been reported in all races (caucasians, blacks and orientals) and both sexes, but may be slightly more common in females and blacks [27]. It is predominantly an adult disease [27], but has been reported in young children [28, 29]. Although EBA has been reported throughout the world [31], its geographic distribution has not been well studied. A recent study suggests that the disease is much less common in Britain than the United States [30]. Some differences in populations might be expected because of the genetic association which will be discussed later.

10.2.2 Cutaneous distribution and morphology of lesions

Clinical features vary greatly from one patient to another so that no distinctive clinical picture emerges for the disease. Variations are seen in the types of skin lesions present, their extent, severity and course. Some patients present as a non-inflammatory mechanobullous disorder, others as an inflammatory blistering disease and others combinations of the two at various times in the course of the disease. Classic EBA is a non-inflammatory mechanobullous disease that presents with marked skin fragility, blisters and erosions at sites of trauma, and heals with scarring and milia (Figure 10.1). In these patients, the extent of the disease may be variable. Some patients have a localized disease that largely affects the dorsum of the hands and arms and closely mimics porphyria cutanea tarda (Figure 10.2). Others have more extensive involvement of the acral sites, especially the arms, hands, feet, knees and elbows, and these patients present a picture similar to dystrophic dominant EB. Still other patients have generalized cutaneous involvement resembling that seen in recessively inherited epidermolysis bullosa dystrophica. Nail dystrophy and scarring alopecia may be seen.

Some patients present with an inflammatory bullous disease in which the blisters arise spontaneously on erythematous skin [20, 21] (Figure 10.3). These patients may resemble bullous pemphigoid, cicatricial pemhigoid or even dermatitis herpetiformis in the clinical disease they manifest. The bullous pemphigoid-like presentation has been the more common where patients manifest a generalized bullous eruption featuring large tense bullae and a predilection for the flexural and/or intertriginous areas. Lesions in this phase may heal without scarring or milia.

During the course of the disease, transitions may be seen from the inflammatory phase to the non-inflammatory mechanobullous phase of the disease. Occasionally, patients undergo a complete transition from inflammatory to non-inflammatory involvement, while other patients exhibit a mixture of inflammatory and non-inflammatory mechanobullous lesions at the same time [23].

10.2.3 Mucous membrane involvement

Mucous membrane involvement is relatively common being present to some extent in an

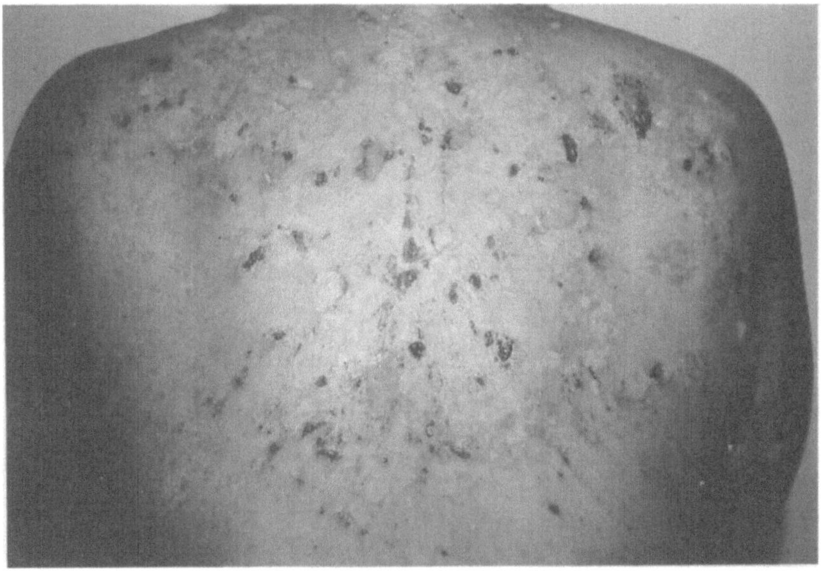

Figure 10.1 Epidermolysis bullosa acquisita (dermolytic pemphigoid). Generalized cutaneous involvement manifests here with blisters, erosions, scarring and milia on the back.

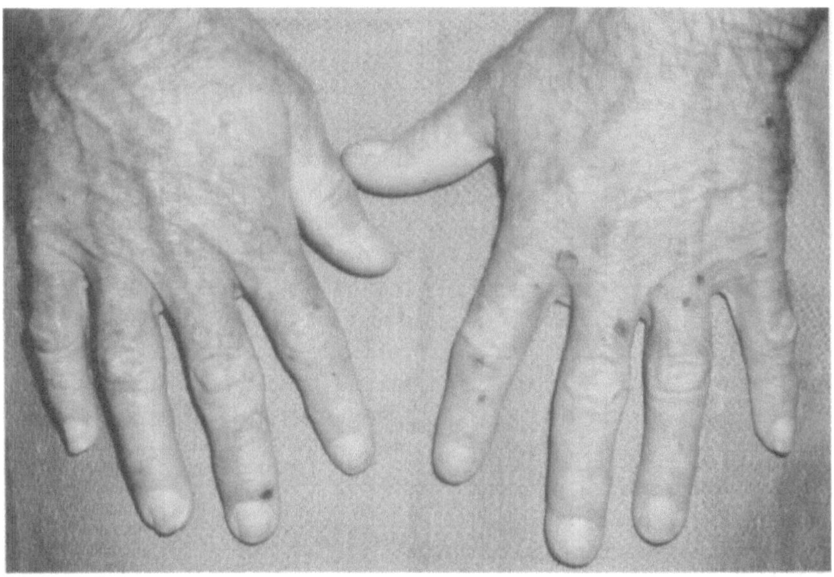

Figure 10.2 Porphyria-like hand involvement is present in this patient with epidermolysis bullosa acquisita.

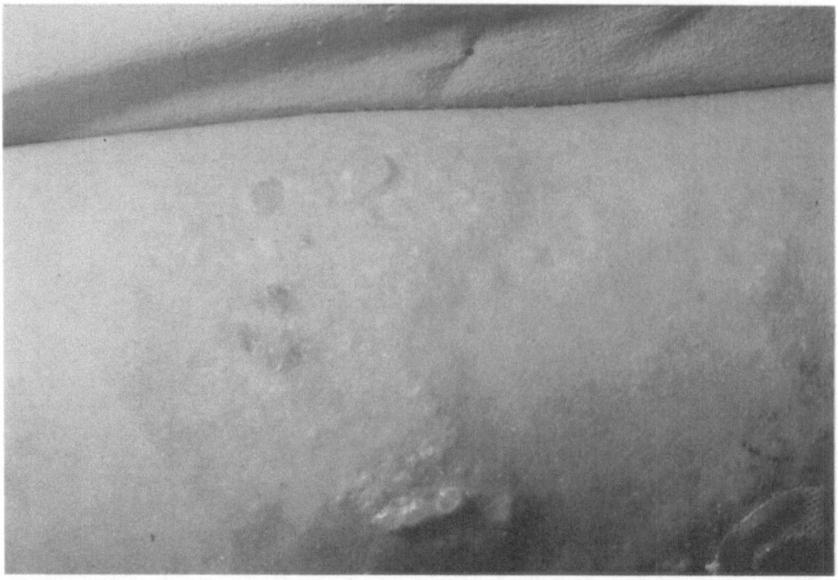

Figure 10.3 Grouped vesicles and bullae on an erythematous base in a patient exhibiting an inflammatory phase of epidermolysis bullosa acquisita.

estimated 50% of cases. The extent of mucous membrane involvement varies from occasional oral lesions to extensive and severe involvement that affects oral, ocular, genital and even oesophageal and laryngeal mucous membranes [32–35]. The latter patients may resemble cicatricial pemphigoid (Figure 10.4). Blisters may lead to scarring, which in turn produce a variety of complications depending on the affected mucous membrane. Conjunctival and corneal scarring may lead to synechia and even blindness [35]. Oesophageal and laryngeal scarring may produce stenosis with symptomatic disability [16, 35].

10.3 GENETICS

An increased frequency of the class II HLA haplotype, DR2, has been identified in patients with EBA. In a recent study, 21 of 29 patients were HLA-DR2-positive [27]. The racial breakdown indicated 12 of 18 black patients and 9 of 11 white patients were DR2-positive which was significant ($P = 0.10$ and $P = 0.001$ levels respectively). These data demonstrate that EBA is strongly HLA class II allele-associated and that genes linked to DR2 may somehow predispose to the development of EBA. Interestingly, bullous SLE is also HLA-DR2-associated [27].

10.4 DIFFERENTIAL DIAGNOSIS

EBA can mimic almost any other chronic vesiculobullous disease. The heterogeneous clinical expression of the disease has been discussed previously. The diagnosis of EBA of the immunopathological form is ultimately dependent upon documentation of IgG immune deposits at the epidermo–dermal junction specifically distributed in and beneath the lamina densa. Bullous SLE represents a special situation that will be discussed later.

10.5 INVESTIGATIONS

10.5.1 Histopathological features

Histopathological findings vary depending upon the inflammatory or non-flammatory nature of the

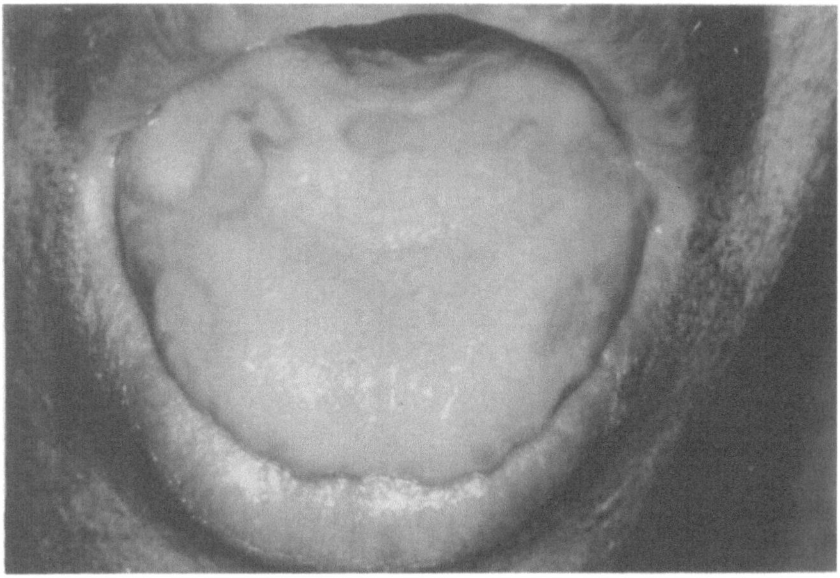

Figure 10.4 Severe oral erosions and scarring in a patient with epidermolysis bullosa acquisita.

lesion biopsied. Inflammatory lesions demonstrate a leucocyte-rich inflammatory reaction at the epidermal junction, especially early. This is usually a neutrophil-predominant infiltrate, although occasionally eosinophils may be admixed. Neutrophils may line the junction in some segment of the biopsy or form neutrophilic microabscesses [20, 21]. The neutrophil-predominant infiltration is helpful in distinguishing EBA from bullous pemphigoid, although it is not definitive. The non-inflammatory mechanobullous skin lesion usually shows epidermal–dermal separation with a sparse or absent inflammatory infiltrate [4].

By electron microscopy, a sublamina densa separation plane can usually be discerned, especially in the non-inflammatory mechanobullous lesions [10, 17, 18, 23]. Depending on a number of factors including the density of the infiltrate, age of the lesion and probably others, more diffuse damage can be seen at the epidermo–dermal junction including damage to the lamina densa and separation in other junctional planes including through the lamina lucida [36]. Because of this, the level of blister separation is not a reliable diagnostic feature of the disease.

In occasional patients a dense amorphous deposit can be seen beneath the lamina densa in the dermis [10, 18]. Sometimes this deposit is quite extensive and thick.

10.5.2 Immunofluorescent studies

Direct immunofluorescence performed on lesional or, even better, on perilesional skin shows a broad linear band of intense IgG deposition [9, 17, 18, 20, 21]. Complement components may also be present. IgA and/or IgM may also be present; however, their frequency is less than IgG and their deposition is less intense.

A circulating IgG anti-BMZ antibody may also be found in these patients (Figure 10.5). The frequency of the circulating antibody varies with the stage of the disease, being present early more frequently than late. Approximately one-half to two-thirds of patients have a circulating antibody sometime in their disease [27].

10.5.3 Immunoelectron microscopy

Direct immunoelectron microscopy usually shows an immune deposit localized to the lamina densa

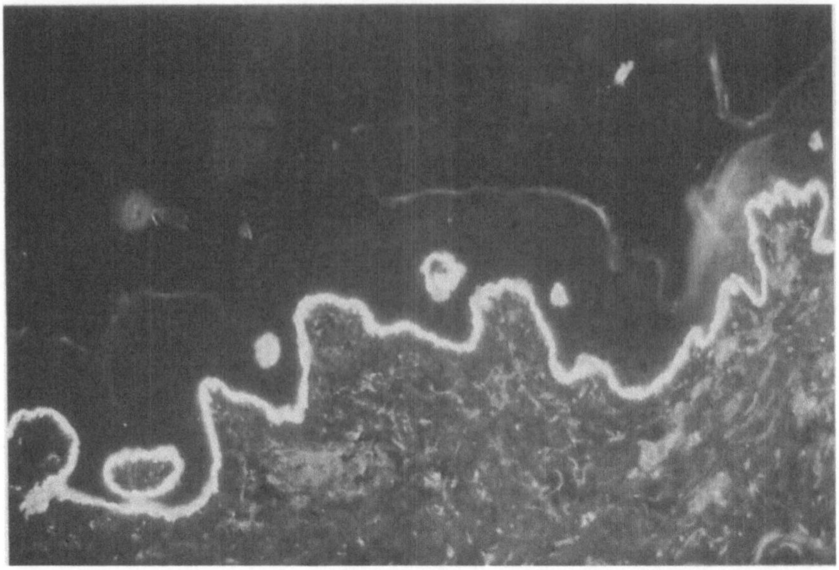

Figure 10.5 Indirect immunofluorescence of EBA antibody on human skin substrate. A broad linear band of fluorescence is present at the epidermal–dermal junction.

and sublamina densa zones [17, 18, 23]. Late in the course of the disease, the deposit may be restricted to the sublamina densa zone only. Circulating IgG anti-BMZ-antibodies from patients with EBA localize to an antigenic site in the lamina densa and sublamina densa area (Figure 10.6). When immunofluorescence is performed with IgG anti-BMZ antibodies from these patients using a 1 M NaCl split-skin substrate [37], the immune deposit is always localized to the dermal side of the split and can be confirmed by immunoelectron microscopy to be on and beneath the lamina densa which goes with the dermal side of the split. These studies indicate that the EBA antigen is a normal component of human skin localized to the lamina densa and sublamina densa area.

10.5.4 Identification of the EBA antigen

Using Western immunoblots, EBA antibodies detect 290- and 145-kDa proteins in crude BMZ extracts [38–40]. Interestingly, circulating antibodies derived from both classic EBA and bullous pemphigoid-like EBA recognize the same antigens in BMZ extracts [20, 21] (Figure 10.7). Monoclonal antibodies were developed to the EBA antigen by initially immunizing animals with BMZ extracts [41]. These antibodies recognize the 145- and 290-kDa proteins on immunoblots and are distributed at the epidermo–dermal junction by immunofluorescence and to the lamina densa and sublamina densa area by immunoelectron microscopy (Figure 10.8). Immunoprecipitation studies carried out using EBA specific antibodies and human keratinocyte and fibroblast cultures as a source of EBA antigen indicate that the EBA antigen is synthesized by both human keratinocytes and fibroblasts and that the 290-kDa EBA antigen is the major biosynthesized protein [42–44]. No 145-kDa protein was detected. Protein degradation studies using bacterial collagenase showed that the 290-kDa protein was progressively degraded to the 145-kDa protein [40]. As a result of these studies, we proposed that the EBA antigen is composed of collagenous and non-collagenous domains of approximately equal size (145-kDa) with the non-collagenous domain in the lamina densa and the collagenous domain in the sublamina densa area [40].

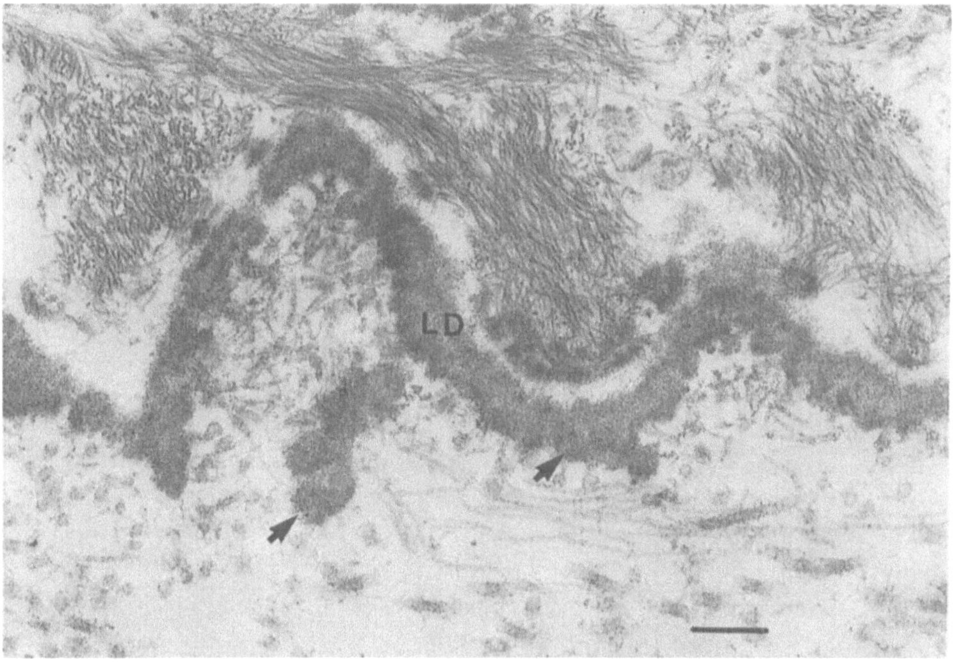

Figure 10.6 Immunoelectron microscopy of EBA antibody on human skin substrate using a multistep immunoperoxidase procedure. Immuno deposits (arrows) are present overlying the lamina densa (LD) and in the sublamina densa region. Calibration bar 0.25 μm.

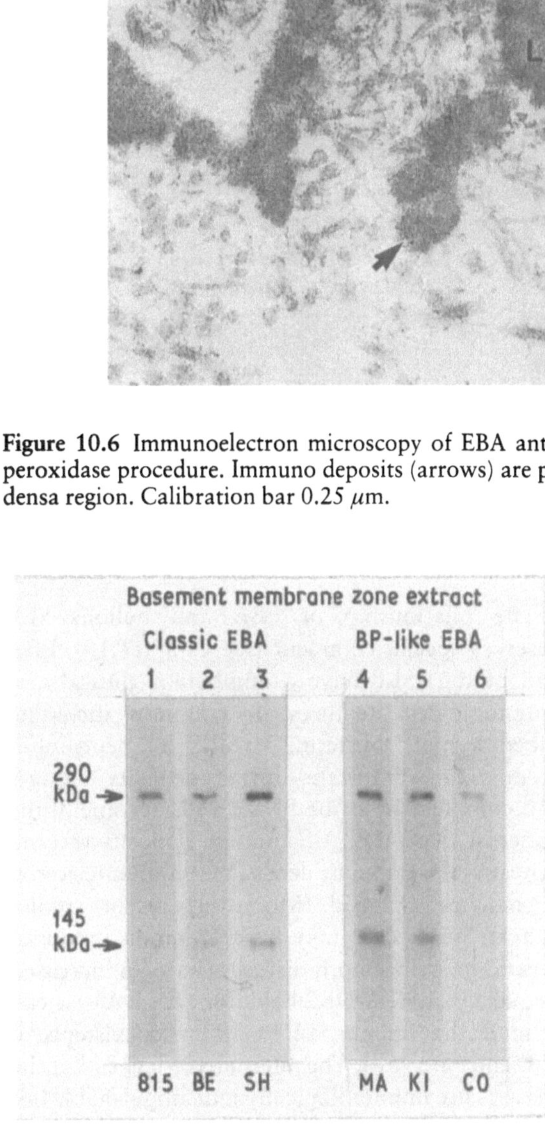

Figure 10.7 Western immunoblot analysis of EBA antibodies from patients with both classic (815,BE,SH) and bullous pemphigoid-like (MA,KI,CO) EBA using a human skin BMZ extract, 290-kDa and 145-kDa bands are present.

Similarities between the EBA antigen and type VII procollagen were then appreciated. Type VII is a recently described collagen that contributes to the structure of anchoring fibrils [45–47]. Anchoring fibrils are composed of the *C*-terminal globular domain and the collagenous domain of type VII procollagen but lack the *N*-terminal globular domain. The *C*-terminal domain is localized to the lamina densa and the collagenous portion to the sublamina densa region. Lateral aggregation of the collagenous domain results in the characteristic central periodicity of the anchoring fibril. As evidence of the identity of the EBA antigen and type VII procollagen, sera from patients with EBA, the monoclonal antibodies to the EBA antigen and to the *C*-terminal domain of type VII procollagen produced identical labelling of both human amnion and skin extracts in immunoblots. Moreover, Western immunoblots of the EBA antigen extracted from skin and of type VII procollagen showed identical labelling with the above antibodies. None of the antibodies labelled Western blots of

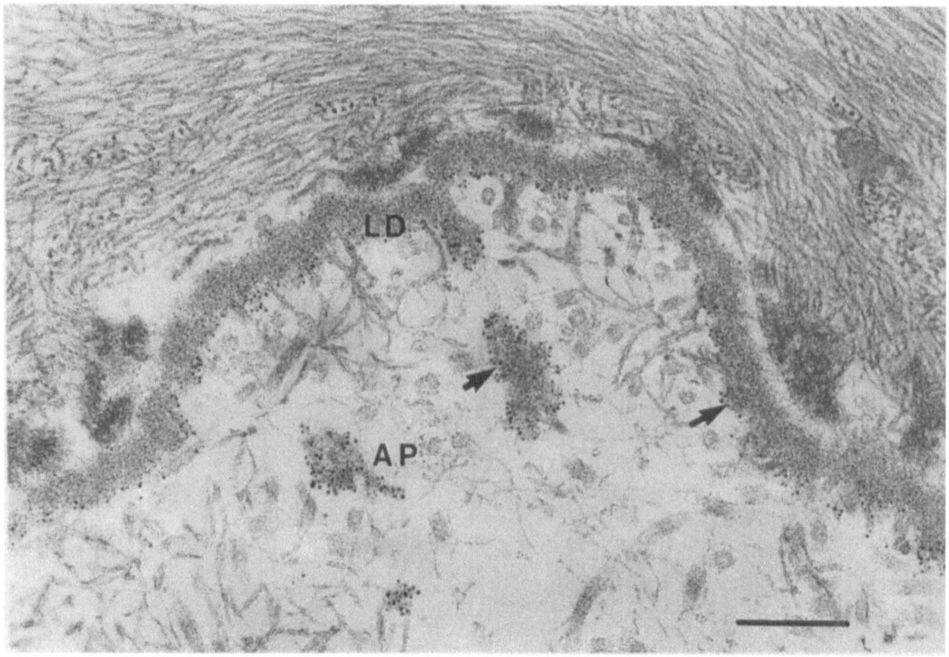

Figure 10.8 Immunoelectron microscopy of anti-EBA monoclonal antibody on human skin substrate using an immunogold procedure. Gold deposits (arrows) are localized to the lamina densa (LD) and anchoring plaques (AP) in the dermis. Calibration bar 0.25 μm.

pepsinized type VII collagen that was missing the globular terminal domains. These data indicate that the EBA antigen is the globular C-terminus of type VII procollagen [48].

10.6 SYSTEMIC MANIFESTATIONS AND ASSOCIATED DISEASES

Epidermolysis bullosa acquisita has been associated with numerous other disorders including rheumatoid arthritis, multiple myeloma, chronic thyroiditis, diabetes mellitus, lymphoma, amyloidosis, inflammatory bowel disease, amoebic dysentery, pulmonary fibrosis, psoriasis, tuberculosis, cancer of the lung, cryoglobulinaemia and multiple endocrinopathy syndrome [49–52]. Some of these associations may be chance occurrences. Nevertheless, some of the associations share a possible autoimmune aetiology and suggest a common link.

The relationship of EBA and bullous SLE deserves special comment (see Chapter 18). EBA and bullous SLE have a number of clinical and immunological features in common including subepidermal blistering with a neutrophil-predominant infiltrate, linear deposits of IgG and complement at the BMZ, and, in some of the patients, deposition of immune deposits on and beneath the lamina densa by immunoelectron microscopy [53–57]. Moreover, recent studies indicate that there may be a common immunogenetic link since both diseases share an increased frequency of HLA-DR2 haplotype [27]. A case can be made that bullous SLE represents coexistence of SLE and EBA [58]. The alternative view is that the diseases are immunologically indistinguishable but otherwise separate diseases each with typical features rarely seen in the other disease. Skin fragility and healing with scarring and milia are not features of bullous SLE. Responsiveness to dapsone, which is characteristic of bullous SLE, is rarely seen in EBA [56]. In addition, not all patients with bullous SLE react immunologically to the EBA antigen [55]. A reasonable view might be that patients with systemic LE react to a broad repertoire of antigens. When these antigens are the EBA antigen or perhaps other antigens at the BMZ, a blistering disease may result which we call bullous SLE.

10.7 PATHOGENESIS

An antibody-mediated complement-dependent mechanism may account for the tissue injury seen in some EBA patients especially those with the inflammatory phase of the disease which is characterized by neutrophil-predominant inflammation. Complement-binding EBA antibodies bind to the BMZ of normal human skin in organ culture and form complement-activating immune complexes that mediate complement-dependent migration and attachment of neutrophils to the BMZ [59]. Tissue injury, even basement membrane separation, can be seen in this model. Complement activation and generation of complement-dependent chemotactic activity for leucocytes was essential to demonstrate neutrophil attachment and tissue injury.

In other studies considerable functional heterogeneity was found in the ability of EBA antibodies from different patients to mediate complement activation and generation of complement-dependent chemotactic activity [60, 61]. The differences were due to varying amounts of complement-activating complexes found at the BMZ and the availability of circulating complement-binding anti-BMZ antibodies. A strong correlation was seen between those patients who demonstrated neutrophil-predominant inflammation and the presence of functional complement-binding antibodies bound in skin. On the other hand, those patients with non-inflammatory mechanobullous lesions lacked functional complement-binding antibodies, suggesting that some other mechanism of tissue injury may also be present in EBA. In these patients it is possible that the antibodies work by some other mechanism or even that a non-immune mechanism is operative. The pathogenesis of the non-inflammatory mechanobullous lesion is not understood at this time.

10.8 TREATMENT

In general, EBA is poorly responsive to therapeutic measures that control other bullous diseases such as bullous pemphigoid and pemphigus. Indeed, its poor response to therapy has been a distinguishing feature of the disease [23]. Some patients, especially those with inflammatory involvement, may respond favourably to relatively high doses of corticosteroids, for example, prednisone 1–2 mg/kg. Cyclophosphamide, azathioprine or methotrexate may be added on theoretical grounds but their benefit is uncertain as steroid-sparing agents. Dapsone is rarely effective either alone or in combination with steroids whereas dramatic responses may be seen in bullous SLE [57]. The non-inflammatory mechanobullous phase is particularly difficult to treat. We have not seen such a patient clear with corticosteroids. Dilantin, gold and vitamin E have all been suggested as therapeutic agents, but we have not seen the disease clear with their use. Cyclosporin A has shown promise in recent reports of successful responses in patients who have failed many other therapeutic approaches [62–64]. Plasmaphaeresis has also been suggested as a means to decrease the circulating antibody concentration in both plasma and tissue [31] and is worthy of more extensive trial.

Non-specific supportive measures should be employed to control cutaneous infection, maintain nutrition and minimize local trauma to the fragile skin.

10.9 PROGNOSIS

Epidermolysis bullosa acquisita follows a protracted chronic course. In some patients, the disease is progressive while in others it smoulders along relentlessly. Periods of relative activity and inactivity may punctuate the course. In some patients, the disease activity may remit for months or even years and reactivate later. The eventual outcome of the disease has not been thoroughly studied and permanent remissions have not been well documented. In any event, EBA may be a serious debilitating disease that results in significant morbidity, disfigurement and severe complications especially to affected mucous membranes.

REFERENCES

1. Elliott, G.T. (1895) Two cases of epidermolysis bullosa. *J. Cutan. Genitourin. Dis.*, **13**, 8–10.
2. Wise, F. and Lautman, M.F. (1915) Epidermolysis bullosa beginning in adult life. The acquired form of the disease, with the report of a case and review of the literature. *J. Cutan. Dis.*, **33**, 44–52.
3. Kablitz, R. (1904) Ein Reitrag Zur Frage der Epidermolysis Bullosa (hereditaria et acquisita) Rostock. (Dissertation).
4. Roenigk, H.H. Jr., Ryan, J.G. and Bergfeld, W.F. (1971) Epidermolysis bullosa acquisita: report of three cases and review of all published cases. *Arch. Dermatol.*, **103**, 1–10.
5. Muller, S.A., Sams, W.M. and Dobson, R.L. (1969) Amyloidosis masquerading as epidermolysis bullosa acquisita. *Arch. Dermatol.*, **99**, 739–47.
6. Beer, W.E. and Cooke, K.B. (1967) Epidermolysis bullosa induced by penicillamine. *Brit. J. Dermatol.*, **79**, 123–5.
7. Harber, L.C. and Bickers, D.R. (1984) Porphyria and pseudoporphyria. *J. Invest. Dermatol.*, **82**, 207–9.
8. Gilchrest, B., Rowe, J. and Mihm, M.C. Jr. (1975) Bullous dermatosis of hemodialysis. *Ann. Intern. Med.*, **83**, 480–3.
9. Kushniruk, W. (1973) The immunopathology of epidermolysis bullosa acquisita. *Can. Med. Assoc. J.*, **108**, 1143–6.
10. Gibbs, R.B. and Minus, H.R. (1975) Epidermolysis bullosa acquisita with electron microscopical studies. *Arch. Dermatol.*, **111**, 215–20.
11. Goodwin, P. and Eady, R. (1977) A case of ? epidermolysis bullosa. *Clin. Exp. Dermatol.*, **2**, 409–12.
12. Krivo, J.M. and Miller, F. (1978) Immunopathology of epidermolysis bullosa acquisita: association with mixed cryoglobulinemia. *Arch. Dermatol.*, **114**, 1218–20.
13. Benedetto, A.R., Bergfeld, W.F. and Guirguis, M. (1978) Epidermolysis bullosa acquisita diagnosed by immunofluorescence and electronmicroscopy. *J. Invest. Dermatol.*, 70, 221 (abstract).
14. Livden, J.K., Nilsen, R., Thunold, S. and Schjonsby, H. (1978) Epidermolysis bullosa acquisita and Crohn's disease. *Acta Dermato. venereol. (Stockholm)*, **58**, 241–4.
15. Provost, T.T., Maize, J.C., Ahmed, A.R., Strauss, J.S. and Dobson, R.L. (1979) Unusual subepidermal bullous diseases with immunologic features of bullous pemphigoid. *Arch. Dermatol.*, **115**, 156–60.
16. Richter, B.J. and McNutt, N.S. (1979) The spectrum of epidermolysis bullosa acquisita. *Arch. Dermatol.*, **115**, 1325–8.
17. Nieboer, C., Boorsma, D.M., Woerdeman, M.J. and Kalsbeek, G.L. (1980) Epidermolysis bullosa acquisita: immunofluorescence, electron microscopic and immunoelectron microscopic studies in four patients. *Brit. J. Dermatol.*, **102**, 383–92.
18. Yaoita, H., Briggaman, R.A., Lawley, T.J., Provost, T.T. and Katz, S.I. (1981) Epidermolysis bullosa acquisita: ultrastructural and immunological studies. *J. Invest. Dermatol.*, **76**, 288–92.
19. Roenigk, H.H. Jr and Pearson, R.W. (1981) Epidermolysis bullosa acquisita. *Arch. Dermatol.*, **117**, 383.
20. Gammon, W.R., Briggaman, R.A. and Wheeler, C.E. Jr (1982) Epidermolysis bullosa acquisita presenting as an inflammatory bullous disease. *J. Amer. Acad. Dermatol.*, **7**, 382–7.
21. Gammon, W.R., Briggaman, R.A., Woodley, D.T., Heald, P.W. and Wheeler, C.E. Jr (1984) Epidermolysis bullosa acquisita – a pemphigoid-like disease. *J. Amer. Acad. Dermatol.*, **11**, 820–32.
22. Caputo, R., Berti, E. and Monti, M. (1982) Pemphigoide bullouse a type d'epidermolyse. *J. Dermatol. Paris*, **114**, 27–8.
23. Briggaman, R.A., Gammon, W.R. and Woodley, D.T. (1985) Epidermolysis bullosa acquisita of the immunopathological type (dermolytic pemphigoid). *J. Invest. Dermatol.*, **85**, 79s–84s.
24. Lacour, J-P., Juhlin, L., El Baze, P. and Ortonne, J-P. (1985) Epidermolysis bullosa acquisita with negative direct immunofluorescence. *Arch. Dermatol.*, **121**, 1183–5.
25. Unis, M.E., Pfau, R.G., Patel, H., Takahashi, Y. and Anhalt, G. (1985) An acquired form of epidermolysis bullosa without immunoreactants. *J. Amer. Acad. Dermatol.*, **13**, 377–80.
26. Woodley, D.T., Briggaman, R.A. and Gammon, W.R. (1988) Review and update of epidermolysis bullosa acquisita. *Semin. Dermatol.*, **7**, 111–22.
27. Gammon, W.R., Heise, E.R., Burke, W.A. *et al.* (1988) Increased frequencies of HLA-DR2 in patients with autoantibodies to epidermolysis bullosa acquisita antigen: evidence that autoimmunity to type VII collagen is HLA class II allele associated. *J. Invest. Dermatol.* (in press).
28. Rubenstein, R., Esterly, N.B. and Fine, J.D. (1987) Childhood epidermolysis bullosa acquisita. Detection in a 5 year old girl. *Arch. Dermatol.*, **123**, 772–6.

29. Borok, M., Heng, M.C. and Ahmed, A.R. (1986) Epidermolysis bullosa acquisita in an 8 year old girl. *Pediatr. Dermatol.*, **3**, 315–22.
30. Logan, R.A., Bhogal, B., Das, A.K., McKee, P.H. and Black, M.M. (1986) Localization of bullous pemphigoid antibody – an indirect immunofluorescence study of 212 cases using a split-skin technique. *Brit. J. Dermatol.*, **115**, (Suppl. 30) 29.
31. Furue, M., Iwata, M., Yoon, H.I. *et al.* (1986) Epidermolysis bullosa acquisita: clinical response to plasma exchange therapy and circulating anti-basement membrane zone antibody titer. *J. Amer. Acad. Dermatol.*, **14**, 873–8.
32. Palestine, R.E., Kossard, S. and Dicken, C.H. (1981) Epidermolysis bullosa acquisita: a heterogenous disease. *J. Amer. Acad. Dermatol.*, **5**, 43–53.
33. Dahl, M.G.C. (1979) Epidermolysis bullosa acquisita – a sign of cicatricial pemphigoid? *Brit. J. Dermatol.*, **101**, 475–83.
34. Nilsen, R., Livden, J. and Thunold, S. (1978) Oral lesions of epidermolysis bullosa acquisita. *Oral Surg.*, **45**, 749–54.
35. Lang, P.G. Jr and Tapert, M.J. (1987) Severe ocular involvement in a patient with epidermolysis bullosa acquisita. *J. Amer. Acad. Dermatol.*, **16**, 439–43.
36. Fine, J.D., Tyring, S. and Gammon, W.R. (1988) The presence of intralamina lucida blister formation in epidermolysis bullosa acquisita: possible role of leukocytes. *J. Invest. Dermatol.* (in press).
37. Gammon, W.R., Briggaman, R.A., Inman, A.O. III, Queen, L.L. and Wheeler, C.E. (1984) Differentiating anti-lamina lucida and anti-sublamina densa anti-BMZ antibodies by indirect immunofluorescence on 1.0 M sodium chloride-separated skin. *J. Invest. Dermatol.*, **82**, 139–44.
38. Woodley, D.T., Briggaman, R.A., O'Keefe, E.J. *et al.* (1984) Identification of the skin basement membrane autoantigen in epidermolysis bullosa acquisita. *New Engl. J. Med.*, **310**, 1007–13.
39. Woodley, D.T., O'Keefe, E.J., Reese, M.J., *et al.* (1986) Epidermolysis bullosa acquisita antigen, a new major component of cutaneous basement membrane, is a glycoprotein with collagenous domains. *J. Invest. Dermatol.*, **86**, 668–72.
40. Yoshiike, T., Woodley, D.T. and Briggaman, R.A. (1988) Epidermolysis bullosa acquisita: relationship between the collagenase-sensitive and -insensitive domains. *J. Invest. Dermatol.* (in press).
41. Paller, A.S., Queen, L.L., Woodley, D.T., *et al.* (1985) A mouse monoclonal antibody against a newly discovered basement membrane component, the epidermolysis bullosa acquisita antigen. *J. Invest. Dermatol.*, **84**, 215–17.
42. Woodley, D.T., Briggaman, R.A., Gammon, W.R. and O'Keefe, E.J. (1985) Epidermolysis bullosa acquisita antigen is synthesized by human keratinocytes cultured in serum-free medium. *Biochem. Biophys. Res. Commun.*, **130**, 1267–72.
43. Woodley, D.T., Briggaman, R.A., Gammon, W.R., *et al.* (1986) Epidermolysis bullosa acquista antigen, a major cutaneous basement membrane component is synthesized by human dermal fibroblasts and other cutaneous tissues. *J. Invest. Dermatol.*, **87**, 227–31.
44. Stanley, J.R., Rubinstein, N. and Klaus-Kovtun, V. (1985) Epidermolysis bullosa acquisita antigen is synthesized by both human keratinocyte and human dermal fibroblasts. *J. Invest. Dermatol.*, **85**, 542–5.
45. Lunstrum, G.P., Sakai, L.Y., Keene, D.R., Morris, N.P. and Burgeson, R.E. (1986) Large complex globular domains of type VII procollagen contribute to the structure of anchoring fibrils. *J. Biol. Chem.*, **261**, 9042–8.
46. Sakai, L.Y., Keene, D.R., Morris, N.P. and Burgeson, R.E. (1986) Type VII collagen is a major structural component of anchoring fibrils. *J. Cell Biol.*, **103**, 1577–86.
47. Keene, D.R., Sakai, L.Y., Lunstrum, G.P., Morris, N.P. and Burgeson, R.E. (1987) Type VII collagen forms an extended network of anchoring fibrils. *J. Cell Biol.*, **104**, 611–21.
48. Woodley, D.T., Burgeson, R.E., Lunstrum, G., *et al.* (1988) The epidermolysis bullosa acquisita antigen is the globular carboxyl terminus of type VII procollagen. *J. Clin. Invest.*, **81**, 683–7.
49. Livden, J.K., Nilsen, R., Thunold, S. and Schjonsby, H. (1978) Epidermolysis bullosa acquisita and Crohn's disease. *Acta Dermatovenereol. (Stockholm)*, **58**, 241–4.
50. Ray, T.L., Levine, J.B., Weiss, W. and Ward, P.A. (1982) Epidermolysis bullosa acquisita and inflammatory bowel disease. *J. Amer. Acad. Dermatol.*, **6**, 242–52.
51. Raab, B., Fretzin, D., Bronson, D., *et al.* (1983) Epidermolysis bullosa acquisita and inflammatory bowel disease. *J. Amer. Med. Assoc.*, **25**, 1746–8.
52. Burke, W.A., Briggaman, R.A. and Gammon, W.R. (1986) Epidermolysis bullosa acquisita in a patient with multiple endocrinopathies syndrome. *Arch. Dermatol.*, **122**, 187–9.
53. Olansky, A.J., Briggaman, R.A., Gammon, W.R. *et al.* (1982) Bullous systemic lupus erythematosus. *J. Amer. Acad. Dermatol.*, **7**, 511–20.
54. Tani, M., Shimizu, R., Ban, M., *et al.* (1984) Systemic lupus erythematosus with vesiculobullous lesions. Immunoelectron microscopic studies. *Arch. Dermatol.*, **120**, 1497–501.
55. Gammon, W.R., Woodley, D.T., Dole, K.C. and Briggaman, R.A. (1985) Evidence that anti-basement membrane zone antibodies in bullous eruption of systemic lupus erythematosus recognize epidermolysis bullosa acquisita autoantigen. *J. Invest. Dermatol.*, **84**, 472–6.
56. Barton, D.D., Fine, J.D., Gammon, W.R. and Sams, W.M., Jr (1986) Bullous systemic lupus erythematosus: An unusual clinical course and

detectable circulating autoantibodies to the epidermolysis bullosa acquisita antigen. *J. Amer. Acad. Dermatol.*, **15**, 369–73.

57. Hall, R.P., Lawley, T.J., Smith, H.R. and Katz, S.I. (1982) Bullous eruption of systemic lupus erythematosus. Dramatic response to dapsone therapy. *Ann. Int. Med.*, **97**, 165–70.
58. Dotson, A.D., Raimer, S.S., Pursley, T.V. and Tschen, J. (1981) Systemic lupus erythematosus occurring in a patient with epidermolysis bullosa acquisita. *Arch. Dermatol.*, **117**, 422–6.
59. Gammon, W.R., Inman, A.O. III and Wheeler, C.E. Jr (1984) Differences in complement-dependent chemotactic activity generated by bullous pemphigoid and epidermolysis bullosa acquisita immune complexes: demonstration by leukocytic attachment and organ culture methods. *J. Invest. Dermatol.*, **83**, 57–61.
60. Gammon, W.R. and Briggaman, R.A. (1987) Functional heterogeneity of immune complexes in epidermolysis bullosa acquisita. *J. Invest. Dermatol.*, **89**, 478–83.
61. Gammon, W.R., Yancey, K.B. and Hammer, C.H. (1988) Generation of C5 dependent biological activity by basement membrane zone immune complexes. *Clin. Res.* (in press).
62. Connolly, S.M. and Sander, H.M. (1987) Treatment of epidermolysis bullosa acquisita with cyclosporine. *J. Amer. Acad. Dermatol.*, **16**, 890.
63. Zachariae, H. (1987) Cyclosporin A in epidermolysis bullosa acquisita. *J. Amer. Acad. Dermatol.*, **17**, 1058–9.
64. Crow, L.L., Finkle, J.P., Woodley, D.T. and Gammon, W.R. (1988) Clearing of epidermolysis bullosa acquisita on cyclosporin A. *J. Amer. Acad. Dermatol.* (in press).

Eleven
Dermatitis herpetiformis

Lionel Fry

11.1 INTRODUCTION

Dermatitis herpetiformis (DH) is certainly one of the skin disorders in which significant advances have been made in our understanding of the cause during the last 20 years. In fact it could be argued that it is one of the few skin disorders where, as a result of the cause being identified, there is now a specific treatment, unlike the majority of skin disorders in which treatment is still empirical.

The study of DH, as with many other diseases, has been complicated by lack of objective diagnostic criteria, and thus many disorders with similar clinical and histological features have been wrongly included in studies of patients with DH. The term DH was first coined by Duhring in 1884 on the basis of the clinical features of the rash. The next significant landmark was in 1940 when Costello [1] showed a dramatic clearing of the rash within days with sulphapyradine; this drug was used because it was thought that DH was an allergic reaction to a bacterial infection. However, the rash recurred equally quickly when sulphapyridine was stopped. In 1950, there was the first report [2] of the beneficial effects of sulphones in controlling the rash, and it was claimed that they were more effective than sulphapyridine. In 1943, Civatte [3] distinguished pemphigus from DH and pemphigoid using histological criteria, and Lever [4] subsequently proposed on clinical grounds that the subepidermal bullous disorders, DH and pemphigoid, were in fact different.

Thus in the 1950s and 60s, DH was considered to be a bullous disease with a characteristic rash, in which histologically the blister was subepidermal, and the rash cleared with dapsone. However, these criteria are not absolute, and it is likely that a significant proportion of patients labelled, by using these criteria, as having DH did not in fact have the disease.

In 1966, Marks *et al.* [5] showed that nine of 12 patients with DH had a small-intestinal enteropathy but they were unable to come to a conclusion as to the cause of this finding. The following year I and my colleagues [6] showed that, in DH patients with an enteropathy, there was a high incidence of iron and folate deficiencies, evidence of splenic atrophy, a low serum IgM and a serum agglutinating factor to *Lactobacillus casei*, all features of coeliac disease. In the following 2 years, we showed by gluten withdrawal and subsequent challenge that the enteropathy was indeed due to gluten, and reported that the rash was gluten dependent [7,8].

The next significant advance was in 1969 when van der Meer [9] reported IgA deposits in the uninvolved skin. It was soon found that there were two patterns of IgA deposition, a so-called granular deposition in the dermal papilla (the common pattern) and a rarer linear deposition along the line of the basement membrane. In 1974, Seah and I [10], reviewing the features of DH, stated that IgA deposition in the uninvolved skin was the most reliable diagnostic criterion and the diagnosis should not be made without the presence of IgA, and this has now become accepted practice.

During the last decade it has been shown that patients with linear IgA deposition appear to form a separate clinical entity from those with dermal papillae deposition. The distribution and morphology of the rash [11], lack of response to gluten withdrawal [12] and HLA studies [13] all suggest two different disorders. Only patients in whom there is papillary deposition of IgA should be considered as having DH, and those in whom the deposition is linear and along the basement membrane are now referred to as having linear IgA disease (see Chapter 8). The patterns of IgA deposition in the uninvolved skin have also enabled DH to be distinguished from other bullous disorders in childhood which is important not only for diagnosis but because of the therapeutic implications.

Thus from being considered as just one of the bullous dermatoses for nearly a century, DH has now been shown to be a specific entity. The disorder is due to gluten sensitivity and we now have a definitive objective criterion, namely IgA deposits in the upper dermis, for establishing the diagnosis.

11.2 CLINICAL FEATURES

11.2.1 Presentation

(a) Age

DH appears to commence at any age. The youngest age of onset reported is 10 months [14] and the oldest over 90 years [15]. In our experience at St Mary's in studying 148 patients, DH is rare in children – in only two patients did the rash start before the age of 10 (Figure 11.1). In the majority of patients the symptoms began in young adults between the ages of 15 and 40, and the mean age of onset was 34 years. Only 18% of our patients developed DH after the age of 50. However, in 5% the disease began in the eighth decade. The average age of onset (Table 11.1) was in the fourth decade in studies from Finland [16], three centres in the UK (Edinburgh [17], Cardiff [18] and St Mary's) and two from Sweden [19,20]. However, in one study from Southern Sweden [15], the average age was higher.

Although in the majority of subjects DH begins in adult life, there have been three reports in children [14,21,22]. There is a suggestion that DH may be more common in children in some countries, e.g. Italy [14] and Hungary [21]. In our experience at St Mary's, where we are a referral centre for DH, we have not seen a patient whose rash began before the age of 6.

Although both DH and coeliac disease (CD) are due to gluten and have a gluten-sensitive enteropathy, patients with coeliac disease present most commonly in childhood in the first 2 years of life, whereas DH in children occurs later, the mean age of onset being approximately 7 years.

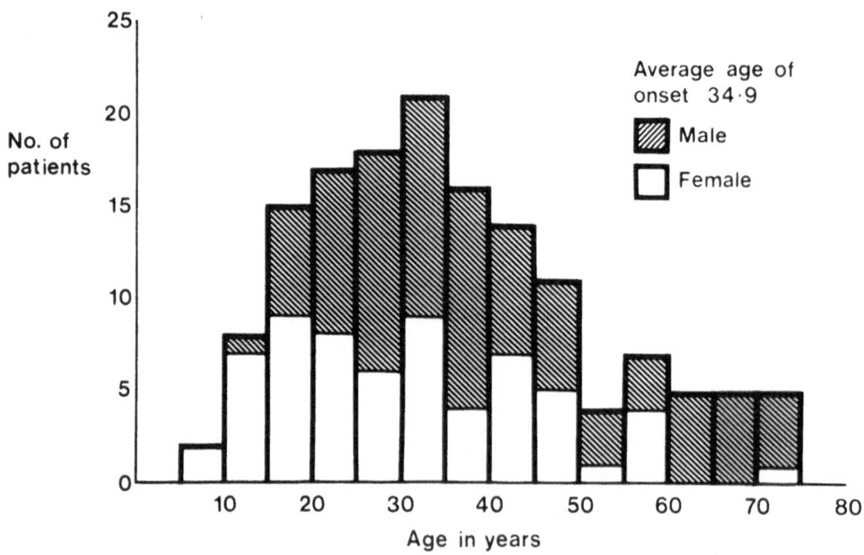

Figure 11.1 Age of onset and sex ratio of DH (St Mary's Hospital data).

Table 11.1 Age of onset of DH

Centre	*No.*	*Range of age (years)*	*Mean (years)*	*Sex ratio M : F*
London (St Mary's)	148	6–74	34.9	1.34 : 1
Western Sweden [19]	84	5–79	37	1.05 : 1
Central Sweden [20]	119	4–80	43.9 (m) 39.9 (f)	2.05 : 1
Southern Sweden [15]	45	Not given	53.1	0.80 : 1
Southern Sweden [15]	51	Not given	45.6	2.00 : 1
Edinburgh [17]	76	12–77	43 (m) 38 (f)	1.81 : 1
Cardiff [18]	42	22*–60	35.0 (m) 35.2 (f)	1.21 : 1
Finland [16]	492	3–77	33.0 (m) 30.6 (f)	1.60 : 1

* Months.

(b) *Sex ratio*

In most large studies DH has been found to be more common in males. The average of the ratios reported in Table 11.1 is approximately M : F, 1.5 : 1. However, an interesting observation is that females tend to have an earlier onset of DH compared to males, and below the age of 40 DH is more common in females. In children with DH there is a predominance of females; in the largest study of children a M : F ratio of 1 : 2 was reported [14]. It is interesting that in childhood DH there is a higher incidence of a severe enteropathy compared to adults, and the M : F ratio is similar to that found in coeliac disease, which has a predominance of females.

(c) *Incidence*

There have only been a few studies of the incidence of DH in the population. In a study from Edinburgh [17] the incidence was 11.5/100 000 and a similar figure (11.4/100 000) was reported from Finland [16]. However, a higher incidence has been found in Swedish studies: 19.6/100 000 in Malmo and 26.8/100 000 in Kristianstad [15]. 39.2/100 000 in central Sweden [20] and 22.9/100 000 in Western Sweden [19]. In a study reported from Northern Ireland [23] the incidence of DH was reported as 1 : 560. However, the author states that if strict criteria are applied, then the incidence fell to 1 : 1700. This report illustrates the confusion that applies to the diagnosis of DH if accepted diagnostic criteria are not adhered to, and have made many earlier studies on DH meaningless. Even in this report from Northern Ireland, the criteria are not described in detail, so it is difficult to know what significance to attach to the findings.

The incidence of DH appears to be less than that of CD. In Edinbugh CD was found to be five times as common as DH, thus the incidence of DH is approximately 1 : 10 000 and CD is 1 : 2000. The figures that are available for Sweden also suggest that CD is more common. However, in Sweden the difference in incidence between the two disorders is nearer 1 : 2.

(d) *Geographical distribution*

CD is often considered to be a disease of Europeans, and is therefore most commonly seen in Europe and countries to which Europeans have emigrated. Although the epidemiological studies on DH are sparse compared to those on CD, it would appear that DH is also essentially a European disease. However, as with CD, it has been reported in the Middle East and Far East although the incidence appears to be considerably lower than in European communities. At St Mary's we have now seen 160 patients with DH, and despite relatively large Asian and Afro-Caribbean communities in the vicinity, we have not seen a case of DH in these races. The only possible exception is a patient of mixed Indian and Portugese parentage.

The highest reported incidence of CD in the world is in Galway, in the west of Ireland, where 1 in 303 of the population is reported to have the disease [24]. It is an impression we have gained in our DH clinic at St Mary's that a very high proportion of our patients are of Irish descent. It would therefore appear that manifestations of gluten sensitivity, CD and DH occur predominantly in the same parts of the world and possibly the ratio of CD to DH is similar in all areas.

11.2.2 Cutaneous distribution

The rash of DH tends to be very symmetrical. The commonest site of involvement is the extensor surfaces of the elbow and proximal forearms (Figure 11.2) with over 90% of patients having lesions at this site [25]. The next most common site is the buttocks (Figure 11.3), occurring in some two-thirds of patients, and the third most common site is the extensor surfaces of the knees (Figure 11.4). Other sites frequently affected are the back, particularly over the scapulae, and face. Involvement of all areas apart from the soles has been described. In some patients the rash may be confined to one or two areas, e.g. elbows and buttocks, whilst in others the eruption is widespread. Lesions also appear, apparently from trauma, under tight clothing, e.g. belts, braces, bras.

In patients whose eruption is treated by drugs, if there is a breakthrough, the face is commonly affected in addition to the elbows and buttocks.

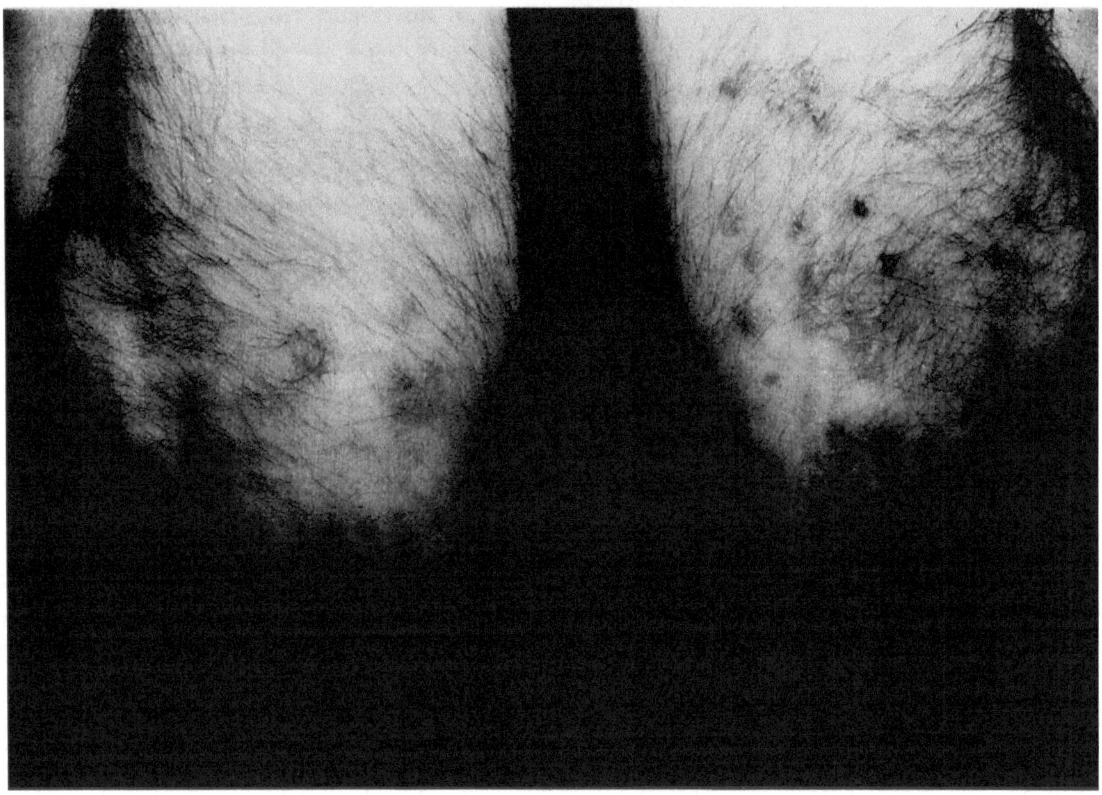

Figure 11.2 The commonest site for DH lesions is the elbow and proximal extensor forearms.

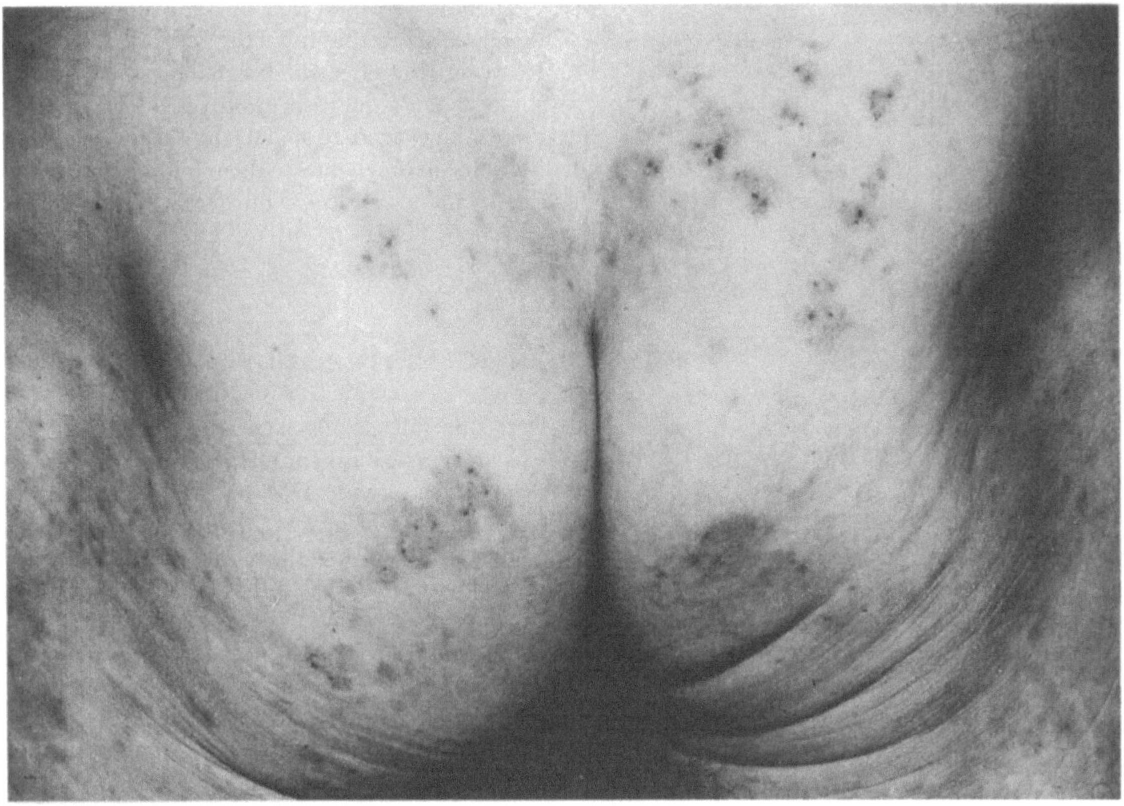

Figure 11.3 Grouped lesions on the buttocks.

When the rash breaks through due to inadequate drug control, it tends to occur in the same sites in an individual each time.

11.2.3 Mucous membrane involvement

In our experience at St Mary's, mucous membrane involvement is rare (occurring in less than 5% of patients). IgA deposition does occur in the oral mucosa [26] but, as with uninvolved skin, does not necessarily lead to clinical lesions. One study [27] reported a high incidence (12 of 15 patients) of oral lesions, but in only two were the lesions symptomatic.

It is possible that in some of the earlier case reports of oral involvement, the patients may not have had DH but linear IgA disease in which over 25% of patients have symptomatic oral lesions.

11.2.4 Morphology of lesions

The classical lesion of DH is a small blister situated on an erythematous urticarial base. The blisters may be grouped (hence the name herpetiformis) on an urticarial plaque. However, in practice it is often rare to find blisters. It has to be stressed that DH is an intensely irritating disorder and patients therefore cannot resist scratching, and the most frequent lesions seen are excoriated and scabbed papules. In fact, if the rash is chronic and well established there are often lichenified patches at the sites of involvement. The absence of blisters (because of scratching) cannot be too strongly emphasized for the practising clinician. The distribution of the rash is far more likely to suggest the diagnosis than the morphology of the rash.

Large blisters (greater than 1 cm in diameter) are rare but do occur. Occasionally blisters and

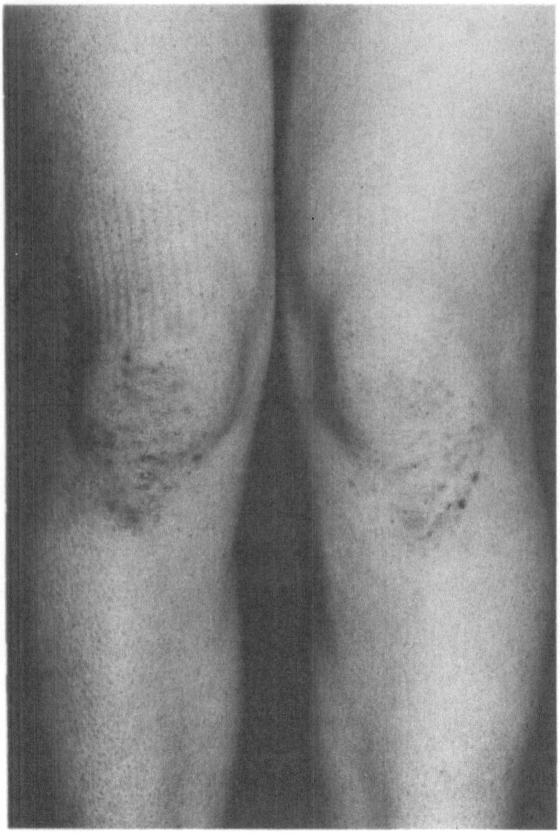

Figure 11.4 Symmetrical lesions on the knees.

excoriations are the only lesions, and no urticarial plaques are present. Alternatively urticarial patches may be the predominant lesion with no clinical blister formation. Thus the rash in DH is of variable morphology.

Scarring is not a feature of DH despite the fact that the primary site of the skin lesion is dermal.

(a) *Variation in severity of the skin lesions*

It has already been mentioned that in some patients the eruption may be widespread whilst in others only a few lesions are present. In a few patients with mild disease, the rash may be of an intermittent nature with periods of clinical remission. However, this presentation occurred in less than 10% of our patients at St Mary's.

There is no doubt that in some female patients there is an exacerbation of the rash premenstrually. However, the effect of pregnancy is variable. In some patients the rash improves whilst in others there is an exacerbation. DH may also occur for the first time in pregnancy with an improvement when the pregnancy is over. Thus female sex hormones appear to have a modifying effect on the disease process.

11.3 GENETIC STUDIES

Until the late 1960s it was thought that there was no genetic basis for DH. However, the finding that patients with DH had a gluten-sensitive enteropathy which was identical to CD led to studies that have now shown a genetic basis. It was first shown in 1950 [28] that in 205 children with clinical CD there was an 8.2% incidence of the disease in relatives; later studies give an overall incidence of approximately 10% in first-degree relatives [29]. The incidence in parents is lower than that of siblings and children of patients with CD, and incidences as high as 33% for children [30] and 25% for siblings [31] have been reported. However, this is based on intestinal biopsy findings, and many of the subjects are asymptomatic. DH cannot be asymptomatic and the incidence of a positive family history is considerably lower than in CD. In our study of 160 patients we have found only two with a first-degree relative with DH. Reunala and his colleagues [32] reported six out of 184 DH patients with first-degree relatives with the disease. There is also an increased incidence of CD in relatives of patients with DH; we have three, and Reunala *et al.* [32] also reported three. Love [23], in a study of 60 DH patients in Ireland reported a higher incidence of DH in relatives, with 11 (2.4% of all first-degree relatives), but the incidence of CD was only three (0.6%). In studying a similar number of CD patients the same author reported 24 (5.5% of all first-degree relatives) with CD but only three (0.6%) with DH.

Two studies [32,33] have been reported in which first-degree relatives of patients with DH had small-intestinal biopsies performed. In the study by

Marks *et al.* [33] seven out of 19 biopsies, and in Reunala's study [32], eight out of 20 biopsies, showed evidence of gluten-sensitive enteropathy. All the patients with enteropathy in both studies were asymptomatic (apart from one who had the rash of DH). This incidence of enteropathy in relatives of patients with DH is even higher than that reported for CD.

Studies on monozygotic twins have shown several examples of concordance for CD, but there have been only two reports of concordance for DH in monozygotic twins [34,35].

Two studies [32,36] have carried out skin biopsies on relatives of patients with DH, but in neither study was IgA found in the skin.

All the above studies imply that genetic factors are important in DH as well as CD. It would appear that the expression of gluten-sensitive enteropathy is high in relatives of both patients with DH and CD, but the genetic expression of the rash may be due to other genes or environmental factors with less penetrance than those for the enteropathy. It is of interest that in the studies from Ireland where there is the highest incidence of CD in the world, there also appears to be the highest incidence of DH, and a higher incidence of DH in relatives of patients with the disease. All these observations support the genetic basis for DH.

11.3.1 HLA antigens

Several studies have shown a significantly increased incidence of the class I antigen HLA-B8 in DH and CD, the incidence being approximately 80% in both diseases. The very early studies reported a slightly lower incidence in DH, but this was probably due to imprecise criteria for establishing the diagnosis resulting in the inclusion of patients who did not have the disease. Studies of the class II DR antigens have shown an even higher incidence of DR3 in both diseases, being approximately 90% [37–40]. In addition to DR3, DR7 has also been found to be significantly increased in patients with CD [38,40,41]. However, DR7 has not been found to be raised in DH [39,40], demonstrating for the first time a genetic difference between DH and CD. In addition, Sachs *et al.* [40] more recently found an increased incidence of DR2 in DH but not in CD.

It has been suggested that CD is primarily determined by the DQ locus [42]. In the study by Sachs *et al.* [40] the incidence of DQw2 was 100% in CD and 95% in DH. However, there are reports of patients with CD who are not DQw2, and thus it is unlikely that DQw2 is the gene product directly involved in disease susceptibility. It is likely that the very high incidence of DQw2 in both groups may be explained by linkage disequilibrium between DR3 and DQw2 which exists in the general population.

It has been suggested that two genes, one associated with DR3 and the other with DR7, code for susceptibility to CD [43]. Sachs *et al.* [40] suggested that DR3 with B8 and DQw2 and DR7 in association with B44 and DQw2 are the gene combinations encoding for CD. It is interesting to note that DQw2 associated with DR3 can be biochemically (although not serologically) distinguished from the DQw2 product associated with DR7: thus different susceptibility genes may be associated with different DQw2 products. Similarly, in DH two susceptibility genes may be involved, one associated with DQw2-DR3, and the other with DQw1-DR2 [40].

More recent studies [44], investigating DNA polymorphism of the class II alpha-chain genes in DH, CD and insulin-dependent diabetes, concluded that the genetic susceptibility for these three conditions is encoded by genes within the DQ-DX subregion of chromosome 6.

Taken together, the familial and HLA antigen studies have demonstrated that the susceptibility to CD and DH is genetically determined. It appears that one susceptibility gene associated with DQw2-DR3 predisposes to gluten sensitivity, and that other susceptibility genes, one associated with DQw2-DR7 and one with DQw1-DR2 determines whether the patient develops CD or DH respectively. However, the susceptibility gene for gluten sensitivity appears to have greater expression than the modifying genes, and this may explain the increased incidence of CD in relatives of patients with DH, and of DH in relatives of patients with CD. It is probable that environmental factors or other genes yet to be determined are also important in disease expression as a high proportion of relatives of both DH and CD patients show evidence of gluten sensitivity on small-intestinal biopsy and yet they are asymptomatic.

11.4 DIFFERENTIAL DIAGNOSIS

The differential diagnosis depends on the duration and nature of the eruption. There are a number of other conditions apart from DH that respond to sulphones, and the beneficial response may lead to the patient being diagnosed incorrectly as having DH. The conditions that respond to sulphones include linear IgA disease (LAD), chronic bullous dermatosis of childhood, subcorneal pustular dermatosis, erythema elevatum diutinium, some forms of vasculitis and some patients with eczema and pemphigus.

In adults the two most common diseases that have to be distinguished from DH are LAD (Chapter 8) and eczema. In LAD the rash does not show a predilection for the elbows, knees and buttocks. In a study from our clinic [45], the commonest diagnosis of patients incorrectly diagnosed as having DH was dapsone-responsive eczema. Pemphigoid tends to occur predominantly in the elderly and does not show a predilection for the extensor surfaces of the limbs. Erythema multiforme may produce similar lesions to DH. However, it is usually acral and self-limiting and shows no response to dapsone. Scabies has in the past been misdiagnosed as DH because of the involvement of the buttocks in both disorders and because of the intense irritation. A trial of a scabicide is advisable if there is any doubt. Chronic papular urticaria, especially if blistered, has certainly been misdiagnosed as DH in the past. Other dapsone-responsive eruptions that may cause confusion are erythema elevatum diutinum, which presents with violaceous plaques on the hands and arms, and some forms of cutaneous vasculitis presenting as urticarial plaques. Subcorneal pustular dermatosis is distinguished by numerous small blisters and pustules. In children, chronic bullous dermatosis of childhood must be distinguished from DH.

The importance of making the correct diagnosis cannot be overemphasized. In the past, dapsone was the suppressive treatment for many chronic bullous disorders mentioned above, but DH can now, and in the majority of patients should, be treated with a gluten-free diet, which is of no value in the other diseases.

11.5 INVESTIGATIONS

11.5.1 Biopsy of uninvolved skin for detection of IgA

This is *the* investigation for establishing the diagnosis of DH. In 1974 we (Fry and Seah [10]) emphasized the presence of IgA in the uninvolved skin as the best criterion for making the diagnosis of DH and the following year [46] proposed that the diagnosis should not be made unless IgA was found. Over the last decade these views have gained acceptance in centres with an interest in DH. IgA is not usually present in established lesions.

(a) Site of biopsy

IgA is found in all uninvolved skin in DH, although there may be some variation in quantity (as assessed by immunofluorescence [47]. The flexor aspect of the forearm is the most convenient site, but the biopsy will leave a small scar and therefore the upper and outer buttock is to be preferred.

(b) Patterns of IgA deposition in the skin

Papillary. This is so called because the IgA deposits are found in the dermal papillae (Figure 11.5). This is the common pattern of IgA deposition in DH. The deposits appear as small 'granules' or are sometimes 'fibrillar'. The appearance probably depends on the plane of section of the reticulin fibres where the IgA is deposited. The granular deposits, however, are not always confined to the dermal papillae but may also be seen in the upper dermis below the rete pegs.

Linear granular. It is most important to be able to distinguish between a linear granular pattern of IgA deposition (Figure 11.6) and a linear homogeneous pattern (Figure 11.7). It has now been shown that the linear granular pattern is DH, whereas the linear homogeneous pattern implies linear IgA disease [11] (Chapter 8). Follow-up

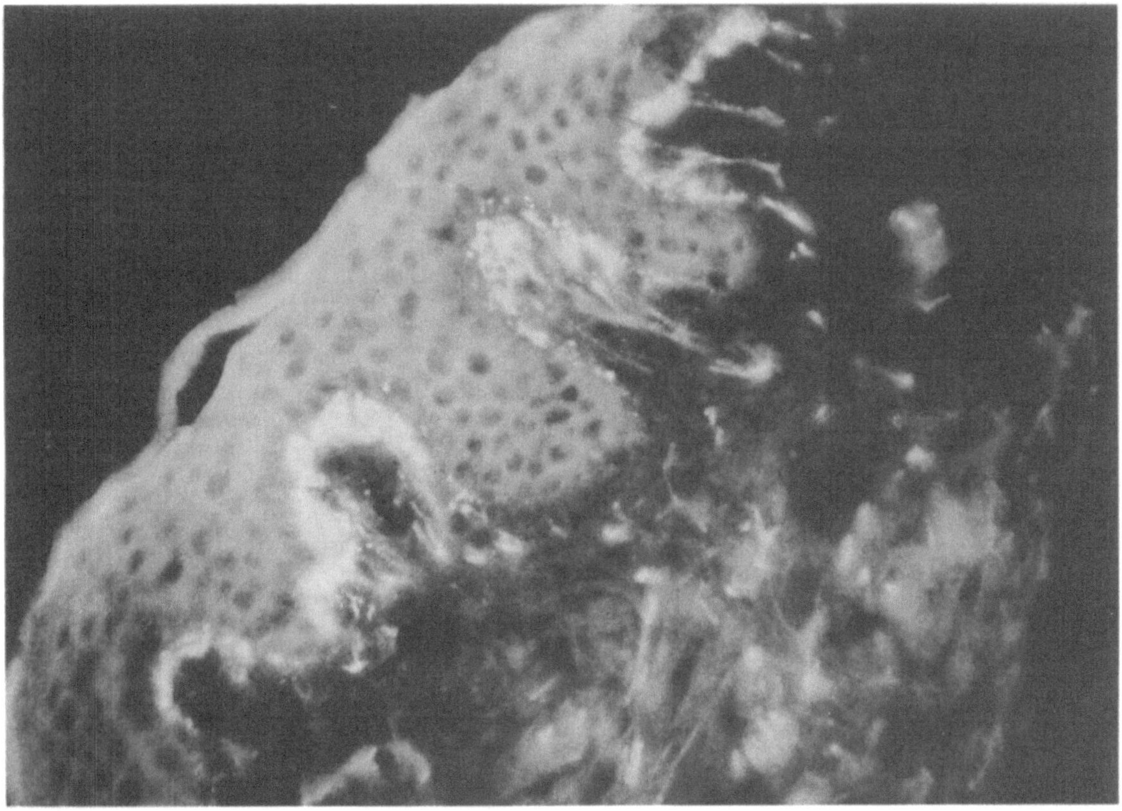

Figure 11.5 Granular IgA deposits in the dermal papillae.

studies in our department have shown that over a period of time the linear granular pattern may revert to a papillary pattern, but the homogeneous pattern does not and implies a different clinical entity.

Treatment of the rash with sulphones or sulphonamides does not alter the IgA deposits in the skin, and therefore biopsies can be taken for diagnostic purposes after the start of drug therapy. A gluten-free diet has no immediate effect on IgA deposition. However, after many years the quantity of IgA does decrease and may eventually disappear [48,49].

(c) Complement

The C3 component of complement is found in approximately two-thirds of patients taking a normal diet [48,50]. The site of deposition of C3 is the same as IgA.

(d) Other immunoglobulins

IgG and IgM may also be present in addition to IgA in the uninvolved skin. IgM is commoner than IgG; the latter was found in 10% of biopsies and IgM in a third [25]. The site of deposition tends to be the same as IgA.

(e) Failure to detect IgA

If the clinical features of the rash and response to sulphones suggest DH but no IgA is detected on the first section of the biopsy, the following course of action should be taken. First, serial sections of the biopsy should be cut and if these are all negative a second biopsy should be taken. In 50 patients

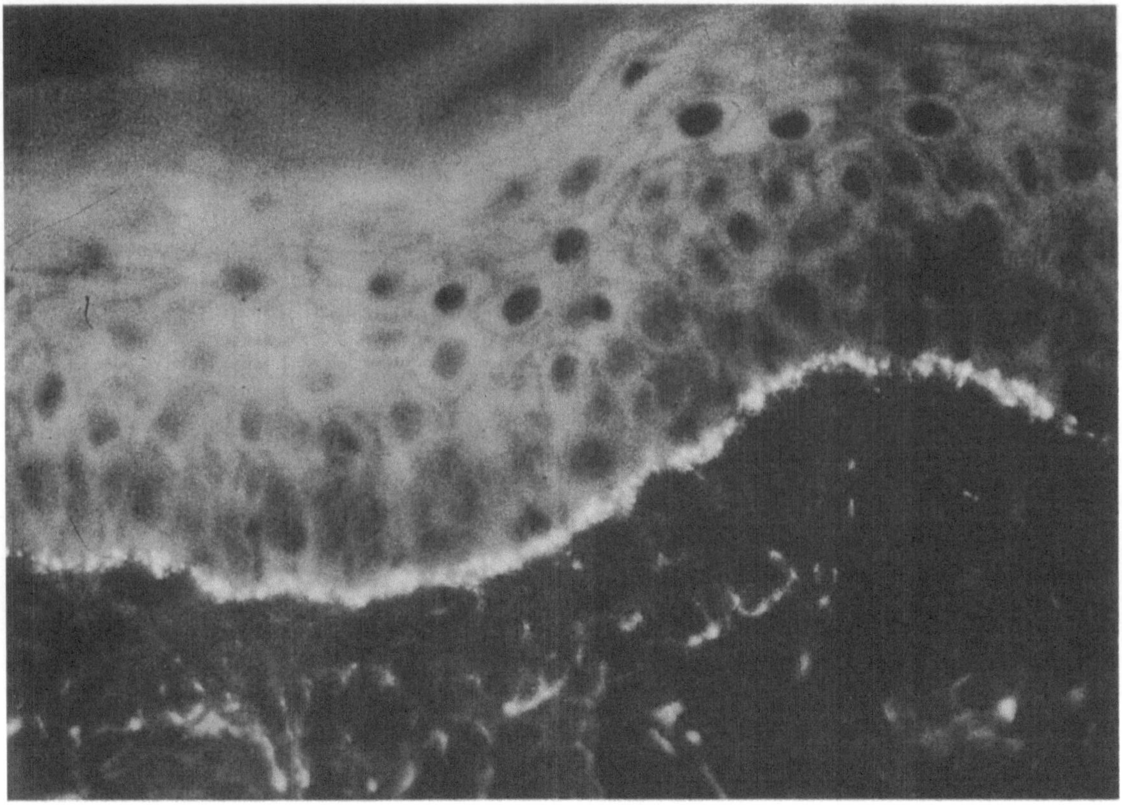

Figure 11.6 Linear granular deposition of IgA along the line of the basement membrane found in DH.

reported by myself and Seah [46] only two required a second biopsy to detect IgA.

11.5.2 Biopsy of lesional skin

Ideally an intact blister with surrounding urticarial skin should be taken for histological study. The characteristic features of DH are a subepidermal blister and microabscesses in the surrounding dermal papillae. Polymorphs are the predominant cell in the bullae and microabscesses, and leucocytoclasis and fibrin deposition is commonly seen. Eosinophils are present in approximately 25% of bullae [51].

Both pemphigoid and linear IgA disease have similar histological features and there is considerable overlap between the three diseases. Thus immunofluorescent studies to detect the class and pattern of immunoglobulin deposition in the uninvolved skin is a more reliable way of establishing the diagnosis with certainty.

11.5.3 Small-intestinal biopsy

Ideally this should be performed in all patients once the diagnosis has been established by the presence of IgA in uninvolved skin. Approximately two-thirds of patients will have an abnormal mucosa as judged by dissecting microscope appearance and routine histology. The features are those of a gluten-sensitive enteropathy, i.e. a flat or convoluted appearance revealed by the dissecting microscope, and partial or subtotal villous atrophy on histological examination. In addition there is a lymphocytic and plasma cell infiltrate of the lamina propria and an increase in the intraepithelial

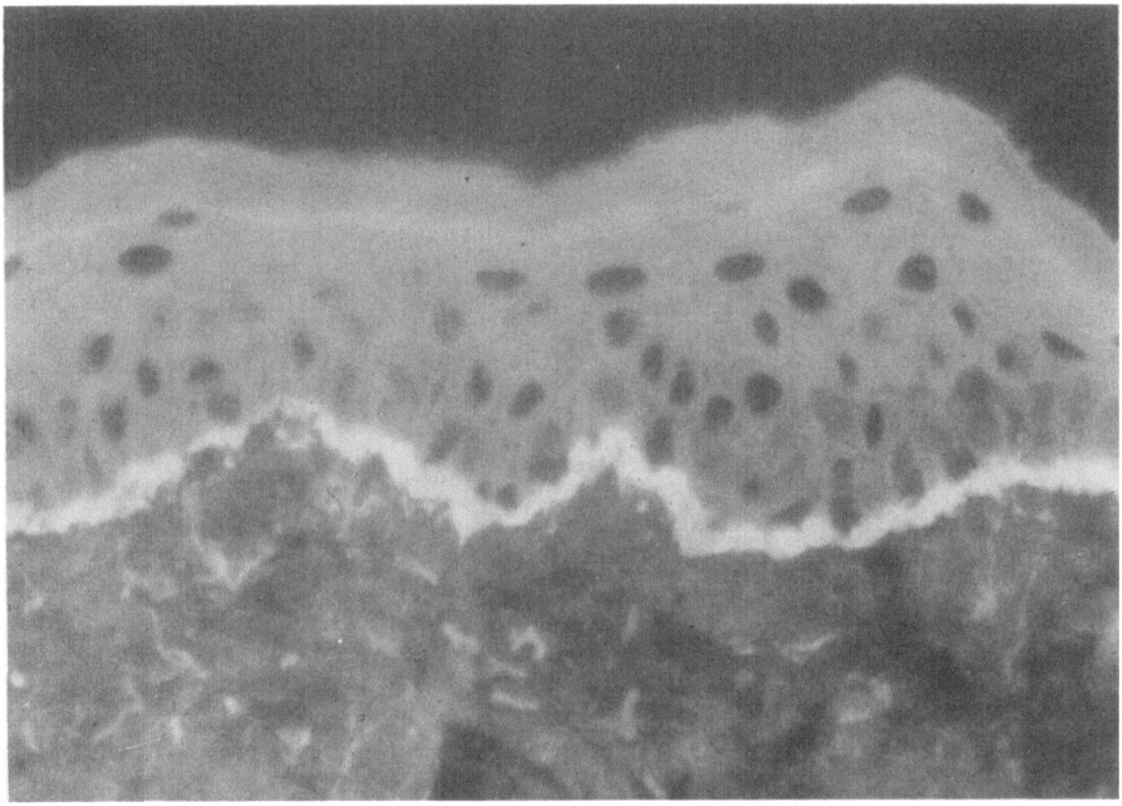

Figure 11.7 Linear homogeneous deposition of IgA along the line of the basement membrane, as found in linear IgA disease.

lymphocytes. The latter is a feature in 90% of patients and is not related to the other histological features [52]. Thus only 10% of patients with DH show no abnormality of the intestinal mucosa with routine tests currently used.

11.5.4 Haematological investigations

(a) Full blood count and peripheral blood film appearance

These are essential. Features of macrocytosis, hypersegmented polymorphs and Howell–Jolly bodies should be looked for. Although anaemia is not a common feature in untreated DH it may occur owing to malabsorption of iron and/or folate. However, in patients treated with dapsone, anaemia is not uncommon due to haemolysis. The presence of Howell–Jolly bodies signifys splenic atrophy and if present would support the diagnosis of gluten sensitivity.

(b) Serum iron

Low serum iron occurs in approximately one-third of patients with DH.

(c) Red cell folate

Folate deficiency may be due to chronic haemolysis from dapsone therapy or due to malabsorption.

(d) *Serum vitamin B_{12}*

If macrocytosis is present, serum vitamin B_{12} should be measured. There is an increased incidence of pernicious anaemia in DH patients.

(e) *Liver function tests*

Abnormal liver function tests have been reported in 17% of patients [53]. In 8% the raised bilirubin was attributed to dapsone therapy. Hepatic injury has been reported in a small proportion of patients with gluten-sensitive enteropathy.

(f) *Urine analysis*

This should be performed yearly as there is an increased incidence of type 1 diabetes mellitus. In addition there are reports of glomerulonephritis in association with DH, but these are extremely rare.

(g) *Autoantibody screen*

There is a highly significant increase of thyroid disease and pernicious anaemia in DH. In addition other autoimmune disorders, including systemic lupus erythematosus, myasthenia gravis and chronic active hepatitis, occur more frequently. If thyroid antibodies are detected it is advisable to perform thyroid function tests yearly.

11.6 SYSTEMIC MANIFESTATIONS AND ASSOCIATED DISEASES

11.6.1 Malabsorption

Despite the fact that approximately two-thirds of patients with DH have a demonstrable enteropathy on small-intestinal biopsy, it is extremely rare for them to have symptoms referrable to the enteropathy. In fact it appears that enteropathy in DH is characterized by its mildness compared to that of CD, and severe and extensive enteropathy is not usually seen in DH particularly in adults. In a study of 13 adults with DH we found that, as a group, their heights and weights were normal, and only one of the patients had increased bowel motions [6]. However, in children the enteropathy does appear to be more severe than in adults, and Ermacora *et al.* [14] reported that 30 (38%) of 76 children with DH had abdominal symptoms. However, only 11 (15%) were below the normal percentile for their weight, and 10 (13%) for their height. Tests of intestinal function are invariably normal, including xylose, folate and vitamin B_{12} absorption in adults [6], but 32% of children had an abnormal xylose test [14]. However, mild steatorrhoea, which is usually symptomless, is not uncommon in adults [6].

Malabsorption of iron and folate does occur in DH and the reported incidence of anaemia is 20–30% but it is invariably mild.

11.6.2 Autoimmune disorders

(a) *Thyroid disease*

This is the most common autoimmune disease associated with DH. The incidence of thyroid antibodies has recently been found to be as high as 48% in a group of 115 patients at St Mary's. However, the incidence of overt thyroid disease is considerably lower, only being present in six (5%). In addition, a further six patients were found to have raised thyrotropin (TSH) levels implying some degree of thyroid failure. A similar incidence for overt thyroid disease was found in two other studies [17,18], although the incidence of thyroid antibodies was lower. In a study from Salt Lake City [54], 34% of 50 DH patients were reported to have thyroid disease, and 38% of the total patients had thyroid antibodies. It is possible that there are local factors in Salt Lake City which predispose to thyroid disease to give this very high incidence of disease compared to that in the UK studies.

(b) *Gastric parietal cell antibodies, gastric function and pernicious anaemia*

In our patients at St Mary's the incidence of gastric parietal cell antibodies is 20%, in a study of 142 patients, and five of them have developed pernicious anaemia. This is slightly higher than the incidence from the Edinburgh study [17] who found 14% of 76 patients who had gastric parietal cell antibodies, but only two patients developed pernicious anaemia.

In a recent study on the gastric morphology and function, achlorhydria was found in 30 (26%) of 116 patients with DH, and 92% of those had atrophic gastritis on biopsy [55]. This report found a good correlation between the presence of gastric parietal cell antibodies and gastric function; 19 of 28 patients with achlorhydria had antibodies, but of 56 patients with normal acid secretion, only four had antibodies.

(c) Other autoimmune diseases

A number of other autoimmume diseases have been found in patients with DH and these include insulin-dependent diabetes, systemic lupus erythematosus, myasthenia gravis and rheumatoid arthritis. However, the incidence of these disorders is lower than that for thyroid disease and pernicious anaemia in our experience.

6.3 Atopy

Davies *et al.* [18] found atopic disease in nine of their 42 DH patients.

11.6.4 Lymphoma

It is well known that there is an increased incidence of lymphoma in patients with CD and this has now been shown to be the case in DH. Leonard *et al.* [56] in a report of 109 patients with DH reported three patients with lymphoma giving a relative risk of 100 for this type of tumour in DH. These authors found that all the lymphomas developed in patients with macroscopic evidence of enteropathy on biopsy, and in patients who were not taking a gluten-free diet. However, Reunala [57] reported four patients with lymphoma, all of whom were on a gluten-free diet.

It has not been established for either CD or DH whether gluten *per se* is the cause of the lymphoma. It is possible that the known immunological abnormality in these patients may itself predispose to the development of lymphoma.

Although the majority of the lymphomas reported in association with DH develop in the gastrointestinal tract, they may arise elsewhere.

11.7 PATHOGENESIS

11.7.1 Gluten

The most significant advance in our understanding of DH has been the observation that the rash is due to gluten. The role of gluten in DH emerged following the finding that a high proportion of patients with DH had an enteropathy which was identical to that found in CD [5,6]. It was soon shown that the enteropathy was indeed due to gluten, as it improved with gluten withdrawal [7,58], and recurred on reintroduction to gluten [8]. It was unfortunate that there was a dispute at this stage as to whether the rash was due to gluten. I and my colleagues were emphatic that the rash was gluten dependent and Shuster and his colleagues and the early reports from the USA [59] were equally emphatic that the rash was not gluten dependent. The fact that the latter workers were wrong was due to the fact that they came to their conclusion after only giving gluten-free diets for a period of up to 6 months which is too early to obtain significant improvement in the rash in the majority of patients. We persisted for longer because of the observation that the small intestine may take many months or even years before becoming normal following gluten withdrawal. Several detailed studies have now confirmed the initial observation that the rash will indeed clear with gluten withdrawal [14,60–62]. The final convincing evidence that gluten causes the rash came from the study of Leonard *et al.* [63] in which gluten was reintroduced to 12 patients whose rash had been controlled with a gluten-free diet for periods ranging from 2 to 12 years (average 7.6). The rash recurred in 11 of the 12 patients.

11.7.2 IgA in the skin

The second most important observation that has been made is the finding of IgA in the uninvolved skin. This has been of significant importance in diagnosis, allowing DH to be distinguished from other bullous diseases. The pathogenic significance of the IgA is unresolved.

In favour of the IgA being involved in the pathogenesis of the skin lesions is the fact that it is the only immunoglobulin found consistently in the skin. In addition, IgA is the principal immunoglobulin produced by the intestine, and it is known that there is a gluten-sensitive enteropathy in patients with DH and the response to the gluten is likely to be the production of an IgA antibody. The IgA in the skin has been shown to be dimeric [64] and therefore it is likely to be derived from the intestine. Finally, complement activation in the skin in DH has been shown to be via the alternative pathway [65,66] and it is known that aggregated IgA can activate complement via this pathway.

However, against the IgA in the skin having a pathogenic role are the following observations: (i) IgA is found in the uninvolved skin; (ii) IgA is still present in the skin of patients with spontaneous remission; (iii) IgA is still present in the skin of patients whose disease has been controlled with a gluten-free diet. However, it has been suggested that it is the quantity of IgA present in the skin that may be important in triggering the pathogenic pathway for a skin lesion. In favour of this suggestion is the observation that the quantity of IgA does appear to fall gradually when the rash is controlled by a gluten-free diet [48], and eventually may disappear only to reappear on the reintroduction of gluten [63].

A study arguing against a possible pathogenic role has shown that the IgA in the skin in DH is IgA1 [67]. This report argued that the IgA produced in the intestine is both IgA1 and IgA2, and therefore questioned whether the IgA in the skin was derived from the intestine. It is possible that only IgA1 has the capacity to bind to the skin or that in the diseased state it is IgA1 that is predominantly produced in the intestine.

11.7.3 Reticulin and the anti-reticulin antibody

It has been shown that the IgA deposits in the skin are bound to the reticulin fibres in the dermal papillae. The anti-reticulin antibody was first described in patients with DH and then was also shown to be present in patients with CD. It was shown that treatment with a gluten-free diet resulted in a fall in the anti-reticulin antibody titre and the eventual disappearance of the antibody from the serum coinciding with the disappearance of the rash. It was suggested that gluten may bind to the reticulin fibres as a gluten–anti-gluten immune complex and damage the reticulin fibres and render them immunogenic [68]. This may explain why it takes so long for the rash to disappear after gluten withdrawal. Some support for this hypothesis came from the observations by Unsworth *et al.* [69] that gliadin does indeed bind non-specifically to reticulin. Further work by Unsworth and his colleagues [70] has shown that gliadin binds to reticulin in a lectin-like manner and this would explain the observation that gliadin will bind to certain other sites in which similar glycoproteins are also present.

11.7.4 Complement

The histological features of the skin lesion are compatible with complement activation, the subsequent production of neutrophil chemoattractants, and tissue damage from proteolytic enzymes produced by the leucocytes. C3 complement component is found in early lesions; Seah *et al.* [65] found it in eight of nine patients. However, C3 is also found in approximately two-thirds of biopsies taken from uninvolved skin [48,50]. As with IgA it has to be explained why C3 is present in the skin (signifying complement activation) and yet no skin lesion is produced. It is possible that the production of a skin lesion may depend on the amount of complement activated, and in the uninvolved skin the quantity is too small. In support of the complement being important in the pathology of the skin lesions is the observation that the incidence of C3 in uninvolved skin falls to 16% in patients on a gluten-free diet, and the longer the patient has been on the diet the lower the incidence of C3 [50]. Thus as the quantity of IgA falls with the gluten-free diet, it appears that complement activation is less likely to occur.

11.7.5 Is gliadin present in the skin?

Although gluten causes the skin lesions in DH, the pathogenic mechanisms are not known. It has been argued that the IgA in skin represents a gluten–anti-gluten IgA immune complex. However, gliadin has not been detected using an anti-gliadin antibody. It is possible that gliadin is surrounded by the IgA and is therefore not 'available' for detection. Studies to elute IgA from the skin to try and detect gliadin in the eluate have not proved successful. It is difficult to elute IgA from the skin with the chemicals usually employed for elution of immune complexes from other tissues. This has led to the suggestion that the IgA may be covalently bound to the tissues. There have been recent reports of successful removal of IgA from DH skin [71,72], but the techniques used have almost certainly damaged the proteins and as yet there are no reports of gliadin in the eluate.

11.7.6 Immune complexes

If gluten is to reach the skin to cause the skin lesions it is most likely to be transported in the form of an immune complex. As IgA is the predominant immunoglobulin in the skin, then it is likely that the immune complex would be an IgA one. Zone *et al.* [73] reported circulating IgA immune complexes in six of 18 patients with DH, and the same group subsequently showed that gluten intake raises the level of these complexes in DH patients [74]. Unfortunately, as yet, gliadin has not been demonstrated in these complexes, but this may be for technical reasons.

11.7.7 Small intestinal pathology in DH

Although both the skin and intestinal lesions in DH are due to gluten, the pathological mechanisms producing the lesions would appear to be different. Whereas the skin lesion appears to be due to immune complex deposition with complement activation leading to an influx of polymorphonuclear white cells and subsequent tissue damage in the dermal papilla, in the intestine the predominant feature is an infiltration of the mucosa, particularly the lamina propria with mononuclear cells (mainly lymphocytes and plasma cells). The damage to the intestine, i.e. the alteration in villous and epithelial cell height, would appear to be mediated via lymphokines produced by the lymphocytes. In support of this suggestion is the finding that the ratio of activated helper to suppressor lymphocytes in the lamina propria is 4 : 1 in DH and CD, whereas in normal subjects it is 1 : 1 [75]. Thus the small intestinal pathology is locally produced via activated lymphocytes which are sensitized to gluten. The skin lesions are probably due to anti-gliadin antibody production in the intestine which then forms an immune complex with gliadin and travels to the skin where it is deposited in the dermal papillae.

11.7.8 Iodine and iodides

It is an interesting yet unexplained observation that potassium iodide, whether taken orally or applied to the skin, will induce lesions of DH in the previously uninvolved skin. In fact, the potassium iodide patch was often used to diagnose DH prior to the more specific tests. The clinical response to iodides is not seen in patients whose rash is controlled by dapsone or a gluten-free diet, even though IgA is still present in the skin [76]. The response is also negative in patients in remission, although they also have IgA in the skin.

The skin lesions produced by iodides in DH patients are identical to the spontaneous ones. It would appear that in some way iodides lower the threshold for activation of the final pathogenic pathways in the production of a DH lesion. This could possibly affect complement activation or production of chemical mediators. Dapsone appears to have the opposite effect to iodides, with its action on the final pathogenic mechanisms. Dapsone does not appear to influence complement deposition or activation, but is more likely to have an effect on chemical mediators involved in production of the lesion, either by blocking their actions or inhibiting their production.

11.7.9 Anti-gliadin antibody

Anti-gliadin antibodies are found in approximately half the patients with DH. Thus the incidence of these antibodies is not high enough to be of value as a diagnostic test for DH. Their presence correlates well with the severity of the enteropathy [77,78]. They are of both IgA and IgG class, with a higher incidence of IgG antibodies; it is therefore likely that the anti-gliadin antibodies detected in the serum are of no pathogenic significance and may simply be an indication of the damaged intestinal mucosa. Further evidence against them having any pathological role in DH is that the incidence and titre bear no relationships to the severity of the rash. Finally there is a higher incidence of anti-gliadin antibodies in CD and yet these patients have no skin lesions.

As the presence of anti-gliadin antibodies appears to correlate well with the severity of the intestinal damage it is likely that the gluten may gain access to the lamina propria due to increased permeability secondary to the damaged mucosa [79]. However, it has been claimed that there is increased permeability of the intestinal mucosa both in DH and CD and this is a primary fault leading to the development of the disease [80]. These researchers found that permeability of the intestine was increased even in those patients treated with a gluten-free diet, and did not correlate with the severity of the enteropathy.

11.7.10 Conclusion of pathogenic mechanisms

Although the cause of both the rash and intestinal pathology has been shown to be gluten dependent, it is not established how gluten produces the lesion at either site. The fact that the majority of the Western World can eat gluten without developing either DH or CD implies an underlying predisposition to the abnormal reaction and there is now strong evidence that this is genetically determined. The high incidence of the genetic phenotype (HLA-B8/DR3) found in both CD and DH is also present in autoimmune disorders and this undoubtedly explains the high incidence of autoimmune diseases associated with DH and CD. However, apart from the genetic similarity between DH and CD it appears that there are also genetic differences between the two disorders which localize the disease to the intestine in CD, but allows the development of skin lesions in DH.

11.8 TREATMENT

Well over 98% of patients with DH require treatment for symptomatic control of the rash and irritation. Patients with very mild disease are the exception and may not even find their way to dermatological clinics. There are two ways of treating DH; one is with drugs and the other with a gluten-free diet. It is imperative to realize that immediate relief of irritation and suppression of the rash can be obtained with drugs, but that control of the rash by diet takes months. Therefore initial treatment is with drugs whether combined with a gluten-free diet or not.

11.8.1 Drugs

There are three drugs effective in controlling the rash of DH. These are sulphapyridine, dapsone and sulphamethoxypyridazine. These drugs have no effect on the enteropathy. Adequate dosage begins to relieve the irritation within 48 h and will clear the rash within days. However, relapse of the irritation and rash is equally rapid when the drugs are stopped. The mechanisms by which these drugs suppress the rash in DH are not known, but it is likely to be at the end stage of the disease process, probably on production, or blocking the action, of chemical mediators.

(a) Dapsone

Dosage. The initial dose for an adult should be 100 mg daily and the patient should be seen 2 weeks later. If the rash is completely controlled the dose should be reduced to 50 mg daily, and if control is still achieved with this dose, subsequent reduction should be advised, increasing the interval of time between taking the drug, i.e. every second day, to third day, etc. until the rash breaks through. In our experience the minimal dose in adults has been 50 mg twice weekly for complete control of the rash. If the eruption is not controlled on 100 mg daily after 2 weeks, the dose should be increased to 200 mg daily for a further period of 2 weeks, and if no control achieved, then the dose may be increased to 300 mg daily. If control is not achieved on this dosage the diagnosis should be reviewed, including another skin biopsy for detection of IgA. In some 160 patients with DH seen at St Mary's over the last 18 years only two required a dose higher than

300 mg daily for suppression of the rash. One required 400 mg daily, and another 700 mg daily, but even then there was not complete control.

It is important that the minimum dose to suppress the rash is found, and that patients do not take a higher dose than required. The incidence and severity of side effects is generally related to dosage. It is important to be aware that there may be variation in the dose of dapsone, required to suppress the rash, in the course of time, and if patients are adequately controlled at their follow-up appointments, then they should always be advised to reduce the dose. In the follow-up of 36 patients, over a mean of 7.4 years, we found the dose of dapsone for control of the rash remained constant in 13, increased in eight and decreased in 15 (five of whom no longer required drugs) [49].

Side effects. Haemolytic anaemia is one of the commonest side effects, and it appears to be dose related. If patients are going to develop severe haemolysis this will usually be apparent at the beginning of treatment. It is imperative that a full blood count is carried out 2 weeks after commencement of treatment and 1 month later. If haemolysis has not developed then subsequent blood tests can be carried out at 3 monthly intervals in the first year, and 6 monthly intervals subsequently. The reticulocyte count is a good indicator of the degree of haemolysis. Methaemoglobinaemia clinically presents as cyanosis. The severity of methaemoglobinaemia is not directly related to the dose of dapsone. The importance of methaemoglobinaemia is that it will reduce the oxygen-carrying capacity. Agranulocytosis is very rare, but has been recorded.

Headache is one of the commonest side effects and may be severe enough to warrant discontinuing the drug. Lethargy, insomnia and depression may occur. Peripheral neuropathy, which is mononeuritis, of the so-called entrapment type, is a rare but well-recognized complication. The neuropathy is reversible when the drug is discontinued.

Anorexia and nausea has been attributed to dapsone, but may in fact be due to the gluten-sensitive enteropathy. In our experience we have not seen this problem due to dapsone. Severe hypoalbuminaemia has been reported with dapsone, but is very rare.

(b) Sulphapyridine

Dosage. The initial dose should be 2.0 g daily. As with dapsone the patient should be reviewed after 2 weeks, and the dose increased or decreased accordingly. The dose should not exceed 4.0 g daily. In the majority of patients the rash will be controlled with a dose of between 1.0 and 4.0 g daily. As with dapsone, the minimum dose to control the rash should be found, and it is important to remember that the dosage may vary in time, and reduction in dosage should always be attempted if there has been no rash or irritation between the consultations.

Side effects. The common ones are nausea, lethargy and depression. Haemolytic anaemia, renal calculi, agranulocytosis and central nervous system abnormalities have been described.

(c) Sulphamethoxypyridazine

Dosage. The initial dose should be 0.5 g daily. The patient should be seen after 2 weeks and the dose decreased or increased as necessary. The maximum dose should not exceed 1.5 g daily.

Side effects. In our experience, in the dose used, side effects are minimal. When they occur, they include skin rashes, nausea and lethargy.

(d) Drug combinations

If adequate control of the rash is not obtained with a high dose of a particular drug, e.g. 300 mg of dapsone, 4.0 g of sulphapyridine or 1.5 g of sulphamethoxypyridazine daily, individually, then by combining two or even three drugs it may be possible to obtain control of the rash, and diminish the incidence of side effects.

(e) Choice of drug

It is our impression, rather than established fact, that dapsone is superior to the two sulphonamides in controlling the rash, and for this reason it is often the first choice of drug. The disadvantage of sulphapyridine is the large number of tablets to be taken daily compared to dapsone. However, the incidence and severity of side effects is higher with dapsone than the sulphonamides. Because most patients taking dapsone will have some degree of haemolysis and methaemoglobinaemia, we do not use dapsone as a first-line drug in patients over 50 years of age. In a number of patients, symptoms of ischaemic heart disease have been precipitated as a result of the fall in haemoglobin concentration and its reduced oxygen-carrying capacity. Sulphamethoxypyridazine is the drug of choice in elderly patients.

11.8.2 Gluten-free diet

It has been established by several centres that a gluten-free diet is effective in controlling the rash of DH. However, it is imperative to remember that for the diet to be effective it must be strict and that the time taken to control the rash is on average 24 months [60]. Reduction in the drug requirements for control of the rash may begin after 3 months, but the average time is 8 months. Patients who do not stick strictly to the diet may obtain some reduction in the dose of their drugs. We found, in a study of 42 patients on a gluten-free diet, that if the diet was completely strict, 96% of patients were able to discontinue their drugs, the time taken for this varying from 6 to 54 months (mean 25) [49]. In patients in whom there was occasional unintentional gluten intake, only 45% were able to stop their drugs and the time taken for this ranged from 6 to 108 months (mean 39). Patients who knowingly took food containing gluten even only once a week were not able to discontinue their drugs.

In our experience, if the gluten-free diet is to be part of the treatment, it should be supervised by a dietician at least initially, and patients should join the Coeliac Society and receive their handbook.

(a) Advantages of a gluten-free diet

First, there is no doubt that patients experience a subjective improvement within weeks of taking the diet. Patients comment they have more energy and have never felt so well. Second, if patients adhere to the diet they will no longer require drugs and be subject to their side effects. Thirdly, not only is the skin pathology being treated, but also the enteropathy which at times may itself give rise to symptoms. It is, however, not known whether the diet will protect against the risk of developing a lymphoma.

(b) Suitability for a gluten-free diet

In our experience, although a gluten-free diet can be considered to be the ideal treatment, it is not advisable in all patients. In elderly patients who are adequately controlled by drugs with no side effects, then the diet seems unnecessary. The diet may be difficult to adhere to for social reasons, e.g. in patients who eat in restaurants a great deal as part of their work or general lifestyle. Some patients of low intelligence find the diet too difficult and therefore ineffective, and in these patients it is doubtful whether it is worth pursuing. As a general rule a gluten-free diet should be advised, but each patient has to be considered individually with regard to suitability.

11.9 PROGNOSIS AND SEQUELAE

DH is a chronic disease with a low incidence of spontaneous remission [17,19,49,81]. Alexander [81] reported spontaneous remission in 17 of 144 (12%) patients in 25 years of experience. We reported an incidence of remission of 14%, five of 36 patients in a follow-up period ranging from 3 to 14 years [49] and Gawkrodger *et al.* [17] had a similar remission rate of two of 25 patients in an 11-year period of follow-up. Both Alexander [81] and ourselves [49], however, commented on the fact that remission was not complete and that patients often had bouts of irritation and a few skin lesions, but they were not severe enough to warrant systemic treatment. We found that the mean time for remission in our five patients was an average of 5.6 years after the commencement of rash. Two studies from Sweden [15,20] both reported that approximately 20% of their patients had mild cutaneous involvement from the onset of the rash which did not require any treatment. However, this has not been our experience at St Mary's, and we have had only two out of 160 patients who required no treatment. In Christensen's study [15], in over a third of their patients the rash began over the age of 60 and the authors themselves comment on the observation that as a rule the older the age of onset the less severe the eruption. There is also a tendency for the rash to be less severe in patients over the age of 60, even if they have had the problem for many years.

Although there is no obvious increase in mortality from the skin involvement of DH itself, the morbidity from the untreated rash and drug therapy is considerable. We found that 26% of patients taking dapsone had side effects [49]. The question often arises as to whether all patients with DH should be treated with a gluten-free diet to prevent complications. The mortality rate of untreated coeliac disease has been reported as 18% but only 0.4% in those treated with a gluten-free diet [29]. However, the enteropathy in DH is less severe and only seldom gives rise to serious medical problems. The obvious advantages of the diet are in a reduction of morbidity from the disease (a significant subjective improvement – apart from control of the rash) and no side effects from drugs. The question as to whether the diet will lessen the incidence of lymphoma in these patients is unanswered.

Apart from the associated gluten-sensitive enteropathy, there is the increased incidence of other associated disorders, particularly thyroid disease and pernicious anaemia, but these should be detected early and respond to appropriate therapy.

ACKNOWLEDGEMENTS

It is a pleasure to acknowledge the following colleagues with whom I have collaborated in the study of DH, and have helped increase our understanding of the disease: R.M.H. McMinn, E.J. Holborow, A.V. Hoffbrand, P.P. Seah, J.N. Leonard, F. Wojnarowska, C.E.M. Griffiths, H. Valdimarsson, D.J. Unsworth, G.P. Haffenden, J.A. Sachs, A. Rutman. Grants from the Medical Research Council, Wellcome Trust and Coeliac Trust are gratefully acknowledged.

REFERENCES

1. Costello, M. (1940) Dermatitis herpetiformis treated with sulphapyridine. *Arch. Dermatol. Syphil.*, **41**, 134.
2. Esteves, J. and Brandao, F.N. (1950) Au sujet de l'action des sulfamides et des sulphones dans la maladie de Duhring. *Trab. Soc. Port. Dermatol.*, **81**, 209.
3. Civatte, A. (1943) Diagnostic histopathologique de la dermatite polymorphe douloureuse ou Maladie de Duhring-Brocq. *Ann. Dermatol. Syphil. (Paris)*, **3**, 1–30.
4. Lever, W.F. (1951) Pemphigus – an histopathological study. *Arch. Dermatol. Syphil.*, **64**, 727–53.
5. Marks, J., Shuster, S. and Watson, A.J. (1966) Small bowel changes in dermatitis herpetiformis. *Lancet*, ii,1280.
6. Fry, L., Keir, P., McMinn, R.M.H., Cowan, J.D. and Hoffbrand, A.V. (1967) Small intestinal structure and function, and haematological changes in dermatitis herpetiformis. *Lancet*, **ii**, 729–34.
7. Fry, L., McMinn, R.M.H., Cowan, J.D. and Hoffbrand, A.V. (1968) Effect of a gluten-free diet on dermatological, intestinal and haematological manifestations of dermatitis herpetiformis. *Lancet*, **1**, 557–61.
8. Fry, L., McMinn, R.M.H., Cowan, J.D. and Hoffbrand, A.V. (1969) Gluten-free diet and re-introduction of gluten in dermatitis herpetiformis. *Arch. Dermatol.*, **100**, 129–35.
9. Van der Meer, J.B. (1969) Granular deposits of immunoglobulins in the skin of patients with dermatitis herpetiformis. An immunofluorescent study. *Brit. J. Dermatol.*, **81**, 493–503.
10. Fry, L. and Seah, P.P. (1974) Dermatitis herpetiformis: an evaluation of diagnostic criteria. *Brit. J. Dermatol.*, **90**, 137–46.
11. Leonard, J.N., Haffenden, G.P., Ring, N.P., *et al.* (1982) Linear IgA disease in adults. *Brit. J. Dermatol.*, **107**, 301–6.
12. Leonard, J.N., Griffiths, C.E.M., Powles, A.V., Haffenden, G.P. and Fry, L. (1987) Experience with

a gluten-free diet in the treatment of linear IgA disease. *Acta Dermatovenereol. (Stockholm)*, **67**, 145–8.
13. Sachs, J.A., Leonard, J.N., Awad, J., *et al.* (1988) A comparative serological molecular biological study of linear IgA disease and dermatitis herpetiformis. *Brit. J. Dermatol.*, **118**, 759–64.
14. Ermacora, E., Prampolini, L., Tribbia, G., *et al.* (1986) Long-term follow-up of dermatitis herpetiformis in children. *J. Amer. Acad. Dermatol.*, **15**, 24–30.
15. Christensen, O.B., Hindsen, M. and Svensson, A. (1986) Natural history of dermatitis herpetiformis in Southern Sweden. *Dermatologica*, **173**, 271–7.
16. Reunala, T. and Lokki, J. (1978) Dermatitis herpetiformis in Finland. *Acta Dermatovenereol. (Stockholm)*, **58**, 505–10.
17. Gawkrodger, D.J., Blackwell, J.N., Gilmore, H.M., *et al.* (1984) Dermatitis herpetiformis: diagnosis, diet and demography. *Gut*, **25**, 151–7.
18. Davies, M.G., Marks, R. and Nuki, G. (1978) Dermatitis herpetiformis – a skin manifestation of a generalised disturbance in immunity. *Q. J. Med.*, **186**, 221–48.
19. Mobracken, H., Kastrup, W. and Nilsson, L.A. (1984) Incidence and prevalence of dermatitis herpetiformis in Western Sweden. *Acta Dermatovenereol. (Stockholm)*, **64**, 400–4.
20. Moi, H. (1984) Incidence and prevalence of dermatitis herpetiformis in a county in central Sweden, with comments on the course of the disease and IgA deposits as diagnostic criterion. *Acta Dermatovenereol. (Stockholm)*, **64**, 144–50.
21. Marsden, R.A., McKee, P.H., Bhogal, B., Black, M.M. and Kennedy, L.A. (1980) A study of benign chronic bullous dermatosis of childhood and comparison with dermatitis herpetiformis and bullous pemphigoid. *Clin. Exp. Dermatol.*, **5**, 159–76.
22. Reunala, T., Kosnai, I., Karpati, S., *et al.* (1984) Dermatitis herpetiformis jejunal findings and skin response to a gluten-free diet. *Arch. Dis. Childh.*, **59**, 517–22.
23. Love, A.H.G. (1981) Epidemiological and genetic aspects of the coeliac syndrome in relation to dermatitis herpetiformis. In *The Genetics of Coeliac Disease* (ed. R.B. McConell), MTP Press, Lancaster, p. 95.
24. Mylotte, M., Egan-Mitchell, B., McCarth, C.F. and McNicholl, B. (1973) Incidence of coeliac disease in the west of Ireland. *Brit. Med. J.*, **i**, 703–5.
25. Leonard, J.N. (1982) Dermatitis herpetiformis – a comparison between adult patients with papillary and linear deposits of IgA. M.D. Thesis, London Clinic.
26. Nisengard, R.J., Chorzelski, T., Mariejowska, E. and Kryst, L. (1982) Dermatitis herpetiformis: IgA deposits in gingiva, buccal mucosa and skin. *Oral Surg.*, **54**, 22–5.
27. Fraser, N.G., Kerr, N.W. and Donald, D. (1973) Oral lesions in dermatitis herpetiformis. *Brit. J. Dermatol.*, **89**, 439–50.
28. Davidson, L.S.P. and Fountain, J.R. (1950) Incidence of sprue syndrome with some observations on the natural history. *Brit. Med. J.*, **i**, 1157–61.
29. Cooke, W.T. and Holmes, G.K.T. (1984) *Coeliac Disease*, Churchill Livingstone, London.
30. Mylotte, M., Egan-Mitchell, B., Fotrell, P.F., McNicholl, B. and McCarthy, C.F. (1974) Familial studies in coeliac disease. *Q. J. Med.*, **43**, 359–69.
31. Gardiner, A.J., Mutton, K.J. and Walker-Smith, J.A. (1973) A family study of coeliac disease. *Austr. Paediatr. J.*, **9**, 18–24.
32. Reunala, T., Salo, O.P., Tiilikainen, A., Selroos, O. and Kuitunen, P. (1976) Family studies in dermatitis herpetiformis. *Ann. Clin. Res.*, **8**, 254–61.
33. Marks, J., Birkett, D., Shuster, S. and Roberts, D.F. (1970) Small intestinal mucosal abnormalities in relatives of patients with dermatitis herpetiformis. *Gut*, **11**, 493–7.
34. Marks, J., May, S.B. and Roberts, D.F. (1971) Dermatitis herpetiformis occurring in monozygous twins. *Brit. J. Dermatol.*, **84**, 417–19.
35. Green, S.T., Natarajan, S., Connor, J.M. and Forrest, J.A.H. (1986) Monozygous twins concordant for duodenojejunal billous atrophy and dermatitis herpetiformis. *Gut*, **27**, 970–1.
36. Leonard, J.N., Haffenden, G.P., Tucker, W.F.G., *et al.* (1983) Skin biopsies in relatives of patients with dermatitis herpetiformis. *Acta Dermatovenereol. (Stockholm)*, **63**, 252–3.
37. Solheim, B.G., Albreschon, D., Thorsby, E. and Thune, P. (1977) Strong association between an HLA-Dw3 associated B cell alloantigen and dermatitis herpetiformis. *Tissue Antigens*, **10**, 114–18.
38. Betuel, H., Gebuhrer, L., Descos, L., *et al.* (1980) Adult coeliac disease associated with HLA-DRw3 and DRw7. *Tissue Antigen*, **15**, 231–8.
39. Pehamberger, H., Holubar, K. and Mayr, W.R. (1981) HLA-DR3 in dermatitis herpetiformis. *Brit. J. Dermatol.*, **104**, 321–4.
40. Sachs, J.A., Awad, J., McCloskey, D., *et al.* (1986) Different HLA associated gene combinations contribute to susceptibility for coeliac disease and dermatitis herpetiformis. *Gut*, **27**, 515–20.
41. De Marchi, M., Borelli, I. and Olivetti, E. (1979) Two HLA-DR alleles are associated with coeliac disease. *Tissue Antigens*, **14**, 309–16.
42. Tosi, R., Vismara, D. and Tanigaki, N. (1983) Evidence that coeliac disease is primarily associated with DC locus allelic specificity. *Clin. Immunol. Immunopathol.*, **28**, 395–404.
43. Scholz, S. and Albert, E. (1983) HLA and disease:

involvement of more than one HLA linked determinant of disease susceptibility. *Immunol. Rev.*, **70**, 77–88.
44. Hitman, G.A., Niven, M.J., Festenstein, H., *et al.* (1987) HLA class ii alpha chain gene polymorphisms in patients with insulin-dependent diabetes, mellitus, dermatitis herpetiformis and coeliac disease. *J. Clin. Invest.*, **79**, 609–15.
45. Fry, L., Walkden, V., Wojnarowska, F., Haffenden, G.P. and McMinn, R.M.H. (1980) A comparison of IgA positive and IgA negative dapsone responsive dermatoses. *Brit. J. Dermatol.*, **102**, 371–82.
46. Seah, P.P. and Fry, L. (1975) Immunoglobulins in the skin in dermatitis herpetiformis and their relevance in diagnosis. *Brit. J. Dermatol.*, **92**, 157–66.
47. Haffenden, G.P., Wojnarowska, F. and Fry, L. (1979) Comparison of immunoglobulin and complement deposition in multiple biopsies from the uninvolved skin in dermatitis herpetiformis. *Brit. J. Dermatol.*, **101**, 39–45.
48. Reunala, T. (1978) Gluten-free diet in dermatitis herpetiformis. *Brit. J. Dermatol.*, **98**, 69–78.
49. Fry, L., Leonard, J.N., Swain, A.F., *et al.* (1982) Long-term follow-up of dermatitis herpetiformis with and without dietary gluten withdrawal. *Brit. J. Dermatol*, **107**, 631–40.
50. Fry, L., Haffenden, G.P., Wojnarowska, F., Thompson, B.R. and Seah, P.P. (1978) IgA and C3 complement in the uninvolved skin in dermatitis herpetiformis after gluten withdrawal. *Brit. J. Dermatol.*, **99**, 31–7.
51. Blenkinsop, W.K., Fry, L., Haffenden, G.P. and Leonard, J.N. (1983) Histology of linear IgA disease, dermatitis herpetiformis and bullous pemphigoid. *Amer. J. Dermatopathol.*, **5**, 547–54.
52. Fry, L., Seah, P.P., Harper, P.G., Hoffbrand, A.V. and McMinn, R.M.H. (1974) The small intestine in dermatitis herpetiformis. *J. Clin. Pathol.*, **27**, 817–24.
53. Wojnarowska, F. and Fry, L. (1981) Hepatic injury in dermatitis herpetiformis. *Acta Dermatovenereol. (Stockholm)*, **61**, 165–8.
54. Cunningham, M.J. and Zone, J.J. (1985) Thyroid antibodies in dermatitis herpetiformis: prevalence of clinical thyroid disease and thyroid antibodies. *Ann. Intern. Med.*, **102**, 194–6.
55. Gillberg, R., Kastrup, W., Mobacken, H., Stockbrugger, R. and Ahren, C. (1985) Gastric morphology and function in dermatitis herpetiformis and in coeliac disease. *Scand. J. Gasteroenterol.*, **20**, 133–40.
56. Leonard, J.N., Tucker, W.F.G., Fry, J.S., *et al.* (1983) Increased incidence of malignancy in dermatitis herpetiformis. *Brit. Med. J.*, **i**, 16–18.
57. Reunala, T., Heling, H., Kuokkanen, K. and Hakala, R. (1982) Lymphoma in dermatitis herpetiformis: report of four cases. *Acta Dermatovenereol. (Stockholm)*, **62**, 343–5.
58. Shuster, S., Watson, A.J. and Marks, J. (1968) Coeliac syndrome in dermatitis herpetiformis. *Lancet*, **i**, 1101–6.
59. Weinstein, W.M., Brow, J.R., Parker, F. and Rubin, C.E. (1971) The small intestinal mucosa in dermatitis herpetiformis: relationship of the intestinal lesion to gluten. *Gastroenterology*, **60**, 362–9.
60. Fry, L., Seah, P.P., Riches, D.J. and Hoffbrand, A.V. (1973) Clearance of skin lesions in dermatitis herpetiformis after gluten withdrawal. *Lancet*, **i**, 288–91.
61. Heading, R.C., Paterson, W.P., McLellond, B.B.I., Barnetson, R. St. C. and Murray, M.S.M. (1976) Clinical response of dermatitis herpetiformis skin lesions to a gluten-free diet. *Brit. J. Dermatol.*, **94**, 509–14.
62. Reunala, T., Blomquist, K., Tarpila, A., Halme, H. and Kankas, K. (1977) Gluten-free diet in dermatitis herpetiformis. *Brit. J. Dermatol.*, **97**, 473–80.
63. Leonard, J.N., Haffenden, G.P., Tucker, W., *et al.* (1983) Gluten challenge in dermatitis herpetiformis. *New Engl. J. Med.*, **308**, 816–19.
64. Unsworth, D.J., Payne, A.W., Leonard, J.N., Fry, L. and Holborow, E.J. (1982) IgA in dermatitis herpetiformis skin is dimeric. *Lancet*, **i**, 478–80.
65. Seah, P.P., Fry, L., Mazaheri, M.R., *et al.* (1973) Alternate pathway complement fixation by IgA in the skin in dermatitis herpetiformis. *Lancet*, **ii**, 175–7.
66. Provost, T.T. and Tomasi, T.B. (1974) Evidence for activation of complement via the alternate pathway in skin diseases. *Clin. Immunol. Immunopathol.*, **3**, 178–86.
67. Olbricht, S.M., Flotte, T.J., Collins, A.B., Chapman, C.M. and Harrist, T.J. (1986) Dermatitis herpetiformis: cutaneous deposition of polyclonal IgA1. *Arch. Dermatol.*, **122**, 418–21.
68. Seah, P.P., Fry, L., Stewart, J.S., *et al.* (1972) Immunoglobulins in the skin dermatitis herpetiformis and coeliac disease. *Lancet*, **i**, 611–14.
69. Unsworth, D.J., Johnson, G.D., Haffenden, G.P., Fry, L. and Holborow, E.J. (1981) Binding of wheat gliadin *in vitro* to reticulin in normal and dermatitis herpetiformis skin. *J. Invest. Dermatol*, **76**, 88–93.
70. Unsworth, D.J., Leonard, J.N., Hobday, C.M., *et al.* (1987) Gliadins bind to reticulin in a lectin-like manner. *Arch. Dermatol. Res.*, **279**, 232–5.
71. Egelrud, T. and Back, O. (1985) Dermatitis herpetiformis: biochemical properties of the granular deposits of IgA in papillary dermis. Characterisation of SDS soluble IgA-like material and potentially antigen-binding IgA fragments released by pepsin. *J. Invest. Dermatol.*, **84**, 239–45.
72. Meyer, L.J., Carioto, L. and Zone, J.J. (1987)

Dermatitis herpetiformis: Extraction of intact IgA from granular deposits in dermal papillae. *J. Invest. Dermatol.*, **88**, 559–63.
73. Zone, J.J., Lasalle, B.A. and Provost, T.T. (1980) Circulating immune complexes of IgA type in dermatitis herpetiformis. *J. Invest. Dermatol.*, **75**, 152–5.
74. Zone, J.J., Lasalle, B.A. and Provost, T.T. (1982) Induction of IgA immune complexes after wheat feeding in dermatitis herpetiformis patients. *J. Invest. Dermatol.*, **78**, 375–80.
75. Griffiths, C.E.M., Barrison, I., Leonard, J.N., *et al.* (1988) Preferential activation of CD4 T-lymphocytes in the lamina propia of gluten-sensitive enteropathy. *Clin. Exp. Immunol.*, **72**, 280–83.
76. Haffenden, G.P., Blenkinsop, W.K., Ring, N.P., Wojnarowska, F. and Fry, L. (1980) The potassium iodide patch tests in dermatitis herpetiformis in relation to treatment with a gluten-free diet and dapsone. *Brit. J. Dermatol.*, **102**, 313–17.
77. Unsworth, D.J., Leonard, J.N., McMinn, R.M.H., *et al.* (1981) Anti-gliadin antibodies and small intestinal mucosal damage in dermatitis herpetiformis. *Brit. J. Dermatol.*, **105**, 653–8.
78. Kilander, A.F., Gillberg, R.E., Kastrup, W., Mobacken, H. and Nilsson, L.A. (1985) Serum antibodies to gliadin and intestinal morphology in dermatitis herpetiformis. *Scand. J. Gastroenterol.*, **20**, 951–8.
79. Hamilton, I., Fairris, G.M., Rothwell, J., *et al.* (1985) Small intestinal permeability in dermatological disease. *Q. J. Med.*, **56**, 559–68.
80. Bjarnason, I., Marsh, M.N., Price, A., Levi, A.J. and Peters, T.J. (1985) Intestinal permeability in patients with coeliac disease and dermatitis herpetiformis. *Gut*, **26**, 1214–19.
81. Alexander, J. O'D. (1975) *Dermatitis Herpetiformis*, W.B. Saunders Co., London.

PART TWO

The genetically determined bullous diseases

Twelve

Diagnosis and diagnostic techniques

Michael J. Tidman and Robin A. J. Eady

12.1 INTRODUCTION

The development of a blistering eruption in a neonate or infant is a potentially serious situation. Some of the genetically determined bullous diseases are life-threatening conditions and others are associated with chronic disability and pain. Parents of affected children may be committed to dedicated nursing care and subject to all the frustrations of having a disabled child. They may also have to live with anxiety over the risk of having further afflicted offspring. Genetic counselling and prenatal diagnosis rely on establishing a correct diagnosis, which may be difficult at the onset of an inherited bullous disorder without resorting to special investigative techniques.

Those genetically determined diseases in which the formation of blisters represent a prominent clinical feature comprise a widely diverse group of conditions that includes epidermolysis bullosa, bullous ichthyosiform erythroderma, incontinentia pigmenti, acrodermatitis enteropathica, pachyonychia congenita, Hailey–Hailey disease (benign familial pemphigus) and certain of the porphyrias. For those that present in the neonatal period, appropriate laboratory investigation may be necessary to exclude non-inherited disorders with blistering as a feature, such as bullous impetigo, staphylococcal scalded-skin syndrome, erythema toxicum neonatorum, transient neonatal pustular melanosis, miliaria crystallina, bullous urticaria pigmentosa and congenital infections, including syphilis, varicella and herpes simplex.

A systematic approach to the diagnosis of inherited bullous diseases involves the construction of a detailed pedigree, analysis of the clinical features, histological examination and, where appropriate, special investigations which include electron microscopy and immunohistochemistry. Prenatal diagnosis is now feasible for some of the potentially severe blistering genodermatoses.

12.2 INHERITANCE PATTERNS

A list of the more significant inherited blistering diseases and the mode of their inheritance is given in Table 12.1. A characteristic of dominantly

Table 12.1 Inheritance patterns of genetically determined bullous disorders

Disease	*Mode of inheritance*
Epidermolysis bullosa simplex	Autosomal dominant
Junctional epidermolysis bullosa	Autosomal recessive
Dystrophic epidermolysis bullosa	Autosomal dominant or recessive
Bullous ichthyosiform erythroderma	Autosomal dominant
Incontinentia pigmenti	Sex-linked dominant*
Hailey–Hailey disease	Autosomal dominant
Acrodermatitis enteropathica	Autosomal recessive
Pachyonychia congenita	Autosomal dominant
Congenital erythropoietic porphyria	Autosomal recessive
Porphyria cutanea tarda	Autosomal dominant
Variegate porphyria	Autosomal dominant

* With lethality of hemizygous males.

inherited conditions is the variability of their clinical expression, to the extent that affected relatives may be unaware of their diagnosis. It is therefore mandatory to examine the parents and siblings thoroughly. In sporadic cases, where neither parent appears to be affected, confirmation of paternity is desirable, but rarely practical.

12.3 CLINICAL FEATURES

The majority of the inherited blistering diseases have characteristic clinical features that allow for a relatively straightforward diagnosis to be made. This includes incontinentia pigmenti, bullous ichthyosiform erythroderma, Hailey–Hailey disease and pachyonychia congenita. The clinical picture may suggest one of the porphyrias, which can be confirmed by demonstrating the appropriate abnormality of porphyrin metabolism (Chapter 19). The underlying defect of zinc absorption in acrodermatitis enteropathica is usually reflected by low serum levels of zinc, but an additional diagnostic test for this condition is the clinical response to a therapeutic trial of zinc supplementation.

Perhaps the group of bullous genodermatoses most beset with problems in the establishment of a precise diagnosis is epidermolysis bullosa (EB). The classification of EB has become complicated by the large number of variants described [1], which is still expanding [2–4]. There are three major types – simplex, junctional and dystrophic – each with specific levels of cleavage in, or adjacent to, the epidermal basement membrane. Each type has certain characteristic clinical features that are detailed in Chapters 14–16, but it may not be possible to make a confident diagnosis on clinical grounds alone, particularly during the early months of life.

12.4 HISTOLOGICAL EXAMINATION

Light microscopic examination of lesional skin will confirm the clinical diagnosis in the majority of the genetic bullous diseases [5].

12.4.1 Incontinentia pigmenti

The vesicular stage of incontinentia pigmenti is characterized histologically by intraepidermal spongiotic vesicles containing eosinophils and the presence of dyskeratotic keratinocytes.

12.4.2 Bullous ichthyosiform erythroderma

Bullous ichthyosiform erythroderma demonstrates the changes of epidermolytic hyperkeratosis in both blistered and non-blistered skin, consisting of prominent vacuolization of cells in the stratum granulosum and upper stratum spinosum, large irregular keratohyaline granules and large clumps of tonofilaments, with intraepidermal bullae forming by the dissolution and separation of oedematous keratinocytes.

12.4.3 Hailey–Hailey disease

The predominant histological feature in Hailey–Hailey disease is suprabasal acantholysis. Dyskeratosis may also be present.

12.4.4 Pachyonychia congenita

Pachyonychia congenita blisters, which are usually confined to the plantar surfaces, arise within the stratum spinosum and have similar histological features to friction blisters.

12.4.5 Porphyria

Porphyria cutanea tarda and variegate porphyria are characterized by subepidermal bullae, with projection of the normal papillae ('festooning') into the cavity of the blister. A prominent perivascular mantle of periodic acid–Schiff-positive material is frequently evident.

12.4.6 Epidermolysis bullosa

The light microscopic differentiation of EB is less satisfactory. In standard sections of paraffin-embedded material the bullae in all three main types may appear to be subepidermal. Staining of the basement membrane by the periodic acid–Schiff reaction is generally unhelpful, as this stains material within and beneath the true epithelial basement membrane [6] and will not, therefore, discriminate between the different types of EB. In EB simplex, blisters result from cytolysis of the basal keratinocytes, leaving a variable amount of cytoplasm attached to an intact dermo–epidermal junction [7, 8]. In semithin (1 μm) sections of resin-embedded material from lesions of EB simplex it may be possible to resolve the cytoplasmic remnants in the floor of the blisters, thereby differentiating it from the junctional and dystrophic forms. A distinct subtype of EB simplex, the Dowling–Meara or herpetiform variant, is distinguished clinically by clustering of blisters and the gradual development of palmo–plantar keratoderma. Prominent aggregation of the epidermal tonofilaments within areas of incipient blister formation is considered to be a specific histological feature of Dowling–Meara EB simplex [9, 10]. This change may be readily visible in semithin resin-embedded material (Figures 12.1 and 12.2).

12.5 ELECTRON MICROSCOPY

Each of the three major types of EB has a specific cleavage level. EB simplex is characterized by cytolysis of the basal keratinocytes, junctional EB by separation through the lamina lucida of the epithelial basement membrane, and dystrophic EB by blister formation beneath the lamina densa (Figure 12.3). The distance separating these three levels of cleavage is approximately 1–2 μm, too small to be adequately resolved by the light

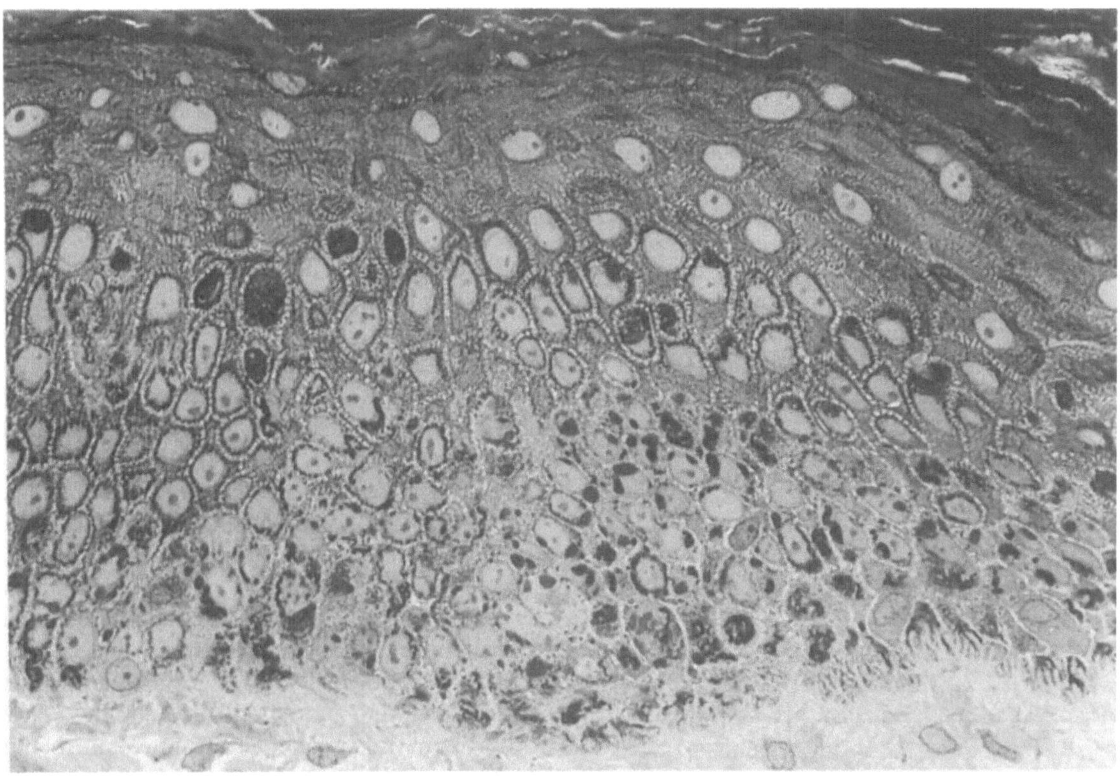

Figure 12.1 Semithin (1 μm) section of perilesional skin in epidermolysis bullosa simplex (Dowling–Meara), demonstrating tonofilament clumping within keratinocytes (Huber stain) (× 160).

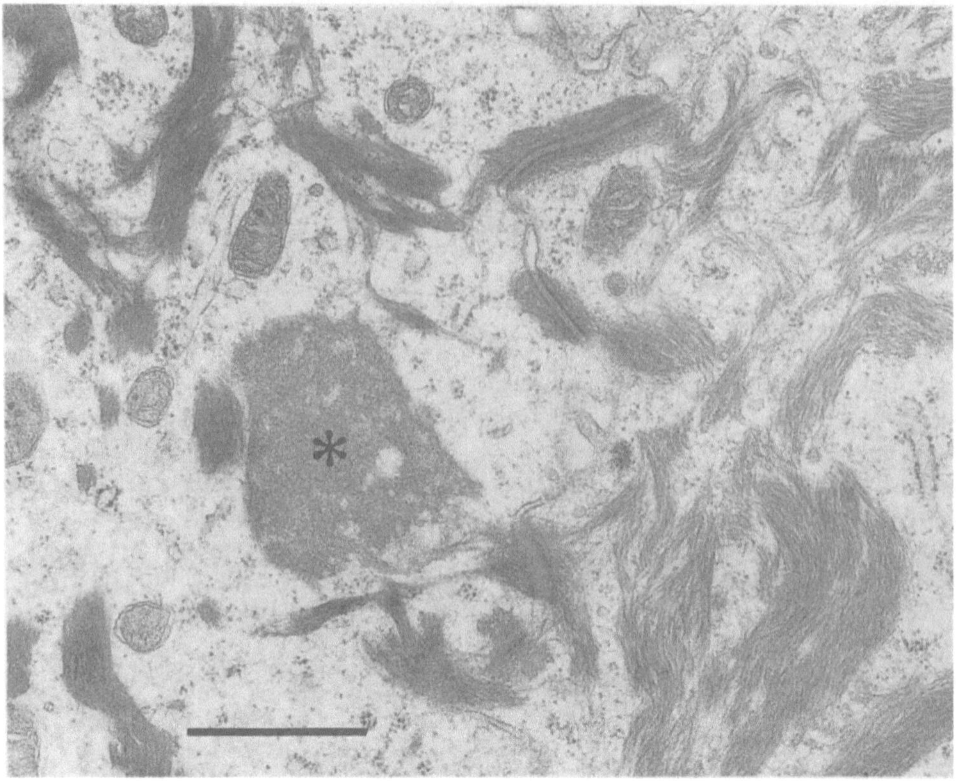

Figure 12.2 Electron micrograph showing clumping of the tonofilaments (*) in epidermolysis bullosa simplex (Dowling–Meara). Calibration bar = 1 μm.

microscope. The definitive diagnosis necessitates either transmission electron microscopy or antigen mapping (see Section 12.6). A fresh blister (preferably less than 12 h old) should be biopsied,

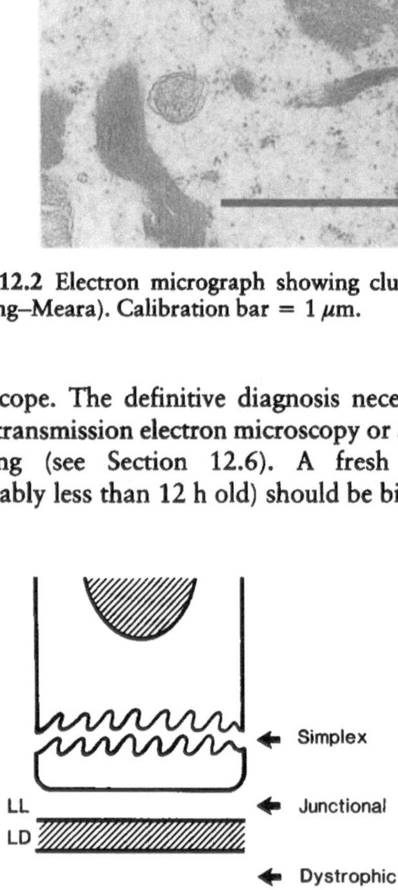

Figure 12.3 Schematic diagram illustrating the levels of cleavage in the three major types of epidermolysis bullosa (LL, lamina lucida; LD, lamina densa).

as the changes that accompany healing may make interpretation difficult. It may be possible to induce a blister by gentle friction in a predilection site with a pencil eraser in the more severe forms of EB [11].

Junctional EB is clinically variable (Chapter 15), and it has been proposed, on the basis of electron microscopical studies [2, 12–14], that a disorder of the hemidesmosomes may be the primary defect. It is true that the hemidesmosomes in junctional EB are usually reduced in number, lack normal sub-basal dense plates and possess rudimentary attachment plaques, but a detailed ultrastructural morphometric analysis has shown there to be a marked heterogeneity of the hemidesmosomes [15], which in some patients may be normal. Unfortunately, the hemidesmosome abnormalities do not correlate precisely with the clinical subtype of junctional EB, and we do not feel that the morphology of the hemidesmosomes in non-lesional skin can be used as an accurate prognostic indicator.

Dystrophic EB is also clinically heterogeneous (Chapter 16) and is associated with a numerical abnormality of the anchoring fibrils. Early reports suggested the anchoring fibrils at the dermo–epidermal junction to be reduced in number [16] and abnormal in structure [17, 18] in dominant dystrophic EB, and diminished [19] or absent [20, 21] in recessive forms of dystrophic EB. Morphometric evaluation of these structures has confirmed a total absence of anchoring fibrils in severe generalized recessive dystrophic EB and reduced numbers in both the dominant and localized recessive forms of dystrophic EB [22]. Thus, an electron microscopic finding that the anchoring fibrils are absent from non-lesional skin would be consistent with a diagnosis of generalized recessive dystrophic EB. However, because of the great variation in the numbers of anchoring fibrils to be found in normal skin [23] it is not feasible to diagnose the localized forms of dystrophic EB solely on an assessment of the anchoring fibrils. Furthermore, it does not appear to be possible to distinguish between the dominant and recessive forms of localized dystrophic EB on purely ultrastructural criteria, and this is, of course, of significance for genetic counselling.

12.6 ANTIGEN MAPPING

If facilities for electron microscopy are not readily accessible, it is possible to determine the precise level of cleavage in EB by antigen mapping [24, 25]. This technique is based on the localization of normal components of the epithelial basement membrane in frozen material from fresh blisters, using an indirect immunohistochemical technique. The three principal levels of blister formation in EB can be distinguished by the use of antibodies to bullous pemphigoid antigen and type IV collagen. Bullous pemphigoid antigen appears to be associated with the cytoplasmic face of the hemidesmosomes [26, 27] and type IV collagen is located within the lamina densa [28]. In EB simplex both antibodies bind to the floor of the blister, in dystrophic EB both are localized to the roof, and in junctional EB the antibody to bullous pemphigoid is to be found in the roof and that to type IV collagen in the floor (Figure 12.4). Proponents of this technique stress the ease and speed with which a diagnosis can be reached, but mistaken interpretations may be made if the blister is not fresh.

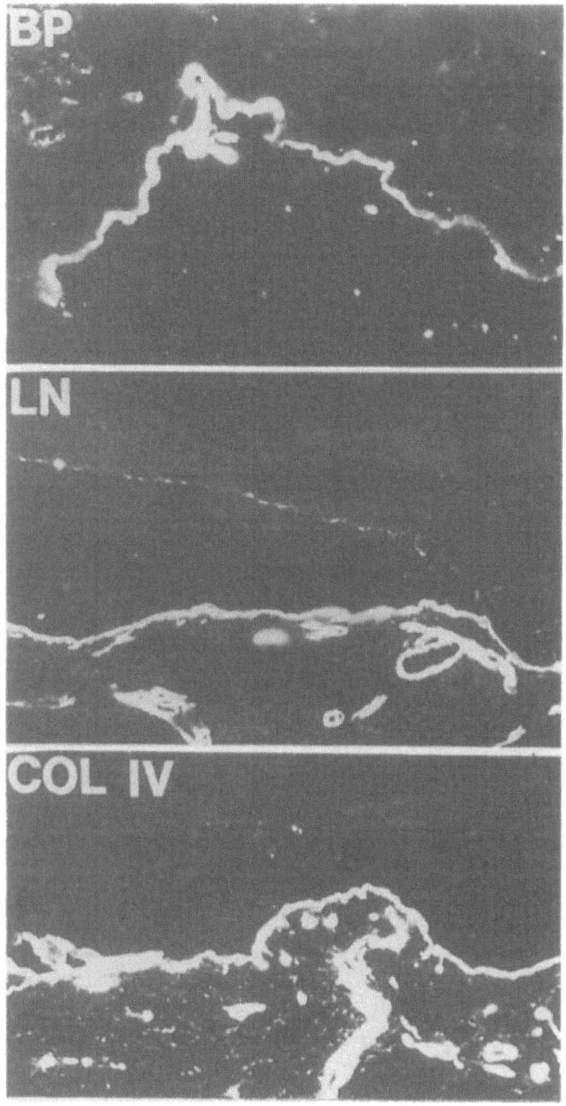

Figure 12.4 Antigen mapping in a case of junctional epidermolysis bullosa. BP: bullous pemphigoid antibody localizing to the blister roof. LN: antibody to laminin localizing principally to the blister floor, with some staining of the roof. COL IV: anti-(type IV collagen) antibody confined to the blister floor.

Electron microscopic examination is less likely to result in an incorrect diagnosis of the level of cleavage, as the suitability, or otherwise, of the specimen is immediately apparent.

12.7 SPECIAL ANTIBODY STUDIES

Within the last few years a number of antibodies have been produced which can be used as immunological probes in the diagnosis of EB. Several of these antibodies, including AF1 and AF2 [21], KF-1 [29] and LH 7:2 [30], identify antigenic components of the lamina densa and anchoring fibrils that are absent from, or markedly deficient in, recessive dystrophic EB. LH 7:2 is a monoclonal antibody to the C-terminus of type VII collagen [31], a major constituent of anchoring fibrils [32], and is particularly useful in the diagnosis of dystrophic EB (Figure 12.5). Staining of the epidermal basement membrane with LH 7:2 is absent in severe generalized recessive dystrophic EB, is only partial in localized recessive dystrophic EB and is normal in dominant dystrophic EB [30]. These observations suggest that LH 7:2 may be of particular value in determining the mode of inheritance in sporadic cases, thus enabling effective genetic counselling.

The human amnion-related antibodies, AA3 and GB3, have been shown to recognize lamina lucida constituents that are deficient in junctional EB [33, 34]. The GB3 antigen has been partially characterized [35].

12.8 SUCTION BLISTER TIMES

The measurement of suction blister times is a straightforward procedure that does not require great expertise or elaborate equipment (see Chapter

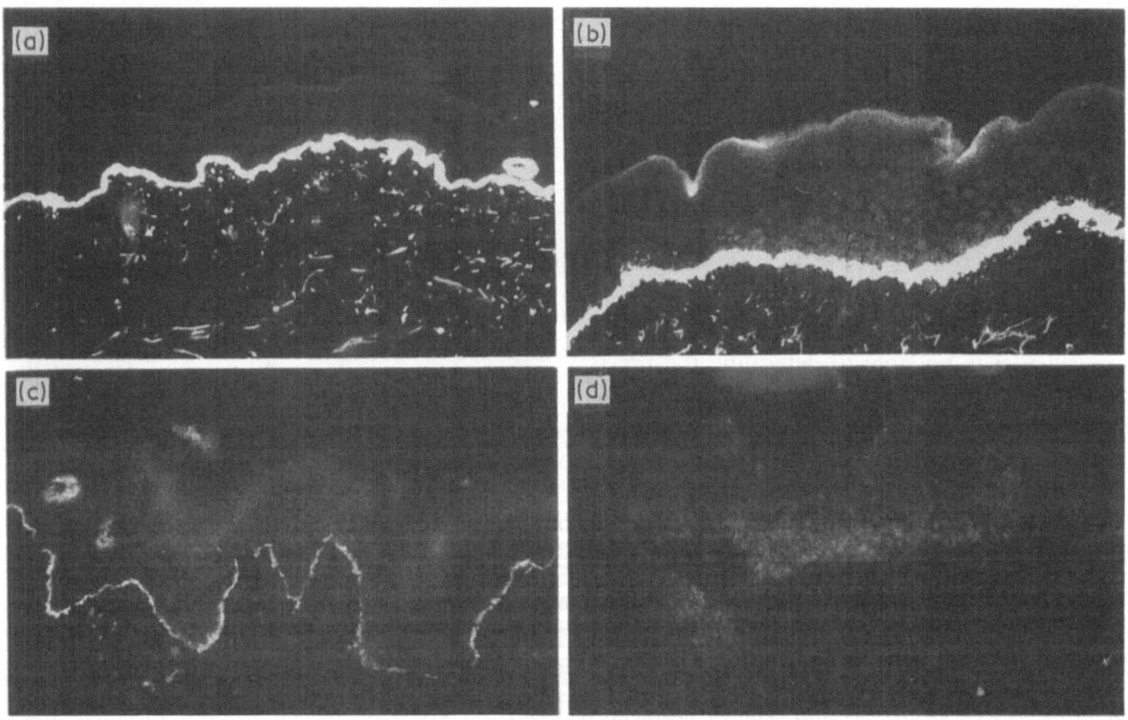

Figure 12.5 Fluorescence staining of the epidermal basement membrane with LH 7:2 [anti-type VII collagen antibody]. (a) Normal skin; (b) non-lesional skin from dominant dystrophic epidermolysis bullosa (DEB); (c) non-lesional skin from localized recessive DEB; (d) non-lesional skin from generalized recessive DEB. (× 240).

2). Suction blisters arise in the lamina lucida of the epidermal basement membrane, and the time taken for them to form has been used as a measure of the cohesive forces within the lamina lucida [36, 37]. Suction blisters develop abnormally rapidly in both junctional EB and in the generalized recessive form of dystrophic EB [38], and we have found that this property may be diagnostically useful [38].

12.9 PRENATAL DIAGNOSIS

Perhaps the most significant recent advance in the management of the inherited bullous disorders is the ability to detect antenatally a number of the more severe blistering diseases in at-risk pregnancies. Prenatal diagnosis, at present, involves a biopsy of the foetal skin using special forceps. The biopsies are taken under both foetoscopic and ultrasonic guidance [39]. Recently, ultrasound has been increasingly used on its own [40]. A predilection site for the condition under consideration should be selected on the foetus and multiple samples obtained. Because this technique requires an adequate volume of amniotic fluid, it is undertaken between 18 and 21 weeks gestation. First-trimester prenatal diagnosis is not yet feasible. Foetoscopy and foetal skin biopsy are relatively safe, with a foetal loss of not more than 5% in experienced hands [41, 42].

Both junctional EB [39] and generalized recessive dystrophic EB [43] have been diagnosed prenatally. The trauma of the biopsy procedure is sufficient in these two conditions (but not in normal foetal skin) to cause dermo–epidermal separation, and subsequent electron-microscopic examination, which can be achieved within 24 h by using a rapid processing method [44], confirms cleavage in the same plane as the natural blisters in the respective conditions. Intrauterine examination of the foetus

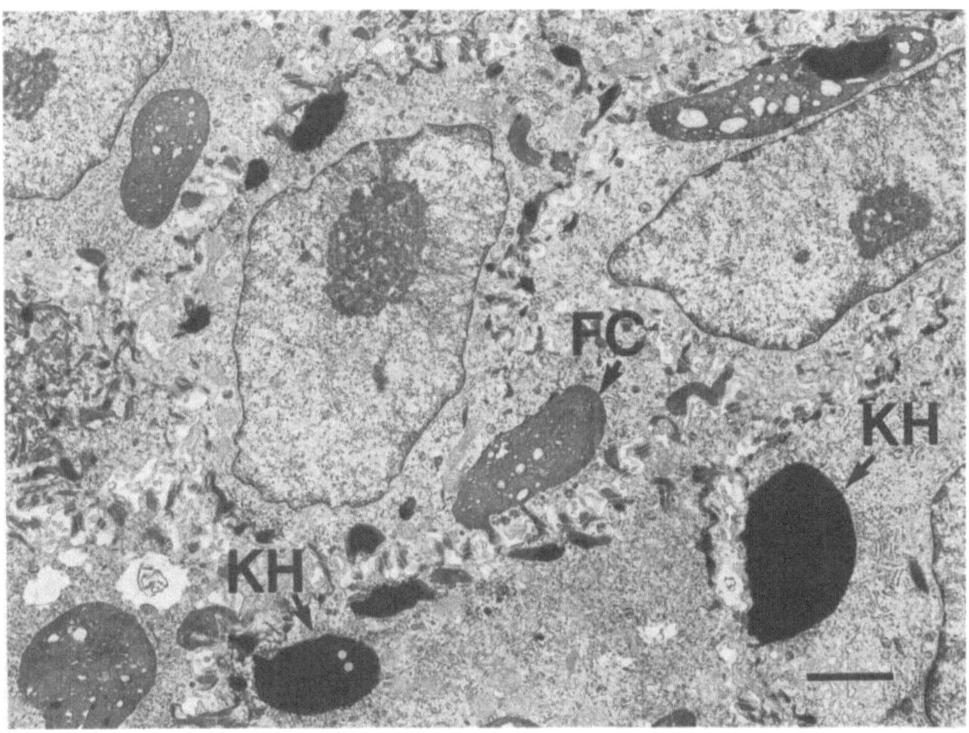

Figure 12.6 Electron micrograph showing tonofilament clumping (FC) and large keratohyaline granules (KH) in bullous ichthyosiform erythroderma. Calibration bar = 1 μm.

with the foetoscope rarely reveals any sign of blistering in affected cases, presumably because of the protected environment afforded by the amniotic fluid.

The antibody probes that identify abnormalities of the epidermal basement membrane in junctional EB and recessive dystrophic EB are now being used in the prenatal diagnosis of these conditions [34, 45], and it is conceivable that they may eventually replace transmission electron microscopy for routine diagnosis. Elevated levels of maternal serum alpha-foetoprotein in pregnancies affected by EB simplex have been recorded [46, 47], but the value of this test in prenatal diagnosis remains to be established.

Bullous ichthyosiform erythroderma can also be successfully diagnosed by foetal skin biopsy [48–50]. Even in the second trimester the histological and ultrastructural (Figure 12.6) features of this condition are evident. A significant proportion of amniotic fluid cells from affected cases have also been shown to contain the characteristic tonofilament aggregates, raising the possibility that prenatal diagnosis may be possible by amniocentesis alone, thereby avoiding the need for a foetal skin biopsy [49, 51].

REFERENCES

1. Gedde-Dahl, T. (1981) Sixteen types of epidermolysis bullosa: on the clinical discrimination, therapy and prenatal diagnosis. *Acta Dermatovenereol. (Stockholm)*, (Suppl.), **95**, 74–87.
2. Hintner, H. and Wolff, K. (1982) Generalized atrophic benign epidermolysis bullosa. *Arch. Dermatol.*, **118**, 375–84.
3. Haber, R.M., Hanna, W., Ramsay, C.A. and Boxall, L.B.H. (1985) Cicatricial junctional epidermolysis bullosa. *J. Amer. Acad. Dermatol.*, **12**, 836–44.
4. Fine, J-D., Osment, L.S. and Gay, S. (1985) Dystrophic epidermolysis bullosa. A new variant characterized by progressive symmetrical centripetal involvement with scarring. *Arch. Dermatol.*, **121**, 1014–17.
5. Lever, W.F. and Schaumburg-Lever, G. (1983) Congenital diseases (genodermatoses). In *Histopathology of the Skin*, 6th edn, J.B. Lippincott, Philadelphia, Chapter 6.
6. Swift, J.A. and Saxton, C.A. (1967) The ultrastructural location of the periodate-Schiff reactive basement membrane at the dermoepidermal junctions of human scalp and monkey gingiva. *J. Ultrastruct. Res.*, **17**, 23–33.
7. Pearson, R.W. (1962) Studies on the pathogenesis of epidermolysis bullosa. *J. Invest. Dermatol.*, **39**, 551–75.
8. Haneke, E. and Anton-Lamprecht, I. (1982) Ultrastructure of blister formation in epidermolysis bullosa hereditaria: V. Epidermolysis bullosa simplex localisata type Weber-Cockayne. *J. Invest. Dermatol.*, **78**, 219–23.
9. Anton-Lamprecht, I. and Schnyder, U.W. (1982) Epidermolysis bullosa herpetiformis Dowling-Meara. Report of a case and pathomorphogenesis. *Dermatologica*, **164**, 221–35.
10. Niemi, K-M., Kero, M., Kanerva, L. and Mattila, R. (1983) Epidermolysis bullosa simplex. A new histologic subgroup. *Arch. Dermatol.*, **119**, 138–41.
11. Eady, R.A.J. and Tidman, M.J. (1983) Diagnosing epidermolysis bullosa. *Brit. J. Dermatol.*, **108**, 621–6.
12. Hashimoto, I., Schnyder, U.W. and Anton-Lamprecht, I. (1976) Epidermolysis bullosa hereditaria with junctional blistering in an adult. *Dermatologica*, **152**, 72–86.
13. Arwill, T., Bergenholtz, A. and Thilander, H. (1968) Epidermolysis bullosa hereditaria. 5. The ultrastructure of oral mucosa and skin in four cases of the letalis form. *Acta Pathol. Microbiol. Scand.*, **74**, 311–24.
14. Hashimoto, I., Gedde-Dahl, T., Schnyder, U.W. and Anton-Lamprecht, I. (1976) Ultrastructural studies in epidermolysis bullosa hereditaria. IV. Recessive dystrophic types with junctional blistering. *Arch. Dermatol. Res.*, **257**, 17–32.
15. Tidman, M.J. and Eady, R.A.J. (1986) Hemidesmosome heterogeneity in junctional epidermolysis bullosa revealed by morphometric analysis. *J. Invest. Dermatol.*, **86**, 51–6.
16. Anton-Lamprecht, I. and Schnyder, U.W. (1973) Epidermolysis bullosa dystrophica dominans. Ein defekt der anchoring fibrils? *Dermatologica*, **147**, 289–98.
17. Hashimoto, I., Anton-Lamprecht, I., Gedde-Dahl, T. and Schnyder, U.W. (1975) Ultrastructural studies in epidermolysis bullosa hereditaria. I. Dominant dystrophic type of Pasini. *Arch. Dermatol. Forsch.*, **252**, 167–78.
18. Hashimoto, I., Gedde-Dahl, T., Schnyder, U.W. and Anton-Lamprecht, I. (1976) Ultrastructural studies in epidermolysis bullosa hereditaria. II. Dominant dystrophic type of Cockayne and Touraine. *Arch. Dermatol. Res.*, **255**, 285–95.
19. Hashimoto, I., Schnyder, U.W., Anton-Lamprecht, I., Gedde-Dahl, T. and Ward, S. (1976) Ultrastructural studies in epidermolysis bullosa hereditaria. III. Recessive dystrophic types with

dermolytic blistering (Hallopeau-Siemens types and inverse type). *Arch. Dermatol. Res.*, **256**, 137–50.
20. Briggaman, R.A. and Wheeler, C.E. (1975) Epidermolysis bullosa dystrophica-recessive: a possible role of anchoring fibrils in the pathogenesis. *J. Invest. Dermatol.*, **65**, 203–11.
21. Goldsmith, L.A. and Briggaman, R.A. (1983) Monoclonal antibodies to anchoring fibrils for the diagnosis of epidermolysis bullosa. *J. Invest. Dermatol.*, **81**, 464–6.
22. Tidman, M.J. and Eady, R.A.J. (1985) Evaluation of anchoring fibrils and other components of the dermal–epidermal junction in dystrophic epidermolysis bullosa by a quantitative ultrastructural technique. *J. Invest. Dermatol.*, **84**, 374–7.
23. Tidman, M.J. and Eady, R.A.J. (1984). Ultrastructural morphometry of normal human dermal–epidermal junction. The influence of age, sex and body region on laminar and non-laminar components. *J. Invest. Dermatol.*, **83**, 448–53.
24. Hintner, H., Stingl, G., Schuler, G., *et al.* (1981) Immunofluorescence mapping of antigenic determinants within the dermal–epidermal junction in mechanobullous diseases. *J. Invest. Dermatol.*, **76**, 113–18.
25. Kero, M., Peltonen, L., Foidart, J-M. and Savolainen, E-R. (1982) Immunohistological localization of three basement membrane components in various forms of epidermolysis bullosa. *J. Cutan. Pathol.*, **9**, 316–28.
26. Westgate, G.E., Weaver, A.C. and Couchman, J.R. (1985) Bullous pemphigoid antigen localization suggests an intracellular association with hemidesmosomes. *J. Invest. Dermatol.*, **84**, 218–24.
27. Mutasim, D.F., Takahashi, Y., Labib, R.S., *et al.* (1985) A pool of bullous pemphigoid antigen(s) is intracellular and associated with the basal cell cytoskeleton–hemidesmosome complex. *J. Invest. Dermatol.*, **84**, 47–53.
28. Yaoita, H., Foidart, J-M. and Katz, S.I. (1978) Localization of the collagenous component in skin basement membrane. *J. Invest. Dermatol.*, **70**, 191–3.
29. Fine, J.-D., Breathnach, S.M., Hintner, H. and Katz, S.I. (1984) KF-1 monoclonal antibody defines a specific basement membrane antigen defect in dystrophic forms of epidermolysis bullosa. *J. Invest. Dermatol.*, **82**, 35–8.
30. Heagerty, A.H.M., Kennedy, A.R., Leigh, I.M., *et al.* (1986) Identification of an epidermal basement membrane defect in recessive forms of dystrophic epidermolysis bullosa by LH7:2 monoclonal antibody: use in diagnosis. *Brit. J. Dermatol.*, **115**, 125–31.
31. Leigh, I.M., Eady, R.A.J., Heagerty, A.H.M., *et al.* (1988) Type VII collagen is a normal component of epidermal basement membrane which shows altered expression in recessive dystrophic epidermolysis bullosa. *J. Invest. Dermatol.*, **90**, 639–42.
32. Sakai, L.Y., Keene, D.R., Morris, N.P. and Burgeson, R.E. (1986) Type VII collagen is a major structural component of anchoring fibrils. *J. Cell Biol.*, **103**, 1577–86.
33. Kennedy, A.R., Heagerty, A.H.M., Ortonne, J-P. *et al.* (1985) Abnormal binding of an anti-amnion antibody to epidermal basement membrane provides a novel diagnostic probe for junctional epidermolysis bullosa. *Brit. J. Dermatol.*, **113**, 651–9.
34. Heagerty, A.H.M., Kennedy, A.R., Eady, R.A.J., *et al.* (1986) GB3 monoclonal antibody for diagnosis of junctional epidermolysis bullosa. *Lancet*, **i**, 860.
35. Verrando, P., Pisani, A., Hsi, B.L., *et al.* (1987) Monoclonal antibody GB3, a new tool for molecular characterization of basement membranes and hemidesmosomes. *J. Invest. Dermatol.*, **89**, 315–16.
36. Kiistala, U. (1972) Dermal–epidermal separation. 1. The influence of age, sex and body region on suction blister formation in human skin. *Ann. Clin. Res.*, **4**, 10–22.
37. Kiistala, U. (1972) Dermal–epidermal separation. II. External factors in suction blister formation with special reference to the effect of temperature. *Ann. Clin. Res.*, **4**, 236–46.
38. Tidman, M.J. and Eady, R.A.J. (1984) Evidence for a functional defect of the lamina lucida in recessive dystrophic epidermolysis bullosa demonstrated by suction blisters. *Brit. J. Dermatol.*, **111**, 379–87.
39. Rodeck, C.H., Eady, R.A.J. and Gosden, C.M. (1980) Prenatal diagnosis of epidermolysis bullosa letalis. *Lancet*, **i**, 949–52.
40. Eady, R.A.J. (1987) Fetoscopy and fetal skin biopsy for prenatal diagnosis of genetic skin disorders. *Semin. Dermatol.* (in press).
41. Rodeck, C.H. and Nicolaides, K.H. (1983) Fetoscopy and fetal tissue sampling. *Brit. Med. Bull.*, **39**, 332–7.
42. Eady, R.A.J. (1987) Prenatal diagnosis. In *Proceedings of XVII World Congress of Dermatology* (in press).
43. Anton-Lamprecht, I., Jovanovic, V., Arnold, M.L., *et al.* (1981) Prenatal diagnosis of epidermolysis bullosa dystrophica Hallopeau-Siemens with electron microscopy of fetal skin. *Lancet*, **ii**, 1077–9.
44. Eady, R.A.J., Gunner, D.B., Tidman, M.J., *et al.* (1984) Rapid processing of fetal skin for prenatal diagnosis by light and electron microscopy. *J. Clin. Pathol.*, **37**, 633–8.
45. Heagerty, A.H.M., Kennedy, A.R., Gunner, D.B. and Eady, R.A.J. (1986) Rapid prenatal diagnosis and exclusion of epidermolysis bullosa using novel antibody probes. *J. Invest. Dermatol.*, **86**, 603–5.
46. Yacoub, T., Campbell, C.A., Gorden, Y.B., *et al.*

(1979) Maternal serum and amniotic fluid concentrations of alphafetoprotein in epidermolysis bullosa. *Brit. Med. J.*, i, 307.

47. Cowton, J.A.L., Beattie, T.J., Gibson, A.A.M., *et al.* (1982) Epidermolysis bullosa in association with aplasia cutis congenita and pyloric atresia. *Acta Paediatr. Scand.*, **71**, 155–60.
48. Golbus, M.S., Sagebiel, R.W., Filly, R.A., *et al.* (1980) Prenatal diagnosis of congenital bullous ichthyosiform erythroderma (epidermolytic hyperkeratosis) by fetal skin biopsy. *New Engl. J. Med.*, **302**, 93–5.
49. Eady, R.A.J., Gunner, D.B., Lamba Carbone, L.D., *et al.* (1986) Prenatal diagnosis of bullous ichthyosiform erythroderma: detection of tonofilament clumps in fetal epidermis and amniotic fluid cells. *J. Med. Genet.*, **23**, 46–51.
50. Anton-Lamprecht, I. (1981) Prenatal diagnosis of genetic disorders of the skin by means of electron microscopy. *Hum. Genet.*, **59**, 392–405.
51. Holbrook, K.A., Dale, B.A., Sybert, V.P. and Sagebiel, R.W. (1983) Epidermolytic hyperkeratosis: ultrastructure and biochemistry of skin and amniotic fluid cells from two affected fetuses and a newborn infant. *J. Invest. Dermatol.*, **80**, 222–7.

Thirteen
Therapy and counselling in epidermolysis bullosa

David J. Atherton

13.1 GENETIC COUNSELLING

Genetic counselling is an essential part of the management of families in whom there is an individual with epidermolysis bullosa. Indeed, it is in my view a serious error to neglect to inform all relevant members of such families of the genetic risks implied by a diagnosis of epidermolysis bullosa in one of its number.

Reliable genetic counselling requires accurate diagnosis. This principle has some very important consequences. For example, if an infant with one of the more serious forms of epidermolysis bullosa dies before a precise diagnosis has been established, it will not be possible to offer the parents reliable counselling or prenatal diagnosis in the mother's next pregnancy. Obvious as this appears, it is a principle that is still frequently neglected in the excitement of caring for a critically ill neonate.

13.1.1 Epidermolysis bullosa simplex

Genetic counselling is generally straightforward in the commoner simplex types of epidermolysis bullosa, as these are transmitted as autosomal dominant traits with a high penetrance and have usually been established in the family for several generations. New mutations for these diseases appear to be relatively uncommon.

Prenatal diagnosis is generally inappropriate in simplex epidermolysis bullosa, with the possible exception of the Dowling–Meara type, which may be severe and disabling [1]. However, although an autosomal dominant mode of inheritance appears probable, very few familial cases have been described. Though prenatal diagnosis seems a theoretical possibility, the author is unaware of any report that this has been successfully accomplished in practice.

13.1.2 Dystrophic epidermolysis bullosa

From a clinical point of view, both dominantly and recessively inherited dystrophic epidermolysis bullosa appear to be heterogeneous, though the subtypes have yet to be fully delineated. Dominant dystrophic epidermolysis bullosa is generally a mild disease not resulting in significant disability; however, occasional individuals are rather severely affected, presenting a clinical picture indistinguishable from generalized recessive dystrophic epidermolysis bullosa. As is usual with dominantly inherited diseases, there may be considerable variability of severity within a single family. Therefore, not knowing the likely level of disability in the as yet unborn child, it is difficult for parents or doctors to feel confident whether termination of pregnancy really would or would not be justified, if the foetus were affected. We have recently cared for a child with extremely severe and disabling disease born into a family in which dominantly inherited dystrophic epidermolysis bullosa of mild degree has occurred for many generations.

The situation is rather different in families where dystrophic epidermolysis bullosa is inherited as an autosomal recessive trait. There are two broad categories of recessive dystrophic epidermolysis bullosa: a localized form, usually clinically mild, and a generalized form, usually more severe but varying considerably in severity between families. The degree of severity within a particular family tends to be fairly constant and predictable, as is usual in recessive disorders. This makes it much easier to counsel parents. If a child is severely affected, parents should be informed of the availability and nature of prenatal diagnostic techniques. The counsellor must take care not to influence the parents too strongly through his/her own prejudices. For example, it would in my view be entirely wrong to deny parents information about prenatal diagnosis because one's own view was that it was indefensible on moral or religious grounds. Equally, we must respect the right of parents to decide against prenatal diagnosis and the concept of termination of an affected foetus.

13.1.3 Junctional epidermolysis bullosa

It is now clear that junctional epidermolysis bullosa is also a heterogeneous disease, comprising several distinct diseases of differing severity. It remains the case, however, that most affected babies have a poor prognosis for survival, even when heroic efforts are made to save them. The majority die within the first 6 months, and few survive beyond the second or third year; yet there are survivors with junctional epidermolysis bullosa who enjoy long lives with relatively mild disease. As with the autosomal recessive types of dystrophic epidermolysis bullosa, the behaviour of the disease in a particular family tends to be rather predictable, and counselling is simplified when one is aware of the form the disease has previously taken in the family. Of course, it could be difficult where a first affected child is only a few months old and parents wish to try for a sibling. In practice, however, few parents do attempt a further pregnancy until the affected child has died or has survived for several years.

13.2 PRENATAL DIAGNOSIS

There is now a wide spectrum of disorders for which prenatal diagnosis is available. This may allow treatments to be undertaken during foetal life, or may provide warning of the need for intervention during the first few hours or days after birth. However, for the present, most prenatal diagnosis is undertaken to permit termination of pregnancy in diseases in which this is considered an appropriate response; this is still the situation with epidermolysis bullosa.

The technique used for the prenatal diagnosis of epidermolysis bullosa is that of foetal skin biopsy [1, 2]. In epidermolysis bullosa the optimum time for foetal skin biopsy is during the 18th week of gestation. The biopsy is taken with very fine forceps that 'pinch off' a piece of skin about 2 mm in diameter. The forceps have a long and very narrow neck, so that the instrument can be passed down a cannula that has been introduced into the amniotic cavity. The biopsy may be taken under direct visual control using a foetoscope, or with ultrasound guidance alone. The procedure may be performed with local or general anaesthesia, and can be done on a day-case basis. Diagnosis depends upon the observation of a split at the dermo–epidermal junction, and determination of the precise level at which this has occurred. Currently this is still most reliably accomplished by electron microscopy, but in time it may become routine to achieve an equally reliable result with the light microscope, using fluorescent monoclonal antibodies which are able to define specific antigenic components of the junction [3]. Using rapid processing techniques, electron-microscopic diagnosis can now be achieved within 24 h [4].

It is important to be aware of the great anxieties faced by parents who have elected to have prenatal diagnosis. By the 18th week, pregnancy is fairly advanced. The mother will have been conscious of foetal movements for some time and will have seen the baby during ultrasound scans. It requires great courage to face the possible loss of the baby at this stage. After the foetal skin biopsy, the wait for the result is an agonizing one. Parents know that termination will take the form of an induced labour. The stresses placed on the medical and nursing staff should also not be neglected. Fortunately, the chances of a normal foetus are 3 to 1, and this makes the whole process feasible and the anxiety bearable.

There is a definite incidence of foetal loss following the procedure of foetal skin biopsy, probably between 0.5 and 1%. Parents must be made aware of this.

Although termination of pregnancy as a way of preventing genetic disease seems to many to be a negative concept, and to others to be an unacceptable one, my own experience has been that its availability provides parents with the confidence to have further children, when otherwise they would not attempt to do so. It allows parents to have the children that they would otherwise not dare to have, and it can provide a normal sibling for a child with epidermolysis bullosa who would otherwise have remained without. It can restore the shattered confience of parents who so often see the birth of a child with a severe genetic disease as a personal failing.

13.3 SKIN BIOPSY IN EPIDERMOLYSIS BULLOSA

Skin biopsy is extremely valuable in epidermolysis bullosa for diagnostic categorization. Biopsy is certainly not necessary in every case, and when a biopsy is to be undertaken, the reasons for it should be clear both to the person taking the biopsy, and to the pathologist who is to interpret it. There is very little point in taking a biopsy if only routine light microscopy is available. Transmission electron microscopy provides the best tool for the interpretation of skin biopsy material in epidermolysis bullosa. Limited interpretation is possible if this facility is not available, by use of appropriate basement membrane zone markers, such as bullous pemphigoid serum, which will allow one to establish whether a split is occurring above or below the lamina densa.

The technique of taking biopsies in epidermolysis bullosa is of the greatest importance if the procedure is to provide useful tissue for the pathologist. The biopsy should be taken from clinically *unaffected* skin. Disruption of the skin should be induced by rubbing the area to be biopsied with a finger for about a minute. There should follow a delay of 5–10 min, after which the biopsy should be taken. We find that the shave technique provides the best quality material, because artefact is minimal, fixation is rapid, orientation is easier and healing is good.

13.4 DIAGNOSIS AND PROGNOSIS OF EPIDERMOLYSIS BULLOSA IN THE NEONATE

Our experience has been that there is no good correlation between the severity of the skin condition in the first 1 or 2 days of life and the precise diagnostic categorization of the infant with epidermolysis bullosa; nor does there appear to be any correlation with prognosis, either for life itself, or for the degree of disability later on. For example, we have found that those neonates with junctional epidermolysis bullosa who die in early infancy are often remarkably mildly affected initially. As far as type of epidermolysis bullosa is concerned, perhaps the most reliable distinguishing sign is hoarseness of the voice, which appears to us to be a very common early feature of the junctional forms of the disease. Almost all other alleged distinguished signs have in our experience at times proved misleading. The later appearance of milia is indicative of dystrophic epidermolysis bullosa, though small numbers of milia can undoubtedly be seen from time to time in non-dystrophic types.

Early diagnostic biopsy is helpful, but is not that valuable in terms of prognosis unless those monoclonal markers are used that enable further diagnostic distinction, for example, between the localized and generalized variants of dystrophic epidermolysis bullosa.

Overall it is wise to avoid making pronouncements regarding prognosis in infants with epidermolysis bullosa unless the situation is fairly clear, as it is with the infant with junctional epidermolysis bullosa who fails to gain weight over a period of several months. After the age of about 6 months, the situation generally becomes much clearer, and some comment can be made on both the risk of mortality and on the likely degree of disability in survivors.

13.5 SKIN CARE IN EPIDERMOLYSIS BULLOSA

Skin care in patients with epidermolysis bullosa must incorporate the twin objectives of protection against trauma and provision of optimal conditions for rapid healing of blisters and erosions. A third objective, relevant in the older patient, is surveillance for epidermal neoplasia.

It is perhaps most convenient to consider skin care separately for the three age groups: neonates, older infants and toddlers, and older children and adults.

13.5.1 Neonates

Some infants with epidermolysis bullosa already have extensive lesions at birth; others develop lesions rapidly during their first few days. Some patients with simplex types of epidermolysis bullosa do not develop their first lesions until later on.

The skin of neonates with epidermolysis bullosa may be extraordinarily sensitive, even to 'normal' handling. We commonly find that infants transferred to our unit have erosions on each side of the trunk where they have been picked up earlier. Sometimes there are five on each side, one for each of the nurse's fingers. Therefore, special handling techniques need to be used in the nursing of these infants. I will describe the way we care for these babies in our unit.

We nurse babies with epidermolysis bullosa on a piece of 1 inch (2.5 cm)-thick foam, measuring about 36 inches (90 cm) square, which is covered by a silk sheet. Using this arrangement, the baby can be held without direct contact, making it possible to feed, comfort and move the baby about safely.

We change dressings twice daily. We like to drain new blisters after puncturing them with a sterile disposable needle, as they will often extend if left alone. The blister roof is left *in situ*. We normally then bath the baby in warm water with a little added potassium permanganate, enough to make the water slightly pink. The baby is dried with a hair drier, after which eroded areas should, if necessary, be gently cleaned with cotton wool balls soaked with sterile normal saline. Vaseline gauze (Sherwood Medical, Greenwich, Connecticut, USA) is now applied to eroded and blistered areas. If eroded areas are obviously infected, we spread stabilized hydrogen peroxide cream (Hioxyl, Quinoderm, Oldham, UK) on to the Vaseline gauze on the side that will come into direct contact with the skin. Great caution must be exercised in the choice of topical antibacterial agents for these children because of the very real danger of induction of bacterial resistance, and because of the danger of toxicity that may follow the systemic absorption which is inevitable when a topical agent is applied to de-epithelialized areas under more or less occlusive dressings. The use of topical antimicrobial agents should not be routine. Vaseline gauze is an extremely fine paraffin gauze, which we find greatly superior to standard paraffin gauze because of its greatly reduced thread diameter and mesh size. This gauze is also available in a ribbon form, which is very useful for weaving between fingers and toes. Over the Vaseline gauze is applied a layer of Melolin roll (Smith & Nephew, Romford, Essex, UK); this comprises wadding, with a non-adherent film applied to the underside. This is now secured by a suitable conforming bandage, e.g. J-Fast (Johnson & Johnson, Slough, UK), and/or a tubular stretch bandage such as Tubifast (Seton, Oldham, UK).

Such dressings will generally not adhere to eroded areas, and their use is associated with a good rate of re-epithelialization, probably reflecting both their occlusive and protective properties. They are, however, not used solely to encourage healing of blistered areas; we use them for protection in any area, whether affected or not at the time, that is in our view liable to blistering. We never nurse babies with epidermolysis bullosa completely naked. Such babies are usually uncomfortable, irritable and restless; they therefore tend to do themselves considerable harm, for example by rubbing together their legs, and their lesions heal relatively slowly. We almost always use these dressings on the arms and legs, and often on the trunk also. Babies wearing such dressings are usually more comfortable and are shielded from external mechanical trauma, particularly that which is self-induced. We encourage parents to learn the technique and use it after they take the baby home.

We aim only to keep the baby in hospital until the clinical situation is improving and the parents feel confident enough to take over in their own home. Generally, babies go home about 3–5 weeks after birth. There is of course a geat deal to be done while the child is in hospital in addition to the basic skin care. Feeding and nutritional problems have to be overcome. Precise diagnosis has to be made, and much time needs to be spent with parents explaining the nature of their child's problems and its care. It is generally necessary to communicate before the child's departure from hospital with community nursing and medical staff, and local social services. A visit to the hospital to see the routines is often welcomed by the community nurse.

The genetic situation needs to be clarified with the parents, and the implications for further offspring must be delineated at this stage. The availability of the means to prevent the birth of a similar child *must* be explained to parents; it is in my view the clear responsibility of the child's doctors to do so whatever their personal views. It is essential, lest the issue subsequently be neglected, to do this during the affected child's first admission.

13.5.2 Older infants and toddlers

Over the months that follow birth, it becomes decreasingly appropriate to employ the type of dressing described above. The danger of self-inflicted trauma decreases as the need for mobility and play gradually increases. However, as the child becomes more mobile, the risk of external trauma from falls and knocks initially increases. As the child slowly learns to become more careful, so the amount of mechanical trauma again diminishes. Sadly, toddlers are notoriously careless, and certain sites tend to become recurrently blistered. In dystrophic epidermolysis bullosa, these sites become permanently scarred, a problem because such areas are less resistant to subsequent trauma than unscarred areas. The sites that are at special risk in the toddler are the elbows, wrists, hands, knees, shins, ankles and feet. Many parents elect to use protective dressings to cushion these sites. An appropriate technique is to use Melolin roll next to the skin, over which is applied J-Fast, then Tubifast, over the area to be protected.

The ideal dressing for erosions and blisters in patients with epidermolysis bullosa beyond infancy has yet to be invented. None of the currently available products seems very precisely to fit these patients' requirements. Patients and their parents generally make up their own minds about the dressing materials that most suit their own needs, and the dermatologist's job is really to ensure firstly that they are properly informed about the range of different types of dressing available, and, secondly, that they are able to secure a supply of their chosen dressings as economically as possible. There can be little question that relatively occlusive dressings are more effective in accelerating healing [5–7].

Different patients use a great variety of topical agents, most of which are antimicrobial in their effects. Secondary bacterial infection is a constant problem in blistered and eroded areas, and it frequently delays healing. We still lack the ideal topical antimicrobial agent to protect the patient from the secondary bacterial infections that tend to be such a major problem for them. Of those preparations that are currently available, the following seem most suitable: 1.5% hydrogen peroxide cream (Hioxyl, Quinoderm, Oldham, UK), 10% povidone–iodine aqueous solution or ointment (Betadine, Napp, Cambridge, UK), 0.5% cetrimide cream (Cetavlex, Care, Wilmslow, UK) and 1% silver sulphadiazine cream (Flamazine, Smith & Nephew). Antibiotics of value in the systemic treatment of serious infections should not be used topically to treat chronic dermatoses such as epidermolysis bullosa, nor should important topical antibiotics, especially mupirocin (Bactroban, Beecham, Brentford, UK), because the selection of resistant bacteria is virtually inevitable; indeed, one of the first reports of mupirocin-resistant *Staphylococcus aureus* relates to a patient with epidermolysis bullosa [8].

Some patients apply various natural substances to ulcerated areas with the aim of accelerating healing. Good examples are honey and sucrose [9], which may discourage micro-organisms by providing a hyperosmolar environment. Unfortunately, the beneficial or other effects of such agents have very rarely been the subject of scientific evaluation and it is therefore difficult to comment upon their possible value.

Clearly, avoidance of trauma is an important facet of treatment of these children. It is extremely difficult, however, for parents to get the balance right between what could be regarded as appropriate avoidance of trauma and over-protection of the developing child. Children with epidermolysis bullosa should be brought up as normally as possible, in order to maximize their physical, manipulative and social skills. They gradually themselves learn to take extra care, and to avoid situations in which trauma is likely to occur. Older children with epidermolysis bullosa learn to stand back when other children scuffle. However, during the toddler phase, they tend to be rather careless, and will benefit from constant vigilance on the part of those who are caring for them. In order to give them the best chance of taking part in normal activities, the emphasis should be on the provision of protective dressings and clothing, rather than on the avoidance of all even remotely physical activities. It is particularly important to provide children with epidermolysis bullosa with footwear which allows them the maximum mobility while providing the best possible protection for their feet. Many children can wear 'off the peg' shoes if these incorporate appropriate design features. Ideally, these shoes are made of very soft leather, with the minimum number of internal seams. There should be plenty of room for the toes, in both the horizontal and vertical planes. Both the uppers and the insock should be made of permeable leather, in order to keep the foot as cool and dry as possible, and the inside of the sole should have a shape which is as anatomically appropriate as possible. Few 'off the peg' shoes fulfil these criteria. Recently, however, we have found certain lines of Elephanten shoes (UK Agents: Intershoe Ltd, Stockton on Tees) more or less ideal. Some children will have mis-shapen feet due to early damage and subsequent scarring with contraction. They will require tailor-made shoes, which will similarly need to incorporate the features listed above.

Socks should be absorbent and should therefore contain a high proportion of cotton. They should also provide additional cushioning; the towelling type of sport sock is ideal. Other clothing needs to be chosen carefully. Before purchase, all items should be inspected to check that they do not have rough internal seams, and that they fit loosely, especially at the neck, wrists and ankles. In the UK, a good range of suitable clothes is available from sources that specialize in clothing for those with skin diseases, such as Cotton-On (29, North Clifton Street, Lytham, FY8 5HW).

13.5.3 Older children and adults

The great majority of patients with epidermolysis bullosa find that new blisters develop less frequently with increasing age. It is unclear whether this is because of a genuinely decreased tendency of the skin to blister or is simply a reflection of more effective avoidance of trauma by older patients. However, in the case of patients afflicted by severe dystrophic epidermolysis bullosa, this gradual improvement is counterbalanced by the steadily increasing fragility of skin that has been repeatedly ulcerated in the past, and is now atrophic and as delicate as tissue paper. Whereas, in the past, ulcerated areas would usually heal rapidly, these atrophic areas may now break down so frequently that they never seem to heal. The neck, axillae, elbows, hands, hips, knees and ankles seem to be among the most troublesome sites from this point of view.

The most sinister late complication of dystrophic epidermolysis bullosa is the tendency for epithe-liomata, predominantly squamous carcinomata, to develop in recurrently ulcerated areas [10–12]. Patients may be unaware of this danger and may therefore fail to bring such lesions to medical attention in good time. Sadly, it is not uncommon for patients with epidermolysis bullosa to become disenchanted with the medical profession; such patients may fail to ask for help with an unfamiliar skin lesion. Even if they do, their doctors may themselves be ignorant of this important and frequently lethal complication. It is of the greatest importance that all patients with dystrophic epidermolysis bullosa be fully aware themselves of this risk. We ask them to report any unusual skin lesion, particularly lumps, nodules or ulcers which seem particularly unwilling to heal.

13.6 SKIN GRAFTING IN EPIDERMOLYSIS BULLOSA

It is perhaps surprising that skin autografts can be

so easily and successfully undertaken in patients with dystrophic epidermolysis bullosa. The main use of such grafts is for reconstructive hand surgery. Grafts can also be used in neonates with severe dystrophic epidermolysis bullosa who have deep ulcerations which developed *in utero*, and which may bleed quite heavily during the days after birth and which may take some time to heal, delaying the baby's departure from hospital. Often, the application of partial-thickness skin grafts to such lesions will dramatically accelerate healing and reduce unwanted loss of blood and serum. The donor sites heal quickly with minimal scarring.

The successful use of partial-thickness grafts to heal persistent ulcerations on the skin in pretibial dystrophic epidermolysis bullosa has also been reported [13].

Attempts to grow therapeutically useful autologous keratinocyte sheets *in vitro* from patients with dystrophic epidermolysis bullosa have been frustrated by the tendency of the cells to separate from one another in culture. However, the successful use of sheets of cultured allogeneic keratinocytes has been reported in a case of dystrophic epidermolysis bullosa [14]. Autologous epidermal grafts have been successfully grown on a collagen matrix and used for the treatment of chronic facial ulceration in junctional epidermolysis bullosa [15]. We have treated such lesions in a child with junctional epidermolysis bullosa with sheets of cultured allogeneic keratinocyte grown from healthy donors. Perhaps the major problem in treating lesions of this type is to prevent traumatization of the grafts once these have been initially positioned. Perhaps the best way of protecting the grafts is by use of a suitable 'helmet', particularly at night.

13.7 SYSTEMIC TREATMENTS FOR EPIDERMOLYSIS BULLOSA

Over the years a number of systemic agents have been reported to have beneficial effects in epidermolysis bullosa; the principal claim for such agents has been accelerated healing. The following have been prominent among these.

13.7.1 Phenytoin

Early ultrastructural studies of recessive dystrophic epidermolysis bullosa suggested that collagen breakdown in the papillary dermis might contribute to the development of blisters in that condition [16]. The subsequent observation that skin fibroblasts cultured from patients with recessive dystrophic epidermolysis bullosa synthesize increased amounts of a structurally altered collagenase [17] appeared to strengthen this view and provided the rationale for the therapeutic use of phenytoin, as this agent appeared able to reduce this collagenase production *in vitro* [18].

The successful use of oral phenytoin in patients with this disease has been reported [18,19], with some patients apparently showing more than 50% reduction in new blister formation, but others showing no benefit. It appeared to be very important to maintain adequate blood levels of the drug, i.e. equal or greater than 8 mcg/ml.

However, the use of oral phenytoin at these levels is contraindicated in infancy because of the theoretical hazard of permanent cerebellar damage and ataxia. After infancy, the rate of new blister formation progressively diminishes, and at any age the question arises whether the likely benefits of long-term oral phenytoin outweigh its undoubted adverse effects, which include megaloblastic anaemia, lymphoma, encephalopathy and choreoathetosis. We have not found phenytoin of great value and do not use it routinely.

There has been an isolated report of the apparently beneficial use of oral phenytoin in an infant with junctional epidermolysis bullosa [20]. No further reports of this type have appeared, and it seems improbable that this drug will turn out to be of real value in this form of epidermolysis bullosa.

13.7.2 Retinoids

Following the demonstration that retinoids are able to inhibit collagenase activity *in vitro* [21], there was interest in their possible therapeutic value in recessive dystrophic epidermolysis bullosa. However, these drugs have not to date turned out to be helpful in practice [22,23].

13.7.3 Corticosteroids

High-dose oral corticosteroids have been proposed for the control of blistering in both dystrophic and junctional epidermolysis bullosa [24], and were at one time rather widely used in the more severely affected, often as a long-term therapy. It is of interest that, more recently, it has been found that corticosteroids appear able to reduce collagenase activity in cultures of normal human fibroblasts [25]. On the other hand, it is established that they also inhibit the re-epithelialization of skin wounds.

We have taken the view that the morbidity associated with oral corticosteroid therapy, particularly in the very young, far outweighs its benefits, and we have not used this approach for several years. In our experience, the mortality of severe epidermolysis bullosa in the neonate is now less than it was when such treatment was in vogue.

Patients with recessive dystrophic epidermolysis bullosa having restorative hand surgery appear to do no better if they are given oral corticosteroids during the months after surgery, and we are similarly unconvinced that this form of treatment is overall beneficial to those with severe dysphagia.

13.7.4 Vitamin E

Over the years, there has been interest in the possible value of vitamin E as a treatment for various types of epidermolysis bullosa [26], but little objective evidence for benefit in any. There have been reports claiming that vitamin E has no effect in dystrophic epidermolysis bullosa [27], and others alleging that it can stop new blister formation [28,29].

13.7.5 Other systemic agents

There have been single, unsubstantiated reports of benefit in epidermolysis bullosa from antimalarials (type of epidermolysis bullosa not recorded) [30], and from the neuroleptic butyrophenone derivative pipamperone in a case of Dowling–Meara-type epidermolysis bullosa simplex [31].

13.8 PREVENTION AND TREATMENT OF THE COMPLICATIONS OF EPIDERMOLYSIS BULLOSA

13.8.1 Complications specific to dystrophic epidermolysis bullosa

(a) Digital fusion and contracture

Most, but not all, children with the severe generalized type of recessive dystrophic epidermolysis bullosa experience increasing digital fusion. This is usually more marked in the hands than the feet. The fusion, often described as 'acquired syndactyly', starts proximally in fissures situated at the apices of the interdigital webs. Very gradually, adjacent digits become fused, until eventually the fingers may become completely encased in a glove-like covering of atrophic, scarred skin. This process is almost invariably accompanied by progressive flexion contracture of the hand. The relative degrees of fusion and contracture vary considerably in different children.

Though one may be surprised by the amount of function that is retained in such hands, it is our view that corrective surgery should be undertaken as soon as function is significantly impaired, and particularly before flexion becomes established. Only one hand should be operated upon at one time. The surgical procedure involves firstly separating the fused digits, and then releasing any contractures as completely as possible. Split-skin grafts are then sewn into place in the resulting defects along the separated surfaces and on the palmar aspect of previously flexed joints. Where the hand is almost completely encased, the whole extremity may be more conveniently 'degloved' before proceeding to separate the fingers completely and release the contractures. Various similar procedures have been described in the literature [32–34].

We do not routinely use Kirschner wires to maintain extension during the immediate post-operative period, though they can be useful to maintain complete separation between thumb and index finger. It is, however, of great importance to splint the hand in a flat position, with all joints extended as fully as possible between plaster-of-

Paris slabs on the front and back of the hand. The dressings are changed under general anaesthesia at 2 and 4 weeks.

At the second dressing change, impressions are taken of the hand to enable technicians to make accurately fitting acrylic gloves to act as longer-term splints, with the aim of retarding recurrence of the fusion and contractures. These gloves are made in two halves, a palm and a dorsum, to enable them to be taken on and off easily. After surgery, children initially wear the splints continuously for three months, then for decreasing periods during the day, until after 6 months they wear them only at night.

Unfortunately, these operations often need to be repeated from time to time. It may be necessary to relieve similar flexion contractures at other joints, especially in the feet, at the knees and hips.

Physiotherapy probably has little part to play in the treatment of established flexion contractures, but is useful for the maintenance of mobility, which should have the effect of slowing down the progression of such contractures. Reasonable levels of physical activity should be encouraged in these children, who may mistakenly be immobilized by well-meaning parents or doctors.

(b) Dysphagia

Dysphagia is a rather common complication of dystrophic epidermolysis bullosa, particularly of the recessive types, though it is certainly not restricted to them. There may be little correlation between the severity of the skin disease and the severity of dysphagia in the individual patient. Many factors contribute to dysphagia in these patients, and although great emphasis has been given to the oesophageal strictures that they may develop, these are certainly not the only cause of the dysphagia. Important contributions are made by oral problems, especially by submucous fibrosis in the oral cavity, contraction of the oral and pharyngeal openings, and by fixation of the tongue. In addition, the teeth are often very poor and many may have been extracted. Extremely painful erosions are frequently present in the mouth and pharynx. Combinations of these problems cause patients great difficulties in chewing and swallowing normal food. Eating is often painful, slow and exhausting, so that only relatively small quantities of food can be coped with at any meal. These oral and pharyngeal conditions are often accompanied by oesophageal strictures and disturbed oesophageal motility.

Babies who are being bottle-fed require the softest available teats (generally those designed for premature infants). The opening can be enlarged by use of a hot needle to make feeding easier. Some babies find it easier to take milk from a spoon than from a bottle.

In children with severe dystrophic epidermolysis bullosa, it is wise to liquidize solid foods from the start. Particularly useful for this purpose is a liquidizer which also heats the food, e.g. Thermomix 3300 (Vorwerk International A.G-Wollerau-Suisse, UK Agents: Barbel Marketing Co., Stanton Old Hall, Stanton-in-Peak, Matlock, Derbyshire DE4 4LE, UK). This probably helps reduce mucosal trauma, as well as providing food that can be more easily eaten when swallowing difficulties are already established.

Many children with severe dystrophic epidermolysis bullosa experience periods when they cannot eat at all due either to pain in the mouth or throat, or to obstruction in the pharynx or oesophagus. If they are also unable to drink, it may be necessary to give fluid intravenously. A short admission for intravenous fluid administration allows the affected part to 'rest', and seems to accelerate recovery. Nasogastric feeding can be used to provide longer periods of rest [35].

Where swallowing difficulties occur, particularly when oesphageal strictures have developed, it is often assumed that the situation will inevitably worsen progressively. This has not been our experience, at least in childhood. Dysphagia is prominent in the 3–7-year age group, but often becomes less of a problem as the child grows. For this reason, any question of highly invasive surgery, such as oesophageal replacement, should be delayed until every chance of spontaneous improvement has passed. Oesophageal involvement should be investigated radiologically using cine or video so that motility disorders can be identified, and endoscopy should be avoided. Fibreoptic endoscopy is contraindicated, as visualization of the lumen is both difficult and hazardous.

Although oral corticosteroids often do help with dysphagia due to pharyngeal and oesophageal disease, relatively high dosage is required and treatment may need to be prolonged. For these reasons, we prefer to avoid this approach, except very occasionally as a short-term measure.

Surgical intervention can certainly help. We have sometimes found it beneficial to release the buccal mucosa, to allow fuller opening of the mouth. Dribbling can be improved at the same time by transplantation of the submandibular ducts back into the tonsillar fossa. Improved access to the mouth is sometimes necessary for anaesthesia and dental work, but because these procedures also mobilize the tongue, they have the additional benefit of making it much easier for the patient to masticate, swallow and talk.

Oesophageal strictures which, seriously reducing the patient's nutritional intake over long periods, may require surgical dilatation. However, difficulties arise where there are more than one stricture, or where there is an atonic segment proximal to a stricture. Solitary strictures respond well to dilatation, though futher dilatations will generally be required. Some surgeons consider the use of inflatable balloons for dilatation preferable to bouginage [35]. The question of whether a post-dilatation course of oral corticosteroids prolongs the benefit of this procedure remains unanswered, but my own prejudice is to believe that it may do so. Oesophageal replacement will need to be considered in patients who require extremely frequent dilatation, or when dilatation is not possible. This situation will only arise very rarely [35–38], and should not be considered before puberty.

13.8.2 Complications specific to junctional epidermolysis bullosa

(*a*) *Laryngeal involvement*

Laryngeal disease is a prominent feature in patients with junctional forms of epidermolysis bullosa, but appears to be infrequent in dystrophic epidermolysis bullosa. Involvement of the larynx in junctional epidermolysis bullosa probably reflects blistering and erosion of the small area of stratified squamous epithelium that is normally found on the vocal cords. Many babies with junctional epidermolysis bullosa become hoarse very early in life; indeed the appearance of this symptom seems to be one of the few relatively reliable features that allow a clinical distinction to be made between junctional and dystrophic epidermolysis bullosa in the first weeks of life. Laryngeal disease is life-threatening [39], and may be one of the principal causes of death in junctional epidermolysis bullosa.

We have found that humidification of the inspired air is valuable in babies with subacute stridor. We believe that the onset of acute laryngeal obstruction in these cases is possibly more likely to reflect the development of granulations on the vocal cords than intact blisters, and we therefore treat more intense stridor by inhalation of nebulized racemic adrenaline (racepinephrine, Vaponephrin, 0.5 ml in 2 ml of normal saline [limited supplies available from Fisons Pharmaceuticals, Loughborough, UK, for named patients]), and corticosteroids, such as beclomethasone dipropionate, 100 mcg (Becotide suspension, Allen & Hanburys, Greenford, UK), both as often as 2 hourly. Although we are keen to know the precise cause of the obstruction, we do not routinely undertake laryngoscopy because this would require that we be prepared if necessary both to intubate the patient acutely, and to undertake tracheostomy later. It is our view that tracheostomies are too difficult to maintain in babies with junctional epidermolysis bullosa because of the ulceration that occurs at the insertion of the tube and along the line of the ties used to hold it in place.

13.8.3 Complications common to dystrophic and junctional epidermolysis bullosa

(*a*) *Anaesthesia*

Despite the delicacy of the oral and pharyngeal mucosa, and anxieties about acute laryngeal obstruction if blistering of the larynx were to occur following intubation, general anaesthesia has proved to be fairly straightforward in patients with epidermolysis bullosa, if certain precautions are taken [40,41].

All those involved in handling these children before, during and after surgery must be made aware of the extreme vulnerability of their skin. Patients must be moved about with great care. Trolleys and operating table should be well padded so that pressure on the skin is kept to a minimum. No-one should lean on the patient during the operation. Plenty of non-adherent soft gauze padding such as Melolin roll should separate blood pressure cuffs and tourniquets from the skin. Sticky tapes and other adhesive materials, such as those used to attach ECG electrodes, must be avoided as the skin will come away when they are removed; elasticated netting, conforming bandages, and sutures if necessary, should be substituted. Heart rate is probably best monitored by the use of pulse oximetry. The corneas should be protected with simple eye ointment BP.

It is particularly important that the anaesthetist gain the trust of the child with epidermolysis bullosa prior to surgery, in order to reduce to the minimum the risk of a struggle at the time of induction of anaesthesia. General anaesthesia is to be preferred to extensive local anaesthesia, because the latter may cause blistering. To avoid undue facial manipulation, intubation is generally preferable, and an uncuffed tracheal tube should be selected, a size smaller than one would normally use. The tracheal tube and laryngoscope blade should be well lubricated. The tube should be fixed using ribbon gauze.

Where the tube touches the lips or skin, Vaseline gauze should be interposed. Occasionally, limitation of mouth opening or dental problems may make intubation difficult; in such cases, and for short procedures, inhalational anaesthesia can be maintained by means of a face mask, which should have a soft air cushion separated from the skin by Vaseline gauze. Vaseline gauze should also be placed against the patients' skin where the underside of the jaw is held by the anaesthetist. Oropharyngeal airways should not be used.

The author is unaware of any reported cases in which laryngeal or tracheal obstruction has occurred following intubation in patients with dystrophic epidermolysis bullosa, or in the smaller number of patients with junctional epidermolysis bullosa who have required surgery.

(b) Anaemia

Anaemia is a major problem in many patients with recessive dystrophic epidermolysis bullosa, in a few with dominant dystrophic epidermolysis bullosa and in most survivors with junctional epidermolysis bullosa. Investigations demonstrate haematological features of both iron deficiency and decreased red cell iron utilization ('anaemia of chronic disease') [42]. The iron deficiency probably reflects both chronic blood loss from skin, mouth, oesophagus and anal canal, and poor iron intake.

Where there is evidence of iron deficiency, oral iron supplements should be given; liquid preparations tend to be most appropriate. Iron therapy alone will be ineffective where 'anaemia of chronic disease' is prominent, and in this situation blood transfusion may be necessary. It has been our policy not to transfuse unless the anaemia is causing significant symptoms or handicap; in these relatively immobile individuals, transfusion is therefore rarely necessary until haemoglobin levels fall below 7 g/dl. It must be borne in mind that iron overload may become a problem if transfusions are given more often than every 6–8 weeks over prolonged periods, and desferrioxamine administration would need to be considered in these circumstances. Every effort should be made to improve the patient's general condition, with particular attention to nutrition and to care of the skin, as these measures may reduce the frequency at which transfusion is required.

(c) Constipation

Constipation is common in patients with the more severe types of epidermolysis bullosa, and especially in recessive dystrophic epidermolysis bullosa. It may be associated with faecal soiling. It appears principally to be a reflection of perianal disease; voluntary faecal retention occurs in order to avoid the pain of defaecation. The tendency to constipation is aggravated by a low dietary fibre intake. It seems probable that the tendency of these patients to take food in frequent small quantities, rather than in discrete meals of reasonable size, leads to a degree of disordered intestinal peristalsis, which will tend to aggravate the constipation still further.

The management of this constipation comprises firstly softening residual faecal material with softeners such as docusate sodium (Dioctyl Paediatric Syrup, Medo Pharmaceuticals, Chesham, UK), then emptying any accumulated faecal load by careful phosphate or sodium citrate enemas, or sodium picosulphate (Picolax, Nordic Pharmaceuticals, Feltham, UK) by mouth. The prior application of topical local anaesthetic makes the procedure much less unpleasant for the patient. It is then worthwhile to encourage once daily defaecation by the regular oral administration of senna; it may be necessary to do this for a period of a few months. The senna dose should then be progressively reduced. In the longer term, it is important to prevent the recurrence of constipation by increasing the dietary fibre content or by the administration of bulk-forming agents, such as methyl cellulose. In many cases, it is also necessary to give a faecal softening agent such as lactulose (Duphalac, Duphar Laboratories, Southampton, UK) which has the additional benefit of increasing bulk. The routine administration of liquid paraffin is in our view contraindicated because of the real risk of its entry into the respiratory tract in these patients.

If possible, as much of the daily dietary intake as possible should occur at definite meals, which will encourage a reflex desire to defaecate.

If constipation persists despite these measures, and where anal pain on attempted defaecation is marked, it may be worth considering an anal stretch under general anaesthesia.

(d) Nutrition

Patients with the more severe types of epidermolysis bullosa tend to have serious nutritional problems [43]. Most prominent among these are:

1. poor nutritional intake, mainly due to a combination of shrinkage and reduced mobility of the tongue, contraction of the mouth, painful oral and pharyngeal ulceration, dental decay, oesophageal stricture, and anorexia secondary to constipation
2. loss of nutrients due to seepage of serum and blood through the skin and mucosae
3. increased nutritional requirements for healing.

Overcoming the combination of nutritional problems presented by these patients is exceedingly difficult. Some patients with dysphagia find it helpful to have their food liquidized, but others never accept this, unless they have been fed nothing else from infancy. However, apart from making it easier for the patient to eat, liquidizing the diet may help prevent further damage to the pharynx and oesophagus, and may reduce the frequency of the episodes of acute dysphagia they often experience. However, liquidizing food usually involves increasing its fluid content and therefore its bulk. If water or gravy is used for this purpose, the calorific value of the food will be reduced, whereas this effect can be minimized by the use of milk or soup. The process may make food blander and less appetizing. Sieving food should be avoided as it removes fibre, which is retained if food is liquidized.

Many patients' diets are heavily dependent upon milk. This dependence upon milk should not be discouraged, but such a diet may be far from complete from a nutritional point of view, and will tend to be short on fibre and iron content. High-fibre foods should be encouraged, yet they tend to have a lower calorie content, and usually require more effort to eat than foods with a low fibre content.

We do not encourage the addition of dextrose polymer to the diet as this will merely increase the calorie intake, without improving overall nutrition. Though sucrose provides a highly effective means of increasing the patient's calorie intake, we like to restrict high-sucrose foods, such as chocolate, to meal times, in order to minimize their harmful effect on the teeth.

Our own experience suggests that the best approach is to inform parents and patients of the nutritional properties of different foods, and to encourage them to focus on those that provide nutrition in its most concentrated and best balanced form. The aim is a well-balanced diet with a higher than normal content of protein, vitamins and minerals. The emphasis is on foods of soft, manageable consistency, with an attractive appearance and flavour.

As has already been emphasized, patients should be encouraged to take their food in discrete meals, rather than be eating small quantities continuously throughout the day. However, many children with epidermolysis bullosa will not be able to eat enough at only three meals, mainly because they find the process of eating both painful and tiring. A system of three or four main meals per day, plus two to three snacks, will often be more appropriate. It is often a good idea to put a limit on the time allowed to each meal or snack to prevent one meal from overlapping with the next.

The first 2 years of life are probably critical to the nutritional status of children with epidermolysis bullosa, and great efforts need to be directed towards improving nutrition during this period. It seems possible that children who show signs of dysphagia from early life should not be encouraged to move on to solid foods at all, but should be maintained on a liquidized diet throughout their life.

Since few patients do succeed in achieving even a normal nutritional intake, vitamin and mineral supplements are advisable. We generally give a complete vitamin supplement such as Ketovite (Paines & Byrne Ltd, Greenford, UK), a liquid iron supplement such as Sytron (Parke-Davis & Co Ltd, Eastleigh, UK), or one in the form of granules that can be dispersed in food, such as Feospan (Smith, Kline & French Laboratories Ltd, Welwyn Garden City, UK), and a zinc supplement such as Z-Span (Smith, Kline & French), which also takes the form of granules that can be dispersed in food. Patients with relatively smaller requirements may find it more convenient to take the contents of one Forceval capsule (Unigreg Ltd, Wimbledon, London, UK) daily; this contains both multivitamins and minerals, including iron and zinc.

(e) Teeth

Dental problems are a prominent feature in patients with severe dystrophic and junctional epidermolysis bullosa. While dental enamel hypoplasia appears to be common in junctional epidermolysis bullosa [44], the teeth are usually structurally normal in dystrophic epidermolysis bullosa [45]. In both forms of the disease, the teeth are prone to severe caries due to several factors, including chronic intraoral infection and gum disease, a high-sucrose intake and the absence of the normal physical cleansing effect of food due to the diet being more or less liquid. The situation is made worse in severe dystrophic epidermolysis bullosa by the loss of the gingivobuccal sulci, causing residual food to remain applied to the buccal surfaces of the teeth for long periods, and by the loss of the normal cleansing of the teeth because of fixation and shrinkage of the tongue.

Appropriate dental care includes the following elements:

1. improvements in the diet, particularly a reduction in sucrose intake and an attempt to confine the eating of sucrose to distinct meal times
2. improved cleaning of the teeth, by the use of a soft brush, or, where this is not possible, gauze on a finger [a fluoride-containing non-abrasive toothpaste should be used or, if this is not feasible, a little antiseptic gel, e.g. chlorhexidine 1% gel (Corsodyl, ICI Pharmaceuticals, Macclesfield, UK)]
3. the regular use of an antiseptic mouthwash after meals to clean away as much of the residual food as possible, e.g. Corsodyl (0.2% chlorhexidine solution, ICI)
4. oral fluoride supplements in areas where it is not adequately present in tap water (these should be started as early in life as possible)
5. regular examination and treatment by an interested dentist.

From the point of view of dental therapy, the problems in dystrophic and junctional epidermolysis bullosa are somewhat different. In dystrophic epidermolysis bullosa, we favour a conservative approach, rather than wholesale extraction as has been recommended elsewhere. Those who propose this approach argue that the patients do not require teeth as their diet is more or less liquid. We believe that the possession of teeth is helpful in giving the patients a more normal facial appearance, since these patients will not tolerate dentures. Furthermore, we have gained the impression that shrinkage of the mouth is accelerated by dental extractions. Undoubtedly, extraction is sometimes the only practical option for severely carious teeth because of the difficulty of doing conservative dental work through the very restricted oral opening of these patients. Where extraction is necessary, healing is rapid. In junctional epidermolysis bullosa, the patients usually tolerate a less liquid diet and, because there is much less mucosal scarring, the teeth are more accessible to the dentist. A normal conservative approach is therefore both more necessary and feasible.

(f) Eyes

Conjunctival bullae, leading to conjunctival ulceration and painful corneal erosions, are frequent in patients with severe dystrophic epidermolysis bullosa and junctional epidermolysis bullosa [46], and have been reported in epidermolysis bullosa simplex [47]. They may lead to conjunctival and corneal scarring, and thus threaten vision in the longer term, both by their direct effects and by interfering with tear film stability and tear production. The use of lubricants such as simple eye ointment BP (10% liquid paraffin, wool fat 10%, in yellow soft paraffin) is valuable when patients have bullae. Topical corticosteroids without preservative may be indicated in the acute phase of ulceration, but their use should not be prolonged unless it is possible to monitor intraocular pressure.

13.9 DYSTROPHIC EPIDERMOLYSIS BULLOSA RESEARCH ASSOCIATION (DEBRA)

DEBRA is an association formed by patients with epidermolysis bullosa and parents of affected children. Despite the name, the association exists to help those with all forms of epidermolysis bullosa. It provides counselling and support, regular meetings and newsletters, and very effectively promotes the interests of those with epidermolysis bullosa, at all levels. It provides information to professionals involved in the care of individuals with epidermolysis bullosa, and creates helpful links between patients and professionals. It provides a stimulus as well as funds for research, and has proved to be one of the most effective of all such patient support groups.

REFERENCES

1. Anton-Lamprecht, I. (1984) Prenatal diagnosis of epidermolysis bullsa hereditaria: a review. *Semin. Dermatol.*, **3**, 229–40.
2. Perry, T.B. (1984) Clinical procedures for prenatal diagnosis of inherited skin disease. *Semin. Dermatol.*, **3**, 155–66.
3. Heagerty, A.H.M., Kennedy, A.R., Gunner, D.B. and Eady, R.A.J. (1986) Rapid prenatal diagnosis and exclusion of epidermolysis bullosa using antibody probes. *J. Invest. Dermatol.*, **86**, 603–5.
4. Eady, R.A.J., Gunner, D.B. and Tidman, M.J., *et al.* (1984) Rapid processing of fetal skin for prenatal diagnosis by light and electron microscopy. *J. Clin. Pathol.*, **37**, 633–8.
5. Gould, D.J., Condon, P. and Cunliffe, W.J. (1977) Porcine dermis dressings in epidermolysis bullosa. *Arch. Dermatol.*, **113**, 1456.
6. Mallory, S.B. (1982) Adjunctive therapy for epidermolysis bullosa. *J. Amer. Acad. Dermatol.*, **6**, 951–2.
7. Eisenberg, M. (1986) The effect of occlusive dressings on re-epithelialization of wounds in children with epidermolysis bullosa. *J. Pediatr. Surg.*, **10**, 892–4.
8. Rahman, M., Noble, W.C. and Cookson, B. (1987) Mupirocin-resistant *Staphylococcus aureus*. *Lancet*, **ii**, 387.
9. Chirife, J., Scarmato, G. and Herszage, L. (1982) Scientific basis for use of granulated sugar in treatment of infected wounds. *Lancet*, **i**, 560.
10. Wechsler, H.L., Krugh, F.J., Domonkos, A.N., *et al.* (1970) Polydysplastic epidermolysis bullosa and development of epidermal neoplasms. *Arch. Dermatol.*, **102**, 374–80.
11. Didolkar, M.S., Gerner, R.E. and Moore, G.E. (1974) Epidermolysis bullosa dystrophica and epithelioma of the skin. *Cancer*, **33**, 198–202.
12. Tidman, M.J., Atherton, D.J. and Eady, R.A.J. (1984) Squamous carcinoma as a complication of dystrophic epidermolysis bullosa. *J. R. Soc. Med.*, **77** (Suppl. 4), 37–9.
13. Furue, M., Ando, I., Inoue, Y., *et al.* (1986) Pretibial epidermolysis bullosa. *Arch. Dermatol.*, **122**, 310–13.
14. McGuire, J., Birchall, N., Cuono, C., *et al.* (1987) Successful engraftment of allogeneic keratinocyte cultures in recessive dystrophic epidermolysis bullosa. *Clin. Res.*, **35**, 702A.

15. Carter, D.M., Lin, A.N., Varghese, M.C., *et al.* (1987) Treatment of junctional epidermolysis bullosa with epidermal autografts. *J. Amer. Acad. Dermatol.*, **17**, 246–50.
16. Pearson, R.W. (1962) Studies on the pathogenesis of epidermolysis bullosa. *J. Invest. Dermatol.*, **39**, 551–75.
17. Bauer, E.A., Gedde-Dahl, T. and Eisen, A.Z. (1977) The role of human skin collagenase in epidermolysis bullosa. *J. Invest. Dermatol.*, **68**, 119–24.
18. Bauer, E.A., Cooper, T.W., Tucker, D.R. and Esterly, N.B. (1980) Phenytoin therapy of recessive dystrophic epidermolysis bullosa. Clinical trial and proposed mechanism of action on collagenase. *New Engl. J. Med.*, **303**, 776–81.
19. Cooper, T.W. and Bauer, E.A. (1984) Therapeutic efficacy of phenytoin in recessive dystrophic epidermolysis. *Arch. Dermatol.*, **120**, 490–5.
20. Rogers, R.B., Yancey, K.B., Allen, B.S. and Guill, M.F. (1983) Phenytoin therapy for junctional epidermolysis bullosa. *Arch. Dermatol.*, **119**, 925–6.
21. Bauer, E.A., Seltzer, J.L. and Eisen, A.Z. (1982) Inhibition of collagen degradative enzymes by retinoic acid *in vitro*. *J. Amer. Acad. Dermatol.*, **6**, 603–7.
22. Fritsch, P., Klein, G., Aubock, J. and Hintner, H. (1983) Retinoid therapy of recessive dystrophic epidermolysis bullosa. *J. Amer. Acad. Dermatol.*, **5**, 766.
23. Tabas, M. quoted by Spraker, M.K. (1985) Report on the First National Epidermolysis Bullosa Conference. *Pediat. Dermatol.*, **3**, 81.
24. Moynahan, E.J. (1982) The treatment and management of epidermolysis bullosa. *Clin. Exp. Dermatol.*, **7**, 665–72.
25. Koob, T.J., Jeffrey, J.J. and Eisen, A.Z. (1974) Regulation of human skin collagenase activity by hydrocortisone and dexamethasone in organ culture. *Biochem. Biophys. Res. Commun.*, **61**, 1083–8.
26. Ayres, S. and Mihan, R. (1969) Pseudoxanthoma elasticum and epidermolysis bullosa. Response to vitamin E (tocopherol). *Cutis*, **5**, 287–94.
27. Unger, W.P. and Nethercott, J.R. (1973) Epidermolysis bullosa dystrophica treated with vitamin E and oral corticosteroids. *Can. Med. J.*, **108**, 1136–8.
28. Sehgal, V.N. and Sanyal, R.K. (1972) Vitamin E therapy in dystrophic epidermolysis bullosa. *Arch. Dermatol.*, **105**, 460.
29. Michaelson, J.D., Schmidt, J.D., Dresden, M.H. and Duncan, W.C. (1974) Vitamin E treatment of epidermolysis bullosa. *Arch. Dermatol.*, **109**, 67–9.
30. Baer, T.W. (1961) Epidermolysis bullosa hereditaria treated with antimalarials. *Arch. Dermatol.*, **84**, 193–4.
31. Bonnetblanc, J.M. and Bouquier, J.J. (1986) Response to pipamperone in case of epidermolysis bullosa herpetiformis. *Lancet*, **i**, 1327–8.
32. Horner, R.L., Wiedel, J.B. and Bralliar, F. (1971) Involvement of the hand in epidermolysis bullosa. *J. Bone Jt. Surg.*, **53A**, 1347–56.
33. Lamesch, A. and Reiffers, J. (1981) Surgical treatment of syndactylia in recessive dystrophic epidermolysis bullosa. *Z. Kinderchir.*, **35**, 118–20.
34. Greider, J.L. Jr and Flatt, A.E. (1983) Care of the hand in recessive epidermolysis bullosa. *Plast. Reconstr. Surg.*, **72**, 222–7.
35. Feurle, G.E., Weidauer, H., Baldauf, G., *et al.* (1984) Management of oesophageal stenosis in recessive dystrophic epidermolysis bullosa. *Gastroenterology*, **87**, 1378–80.
36. Orlando, R.C., Bozymski, E.M., Briggaman, R.A. and Bream, C.A. (1974) Epidermolysis bullosa: Gastrointestinal manifestations. *Ann. Intern. Med.*, **81**, 203–6.
37. Fonkalsrud, E.W. and Ament, M.E. (1977) Surgical management of esophageal stricture due to dystrophic epidermolysis bullosa. *J. Pediatr. Surg.*, **12**, 221–6.
38. Harmel, R.P. Jr (1986) Esophageal replacement in two siblings with epidermolysis bullosa. *J. Pediatr. Surg.*, **21**, 175–6.
39. Davies, H. and Atherton, D.J. (1987) Acute laryngeal obstruction in junctional epidermolysis bullosa. *Pediatr. Dermatol.*, **4**, 98–101.
40. James, I. and Wark, H. (1982) Airway management during anaesthesia in patients with epidermolysis bullosa dystrophica. *Anesthesiology*, **56**, 323–6.
41. Katz, J. and Stewart, D.J. (1987) Epidermolysis bullosa. In *Anesthesia and Uncommon Pediatric Diseases*, W.B. Saunders, Philadelphia, pp. 384–7.
42. Hruby, M.A. and Esterly, N.B. (1973) Anemia in epidermolysis bullosa letalis. *Amer. J. Dis. Childn.*, **125**, 696–9.
43. Lechner-Gruskay, D., Honig, P.J., Pereira, G. and McKinney, S. (1988) Nutritional and metabolic profile of children with epidermolysis bullosa. *Pediatr. Dermatol.*, **5**, 22–7.
44. Brain, E.B. and Wigglesworth, J.S. (1968) Developing teeth in epidermolysis bullosa hereditaria letalis. *Brit. Dental J.*, **124**, 255–60.
45. Crawford, E.G., Burkes, E.J. and Briggaman, R.A. (1976) Hereditary epidermolysis bullosa: Oral manifestations and dental therapy. *Oral Surg.*, **42**, 490–500.
46. Hammerton, M.E., Turner, T.W. and Pyne, R.J. (1984) A case of junctional epidermolysis bullosa (Herlitz-Pearson) with corneal bullae. *Austr. J. Ophthalmol.*, **12**, 45–8.
47. Granek, H. and Baden, H.P. (1980) Corneal involvement in epidermolysis bullosa simplex. *Arch. Ophthalmol.*, **98**, 469–72.

Fourteen
Epidermolysis bullosa simplex (intraepidermal epidermolysis bullosa) and allied conditions

Tobias Gedde-Dahl Jr

14.1 INTRODUCTION

Thirty years before the rediscovery of Mendel's laws of inheritance intraepidermal non-scarring blistering was called Erblichen Pemphigus by von Hebra [1]. Köbner in 1886 called the same condition epidermolysis bullosa hereditaria (EBH) [2]. Since the latter term soon became adopted for several congenital traumatic blistering diseases, Hallopeau [3] found it necessary to call the original type 'simple', i.e. epidermolysis bullosa simplex (EBS). By 1908 EBS was recognized as a dominant Mendelian trait [4]. Incidentally, Köbner's cases had mainly blisters of the hands and feet with only occasional blisters elsewhere. Many similar families were later called localized EBS (Weber–Cockayne) named after Weber's (1926) solitary 'recurrent bullous eruption of the feet' case [5] and Cockayne's (1938) two dominant families with blistering feet only [6]. Such cases had previously [7] been called EBS, but Cockayne distinguished them from EBS. Since 1957 [8], EBS (Weber–Cockayne) has been used for cases of blistering of the feet or hands and feet, and EBS (Köbner) for more generalized blistering. One of Cockayne's families had the additional feature of 'easily bruising skin' and may therefore represent a different disease (EBS Ogna) first distinguished in 1970 [9].

The blistering neonate cannot be diagnosed properly without a biopsy. Intraepidermal (this chapter), junctional (Chapter 15) and dermal (Chapter 16) types of blister formation can be discriminated between by using immunostaining for basement membrane zone antigens [10, 11]. Electron microscopy will give the same information and allow further differentiation as to primary type, i.e. for intraepidermal diseases whether they have initial cytolytic changes (epidermolysis bullosa simplex proper) or tonofibril changes (in suprabasal cells for epidermolytic hyperkeratosis or in basal cells for epidermolysis bullosa herpetiformis and others). Antibodies showing specificity for dermal and junctional EB types have been identified, but the use of antibodies to differentiate between types of intraepidermal EB is still exploratory [12].

The severity in infancy and early childhood and frequency of epidermolysis bullosa herpetiformis Dowling-Meara (D-EBH-DM) make it the most important of the intraepidermal EBS from the clinical point of view. It is therefore a paradox that it was recognized as a distinct disease only in the last decade. The reason is that its drastically changing phases make it easily clinically confused with any EB type. The unique clinical features in childhood were first recognized by Dowling and Meara in 1954 [13] and Polano in 1958 [14], but both reports misinterpreted the blisters as subepidermal recessive. Its recognition as a dominant disease [15] and its unique electron microscopical sign of basal cell tonofibrillar clumping were made independently [16–19]. It now seems that basal cell tonofibrillar EB is heterogeneous; this will be discussed below.

Very recently the first recessive type of intraepidermal EB was defined. As it shares some clinical features with junctional EB, the name proposed is pseudojunctional EB (R-EBPJ).

Since neither D-EBH-DM nor R-EBPJ are as yet properly described in the literature, they will be discussed here in some detail. The last paradox of our continued confusion about intraepidermal EB is that they represent temperature-sensitive mutants in man, EB simplex aggravating and EB herpetiformis improving with prolonged heating of the skin. This underlines the necessity of correct diagnosis from the neonatal stage on.

In none of the intraepidermal inherited bullous diseases is the primary gene product of the mutated gene known. Thus genetic entities must be defined by the chromosomal location of the mutated gene. Only one locus is known, the *EBS1* locus on chromosome 8, having a mutational variant causing EB Simplex Ogna (D-EBS-O).

The following diseases will be discussed:

1. epidermolysis bullosa simplex (cytolytic)
   (a) generalized (Köbner) (D-EBS-K)
   (b) localized (Weber–Cockayne) (D-EBS-WC)
   (c) with epidermal bruising, Ogna type (D-EBS-O)
   (d) with mottled pigmentation (D-EBS-M)
   (e) atypical variants
2. epidermolysis bullosa with basal cell tonofibrillar involvement
   (a) herpetiform (Dowling–Meara) type (tonofibrillar clumping) (D-EBH-DM)
   (b) other basal cell tonofibrillar anomalies
3. epidermolytic hyperkeratoses with suprabasal tonofibrillar involvement
   (a) generalized: bullous ichthyosiform erythroderma (D-BIE)
   (b) localized: bullous palmoplantar keratoderma (D-BKPP) and other variants
   (c) generalized epidermolytic hyperkeratosis without tylosis?
4. recessive pseudojunctional epidermolysis bullosa (R-EBPJ)
5. rare reports
   (a) Bart's type
   (b) Dystrophia bullosa (Mendes da Costa) (X-DB-MC).

14.2 EPIDERMOLYSIS BULLOSA SIMPLEX (KÖBNER) (D-EBS-K) AND EPIDERMOLYSIS BULLOSA SIMPLEX (WEBER–COCKAYNE) (D-EBS-WC)

14.2.1 Clinical signs and course of disease

The single clinical feature is non-scarring blistering elicited by continuous trauma or friction of the skin, with particular preference for toes, heels, soles, and also for fingers and palms, and with a clear aggravation of the blistering tendency in warm temperatures. The generalized type, D-EBS-Köbner, begins at birth or within the first week of life, and blisters may be widespread on extremities and trunk and, exceptionally, also in the oral and vaginal mucosa. The widespread blistering is always most evident in early infancy, and many D-EBS-K families later have mostly localized blistering of hands and feet. The more severely affected families continue to show generalized blisters, e.g. blisters of the neck due to friction of clothes, of the trunk due to friction of bras or belts, and any site given sufficient friction (Figure 14.1). Often aggravation by psychical stress (warm, sweating skin?) and premenstrually, and improvement during pregnancy, are reported. On the whole, however, the blistering tendency seems to remain constant and only to fluctuate with the average ambient temperature (rare or no blisters below 0°C).

If the onset of blisters is after the first week of life, the diagnosis will be localized EBS, i.e. D-EBS-WC. Feet are invariably much more involved than hands (Figure 14.2). Blisters are rare in the winter but recur when the average outdoor temperature has passed a critical (family-specific) level in the spring. Many families with strictly localized D-EBS-WC start with blistering feet the first summer after the child has learned to walk. In some families blisters recur annually throughout life, with a gradual decrease in late adult life. In other families the

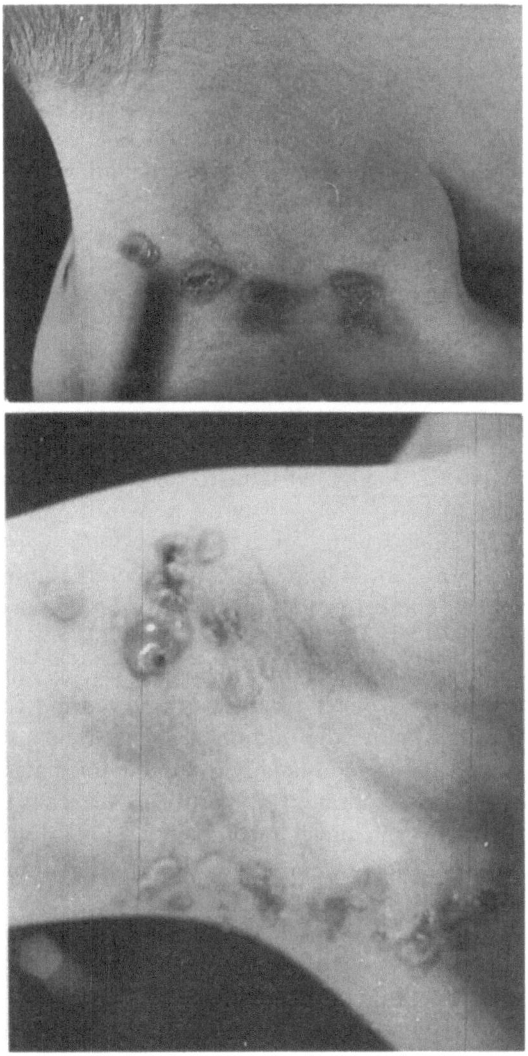

Figure 14.1 Epidermolysis bullosa simplex Köbner (D-EBS-K). Blistering neck and axilla in two cousins [9].

blistering ceases at young adult age or, exceptionally, during childhood.

Onset of recurrent summer blistering of the feet after the third year has a peak at adolescence, and tends to be restricted to a limited number of seasons. The possibility of a spectrum towards 'normal variation' of blister tendency, i.e. during military service, was pointed out in the 1920s [9].

The clinical features of D-EBS-K and D-EBS-WC differ quantitatively rather than qualitatively.

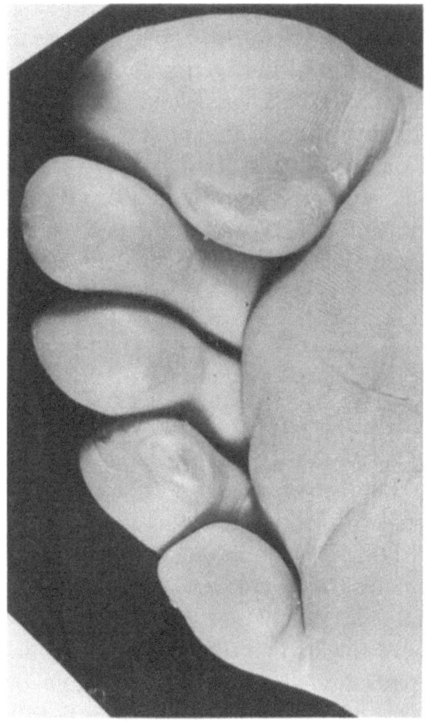

Figure 14.2 Epidermolysis bullosa simplex Weber–Cockayne (D-EBS-WC) [9].

14.2.2 Morphology

The intraepidermal blister is seen by electron microscopy to develop by primary cytolysis of the basal keratinocyte without disturbance of the structural tonofibrils or organelles. This pertains to both D-EBS-K [20] and D-EBS-WC [21] if a freshly induced friction blister is examined. Old blisters may be suprabasal due to regrowth of the blister floor. Pearson [20] found suprabasal blister formation in D-EBS-WC. There are rare families with initial suprabasal cytolysis [22].

14.2.3 Genetics

Autosomal dominant inheritance is the only one proven for D-EBS-K and D-EBS-WC [4, 6, 23]. In reviewing 42 D-EBS-K families, Gedde-Dahl [9] found a single one with 'skipping' of generations [24]. Gonadal mosaicism giving more D-EBS-K cases in the first generation can occur [9].

Extensive genetic linkage studies of D-EBS [9, 25–27] have failed to map any gene locus [27], but the absence of linkage to glutamate–pyruvate transaminase (*GPT*) has shown non-identity with the *EBS1* locus (see Section 14.3.3) [15].

In Norway a prospective study revealed one D-EBS-K mutant per 5000 000 births and a frequency of D-EBS-WC mutants at least three times higher [19].

14.2.4 Differential diagnosis

Infants with severe D-EBS-K may be clinically confused with those with D-EBH-Dowling–Meara, bullous ichthyosiform erythroderma or severe junctional EB. Mild D-EBS-K is also confused with D-EBH-DM. The childhood-onset D-EBS-WC can be distinguished from late-onset dominant dermolytic EB since the latter causes blisters on the dorsum of fingers and toes and leaves milia. R-EB progressiva (junctional) with its benign onset at school age can be differentiated from D-EBS by its preceding nail dystrophy.

14.2.5 Systemic and associated manifestations

There are no systemic and associated manifestations.

14.2.6 Pathogenesis

Fine and Griffith [28] found that fluorescein-labelled soybean agglutinin, reacting with *N*-acetylgalactosamine groups on cell surfaces, gave irregular focal membrane staining of basal keratinocytes in biopsies from two D-EBS-K and six D-EBS-WC patients contrary to the uniformly crisp membrane staining in biopsies from 12 other EB-type patients and seven normal controls. Since other lectins stained the same specimens normally, they suggested a specific defect in glycosylation of D-EBS epidermal cell membranes.

This has no relationship to the association of deficiency of galactosylhydroxylysine glucosyltransferase in most, but not all, D-EBS-K members of a single Finnish family [29] which is due to either chance or a loose genetic linkage [30].

Gelatinase expression in fibroblasts from patients with D-EBS-WC and D-EBS-K may be reduced [31], normal or high [30] and may be genetically linked to the *EBS* gene(s).

Induction of blisters in control skin explants by EBS blister fluid [32] has subsequently been shown to be non-specific [33].

14.2.7 Treatment

A cool environment is the best preventive measure. One patient found it useful to keep a bunch of insoles in his freezer and put a pair in his shoes before taking a walk. Since hyperhidrotic patients suffer more, antihidrotic measures may be helpful for them. Some, but not all, members of the same D-EBS-WC kindreds claim that sea (salt water) bathing is beneficial; they may then tolerate the warm weather. The burning sensation of the soles of the feet before the outbreak of blisters is also partly relieved by salt foot baths immediately after exercise. Vitamin E has been extensively tried, but is no longer recommended [34]. Kero [34] also made a systematic trial of the effect of hydroxychloroquine in four D-EBS-K patients without any improvement recorded. Retinoid (etretinate) treatment has been tried in one D-EBS-K and two unrelated D-EBS-WC patients; the condition was made worse rather than improved [35].

14.2.8 Genetic counselling and prenatal diagnosis

Parents of new D-EBS mutants have a low recurrence risk, whereas all patients have a 50% risk at each pregnancy. Prenatal diagnosis may be relevant for the families with more severe D-EBS-K, but it is not yet available. One observation of transiently raised maternal serum alphafoeto-protein level in a D-EBS pregnancy suggests intrauterine blisters [36]. When the gene locus is known, prenatal diagnosis may be possible via chorion villi DNA typing.

14.3 EPIDERMOLYSIS BULLOSA SIMPLEX OGNA (D-EBS-O)

14.3.1 Clinical signs and course of disease

Serous summer blistering of the feet and hands with a clear relation to ambient temperature appears at age 2–5 years, to recur for several summers up to adult life [9]. Clinically this symptom is difficult to distinguish from D-EBS-WC except that small blisters also appear on the dorsum of the hands and in exceptional cases elsewhere. The most striking feature in all those affected is bruising and fragility of the epidermis (Figure 14.3), evident on the face when the infant hits itself, and after the first year giving constant small erosions on the back of the hands and fingers. Trauma reveals that all the skin is affected. Erosions dry up and heal very quickly, often within a day. Small blood blebs readily appear on the palms and fingers when the skin is squeezed. Affected adults may develop onychogryphoses of the big toes.

One of Cockayne's (1938) two families with recurrent bullous eruption of the feet was reported to bruise easily. Despite the report of a family with D-EBS-Ogna in 1970 [9], no further families have been reported.

14.3.2 Morphology

Electron microscopy reveals initial cytolytic basal cell blistering indistinguishable from that

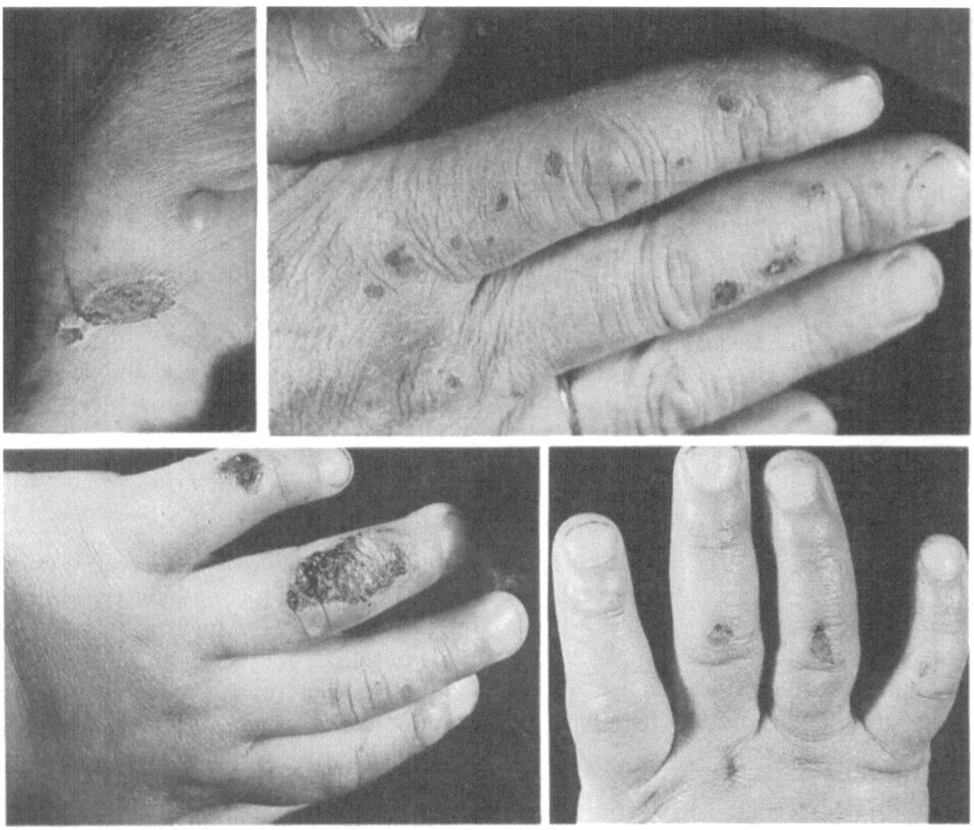

Figure 14.3 Epidermolysis bullosa simplex Ogna (D-EBS-O). Examples of bruised skin in members of a single family [9].

in D-EBS-K or D-EBS-WC. A blind study of volar forearm skin from ten (of 12) siblings, with and without D-EBS-O, did not reveal any difference in ultrastructural morphology [22].

14.3.3 Genetics

In 1987, 106 descendants of a couple married in 1813 in the community of Ogna in South Norway were known to be affected. Inheritance is autosomal dominant. Affected females have a deficiency of affected children relative to normal (and relative to the number of offspring of affected males) [9, 37], but unrelated to sex of offspring [37]. Olaisen and Gedde-Dahl [37] discovered close genetic linkage to the enzyme polymorphism of glutamate–pyruvate transaminase (*GPT*) and named the gene locus *EBS1* and the mutant gene giving the D-EBS-O trait $EBS1^{Ogna}$. This linkage group is assigned to the long arm of chromosome 8.

14.3.4 Differential diagnosis

It can be clinically confused with D-EBS-WC and generalized basal cell tonofibrillar anomalies (see Section 14.4).

14.3.5 Systemic and associated manifestations

None have been reported.

14.3.6 Pathogenesis

The pathogenesis of this disease is unknown.

14.3.7 Treatment

Apart from blister care, as for D-EBS-WC, and occasional taping of erosions, none seems necessary. The patients live normal lives with all sorts of occupations (e.g. carpentry).

14.3.8 Genetic counselling and prenatal diagnosis

No counselling seems necessary. The task must be to identify severe EB cases due to other mutations at the *EBS1* locus and then use the genetic map information to provide prenatal diagnosis (see Section 14.3.3).

14.4 EPIDERMOLYSIS BULLOSA SIMPLEX WITH MOTTLED PIGMENTATION (D-EBS-M)

14.4.1 Clinical signs and course of disease

Congenital onset, generalized serous blistering indistinguishable from mild D-EBS-K associated with mottled pigmentation (Figure 14.4), inconstant slender, curved and variably thickened nails, focal keratotic pits and plugs of palms, and mild and late-onset thinning or premature atrophy of the skin of the extremities was found in a family described by Fischer and Gedde-Dahl [38]. The mottling appeared as small dark and light spots with ill-defined margins giving the skin a dirty appearance; it was usually visible from the neonatal period. The mottled appearance was more clearly seen on the extremities than on the trunk and it gradually faded in adult life making it unnoticeable in the great-grandmother when examined after the age of 50. Two similar sporadic cases have been observed [39]. In the two dominant families studied by Boss *et al.* [40], blistering appeared only at childhood, but a speckled hyperpigmentation appeared at 1 year of age and a more severe palmoplantar punctate keratosis developed. Hence there is some heterogeneity between these families.

14.4.2 Morphology

Light microscopy revealed basal cell intraepidermal localization of a friction-induced blister on the thigh [38]. Electron microscopy [41] revealed cytolytic blister formation and increased amount of lipid droplets in the basal keratinocytes and normal melanocytes and melanosomes. The pigmented areas showed increased melanin in the keratinocytes.

By using immunostaining with antibodies against laminin, type IV and type VII collagen, Bruchner-Tuderman [39] discovered a highly unusual disruptive staining pattern along the basal membrane in her sporadic male case. A disrupted

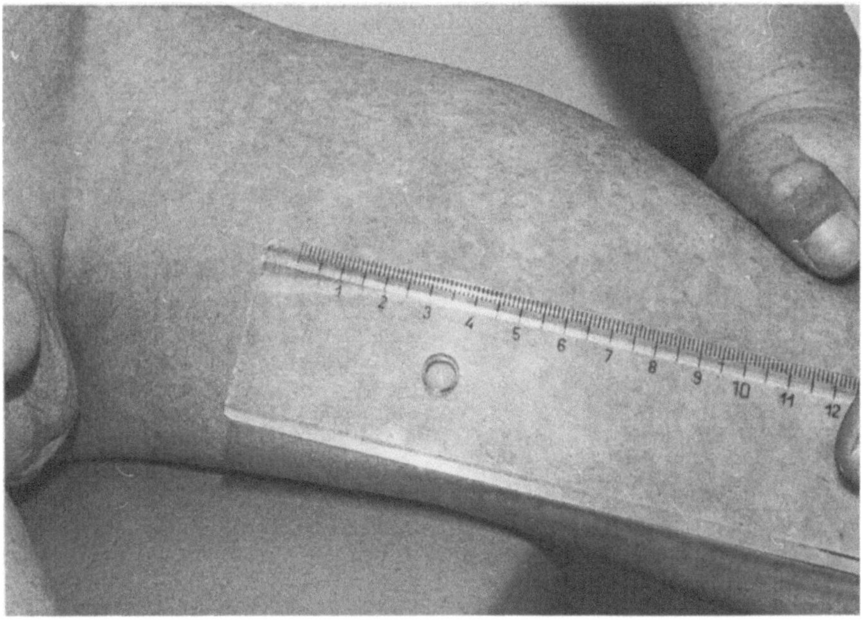

Figure 14.4 Epidermolysis bullosa simplex with mottled pigmentation (D-EBS-M) in a child aged 7 years [38].

dermal membrane was also seen by electron microscopy.

14.4.3 Genetics

Studies of four generations suggest autosomal dominant inheritance [38]. Unpublished genetic linkage studies on the family have excluded close linkage to *GPT(EBS1)* but possible linkage to the *PGM3* marker on chromosome 6.

14.4.4 Differential diagnosis

D-EBS-M can be confused with D-EBS-K if the dyspigmentation is overlooked or after it has faded at adult age.

14.4.5 Systemic and associated abnormalities

All are mentioned under clinical features.

14.4.6 Pathogenesis

Gedde-Dahl and Fischer [42] proposed that the mottled appearance could be due to clonal inactivation of one gene in a gene pair (autosomal inactivation). The cytolytic basal cell blistering, the dyspigmentation and abnormal type VII collagen expression may be effects of a single gene expressed in the keratinocytes [39].

14.4.7 Treatment, genetic counselling and prenatal diagnosis

See Sections 14.4.3 and 14.2.7.

14.5 ATYPICAL VARIANTS OF EPIDERMOLYSIS BULLOSA SIMPLEX

A typical D-EBS-WC family with regard to summer blistering of the feet had, in addition, painful localized hyperkeratoses of the soles and palms. The distinctiveness of this variant was verified by improvement of keratoses and disappearance of blistering during retinoid treatment [43].

Not infrequently patients present with recurrent desquamation of the soles, often heat-related, sometimes familial, without regular blister formation, clinical features that do not satisfy the

D-EBS-WC criteria. The aetiology is unknown and probably heterogeneous.

Corneal involvement with basal cell vacuolization in Bowman's membrane was recorded in a dominant family which represents either D-EBS or D-EBH-DM [44].

14.6 EPIDERMOLYSIS BULLOSA HERPETIFORMIS DOWLING–MEARA (D-EBH-DM)

14.6.1 Clinical signs and course of disease

Blisters appear at birth or within the first days of life either mainly on fingers and toes or more widespread (Figures 14.5–14.7). The onset can simulate other types of EB and even epidermolytic hyperkeratosis, but has so far not presented with congenital ulceration, generalized erythema or syndactyly. Oral mucosal blisters are absent or minor. Initially the nails are normal, but as blisters occur in the nail bed, occasionally nails may be shed to regrow normally. Owing to the intensity of blistering, the fingertips may appear red with healing blisters, but they are normally slender in contrast to the swollen paronychia-resembling fingertips observed in recessive junctional EB. The majority of blisters are clear, but some are haemorrhagic. They heal without sequelae and only occasional transitory milia are formed.

No other EB type shows such a drastic change in clinical features and course of the disease. The typical case commences with blistering extremities for weeks or months. Blisters on hands and feet are often large, tense and may cover the whole palm or sole. Figure 14.8 illustrates the detailed course of blistering during the first year in a typical female case.

After the first month more specific signs appear (Figure 14.6). First, there may be outbreaks of 'spontaneous' smaller vesicular serous blisters,

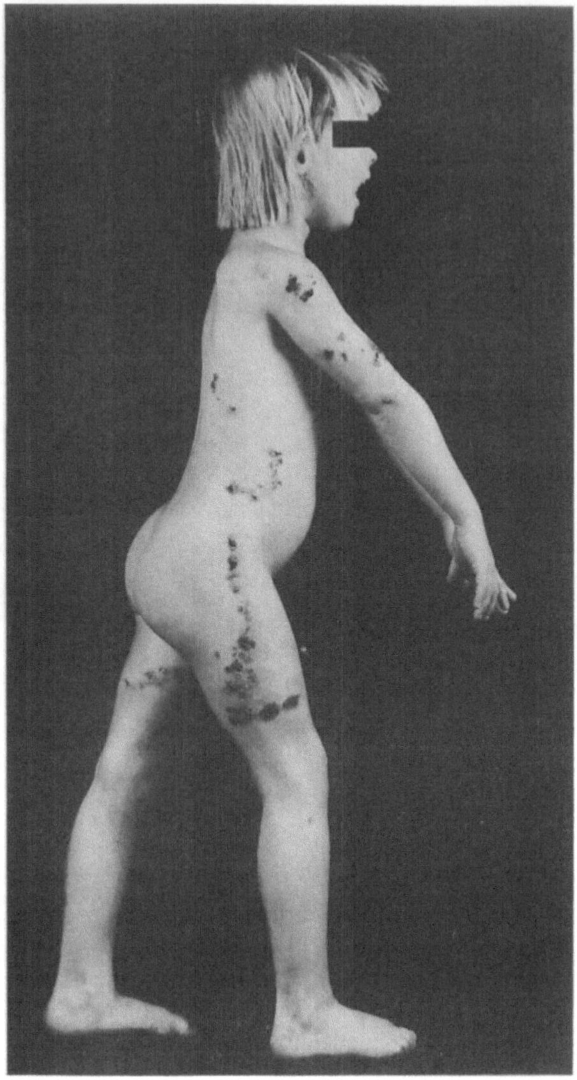

Figure 14.5 Epidermolysis bullosa herpetiformis Dowling–Meara (D-EBH-DM). Pathognomonic groups of blisters in a 5-year-old female mutant (courtesy of Dr Stefan Aronson, Sweden).

Figure 14.6 D-EBH-DM with a benign onset simulating localized dystrophic epidermolysis bullosa in the first month of life (notice milia formation on malleolus, which was not recorded later). The spreading of herpetiform blister became apparent within the first 6 months. Early childhood involvement is particularly severe on hands and feet. This patient is the daughter of the mutant shown in Figure 14.7.

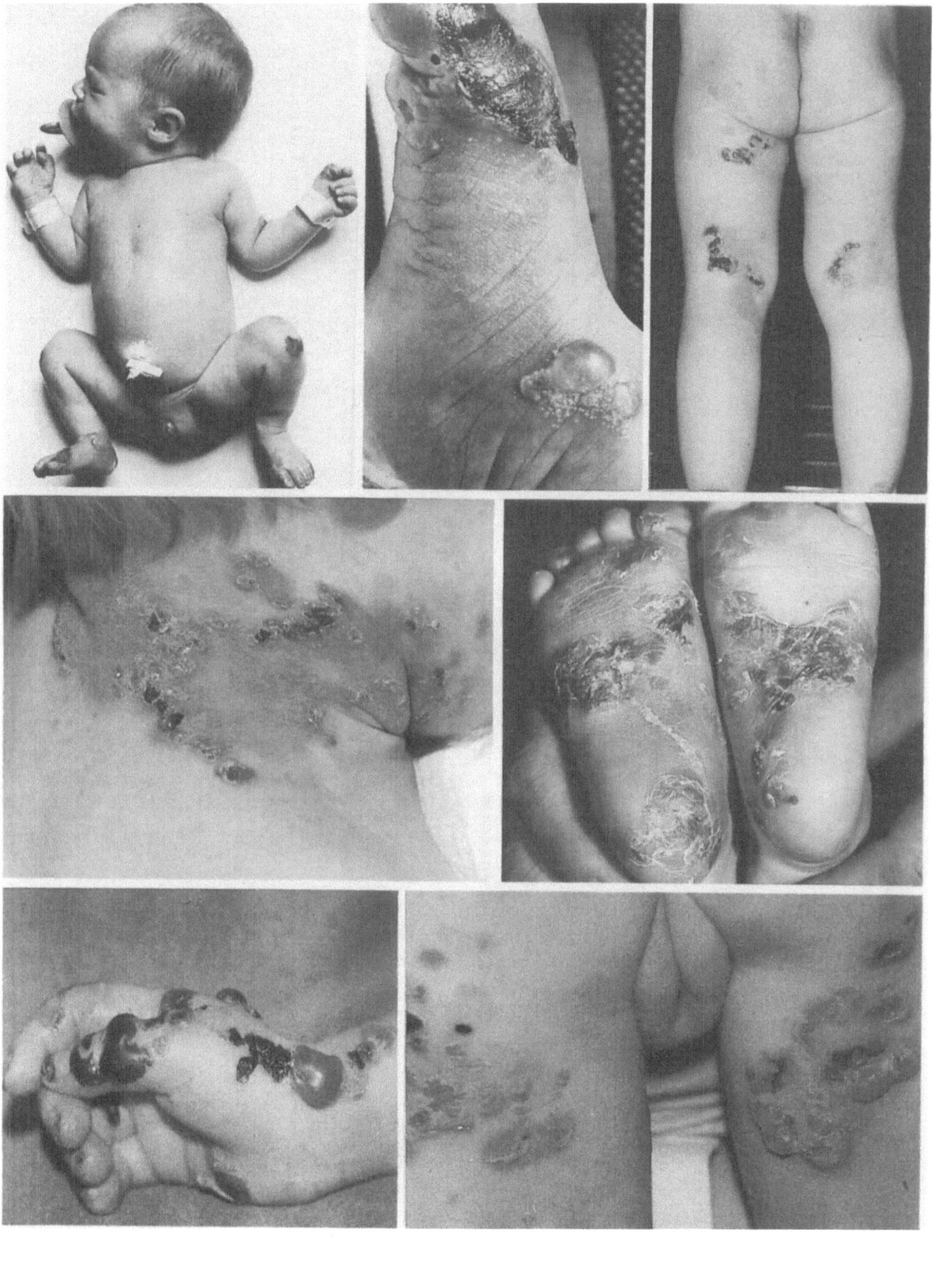

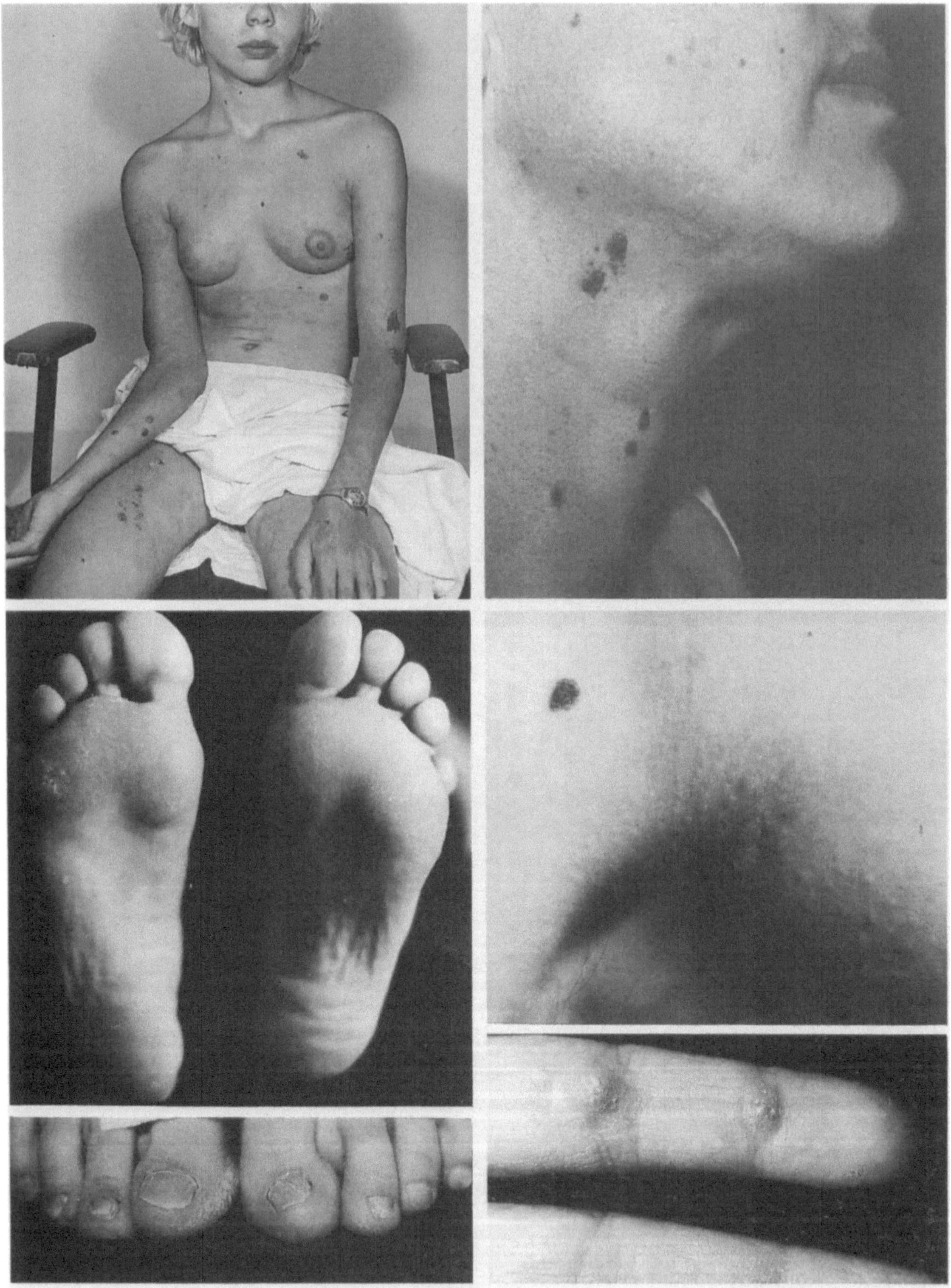

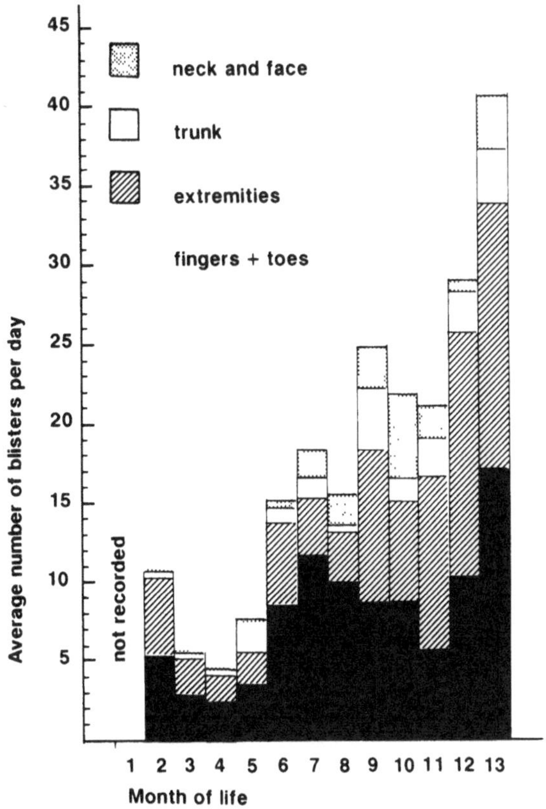

Figure 14.8 Epidermolysis bullosa herpetiformis Dowling–Meara. Distribution of the 5957 blisters recorded from the second to the thirteenth month of life in an average severe female (mutant) case born January 2nd 1987.

typically on the neck (submandibular) or face. Secondly, groups of blisters proximal to hands and feet appear between 2 and 6 months. From this age to school age the herpetiform grouping of blisters (with central healing) on extremities, and after the first year also on the trunk, is a pathognomic feature (Figure 14.5). Often an erythematous area remains for days and even weeks after the herpetiform blistering, and this may persist with crops of blisters recurring in the same place. However, eventually the skin always returns to normal except for a variable tendency to develop benign pigmented nevi (Figure 14.7) at sites of erosions. Although the fingers and toes may improve, hands and feet continue to blister, worsening with walking. In many cases walking has been delayed because the infant will not put pressure on the blistered soles, and some underutilize their hands. Prolonged hyperthermia (over 1 day) improves or even 'clears' the skin of blisters which then recur within a few days after the temperature has dropped to normal. Polano [14] was the first to point out this striking phenomenon. However, it is not easy to determine if the blistering tendency varies with external temperature; in addition, the flexural preponderance of blisters and individual case histories indicate that sweating aggravates the condition (see Section 14.6.7). Seasonal variation is variably reported and seems more related to change of clothing than external temperature (in contrast to EB simplex proper), springtime being most often mentioned as the worst season. There are cases, however, where no improvement with fever is noticeable (see Section 14.6.3). Severe cases have generalized blisters from birth (Figure 14.9) and may be fatal [44, 46].

During early childhood it becomes apparent that palms and soles very gradually become permanently hyperkeratotic. Yellowish tylosis is the only constant sign of the disease in adults. The improvement with age may be noticeable from around the 5th year on, and was described as relatively abrupt in the 6th–7th year in one case [13]. Others show a more gradual improvement at school age (Figure 14.7). Blisters may be friction-related or adhesive-tape-induced, but 'spontaneous' blisters show irregular periodicity.

In adulthood blisters either cease, or appear sporadically, particularly the small vesicular type outbreaks. A burning sensation in the hyperkeratotic soles is elicited by prolonged walking or standing. Toe nails may become dystrophic after multiple regrowths, but finger

Figure 14.7 D-EBH-DM at adolescence (14 years) and at adult age in a dominant mutant [9]. Scattered blisters and multiple post-eruptional benign junctional nevi associated with diffuse yellowish plantar keratosis and minimal nail dystrophy. See Figure 14.6 for her affected daughter.

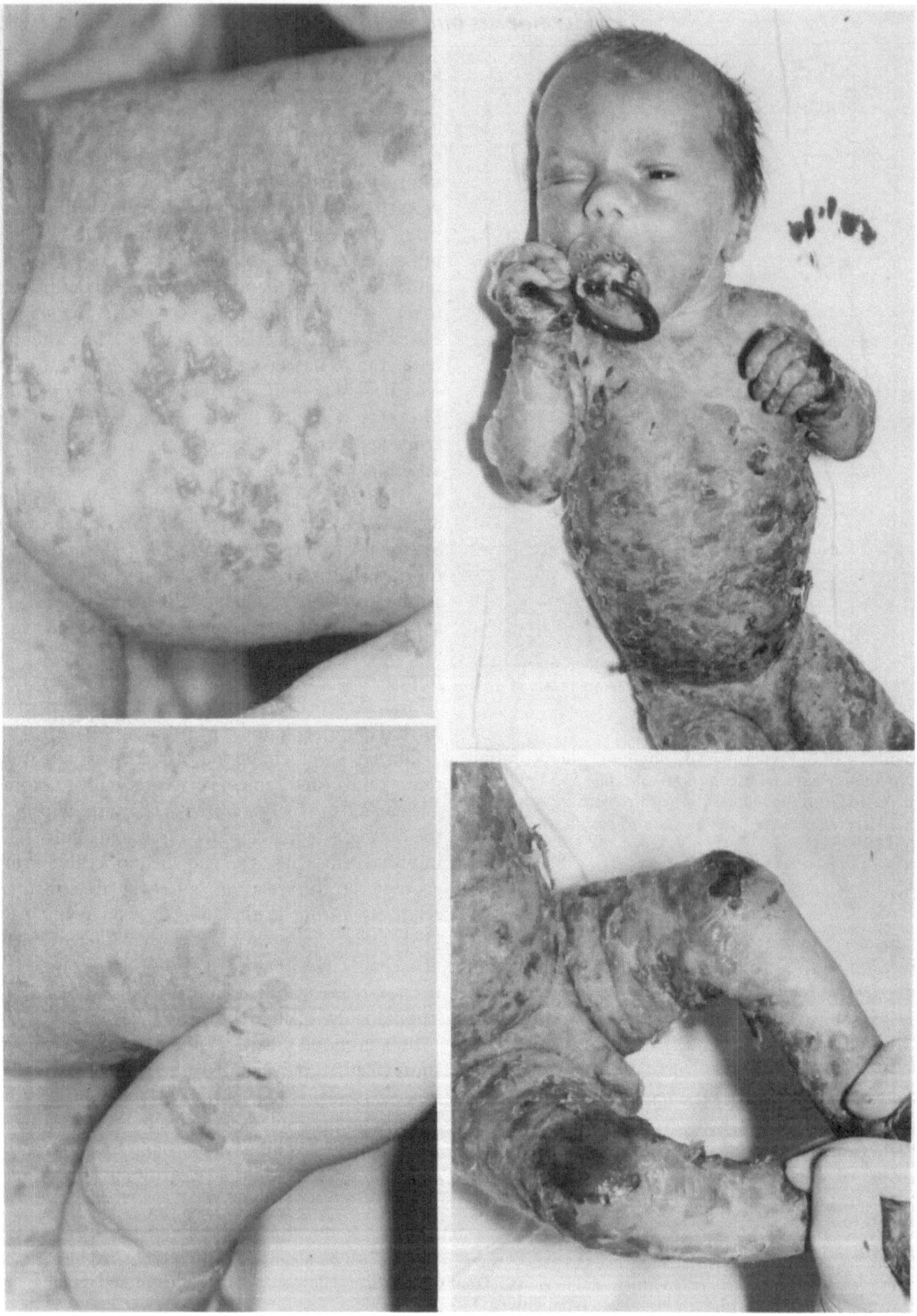

nails often remain normal. The teeth have normal white-appearing enamel [18, 35] unlike the enamel defect observed in junctional EB and the yellowish dentine defects in recessive dermolytic EB. However, enamel defects and loss of small shells of the enamel have been described [35].

14.6.2 Morphology

The blisters appear to form by initial tonofilament clumping followed by cytolysis in the basal parts of the basal keratinocytes. By ordinary light microscopic examination the blister appears to be subepidermal [9, 13, 14, 17, 47]. Biopsy of a fresh blister may show remnants of the basal cell on the blister floor at the edge of the blister. In the immediately adjacent perilesional skin the keratinocytes are elongated with holes or fractures in the subnuclear cytoplasm (at variance with the EB simplex type of blister).

Under the electron microscope the tonofilaments show aggregation or clumping in the basal part of the basal keratinocytes [16–18], most conspicuously immediately above their anchorage to the attachment plate of the hemidesmosomes (Figure 14.10). Occasional suprabasal cells have tonofibrillar clumps, but generally the spinosum layer have normal appearing tonofibrils. The basal cell tonofibrillar abnormality is also found in cells without cytolysis in the perilesional skin. In the classical patient, no tonofibril or other changes can be seen in biopsies of normal non-active skin areas under the electron microscope [17]. The fresh blister roof has occasional dyskeratotic cells with tonofibrillar clumping, but is otherwise normal except for the intraepidermal split.

Eosinophils are abundant in many biopsies, and, in blister fluid, high mitotic activity has been noticed in the keratinocytes [16, 17]; atypical mitoses in neonatal skin were reported by Niemi [18].

The pathognomonic electron microscope findings were discovered independently by Anton-Lamprecht *et al.* [16] and Niemi [18].

14.6.3 Genetics

Dominant inheritance was first revealed in an infant born to an unclassifiable mild 'dominant mutant' case of Gedde-Dahl [9]. Since then, numerous cases have been proven by electron microscopy. The majority of DM cases have been sporadic (normal siblings and parents), and a minority have had an affected parent or other relative, hence autosomal dominant inheritance must be assumed. However, the autosomal dominant inheritance does not explain the apparent excess of females [13, 14, 17, 22, 31, 34, 45–53].

On the basis of several large studies [34, 54], one may wonder if DM cases are genetically heterogeneous, one being X-linked dominant, another autosomal dominant. The observation of an extremely severe male (mutant) case (Figure 14.9) as opposed to the female mutants (Figures 14.5–14.7) with mother–daughter transmission only could corroborate an X-linked form. However, very severe female cases are also known [22,45,46]. With respect to tonofibrillar clumping, herpetiform blistering, site of blistering and improvement with age, the X-linked dominant families do not differ from the classical DM description given in Section 14.6.1. So far, the 'improvement by fever' is not reported for verified autosomal families with father–son transmission.

14.6.4 Differential diagnosis

In the first few months of life D-EBH-DM is difficult to distinguish from most other types of epidermolysis bullosa. Between 6 months and 7 years of age the clinical picture is pathognomonic. Without a history, juvenile dermatitis herpetiformis is a differential [55].

From school age on, epidermolysis bullosa simplex and benign junctional epidermolysis bullosa types may be diagnosed, and at adult age any diffuse type of palmoplantar hyperkeratosis.

14.6.5 Systemic and associated manifestations

None have been reported.

Figure 14.9 D-EBH-DM. A very severe male mutant case at age 2 weeks and 13 months. The extensive exfoliation of skin at age 3 days is shown in ref. [77]. A neonatal biopsy raised the suspicion of D-EBS-K, but when fully worked up disclosed the basal cell tonofibrillar aggregation typical of D-EBH-DM. Clinical discrimination was difficult due to the intensity of blistering everywhere.

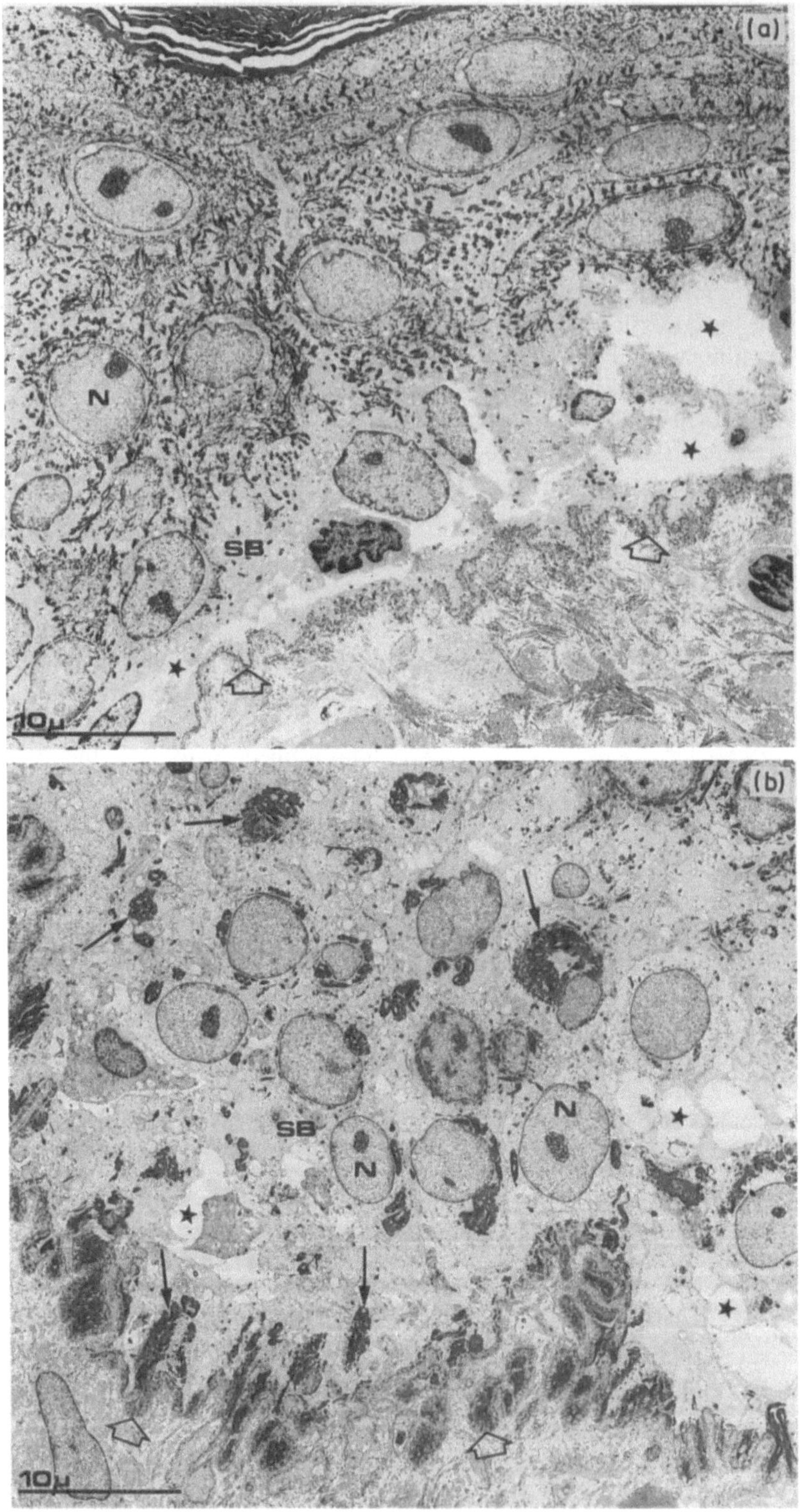
(a)
N
SB
10µ
(b)
SB
N
N
10µ

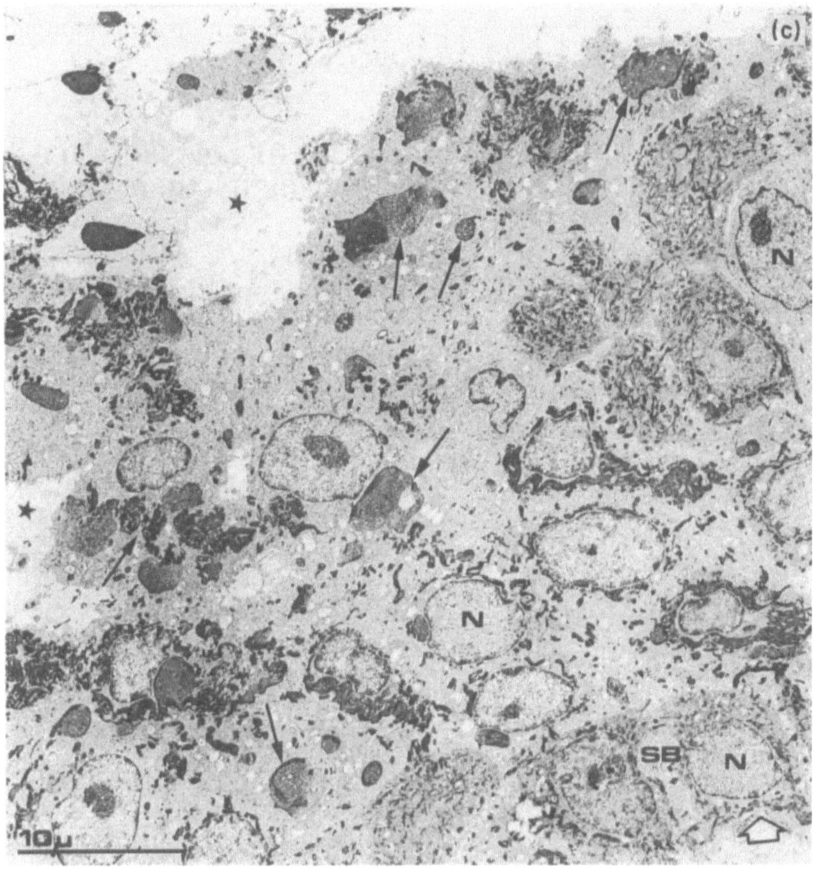

Figure 14.10 Electron microscopic diagnosis. Initial stages of blister formation in (a) EBS (Köbner) via cytolysis of morphological normal appearing basal cells, (b) EBH Dowling–Meara via cytolysis of basal cells following clumping and aggregation of keratins within the cytoplasm of basal and suprabasal cells and along the dermo–epidermal junction, (c) bullous congenital ichthyosiform erythroderma (epidermolytic hyperkeratosis) via cytolysis and acantholysis of high-level keratinocytes, while basal cells remain spared and appear morphologically normal. SB, basal cell layer; N, nuclei; asterisk, focal areas of initial blistering; arrows, clumps and aggregation of keratin filaments; open arrows, dermo–epidermal junction. (× 2282). The electron micrographs were provided by I. Anton-Lamprecht and co-workers.

14.6.6 Pathogenesis

No biochemical abnormality has so far been found. Tidman *et al.* [53] were unable to show abnormal keratin expression and concluded that the tonofilament clumping might be the result of post-translational modification of the keratin filaments. However, mutations in keratin genes are not excluded. Interaction with saprophytic bacterial or viral infection has not been thoroughly studied (see Section 14.6.7).

In a few instances serum zinc levels have been found to be low [18, 35, 56] (see Section 14.6.7), but there are no abnormalities of zinc absorption and most patients have normal levels.

On the basis of genetic heterogeneity hypothesis (Section 14.6.3), one possibility could be than an essential protein is a heteropolymer consisting of one polypeptide coded by X and another polypeptide coded by an autosome. Mutations in any of these polypeptides could lead to similar diseases.

14.6.7 Treatment

Trauma prophylaxis, so essential for other EB types, seems to be of very limited value except for hands and feet in early infancy. Blisters should be punctured by sterile needles and the collapsed blister roof left in place unless there is secondary infection, which is not usually a problem when regular antiseptic baths are used. Oral zinc supplements were found beneficial in one case [56]. Our case with an initial subnormal zinc level was treated for 2 years, the mother claiming more rapid healing, but the blistering rate was not reduced. The improvement was not sufficiently dramatic to prevent discontinuation because of nausea.

Cases that improve during hyperthermia also show improvement in a hot dry climate and as a result of sea bathing. Scandinavian patients have improved during Mediterranean holidays/ treatment trips, but with recurrence shortly after returning home [34,35]. Long (over 1 h) 32° C baths also improve the skin, but are impractical for small children.

Improvement during treatment with antibiotics in non-febrile patients has not been systematically studied.

Hashimoto *et al.* [49,50] obtained a long-lasting (7 months) improvement after local low-dose PUVA treatment, using the contralateral side of the body as a control in three D-EBH-DM girls. Other EB types do not respond.

14.6.8 Genetic counselling and prenatal diagnosis

Parents of a new mutant case have a very low recurrence risk with future pregnancies, but higher than the average population in view of the possibility of gonadal mosaicism for the mutant gene. It is important to convey this low risk to the parents because the state of their affected child often makes them hesitant to have further children [49]. Affected cases have a 50% risk in each pregnancy of an affected baby. At present, no prenatal diagnosis is safe since unaffected non-blistered skin may show no tonofibrillar clumping and tonofibrils are sparse around the 20th gestational week. In a critical case, foetoscopy and foetal skin biopsy may be offered provided these reservations are properly communicated.

14.7 OTHER BASAL CELL TONOFIBRILLAR ANOMALIES

One family [34, 57, 58] had hypoplasia of basal cell tonofibrils associated with intraepidermal (basal cell) blistering in a father and daughter, with severe childhood blistering improving from the sixth year. Clinically it differed from the Dowling-Meara type by abnormal fragility of the skin (see Section 14.3), strongly trauma-related blistering, progressive alopecia, and gradual atrophy of the skin with pigmented spots. Owing to the congenital absence of skin in patches on the extremities, Kero [34] named it D-EB-Bart; however, Bart's family were otherwise clinically different and has never been studied morphologically [59]. In the electron microscope report (abstracts), the authors called this case EB simplex with a new tonofilament defect. A recent trunk-skin biopsy of the father showed normal tonofibrils. The name D-EB-Kero–Niemi (D-EB-KN) is suggested.

A male sporadic case with generalized fragility of the skin and scattered trauma-related congenital-onset serous blistering, clinically diagnosed as a new dominant mutant of the D-EBS-Ogna category [9], was shown by electron microscopy to have tonofibrillar clumping classical for the Dowling-Meara type [22]. His blistering was never herpetiform but improved at school age, and he did not develop the summer blistering of feet and hands seen with D-EBS-Ogna. The striking bruising tendency of the skin is the only persisting clinical sign. It is a peculiar clinical observation that some D-EBH-DM cases do have bruising of the skin, while others have not. This adds to the large variation in severity among these cases. Again, it is unknown if these apparently different mutations occur at the same gene locus, thereby explaining the morphological similarity.

Presumably generalized abnormalities of basal cell tonofibrils give 'bruising epidermis' which is lacking in D-EBH-DM proper.

14.8 EPIDERMOLYTIC HYPERKERATOSES AND SUPRABASAL TONOFIBRILLAR DISEASES

14.8.1 Bullous ichthyosiform erythroderma (D-BIE)

(a) Clinical signs and course of disease

Congenital-onset generalized non-scarring blistering is easily mistaken for generalized EBS (Köbner) (see Section 14.2), until the development of the severe diffuse palmoplantar hyperkeratosis at the end of the first year, gradually associated with greasy-looking hyperkeratosis over the knees, elbows and axillary folds. However, from the onset, the skin is variably erythematous and blisters are more flaccid and easily broken than in EBS, and direct desquamation without blister formation is also seen. Whereas in severe cases the blistering is lifelong and particularly painful under the keratotic layers of soles and palms, other cases cease to blister during infancy, and later only the hyperkeratosis remains, which may be diffuse or irregular, but is always worse on palms and soles, followed by the joints. The clinical picture (Figure 14.11) is strikingly different from the non-bullous ichthyoses.

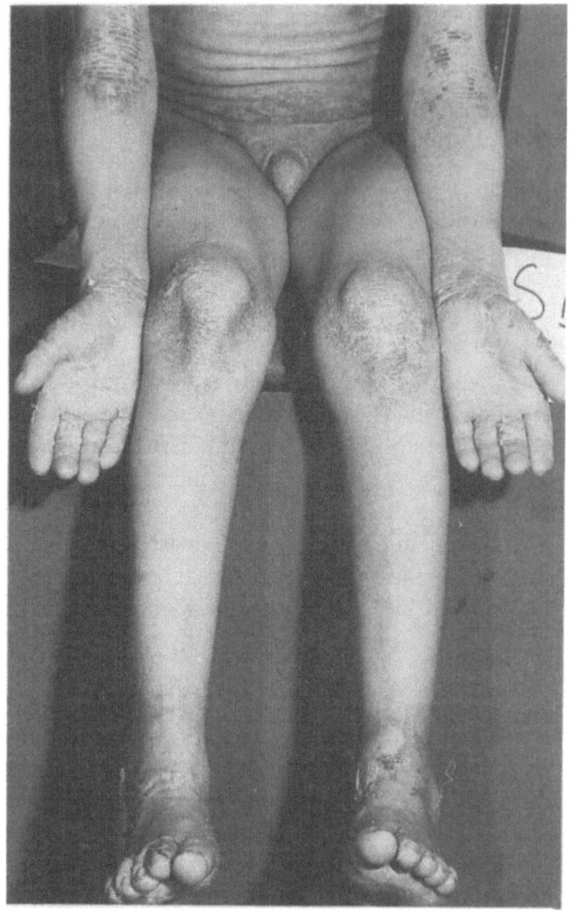

Figure 14.11 Bullous ichthyosiform erythroderma (D-BIE) in a 6-year-old boy (unpublished).

(b) Morphology

Light microscopy reveals cell vacuolization ('balloon cells') of the granular and upper Malpighian layer, hyperkeratosis, papillomatosis and acanthosis [60]. Electron microscopy reveals tonofibrillar clumping or shells of tonofibrillar material near the cell membrane and around the nucleus while the intervening cytoplasm is 'clear' [61]. The connection between tonofibrils and desmosomes is disturbed. Acanthokeratolysis and cytolysis is responsible for the blister formation. The tonofibrils of the basal cells look essentially normal.

(c) Genetics

Bullous ichthyosiform erythroderma is an autosomal dominant [60, 62].

The frequency of D-BIE is quoted as 1 in 300 000 births [60]. In a 1963–1987 prospective study in Norway, the author found one new mutant among 1.44 million births.

(d) Differential diagnosis

In the neonatal period generalized EB, particularly D-EBS-K, and occasional severe cases of D-EBH-DM (cf. Figure 14.9) pose a problem, and cases have been mistaken for EB for years. Patients of low severity who cease to blister in infancy or early childhood may be mistaken for severe non-bullous types of palmoplantar keratoses.

(e) Systemic and associated manifestations

None have been reported.

(f) Pathogenesis

Apart from what can be deduced from morphology, the pathogenesis is unknown. One possibility is a mutation of keratin genes.

(g) Treatment

The keratotic skin is often malodorous due to secondary infection, and disinfectants are needed. Keratolytic agents are needed, particularly on the soles and palms. Retinoid treatment is effective for the hyperkeratosis, but erythema and tender skin is aggravated and, in cases with persistent blistering, the blister formation increases. Hence, retinoids may not be able to be used for the most severe cases.

(h) Genetic counselling and prenatal diagnosis

Parents of new mutants have a very low recurrence risk (see Sections 14.6 and 14.8.2). The patients themselves have a 50% risk at each pregnancy of having an affected baby. Prenatal diagnosis is made by foetoscopy and electron microscopy of foetal skin at the 20th–21st gestational week. Because of the late development of keratinization, too few tonofibrils may be found to verify clumping, but vacuolization in the suprabasal cells is more easily seen. This expression varies between families, as does the inconstant tonofibrillar clumping in amnion cells [63–65]. If D-BIE should turn out to reflect mutations in keratin genes, these have been cloned and can be used in future chorionic villus sample DNA diagnosis.

14.8.2 Epidermolytic palmoplantar keratoderma (D-EPPK) and other localized variants

Inherited localized hyperkeratosis with the typical epidermolytic hyperkeratosis morphology (cytolysis and clumps of tonofilaments) is as frequent as the generalized (D-BIE) form but is rarely associated with clinical blistering [66]. Dominant inheritance (D-EPPK) is one form.

14.8.3 General epidermolytic hyperkeratosis without tylosis?

A mother (dominant mutant) and three sons showed typical clinical features of a mild generalized D-BIE, but they all lacked palmoplantar hyperkeratosis. Bruising skin and flaccid blisters were more evident on the trunk than on extremities. Morphological studies need to be done [35].

14.9 INTRAEPIDERMAL PSEUDOJUNCTIONAL EPIDERMOLYSIS BULLOSA (R-EBPJ)

14.9.1 Clinical signs and course of disease

These patients, in this case a Dutch and a Finnish family, display an unusual clinical picture most reminiscent of benign junctional EB [34, 67, 68]. They have blisters on the fingers at birth and variable generalized blistering. The buttocks have sores and lifting up the babies results in blisters showing the pattern of the finger grip. They may die in infancy. The blisters do not scar or form milia. Conjunctival and laryngeal involvement are reported. Muscular dystrophy becomes apparent in childhood or teens and progresses to wheelchair dependence. Later there is diffuse mild skin atrophy over elbows, knees, shin and dorsum of fingers, associated with variable dyspigmentation, e.g. albostriate white elevations on lower back skin resembling those transitorily seen in junctional R-EBA-inversa [69]. Nails may be lost or dystrophic (Figure 14.12). Teeth may be shed and discoloured.

A similar Sudanese kindred had not developed muscular dystrophy by late childhood [70], though seemingly with the same skin disease.

14.9.2 Morphology

Light microscopy reveals apparent subepidermal cleavage. However, electron microscopy demonstrates remnants of basal cells at the blister floor, and cytolytic as well as acantholytic cells in the blister roof. The blister floor is partly covered by cytoplasm and plasma membrane remnants of the basal cells, partly devoid of it revealing a clean

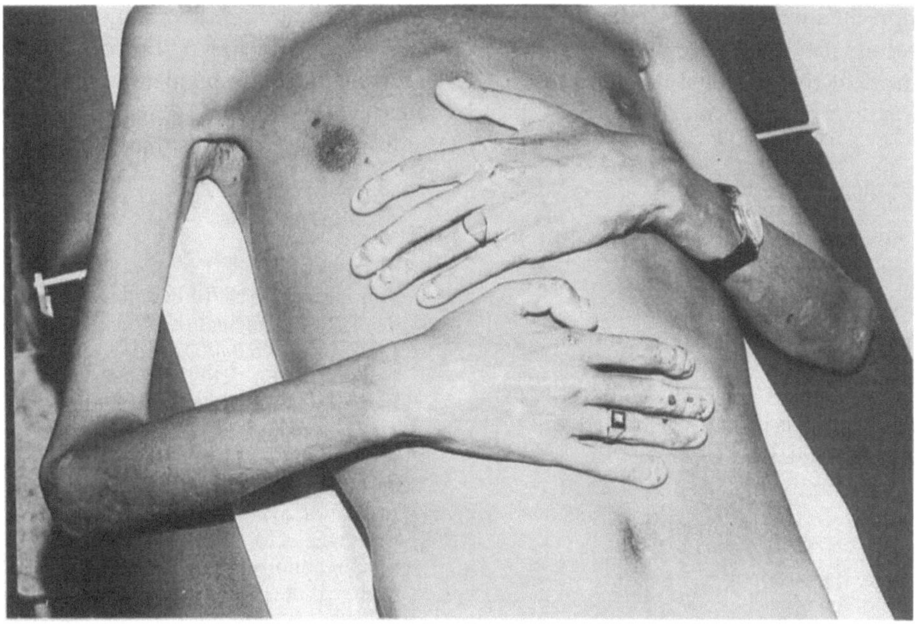

Figure 14.12 Pseudojunctional epidermolysis bullosa (R-EBPJ) and limb-girdle muscular dystrophy in a patient aged 33 years [67]. Note dystrophic nails, blood blister on finger and scattered apigmented atrophic skin areas on hands and forearms. See text for ultrastructural findings.

'junctional' surface of basal lamina and anchoring fibrils only (pseudojunctional) [22, 68, 70]. Hemidesmosomes and tonofibrils may be normal or abnormal in different kindreds [22, 68, 70].

14.9.3 Genetics

The European families apparently both have the same unusual autosomal recessive intraepidermal pseudojunctional type of epidermolysis bullosa (R-EBPJ). More unpublished cases with the same electron microscopical findings are now known, but muscular dystrophy has not yet been reported for these [22, 71]. Only when they and the Sudanese family have been followed until adult age can the development of muscular dystrophy be excluded. If it does not develop, the European families may be explained by close linkage between two recessive diseases. The existence of this combination in two separate populations is unlikely unless the genes are so close as to be affected (deleted) by a single mutational event. The possibility of both traits being pleiotropic effects of a single recessive gene is still open.

An extensive number of genetic markers are being tested in the Dutch family to determine the chromosomal assignment of this (these) gene locus (loci).

14.9.4 Differential diagnosis

R-EBPJ can be confused with junctional epidermolysis bullosa atrophicans and epidermolysis bullosa simplex.

14.9.5 Systemic and associated manifestations

Deafness in one ear and high-tune hypoacusis in the other was present in one case [67], and mental subnormality and lactose intolerance have also been reported [68]. Limb-girdle-type muscular dystrophy is discussed above.

14.9.6 Pathogenesis

The pathogenesis of blistering is unknown. The gradual development of atrophy can, according to

Anton-Lamprecht's hypothesis, be associated with variable secondary destruction, inhibition of formation or defective repair of hemidesmosomes in connection with blister formation.

14.9.7 Treatment

See Chapter 15 on junctional epidermolysis bullosa.

14.9.8 Genetic counselling and prenatal diagnosis

Parents of affected cases have a 25% recurrence risk. Prenatal diagnosis has not been tried, but may be possible by foetal skin biopsies provided the index case of the family has been examined.

14.10 RARE REPORTS

14.10.1 Bart's type

Bart's type of epidermolysis bullosa refers to a dominant kindred in which a majority of the affected had congenital localized absence of skin on the feet or legs, many had congenital absence, loss or dystrophy of the nails of the thumbs and big toes (rarely others), and infrequent non-scarring blistering of hands and feet, and occasionally legs, elbows or other areas [59]. Sporadic cases assumed to be of this type have been reported [72], and in two instances intraepidermal blisters have been demonstrated [22, 73]. However, Bart's original family [59] has not been examined morphologically and no clinically similar dominant families with intraepidermal blistering have been verified. Congenital ulceration, on the other hand, has been repeatedly reported in very mild dominant-dystrophic families [9, 74] (Chapter 15). The justification for distinguishing a specific D-EB-Bart type is therefore in doubt. With congenital ulceration, the early childhood phase of recessive-dystrophic EB of the inversa type may clinically simulate Bart's type for years [35].

14.10.2 Dystrophia bullosa (Mendes da Costa)

A single Dutch family with X-linked recessive inheritance is on record [75, 76]. Blisters are intraepidermal, appear mainly on extremities and mainly within the first 3 years of life. Microcephaly and reticulated dyspigmentation are among the much more striking manifestations of this syndrome. The chromosomes are normal.

REFERENCES

1. von Hebra, J. (1870) Pemphigus, Ärztlicher Bericht des k.k. allgemeinen Krankenhauses zu Wien vom Jahre 1870. *Vienna*, 363–4.
2. Köbner, H. (1886) Hereditäre Anlage zur Blasenbildung (Epidermolysis bullosa hereditaria). *Dtsch Med. Wschr.*, **12**, 21–2.
3. Hallopeau, M.H. (1898) Nouvelle note sur la dermatose bulleuse hereditaire et traumatique. *Ann. Dermatol. Syphil.*, **9**, (Ser. 3), 721–8.
4. Gossage, A.M. (1908) The inheritance of certain human abnormalities. *Q. J. Med.*, **1**, 331–46.
5. Weber, F.P. (1926) Recurrent bullous eruption on the feet in a child. *Proc. R. Soc. Med.*, **19**, 72.
6. Cockayne, E.A. (1938) Recurrent bullous eruption of the feet. *Brit. J. Dermatol.*, **551**, 358–62.
7. Elliot, G.T. (1895) Two cases of epidermolysis bullosa. *J. Cutan. Genit. Urin. Dis.*, **13**, 10–18.
8. Wesener, G. (1957) Beitrag zur Kenntnis der sogenannten residivierenden Blasenruption an den Füssen bei heissem Wetter (Weber–Cockayne). *Dermatol. Wschr.*, **136**, 1133–7.
9. Gedde-Dahl, T. Jr (1971) *Epidermolysis Bullosa. A Clinical, Genetic and Epidermiological Study*, Universitetsforlaget, Oslo; The Johns Hopkins Press, Baltimore.
10. Hintner, H., Stingl, G., Schuler, G., *et al.* (1981) Immunofluorescence mapping of antigenic determinants within the dermal–epidermal junction in mechanobullous diseases. *J. Invest. Dermatol.*, **76**, 113–18.
11. Fine, J.-D. (1985) Review: monoclonal antibodies and the skin biopsy: current and potential applications. *Amer. J. Med. Sci.*, **290**, 143–51.
12. Fine, J.-D., Breathnach, S.M., Fox, P.A., *et al.* (1985) Monoclonal antibodies in dermatological research: Studies with a unique keratinocyte-specific cell surface antigen defined by a monoclonal antibody. *Amer. J. Dermatopathol.*, **7**, 171–9.
13. Dowling, G.B. and Meara, R.H. (1954) Epidermolysis bullosa resembling juvenile dermatitis herpetiformis. *Brit. J. Dermatol.*, **66**, 139–43.
14. Polano, M.K. (1958) Naar anleiding van een patientje met hardnekkige blaarvorming. *Maandschr. Kindergeneesk*, **26**, 145–53.
15. Gedde-Dahl, T. Jr (1978) Classification of epidermolysis bullosa. In *Pädiatrische Dermatologie*

(ed. J.J. Herzberg), F.K. Schattauer, Stuttgart, New York, pp. 65–91.
16. Anton-Lamprecht, I., Gedde-Dahl, T. Jr and Schnyder, U.W. (1979) Ultrastructural characterization of a new dominant epidermolysis genotype. *J. Invest. Dermatol.*, **72**, 280 (abstr.).
17. Anton-Lamprecht, I. and Schnyder, U.W. (1982) Epidermolysis bullosa herpetiformis Dowling–Meara. Report of a case and pathomorphogenesis. *Dermatologia*, **164**, 221–35.
18. Niemi, K.-M., Kero, M., Kanerva, L. and Mattila, R. (1983) Epidermolysis bullosa simplex. A new histological subgroup. *Arch. Dermatol.*, **119**, 138–41.
19. Gedde-Dahl, T. Jr and Anton-Lamprecht, I. (1983) Epidermolysis bullosa. In *Principles and Practice of Medical Genetics* (eds A.E.H. Emery and D.L. Rimoin), Edinburgh, Churchill Livingstone, Vol. 1, pp. 672–87.
20. Pearson, R.W. (1971) The mechanobullous diseases (epidermolysis bullosa). In *Dermatology in General Medicine* (eds T.B. Fritzpatrick, K.A. Arndt, W.H. Clark, *et al.*), McGraw-Hill, New York, pp. 621–47.
21. Haneke, E. and Anton-Lamprecht, I. (1982) Ultrastructure of blister formation in epidermolysis bullosa hereditaria: V. Epidermolysis bullosa simplex localisata type Weber–Cockayne. *J. Invest Dermatol.*, **78**, 219–23.
22. Anton-Lamprecht, I. (1987) Personal communication.
23. Siemens, H.W. (1922) Studien über Vererbung von Hautkrank-heiten. I. Epidermolysis bullosa hereditaria (Bullous mechanica simplex). *Arch. Dermatol. Syphil.*, **139**, 45–56.
24. Tilsley, D.A. and Beard, U.T.C. (1963) Epidermolysis bullosa simplex in Tasmania. *Lancet*, **ii**, 905–7.
25. Hauge, M. (1962) Om blodtypenes anvendelse i den humane genetikk. Med særlig henblikk på koblingsanalyser og zygotidiag-nostik. Copenhagen (Aarhuus Stiftsbogstrykkerie). Thesis.
26. Davison, B.C.C. (1965) Epidermolysis bullosa. *J. Med. Genet.*, **2**, 233–42.
27. Mulley, J.C., Nicholls, C.M., Propert, D.N., *et al.* (1984) Genetic linkage analysis of epidermolysis bullosa simplex, Köbner type. *Amer. J. Med. Genet.*, **19**, 573–7.
28. Fine, J.-D. and Griffith, R.D. (1985) A specific defect in glycosylation of epidermal cell membranes. Definition in skin from patients with epidermolysis bullosa simplex. *Arch. Dermatol.*, **121**, 1292–6.
29. Savolainen, E.-R., Kero, M., Pihlajaniemi, T., *et al.* (1981) Deficiency of galactosylhydroxylysyl glucosyltransferase, an enzyme of collagen synthesis, in a family with dominant epidermolysis bullosa simplex. *New Engl. J. Med.*, **304**, 197–204.
30. Winberg, J.-O. and Gedde-Dahl, T., Jr (1986) Gelatinase expression in generalized epidermolysis bullosa simplex fibroblasts. *J. Invest. Dermatol.*, **87**, 326–9.
31. Sanchez, G.F., Seltzer, J.L., Eisen, A.Z., *et al.* (1983) Generalized dominant epidermolysis bullosa simplex: decreased activity of a gelatinolytic protease in cultured fibroblasts as a phenotypic marker. *J. Invest. Dermatol.*, **81**, 576–9.
32. Takamori, K., Naito, K. and Ogawa, H. (1983) Epidermolysis bullosa simplex blister fluid induces an intra-epidermal blister in cultured normal skin. *Brit. J. Dermatol.*, **109**, 643–6.
33. Fine, J.-D., Stewart, B. and Austin, R. (1986) Epidermolysis bullosa blister fluid and human skin organ culture: an unreliable *in vitro* model for the disease. *ESDR and JID 5th Joint Meeting*, June 22–25, Geneva, Abstr. 193, p. 114.
34. Kero, M. (1984) Epidermolysis bullosa in Finland. Clinical features, morphology and relation to collagen metabolism. *Acta Dermatovenereol. (Stockholm), Suppl.* 110.
35. Gedde-Dahl, T. Jr (1987) Unpublished observations.
36. Yacoub, T., Campbell, C.A., Gordon, Y.B., *et al.* (1979) Maternal serum and amnion fluid concentrations of alphafetoprotein in epidermolysis bullosa simplex. *Brit. Med. J.*, **1(6159)**, 307.
37. Olaisen, B. and Gedde-Dahl, T. Jr (1973) GPT-epidermolysis bullosa simplex (EBS Ogna) linkage in man. *Hum. Hered.*, **23**, 189–96.
38. Fischer, T. and Gedde-Dahl, T. Jr (1979) Epidermolysis bullosa simplex and mottled pigmentation: A new dominant syndrome. I. Clinical and histological features. *Clin. Genet.*, **15**, 228–38.
39. Bruckner-Tuderman, L., Vogel, A., Rüegger, S., *et al.* (1988) Basal cell and basement membrane defect in epidermolysis bullosa simplex with mottled pigmentation. *J. Am. Acad. Dermatol.*
40. Boss, J.M., Matthews, C.N.A., Peachey, R.D.G. and Summerly, R. (1981) Speckled hyperpigmentation, palmo-plantar punctate keratoses and childhood blistering: a clinical triad, with variable associations. *Brit. J. Dermatol.*, **105**, 579–85.
41. Gedde-Dahl, T. Jr, Anton-Lamprecht, I. and Fischer, T. (1980) Ultrastructural studies of a new syndrome: Epidermolysis bullosa simplex and mottled pigmentation. *7th European Meeting of the Society for Cutaneous Ultrastructural Research*, Vienna, May 9–10 (Abstr.).
42. Gedde-Dahl, T. Jr and Fischer, T. (1977) Autosomal inactivation? Epidermolysis bullosa simplex with mottled pigmentation. *Eur. Soc. Hum. Genet., Oslo (Abstr.), Clin. Genet.*, **13**, 116–17.
43. Bjerke, J.R. and Gedde-Dahl, T., Jr (1986) Treatment of a hereditary palmoplantar keratoderma with etretinate. *ESDR Symposium on*

Genodermatoses and Genetics of Skin Diseases, Oslo Feb. 7–8, (Abstr.).
44. Granek, H. and Baden, H.P. (1980) Corneal involvement in epidermolysis bullosa simplex. *Arch. Ophthalmol.*, **98**, 469–72.
45. Blanchet-Bardon, C., Nazzaro, V., Raynaud, F., *et al.* (1987) Dominant epidermolysis bullosa, Dowling-Meara type: three observations of an intraepidermal epidermolysis bullosa with varying prognosis (Fr.). *Ann. Dermatol. Venereol.*, **114**, 341–8.
46. Fine, J.-D. (1987) Personal communication.
47. Mizuguchi, M., Kaneko, K. and Kawakami, M. (1983) A Case of Epidermolysis Bullosa Hereditaria – Dowling Meara's Type? – (Jap.) *The Nishinihon Journal of Dermatology* (Fukuoka, Japan) **45**, 365–71.
48. Anton-Lamprecht, I. (1986) Klassifikation und diagnostische zuordnung der verschiedenen typen der hereditären epidermolysen. I. Symposium *Humangenetik in der Dermatologie*, Magdeburg, Nov. 6–8.
49. Hashimoto, I., Katabira, Y. and Mitsuhashi, Y. (1983) PUVA therapy of epidermolysis bullosa herpetiformis Dowling-Meara and its influence on genetic counseling. *Med. Genet. Res.*, **5**, 150–6.
50. Hashimoto, I., Katabira, Y., Mitsuhashi, K. *et al.* (1987) Treatment of epidermolysis bullosa with PUVA therapy. *Congressus Mundi Dermatologiae Berlin*, May 24–29. (Abstr.).
51. Blanchet-Bardot, C. (1987) Personal communication.
52. Eady, R.A.J. (1987) Personal communication.
53. Tidman, M.J., Allen, M.H., Leigh, I.M. *et al.* (1986) Epidermolysis bullosa simplex (Dowling-Meara): An immunohistochemical study of keratin expression. ESDR and JID 5th Joint Meeting, June 22–25, Geneva (Abstr. 253, p. 149).
54. Hacham-Zadeh, S., Rappensberger, K., Livshin, R. and Konrad, K. (1986) Epidermolysis bullosa herpetiformis Dowling-Meara in a large family. ESDR Symposium on Genodermatoses and Genetics of Skin Diseases, Oslo Feb. 7–8 (abstr.).
55. Søby, P. (1946) Herpetiform dermatitis in children. *Acta Derm. Venereol. (Stockh.)*, **26**, 397.
56. Michaelsson, G. (1987) Personal communication.
57. Kero, M., Niemi, K.-M. and Kanerva, L. (1983) Epidermolysis bullosa simplex with tonofilament deficiency (abstr.). Nordiske Dermatologkongress. Oslo, Juni 12–16, 217.
58. Niemi, K.-M., Kero, M. and Kanerva, L. (1986) Epidermolysis bullosa simplex – a new tonofilament defect. ESDR Symposium on Genodermatoses and Genetics of Skin Diseases, Oslo Feb. 7–8, (abstr.).
59. Bart, B.J., Gorlin, R.J., Anderson, V.E. and Lynch, T.W. (1966) Congenital localized absence of skin and associated abnormalities resembling epidermolysis bullosa. A new syndrome. *Arch. Derm.*, **93**, 296–304.
60. Baden, P. and Hooker, P. (1983) Ichthyosiform dermatoses. In *Principles and Practice of Medical Genetics* (eds A.E.H. Emery and D.L. Rimoin), Churchill Livingstone, Edinburgh, New York, pp. 653–71.
61. Anton-Lamprecht, I. and Schnyder, U.W. (1974) Ultrastructure of inborn errors of keratinization. *Arch. Dermatol. Forsch.*, **250**, 207–27.
62. Gasser, V. (1964) Zur Klinik, Histologie und Genetik der "Erythrodermie congenitale ichthyosiforme bulleuse (Brocq.)". *Arch. Klaus Stift. Verebungsforsch.*, **38**, 23–59.
63. Golbus, M.S., Sagebiel, R.W., Filly, R.A., *et al.* (1980) Prenatal diagnosis of congenital bullous ichthyosiform erythroderma (epidermolytic hyperkeratosis) by fetal skin biopsy. *New Engl. J. Med.*, **302**, 93–5.
64. Holbrook, K., Dale, B.A., Sybert, V.P. and Sagebiel, R.W. (1983) Epidermolytic hyperkeratosis: ultrastructure and biochemistry of skin and amnion fluid cells from two affected fetuses and a newborn infant. *J. Invest. Dermatol.*, **80**, 222–7.
65. Anton-Lamprecht, I. and Arnold, M.-L. (1987) Prenatal diagnosis of severe genetic disorders of the skin. In *Pediatric Dermatology* (eds R. Happle and E. Grosshans), Springer-Verlag, New York, Berlin, Heidelberg, pp. 3–22.
66. Blanchet-Bardon, C. and Nazzaro, V. (1987) Use of morphological markers in carriers as an aid in genetic counselling and prenatal diagnosis. *Curr. Probl. Dermatol.*, **16**, 109–19.
67. de Weerdt, C.F. and Castelein, S. (1972) Het voorkomen van epidermolysis bullosa hereditaria dystrophica en progressieve spierdystrofie in één gezin. *Ned. T. Geneesk. (Amsterdam)*, **116**, 1264–8.
68. Niemi, K.-M., Somer, H., Kero, M., *et al.* (1988) Epidermolysis bullosa simplex associated with muscular dystrophy with recessive inheritance.
69. Gedde-Dahl, T. (1981) Sixteen types of epidermolysis bullosa. On the clinical discrimination, therapy and prenatal diagnosis. *Acta Dermatovenereol. (Stockholm), Suppl.* **95**, 74–87.
70. Salih, M.A.A., Lake, B.D., El Hag, M.A., *et al.* (1985) Lethal epidermolytic epidermolysis bullosa: A new autosomal recessive type of epidermolysis bullosa. *Brit. J. Dermatol.*, **113**, 135–43.
71. Bauer, E.A. (1987) Personal communication.
72. Smith, S.Z. and Cram, D.L. (1978) A mechanobullous disease of the newborn. Bart's syndrome. *Arch. Dermatol.*, **114**, 81–4.
73. Bart, B.J. (1970) Epidermolysis bullosa and congenital localized absence of skin. *Arch. Dermatol.*, **101**, 78–82.
74. Joensen, H.D. (1973) Epidermolysis bullosa dystrophica dominans in two families of the Faroe

islands. *Acta Dermatovenereol. (Stockholm)*, 53, 53–60.

75. Woerdeman, M.J. (1957) Dystrophia bullosa hereditaria. Typus maculatus. Proceeding of the Second International Congress for Dermatology. *Acta Dermatovenereol. (Stockholm)*, **678**, 111–16.

76. Hassing, J.H. and Doeglas, H.M.G. (1980) Dystrophia bullosa hereditaria, typus maculatus (Mendes da Costa-van der Valk): a rare genodermatosis. Netherlands' Society Proceedings. *Brit. J. Dermatol.*, **102**, 474–6.

77. Gedde-Dahl, T. Jr (1987) Epidermolysis bullosa syndromes. *Curr. Probl. Dermatol.*, **16**, 129–45.

Fifteen

Junctional epidermolysis bullosa

Robin A.J. Eady and Michael J. Tidman

15.1 INTRODUCTION

In 1935, Herlitz [1] recognized the existence of a distinct hereditary blistering disease that was lethal in early infancy. Since then, the 'hereditary lethal' form of epidermolysis bullosa (EB) has borne his name, but there was no certain means of delineating Herlitz disease from the more common dystrophic forms, which could be clinically confusing, especially in the neonatal period, until Pearson [2] showed by electron microscopy that the level of blistering, in the various types of EB, was at different layers in or around the dermo–epidermal zone. In Herlitz disease blistering is at the level of the lamina lucida of the epidermal basement membrane (EBM). Thus we were introduced to the term junctional bullous epidermatosis or junctional EB (JEB), which could now be clearly distinguished from simplex (epidermolytic) and dystrophic (dermolytic) forms.

It then became evident that not all patients with JEB died of their disease so the 'lethal' part of the description was dropped, or changed to 'non-lethal' [3, 4]. It was also noted that patients, with the 'lethal' or 'non-lethal' varieties of JEB, tended to have atrophic skin – as opposed to scarring which was a feature of the dystrophic disease. In fact, patients with all types of EB may produce scarring, but the nature of the scar tissue will vary. The term 'EB atrophicans' [5] has therefore been used as an alternative for JEB.

Table 15.1 Types of junctional (atrophic) EB

Lethal (Gravis, Herlitz)
Non-lethal (Mitis)
Generalized benign (atrophicans generalisata mitis)
Inverse
Localized
Progressive
Scarring

15.2 CLASSIFICATION OF JUNCTIONAL (ATROPHIC) EB

All forms are recessively inherited [6], therefore unlike dystrophic EB, no major distinction can be made on the basis of dominant or recessive modes of transmission. Given that any classification is deficient, and will remain so until the molecular and biochemical defects have been elucidated, we will follow the somewhat descriptive categories of the disease that others have already proposed, knowing that they have merit in pointing out the clinical heterogeneity [5]. A suggested classification of JEB subtypes is included in Table 15.1.

15.2.1 Lethal JEB (Herlitz disease; EB atrophicans gravis)

Blisters or erosions are noted at or soon after birth. Large areas of skin may be absent [7]. The whole skin is abnormally fragile and the simple acts of lifting or turning the baby may result in blistering or peeling away of the epidermis. The disease will follow a relentless course of repeated blistering, especially in sites that are continually rubbed by the baby (such as the heel or shin). Characteristically lesions are seen on the finger tips around the nails, which are usually shed (Figure 15.1) and buttocks (Figure 15.2), in the mouth (Figure 15.3), and on the back of the scalp. Death often occurs within the first 3–6 months, but some children have survived longer [8–10] probably owing to improved medical and nursing care. In these survivors persistent erosions of the central face associated with exuberant granulation tissue is highly characteristic (Figure 15.4). Chronic anaemia is common [11]. Laryngeal oedema or stenosis [12] may make tracheostomy necessary. There have been many reports of pyloric atresia associated with Herlitz disease (see [13] for review). The dental abnormality has been studied in the Herlitz and non-lethal forms of JEB. The common abnormality seems to be a hypoplasia with an enamel defect [14–16].

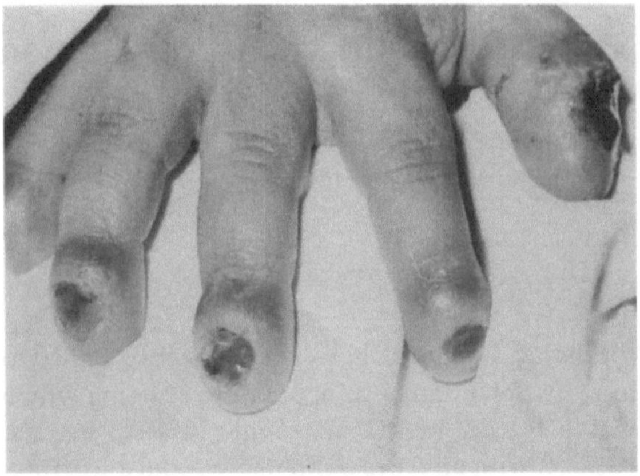

Figure 15.1 Fingertips of a patient with junctional epidermolysis bullosa (JEB) of the Herlitz type. Repeated blistering has led to 'drum-stick' appearances with shedding of the nails.

The precise cause of death in JEB is often undetermined. Pneumonia with septicaemia is frequently a terminal event. At *post mortem*, epithelial separation has been found in several internal organs [8, 13, 17], but the extent of involvement during life has yet to be determined.

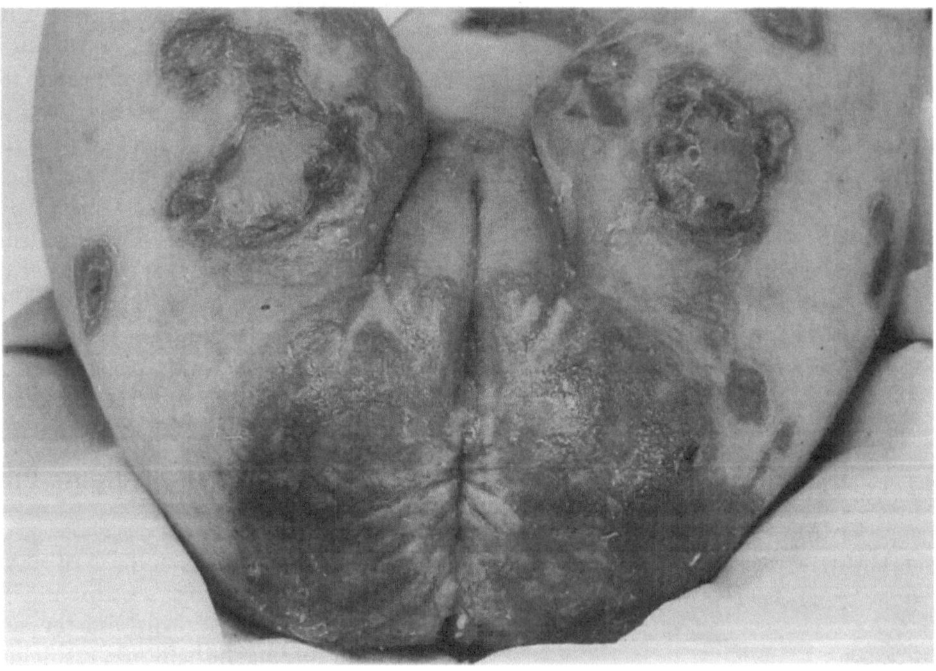

Figure 15.2 Lesions on the buttocks of a baby with lethal (Herlitz) JEB.

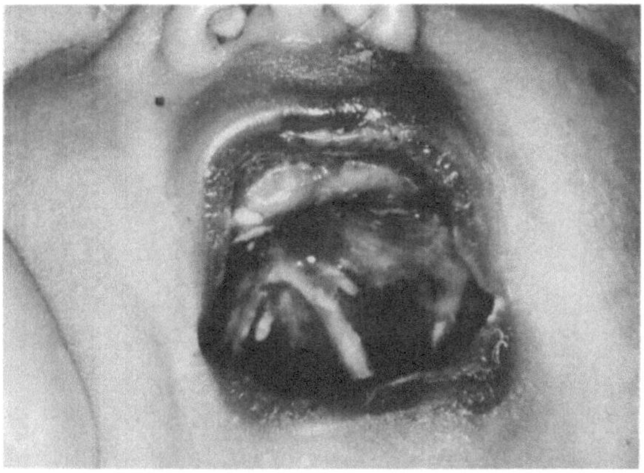

Figure 15.3 Oral lesions in a Herlitz baby. There is severe blistering of the mucosa as well as the lips. [Photograph courtesy of Dr W.P de Groot. First published in S. Hurwitz and R.A.J. Eady (1986) Epidermolysis bullosa. In *Practical Management of the Dermatologic Patient* (eds A. Rook, L.C. Parish and J.M. Beare), J.B. Lippincott, Philadelphia. Reproduced with permission.]

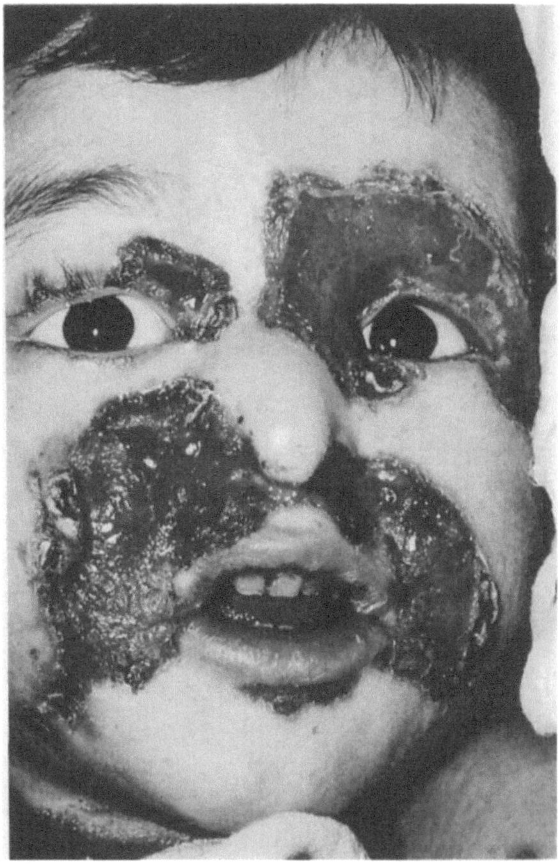

Figure 15.4 Central facial erosions with characteristic exuberant granulation tissue in a 2-year-old boy with Herlitz disease. (Photograph courtesy of Drs W. Cunliffe and J. Norris.)

15.2.2 Non-lethal junctional EB

This term encompasses a group of patients who have certain features in common with Herlitz disease but who tend to develop normally and survive into adulthood.

Generalized atrophic benign EB (EB atrophicans generalisata mitis)

Hashimoto *et al.* [18] and Schnyder and Anton-Lamprecht [19] described a few patients with some of the features of Herlitz disease who survived beyond infancy and to adulthood. Hintner and Wolff [20] coined the term 'generalized atrophic benign EB' to describe eight patients aged between 3 and 40 years with generalized junctional blistering in a disease that ran a relatively benign course. The patients have alopecia (Figure 15.5), scant axillary and pubic hair, dysplastic teeth and dystrophic nails (Figure 15.6). Blisters result in atrophic changes instead of the more obvious scarring associated with milia which characterizes dystrophic EB. A patient who probably had this variety of JEB [21] was found, after death, to have widespread amyloidosis.

Reports on other patients with many of the same features have since been published [22–24].

Inverse junctional EB (EB atrophicans inversa). The so-called 'inverse' distribution of the lesions was first noted by Gedde-Dahl [3] in patients with recessive dystrophic EB. It later became evident that a similar pattern could also occur in JEB [5]. The disease starts at birth and blisters and erosions predominantly involve the buttocks (Figure 15.7), perineum, groins and axillae. Corneal erosions, dysplastic teeth and nail dystrophy are also

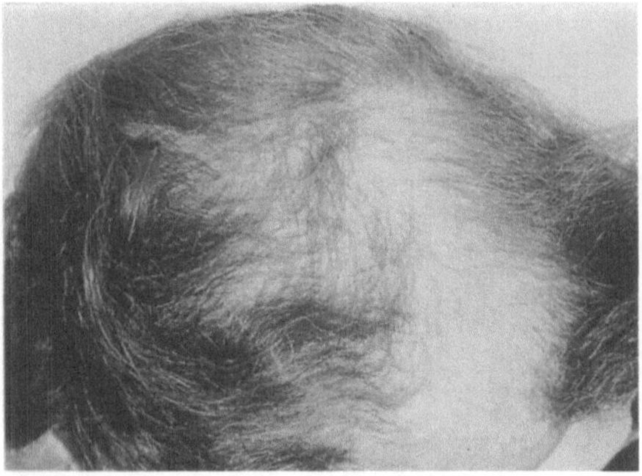

Figure 15.5 Longstanding alopecia in a 65-year-old patient with non-lethal JEB (inverse type).

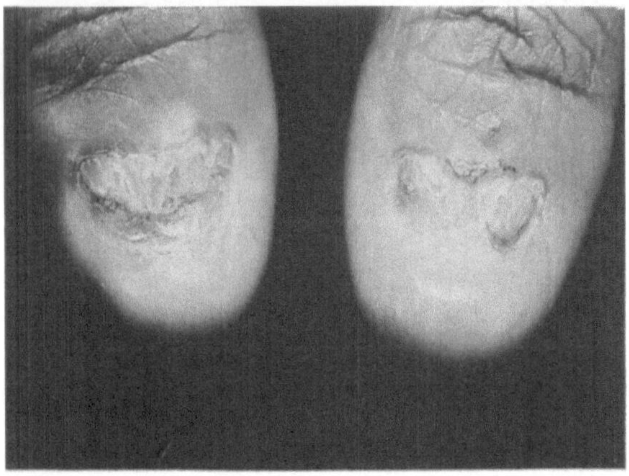

Figure 15.6 Nail dystrophy in a 21-year-old female patient with non-lethal JEB.

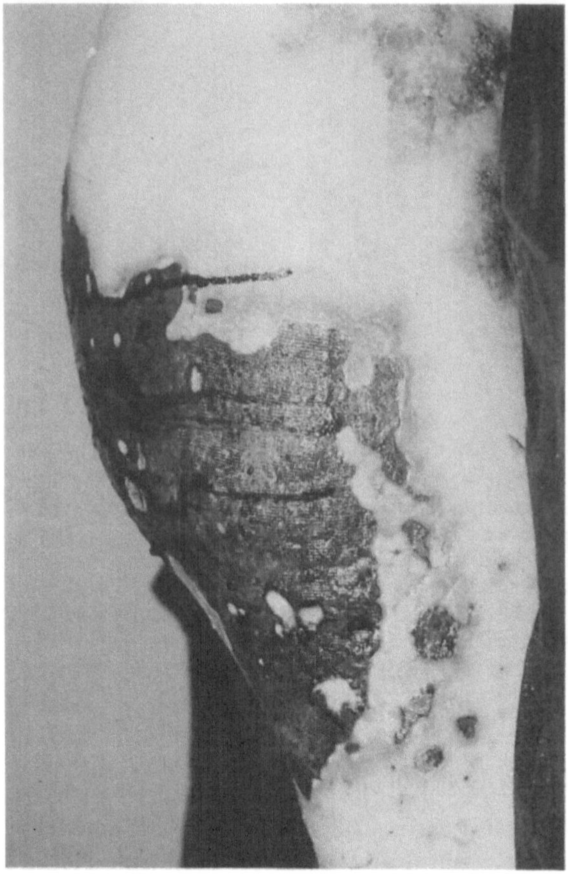

Figure 15.7 Large erosions affecting the buttocks, thighs and hips in a 65-year-old patient with non-lethal JEB (inverse variety).

characteristic. In women, the disease may improve during the reproductive years. The case originally described by Ridley [25] has junctional blistering [26] and therefore exhibits many of the features of this disease.

(b) Localized junctional EB (EB atrophicans localisata)

It is not clear whether this variant [19] is a mild form of generalized atrophic JEB or a separate entity. We [27] have reported on two affected sisters with non-lethal JEB whose disease is mainly confined to the legs (Figure 15.8), although blistering can occur anywhere on the body and involve the mouth [27]. Hyperkeratosis with painful erosions affects the soles (Figure 15.9) with highly similar or identical appearances to those found in the generalized benign or inverse forms of the disease. The scalp and pubic hair are normal and the teeth are not dysplastic.

(c) Cicatricial junctional EB

Haber and colleagues [28] described three cases with electron microscopically proven JEB whose

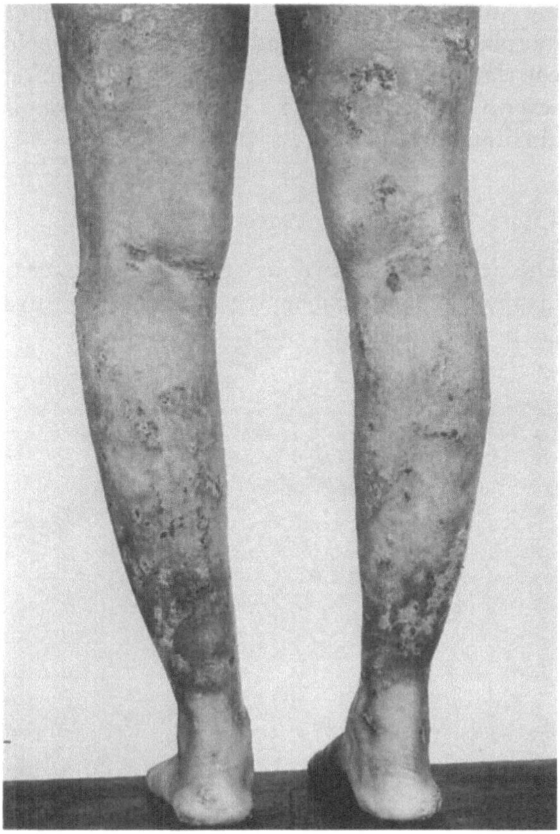

Figure 15.8 Extensive atrophy associated with blisters, erosions and pigmentary changes affects mainly the legs of this 21-year-old woman with non-lethal JEB.

blisters resulted in scarring as opposed to atrophy. There were no milia. In addition, the teeth were dysplastic and the nails absent. In all, the diagnosis of dystrophic EB was made initially. The question has been raised whether these cases fall into the generalized benign atrophic category [29].

(d) Progressive junctional EB (EB atrophicans progressiva)

Originally described by Gedde-Dahl [3] as EB dystrophica neurotrophica, this rare condition has recently been shown in a single case to have junctional blisters [30]. It starts after birth and

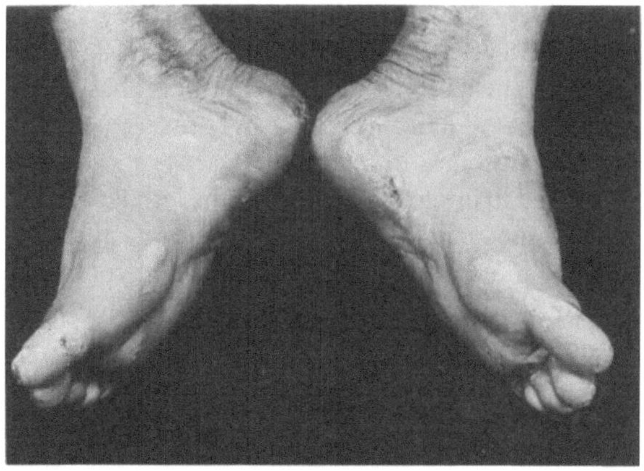

Figure 15.9 The feet of the same patient shown in Figure 15.8. Painful hyperkeratotic plaques have developed at points of friction and repeated blistering.

progresses to leave atrophic scars. Hearing defects may occur.

15.3 DIAGNOSIS OF JUNCTIONAL EB

In the neonatal period, the extensive involvement and severity of the disease often suggest the diagnosis. However, the simplex and recessive dystrophic forms may also present with widespread blistering. As mentioned above, involvement of the mouth, buttocks and periungual sites in a neonate is suggestive if not diagnostic of Herlitz disease. All forms of JEB are recessive, so the involvement of siblings with unaffected parents should be sought. A skin biopsy should be taken from the edge of a fresh blister (less than 12 h old) and preferably one that has been deliberately induced by gentle friction. The sample should be divided for light and electron microscopy and for indirect immunofluorescence (see Chapter 12).

15.3.1 Light and electron microscopy

Light microscopy of a fresh blister will show a sub-epidermal cleft. Usually the epidermis separates cleanly from the dermis. There is little or no evidence of dermal inflammation.

In *all* types of JEB, electron microscopy shows that the level of separation occurs through the lamina lucida of the epidermal basement membrane (Figure 15.10). Wherever possible hemidesmosome ultrastructure [26] should be examined in unseparated skin. In the lethal variant, hemidesmosomes are usually hypoplastic and reduced in number (Figure 15.11). The hypoplasia is characterized by small attachment plaques and diminutive or absent sub-basal plates [26; 2–34]. In non-lethal JEB, the hemidesmosome morphology may be normal [26, 30]. No correlation has yet been found between the clinical severity of JEB and the hemidesmosome abnormality [26].

15.3.2 Immunofluorescence

The technique known as 'immunofluorescence mapping' or 'antigen mapping' offers an alternative

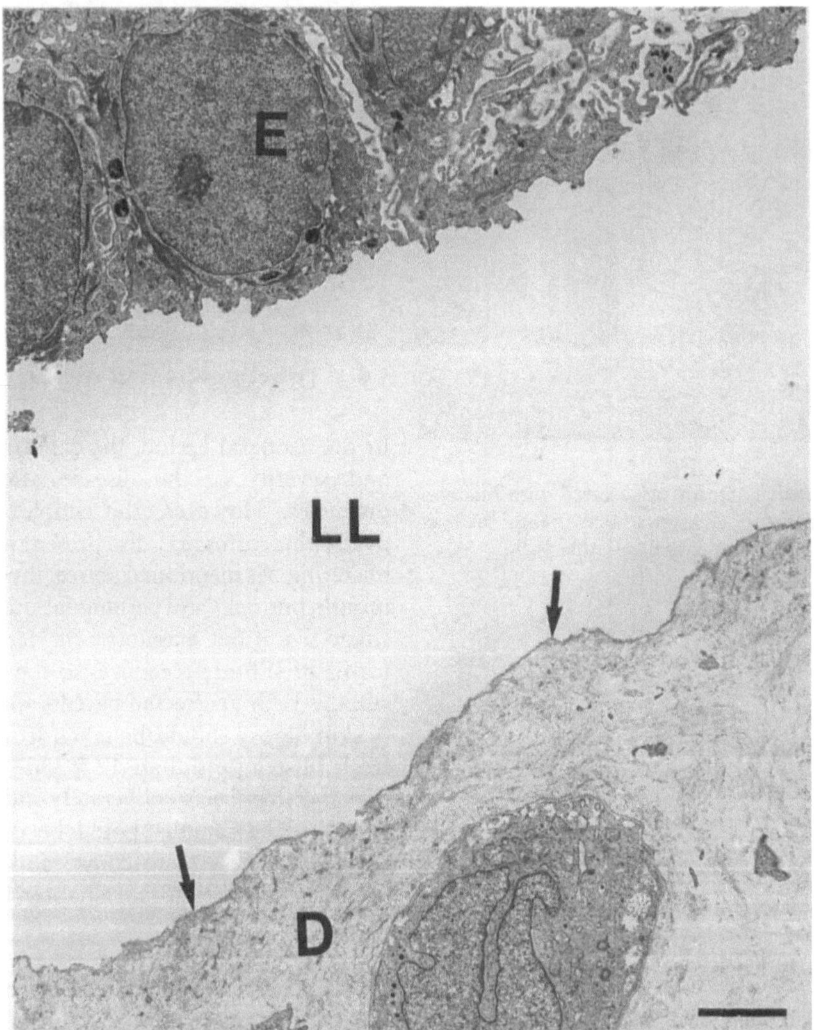

Figure 15.10 Electron micrograph demonstrating the level of blistering in all cases of JEB. The epidermis (E) has cleanly separated from the dermis (D) at the level of the lamina lucida (LL) of the epidermal basement membrane. Arrows point to the lamina densa which remains as a continuous sheet on the blister floor. Bar = 2 μm.

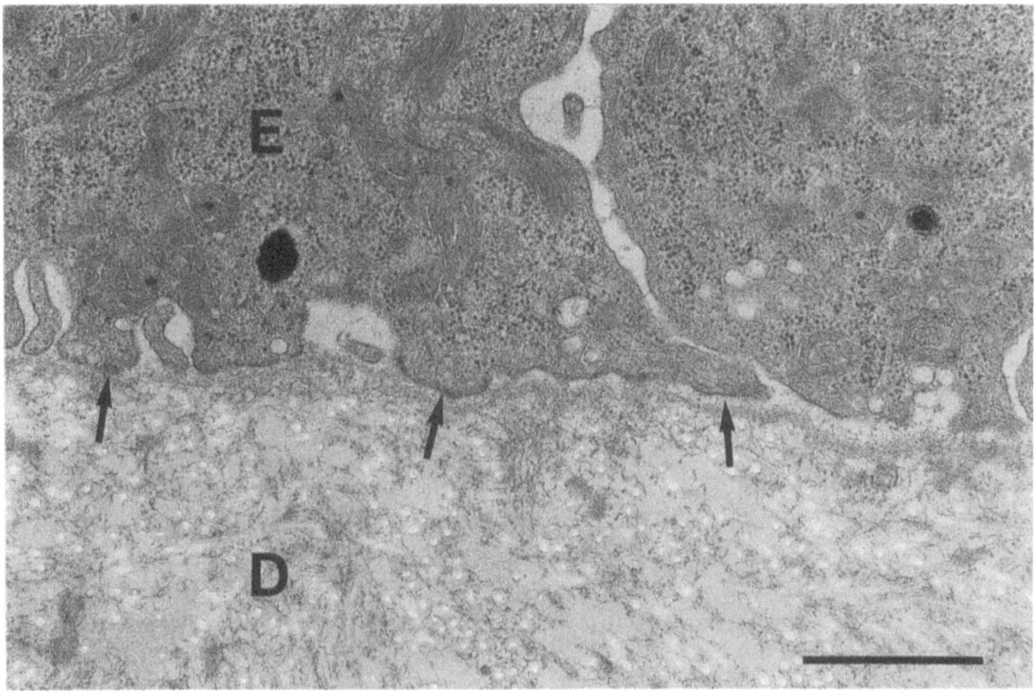

Figure 15.11 Electron micrograph showing hypoplastic hemidesmosomes (arrows) at the base of an epidermal basal keratinocyte (E). For a review of normal hemidesmosome ultrastructure see [26, 31]. Bar = 2 μm.

to electron microscopy and may be used where electron microscope facilities are not available [35, 36] (see Chapter 12).

15.3.3 Special antibody studies

It has recently been shown that the antibodies AA3 and GB3 may be especially useful in the diagnosis of JEB [37, 38]. The antibodies were raised against extracts of human amnion [39, 40]. AA3 is a polyclonal antiserum and GB3 is a monoclonal antibody. Both antibodies recognize normal components of the epidermal basement membrane and the epitopes may be associated with hemidesmosomes [41–43]. In lethal JEB immunofluorescence staining with both AA3 and GB3 is characteristically and consistently abnormal. Staining with AA3 is always present but reduced in intensity, whereas GB3 staining is either markedly reduced or absent (Figure 15.12). In non-lethal JEB, staining with these antibodies is either reduced or normal. Preliminary data suggest that the intensity of staining may correlate inversely with the severity of disease [37] but this observation needs to be confirmed by a larger study. Both AA3 and GB3 have been used in prenatal diagnosis and exclusion of JEB (see below).

15.3.4 Prenatal diagnosis

The procedure used for obtaining skin samples from foetuses at risk for JEB has been described elsewhere [44] and is outlined in Chapter 12. Since the whole skin is abnormal in lethal JEB the foetal buttock or thigh is usually chosen for sampling. For other forms of the disease, such as inverse JEB, the site of biopsy may be more crucial.

In our experience of about 40 pregnancies at risk for lethal JEB, nine have been affected [45]. In all affected cases the diagnosis posed no difficulty since there was extensive separation of the dermis and epidermis which was visible by light microscopy. Electron microscopy confirmed that the ultrastructural level of separation was in the

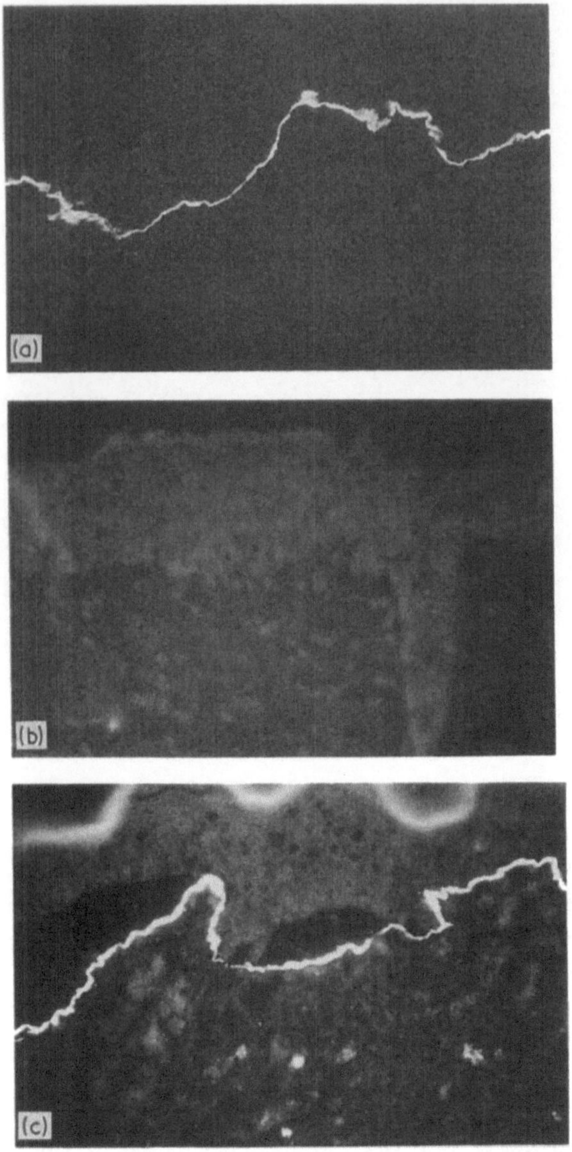

Figure 15.12 Immunofluorescence photomicrographs showing reactivity of GB3 monoclonal antibody which binds to a newly discovered basement membrane antigen [38, 40, 43]. (a) Bright linear staining in normal control skin (× 570). (b) Absence of staining in skin of a neonate with lethal JEB. Arrows indicate dermo–epidermal junction (× 570). (c) Normal staining in skin of a patient with a mild form of non-lethal JEB. Note immunolocalization at the base of a blister (× 570).

lamina lucida. The hemidesmosome abnormality is also evident [44, 45] (Figure 15.11), but very often there is insufficient intact dermo–epidermal junction to make a proper assessment of hemidesmosomes.

The antibodies AA3 and GB3 have been used to detect or exclude lethal JEB in prenatal studies [46, 47] and we have recommended that GB3 be used concurrently with electron microscopy whenever possible. GB3, in particular, has given clear-cut results (absent or much reduced immunofluorescence staining) in all foetal samples shown conclusively by electron microscopy to be affected.

15.4 PATHOGENESIS OF JUNCTIONAL EB

The disease is transmitted by an autosomal recessive gene. The primary abnormality is not known. Whether the different forms are due to mutations affecting different genes or the same gene remains an important question. Electron microscopy suggests that in most patients with JEB there is a structural abnormality of hemidesmosomes. We still do not know which gene or genes is (or are) associated with the proteins comprising the hemidesmosomes. GB3 antigen can be extracted from normal human keratinocytes and has been shown by immunoprecipitation to comprise a group of polypeptides of 93.5–110 kDa [43]. The abnormal binding of GB3 monoclonal antibody to the basement membrane in JEB possibly provides the best clue to tracing a biochemical defect. GB3 antibody binding has been shown to be reduced or absent in both foetal skin and amnion from pregnancies affected by lethal JEB [48]. The question whether this abnormality is primary or secondary has to be addressed.

Lethal JEB fibroblasts, unlike recessive dystrophic EB cells, make normal amounts of collagenase *in vitro* [49, 50]. Kero *et al.* [51] found increased levels of collagenase released from fibroblasts of one patient with non-lethal JEB, and Bauer and Tabas [52] showed that dermal fibroblasts from a group of patients with benign atrophic JEB synthesized abnormally high amounts of collagenase and responded abnormally to colchicine stimulation.

Altered adhesive properties have been shown in JEB keratinocytes *in vitro* [53] and JEB epidermis *in vivo* [54]. Matsumoto and Hashimoto [55] incubated normal skin in organ culture with blister fluid from patients with JEB and found that cleavage occurred in the lamina lucida. Because the *in-vitro* 'blistering' could be prevented by proteinase inhibitors, the authors concluded that proteinases may have a primary role in the blistering process.

15.5 TREATMENT

No specific treatment is known to have a sustained beneficial effect on any form of JEB. Reports on the effectiveness of systemic corticosteroids are anecdotal and in many cases the diagnosis was not established using electron microscopy or antigen mapping. A controlled trial is needed because these drugs may have a place in the management of patients who become acutely ill with laryngeal obstruction. One patient has been reported to improve during phenytoin therapy [56] which more often is used for the treatment of recessive dystrophic EB [57].

The mainstay in the treatment of JEB rests on meticulous attention to protecting the extremely fragile skin and mucosae, avoiding all circumstances which might provoke blisters, and promptly dealing with blisters and erosions once they have arisen [58]. Great care should be taken in lifting and turning babies and small children. Adhesive tape or other sticky substances used to secure electrodes or cardiac monitors should never be applied directly to the skin. Fresh blisters should be punctured and gently drained leaving the blister roof in place. Lesions with a purulent discharge should be swabbed for microbiological examination. Infection is often best dealt with by systemic antibiotic therapy, but topical antimicrobials such as 1% silver sulphadiazine cream, 1.5% hydrogen peroxide cream or mupirocin ointment may help to eradicate micro-organisms. Care should be taken in using topical treatment, especially in babies, because transcutaneous absorption may cause systemic side effects. Fresh erosions can be cleaned with physiological saline soaks. Non-adherent dressings can then be applied. These in turn may need to be kept in place with gauze padding and elasticated bandages. We have found that some of the newer dressings such as Geliperm (Geistlich Sons Ltd) are useful. This can be applied in a hydrated state and has been found soothing and therefore acceptable by the patients. Experimental therapy includes the use of cultured keratinocytes, sheets of which can be placed over the erosions [59]. This treatment was first used for burn victims [60]. Oral blistering in neonates can be reduced by the use of a teat with an extra-large hole which will lessen the need for energetic sucking during feeding. Anaemia may require treatment with oral or parenteral iron or blood transfusion. Special care should be taken if patients need a general anaesthetic. Intubation may lead to blistering in the mouth and upper respiratory tract. The endotracheal tube should be well lubricated and possibly a size smaller than would normally be considered necessary.

REFERENCES

1. Herlitz, G. (1935) Kongenitaler, nicht syphilitischer pemphigus. Eine ubersicht nebst beschreibung einer neuen krankheitsform. *Acta Paediatr.*, **17**, 315–71.
2. Pearson, R.W. (1962) Studies on the pathogenesis of epidermolysis bullosa. *J. Invest. Dermatol.*, **39**, 551–75.
3. Gedde-Dahl Jr, T. (1971) *Epidermolysis bullosa. A Clinical, Genetic and Epidemiological Study,* John Hopkins Press, Baltimore and London.
4. Eady, R.A.J. and Tidman, M.J. (1983) Diagnosing epidermolysis bullosa. *Brit. J. Dermatol.*, **108**, 621–6.
5. Gedde-Dahl, Jr, T. and Anton-Lamprecht, I. (1983) Epidermolysis bullosa. In *Principles and Practice in Medical Genetics* (eds A.E.H. Emery and D.L. Rimoin), Churchill Livingstone, Edinburgh, pp. 672–87.
6. Cross, H.E., Wells, R.S. and Esterly, N. (1968) Inheritance in epidermolysis bullosa letalis. *J. Med. Genet.*, **5**, 189–96.
7. Skoven, I. and Drzewiecki, K.T. (1976) Congenital localized skin defect and epidermolysis bullosa hereditaria letalis. *Acta Dermatol. Venereol.*, **59**, 533–7.

8. Pearson, R.W., Potter, B. and Strauss, F. (1974) Epidermolysis bullosa hereditaria letalis: clinical and histological manifestations and course of the disease. *Arch. Dermatol.*, **109**, 349–55.
9. Turner, T.W. (1980) Two cases of junctional epidermolysis bullosa (Herlitz-Pearson). *Brit. J. Dermatol.*, **102**, 97–107.
10. Silver, H.K. (1957) Epidermolysis bullosa hereditaria letalis: report of a case surviving for two and a half years. *Arch. Dis. Childh.*, **32**, 216–19.
11. Hruby, M.A. and Esterly, N.B. (1973) Anemia in epidermolysis bullosa letalis. *Amer. J. Dis. Child.*, **125**, 696–9.
12. Davies, H., and Atherton, D.J. (1987) Acute laryngeal obstruction in junctional epidermolysis bullosa. *Pediatr. Dermatol.*, **4**, 98–101.
13. Peltier, F.A., Tschen, E.H., Raimer, S.S., *et al.* (1981) Epidermolysis bullosa letalis associated with congenital pyloric atresia. *Arch. Dermatol.*, **117**, 728–31.
14. Crawford, E.G., Jefferson Burkes, E., and Briggaman, R.A. (1976) Hereditary epidermolysis bullosa: oral manifestations and dental therapy. *Oral Surg. Oral Med. Oral Pathol.*, **42**, 490–500.
15. Brain, E.B. and Wigglesworth, J.S. (1968) Developing teeth in epidermolysis bullosa hereditaria letalis: A histological study. *Brit. Dent. J.*, **124**, 255–60.
16. Hill, F.J. and Winter, G.B. (1986) The teeth in dermatological disease. In *Recent Advances of Dermatology*, 7th ed (ed. R.H. Champion), Churchill Livingstone, Edinburgh, pp. 103–25.
17. Schachner, L., Lazarus, G.S. and Dembitzer, H. (1977) Epidermolysis bullosa hereditaria letalis. *Brit. J. Dermatol.*, **96**, 51–8.
18. Hashimoto, I., Schnyder, U.W. and Anton-Lamprecht, I. (1976) Epidermolysis bullosa hereditaria with junctional blistering in an adult. *Dermatologica*, **152**, 72–86.
19. Schnyder, U.W. and Anton-Lamprecht, I. (1979) Zur klinik der epidermolysen mit junktionaler blasenbildung. *Dermatologica*, **159**, 402–6.
20. Hintner, A. and Wolff, K. (1982) Generalized atrophic benign epidermolysis bullosa. *Arch. Dermatol.*, **118**, 375–84.
21. Ridley, C.M. and Levy, I.S. (1968) Epidermolysis bullosa and amyloidosis. *Trans. St. John's Hosp. Dermatol. Soc.*, **54**, 75–82.
22. Tidman, M.J., Eady, R.A.J. and Marsden, R.A. (1985) Non-lethal junctional epidermolysis bullosa. *Brit. J. Dermatol.*, **109**, (Suppl.), 83.
23. Zortea-Caflisch, C. (1985) Epidermolysis bullosa atrophicans generalisata mitis. *Hautarzt*, **36**, 176–8.
24. Paller, A.S., Fine, J-D., Kaplan, S., *et al.* (1986) The generalized atrophic benign form of junctional epidermolysis bullosa: Experience with four patients in the United States. *Arch. Dermatol.*, **122**, 704–10.
25. Ridley, C.M. (1977) Epidermolysis bullosa with unusual features: ? Inversa type. *Proc. R. Soc. Med.*, **70**, 576–7.
26. Tidman, M.J. and Eady, R.A.J. (1986) Hemidesmosome heterogeneity in junctional epidermolysis bullosa revealed by morphometric analysis. *J. Invest. Dermatol.*, **86**, 51–6.
27. Heagerty, A.H.M., Tidman, M.J., Bor, S., *et al.* (1985) Non-lethal junctional epidermolysis bullosa in two adult sisters. *J. R. Soc. Med. Suppl.*, **11**, 32–3.
28. Haber, R.M., Hanna, W., Ramsay, C.A., *et al.* (1985) Cicatricial junctional epidermolysis bullosa. *J. Amer. Acad. Dermatol.*, **12**, 836–44.
29. Tabas, M., Gibbons, S. and Bauer, E. (1987) The mechanobullous diseases. *Dermatol. Clin.*, **5**, 123–36.
30. Haber, R.M. and Hanna, W. (1987) Epidermolysis bullosa progressiva. *J. Amer. Acad. Dermatol.*, **16**, 195–200.
31. Briggaman, R.A. and Wheeler, C.E. (1975) The epidermal–dermal junction. *J. Invest. Dermatol.*, **65**, 71–84.
32. Arwill, T., Bergenholtz, A. and Thildander, H. (1968) Epidermolysis bullosa hereditaria. 5. The ultrastructure or oral mucosa and skin in four cases of the letalis form. *Acta Pathol. Microbiol.*, **74**, 311–24.
33. Hashimoto, I., Gedde Dahl Jr, T., Schnyder, U.W., *et al.* (1976) Ultrastructural studies in epidermolysis bullosa hereditaria: IV. Recessive dystrophic types with junctional blistering. *Arch. Dermatol. Res.*, **257**, 17–32.
34. Hanna, W., Silverman, E., Boxall, L., *et al.* (1983) Ultrastructural features of epidermolysis bullosa. *Ultrastruct. Pathol.*, **5**, 29–36.
35. Hintner, H., Stingl, G., Schuler, G., *et al.* (1981) Immunofluorescence mapping of antigenic determinants within the dermal–epidermal junction in mechanobullous diseases. *J. Invest. Dermatol.*, **76**, 113–18.
36. Kero, M., Palotie, A. and Peltonen, L. (1982) Immunohistological localization of three basement membrane components in various forms of epidermolysis bullosa. *J. Cutan. Pathol.*, **9**, 316–28.
37. Kennedy, A.R., Heagerty, A.H.M., Ortonne, J-P., *et al.* (1985) Abnormal binding of an anti-amnion antibody to epidermal basement membrane provides a novel diagnostic probe for junctional epidermolysis bullosa. *Brit. J. Dermatol.*, **113**, 651–9.
38. Heagerty, A.H.M., Kennedy, A.R., Eady, R.A.J., *et al.* (1986) GB3 monoclonal antibody for diagnosis of junctional epidermolysis bullosa. *Lancet*, **i**, 869.
39. Hsi, B-L., Yeh, C-J., and Faulk, W.P. (1984) Characterization of antibodies to antigens of the human amnion. *Placenta*, **5**, 513.
40. Hsi, B-L and Yeh, C-J.G. (1986) Monoclonal antibodies to human amnion. *J. Reprod. Immunol.*, **9**, 11–21.

41. Verrando, P., Ortone, J-P., Pautrat, G., *et al.* (1986) Identification of a 37 kilodalton protein at the epidermal basement membrane by an antiserum to human amnion. *J. Invest. Dermatol.*, **87**, 190–6.
42. Eady, R.A.J., Tidman, M.J., Heagerty, A.H.M., *et al*, (1987) Approaches to the study of epidermolysis bullosa. In *Current Problems in Dermatology* (eds. K.D. Wuepper, and T. Gedde-Dahl, Jr, Karger, Basel, pp. 127–41.
43. Verrando, P., Hsi, B-L., Yeh, C-J., *et al.* (1987) Monoclonal antibody GB3, a new probe for the study of human basement membranes and hemidesmosomes. *Exp. Cell. Res.*, **170**, 116–28.
44. Rodeck, C.H., Eady, R.A.J. and Gosden, C.M. (1980) Prenatal diagnosis of epidermolysis bullosa letalis. *Lancet*, i, 949–52.
45. Eady, R.A.J. (1987) Fetoscopy and fetal skin biopsy for prenatal diagnosis of genetic skin disorders. *Semin. Dermatol.* (in press).
46. Heagerty, A.H.M., Kennedy, A.R., Gunner, D.B., *et al.* (1986) Rapid prenatal diagnosis and exclusion of epidermolysis bullosa using novel antibody probes. *J. Invest. Dermatol.*, **86**, 603–5.
47. Heagerty, A.H.M., Eady, R.A.J., Kennedy, A.R., *et al.* (1987) Rapid prenatal diagnosis of epidermolysis bullosa letalis using GB3 monoclonal antibody. *Brit. J. Dermatol.*, **117**, 271–5.
48. Eady, R.A.J., Heagerty, A.H.M., Kennedy, A.R., *et al.* (1986) Abnormal expression of basement membrane related antigens in amnion and skin from fetuses with epidermolysis bullosa (abstract). *J. Invest. Dermatol.*, **87**, 137.
49. Bauer, E.A. and Eisen, A.Z. (1978) Recessive dystrophic epidermolysis bullosa: evidence for increased collagenase as a genetic characteristic in cell culture. *J. Exp. Med.*, **148**, 1378–87.
50. Oakley, C.A., Wilson, N., Ross, J.A., *et al.* (1984) Junctional epidermolysis bullosa in two siblings: clinical observations, collagen studies and electron microscopy. *Brit. J. Dermatol.*, **111**, 533–42.
51. Kero, M., Palotie, A. and Peltonen, L. (1984) Collagen metabolism in two rare forms of epidermolysis bullosa. *Brit. J. Dermatol.*, **110**, 177–84.
52. Bauer, E.A. and Tabas, M. (1987) Colchicine as a probe for aberrant collagenase expression in recessive junctional epidermolysis bullosa. In *Biology of Heritable Skin Diseases* (eds K.D. Wuepper and T. Gedde-Dahl, Jr,) Karger, Basel, pp. 142–52.
53. Leigh, I.M., Tidman, M.J. and Eady, R.A.J. (1984) Epidermolysis bullosa: preliminary observations of blister formation in keratinocyte cultures. *Brit. J. Dermatol.*, **111**, 527–32.
54. Tidman, M.J. and Eady, R.A.J. (1984) Evidence for a functional defect of the lamina lucida in recessive dystrophic epidermolysis bullosa demonstrated by suction blisters. *Brit. J. Dermatol.*, **111**, 379–87.
55. Matsumoto, M. and Hashimoto, K. (1984) Blister fluid from epidermolysis bullosa letalis induces dermal–epidermal separation at lamina lucida. *J. Invest. Dermatol.*, **82**, 392–3.
56. Rogers, R.B., Yancay, K.B., Allen B.S., *et al.* (1983) Phenytoin therapy for junctional epidermolysis bullosa. *Arch. Dermatol.*, **119**, 925–6.
57. Bauer, E.A. and Cooper, T.W. (1981) Therapeutic considerations in recessive dystrophic epidermolysis bullosa. *Arch. Dermatol.*, **117**, 529–30.
58. Hurwitz, S. and Eady, R.A.J. (1986) Epidermolysis bullosa. In *Practical Management of the Dermatologic Patient* (eds A. Rook, L.C. Parish and J.M. Beare), J.B. Lippincott, Philadelphia, p.62.
59. Carter, D.M., Lin, A.N., Varghese, M.C., *et al.* (1987) Treatment of junctional epidermolysis bullosa with epidermal autografts. *J. Amer. Acad. Dermatol.*, **17**, 246–50.
60. Gallico, G.G., O'Connor, N.E., Compton, C.C., *et al.* (1984) Permanent coverage of large burn wounds with autologous cultured human epithelium. *New Engl. J. Med.*, **331**, 448–51.

Sixteen

Epidermolysis bullosa dystrophica

Robert A. Briggaman and Eugene A. Bauer

16.1 INTRODUCTION

Epidermolysis bullosa dystrophica (EBD) is a heterogeneous group of inherited mechanobullous diseases that produce separation in the deep portion of the basement membrane zone beneath the lamina densa (dermolytic separation) [1, 2] (Figure 16.1). Dystrophic scarring results from repeated blistering and serves as a clinical marker of these diseases. Traditionally, EBD is subdivided into autosomal recessive and autosomal dominant types. Cases of recessively inherited epidermolysis bullosa dystrophica vary significantly in the severity and extent of the disease that they manifest.

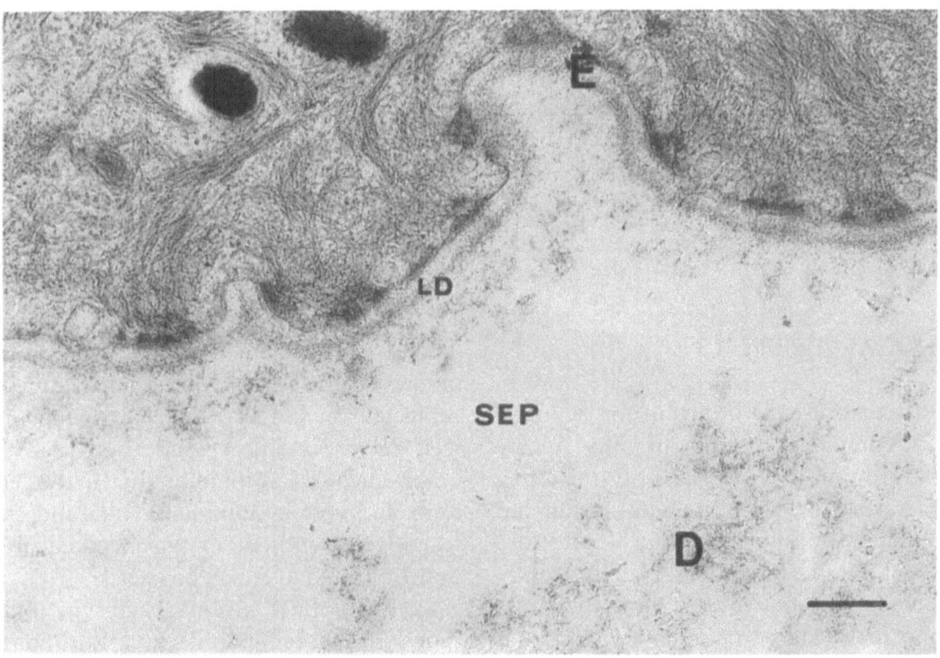

Figure 16.1 Epidermolysis bullosa dystrophica-recessive of the severe generalized subtype. Dermolytic separation (SEP) is present beneath the lamina densa (LD). No anchoring fibrils are seen under the lamina densa. E, epidermis; D, dermis. Calibration bar = 0.25 μm.

Table 16.1 Classification of epidermolysis bullosa dystrophica

Scarring epidermolysis bullosa with dermolytic separation and recessive inheritance (epidermolysis bullosa dystrophica – recessive group)
Epidermolysis bullosa dystrophica recessive (Hallopeau–Siemens)
Generalized gravis (Sublethal, mutilans)
Generalized mitis type
Localized type
Epidermolysis bullosa dystrophica inversa
Scarring epidermolysis bullosa with dermolytic separation and dominant inheritance (epidermolysis bullosa dystrophica – dominant group)
Epidermolysis bullosa dystrophica, hyperplastica (Cockayne–Touraine)
Epidermolysis bullosa dystrophica, albopapuloidea (Pasini)

This has led to a recent trend to subclassify dystrophic recessive EB further (Hallopeau–Siemans) on the basis of clinical findings into severe generalized (gravis), more mild generalized (mitis), localized and inverse subtypes. The distinction among these subtypes is somewhat arbitrary. Autosomal dominant EBD is also subdivided into two forms – an albopapuloid form (Pasini) and a hyperplastic form (Cockayne–Touraine). A current classification of dystrophic EB is found in Table 16.1 [3]. Characteristic clinical features of these diseases are sketched below [4–9].

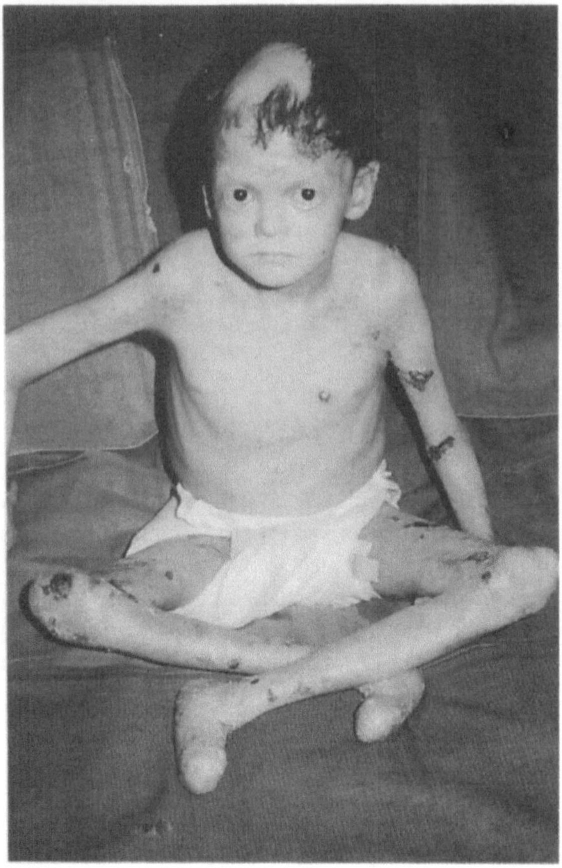

Figure 16.2 Epidermolysis bullosa dystrophica-recessive of severe generalized subtype. Severe scarring complications are evident including cicatricial alopecia, joint contractures, digital fusion and mutilating hand and foot deformities.

16.2 CLINICAL FEATURES

Generalized recessive EBD begins in the neonatal period and continues throughout life. Severe scarring leads to multiple complications including joint contractures (Figure 16.2), digital fusion and eventually mutilating hand and foot deformities (Figure 16.3). Milia are prominent. Nail dystrophy or loss is always present. Mucosal involvement is constant and may lead to oesophageal and anal stenosis as well as ocular complications. Systemic manifestations with growth retardation and anaemia are common.

Localized recessive EBD usually begins in infancy. Cutaneous involvement is limited to areas subject to maximal trauma involving the hands, feet, elbows, knees and buttocks. Mucosal involvement is less common than in the generalized form and may be minimal. Milia and dystrophic scarring are present in the involved areas. Nail dystrophy and loss may be seen.

Recessive EBD inversa begins in infancy and shows a marked predilection for intertriginous areas, especially the groin, axillae and neck. Milia are absent. Mucosal involvement is usually frequent and severe leading to a variety of disabling sequelae including corneal erosions and opacities,

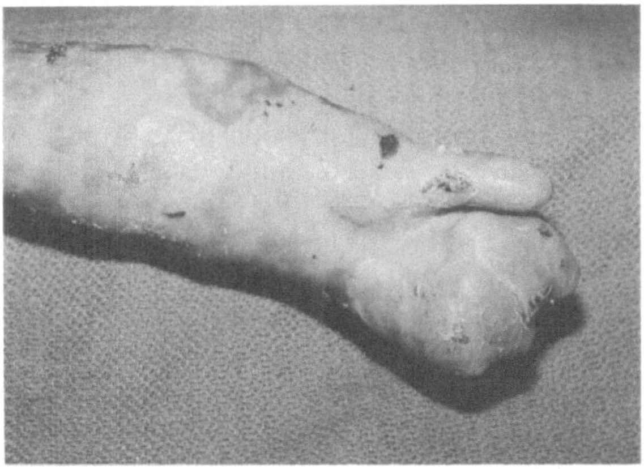

Figure 16.3 Characteristic hand deformity in a patient with severe dystrophic epidermolysis bullosa dystrophica-recessive. A mitten-like encasement surrounds the second to fifth digits.

oesophageal stenosis, lingual scarring with decreased mobility of the tongue, and anal stricture. Extremities are relatively spared.

Dominant EBD-hyperplastic (Cockayne–Touraine) has its onset in infancy or early childhood. Distribution of skin involvement is limited to the extremities, especially the extensor areas. Milia and hyperplastic scarring are common. Mucosal involvement is rare. Teeth are normal. Nails may be dystrophic, especially with hyperplastic nails. In general, this disease is more mild than the albopapuloid type.

Dominant EBD-albopapuloid (Pasini) also has its onset in infancy or early childhood. The cutaneous involvement tends to be more extensive early, but may evolve toward a more limited disease affecting trauma-prone areas of the hands, feet, elbows, knees and buttocks. Albopapuloid lesions characterize this subtype but are not seen in all patients even within the same dominantly inherited kindred. These lesions are lichenoid papules or small flat-topped plaques, usually present on the trunk and less often on the extremities (Figure 16.4).

16.2.1 Presentation

Most patients with dystrophic EB present in infancy. The more severe recessive forms are nearly always manifest at birth or soon thereafter.

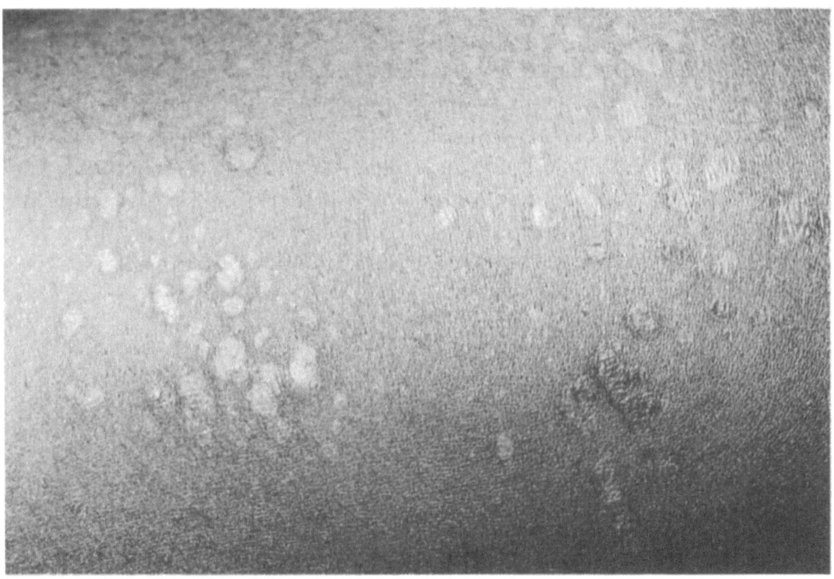

Figure 16.4 Albopapuloid lesions are present on the trunk of a patient with epidermolysis bullosa dystrophica-dominant of the Pasini subtype.

Occasional cases of more mild dominant EBD begin in early childhood.

Dystrophic EB has been reported throughout the world. However, very little is known regarding the distribution of specific types in selected populations on a worldwide basis. Prevalence studies indicate a frequency of the recessive dystrophic type of 1 : 200 000 in Norway [10] and 1 : 300 000 in Britain [11]. Dominant dystrophic cases have a reported prevalence in Norway of 1 : 500 000 [10]. The prevalence of dystrophic EB in the United States is unknown.

The sex incidence of dystrophic EB is equal as would be expected since all of the diseases in this category are autosomal.

16.2.2 Cutaneous distribution

The distribution of skin lesions represents one of the major distinguishing features of the different subtypes of dystrophic EB as noted in the above disease descriptions. Some aspects of cutaneous distribution are worth additional attention. In recessive EBD, the entire cutaneous surface is subject to blistering, although trauma-prone areas bear the brunt of the disease. Knees, elbows, hands and feet are commonly involved in both recessive and dominant forms. In the infant, the ankles and medial aspects of the legs and shins are affected where the infant kicks and rubs the legs together. Similarly, the medial aspects of the arm and the lateral torso are affected more than other areas of skin. Nail involvement is characteristic of all forms of EBD. The nail plate detaches from the underlying nail bed resulting in either lost or dystrophic nails. Scalp involvement is very frequent in more severe forms of EBD-R and leads to scarring alopecia.

16.2.3 Mucous membrane involvement

Mucous membrane involvement is a constant feature of the severe generalized and inversa forms of recessive EBD. Oral and pharyngeal mucous membranes are affected early and the involvement continues throughout life. The characteristic sequence of blisters, ulceration and scarring lead to a variety of complications including microstomia, loss of papillae on the tongue and limited mobility of the tongue [12, 13]. Gingival erosions and scarring may produce gingival retraction around the teeth with the development of marginal dental caries and eventual destruction of teeth [12]. A specific defect in cementum has also been demonstrated in EBD-R [14]. Oesophageal involvement is very frequent and a major source of disability [15–22]. The upper third of the oesophagus is most commonly affected, next most is the lower third toward the gastro-oesophageal junction. Boluses of food probably cause mucosal detachment and ulcer formation. Repeated involvement leads to scarring and narrowing of the lumen (Figure 16.5). Areas of oesophageal stenosis may be narrow or broad involving many centimetres. On some occasions, the entire oesophagus may be involved. Eventually, the obstruction may become very tight and produce complete oesophageal obstruction. Sometimes the areas of stenosis are band-like or webbed. Oesophageal webs are probably more common than previously recognized [6, 21, 22].

Involvement of the mucous membranes of the eye and periocular skin may lead to a variety of problems [6, 23]. Direct involvement of the cornea produces erosion, scarring and corneal opacification. The lids may also be involved. Scarring of the lower lid produces ectropion with the potential for further corneal damage [23]. Involvement of the anal canal and perianal skin is common in severe generalized and inversa forms of recessive EBD. Painful defaecation results and may lead to chronic constipation. Anal stenosis from repeated erosions and scarring may be a further complication. Involvement of the genital mucous membranes and surrounding skin may also occur. Perineal and mucosal involvement around the vaginal introitus may also lead to scarring and vaginal stenosis [24].

16.2.4 Morphology of lesions

Blisters and ulcers result from skin fragility when the skin is subjected to minimal trauma, even the rubs and scuffs of everyday life. Blisters may be haemorrhagic or clear. Intact blisters tend to extend laterally and may become huge. Once formed, ulcers heal slowly. In some skin areas subject to

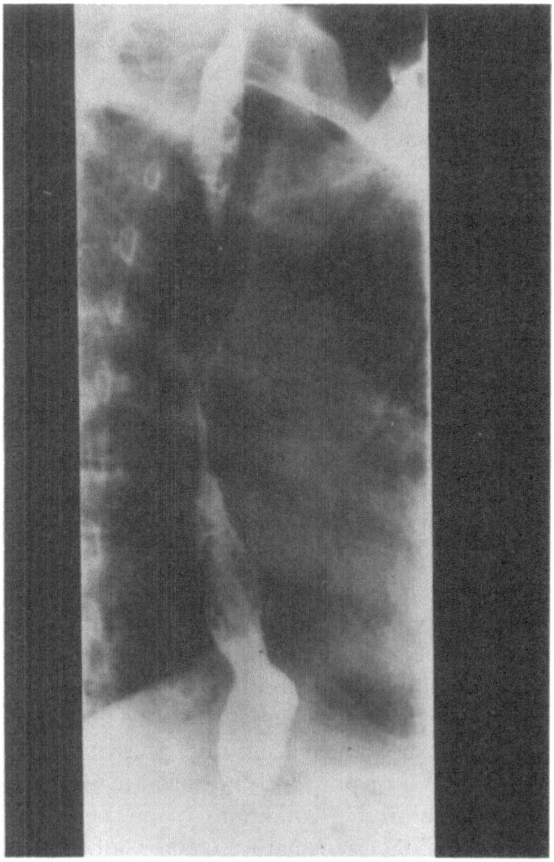

Figure 16.5 Oesophageal stenosis is present in the upper and mid-portion of the oesophagus in a patient with epidermolysis bullosa dystrophic-recessive.

sustained trauma, ulcers may persist for prolonged periods. Repeated cycles of blisters, ulcers and healing with residual scarring at the same site characterize all forms of EBD.

(a) Congenital localized absence of skin

A skin defect in the form of an ulceration may be present at birth in association with various forms of epidermolysis bullosa and has been termed congenital localized absence of skin or aplasia cutis congenita. The former is the better term and will be used here but neither is truly accurate. Congenital localized absence of skin can be classified according to the distribution of lesions, depth of the defect, presence of associated gastrointestinal atresias, and the association with various types of epidermolysis bullosa [6]. The following types of EB have been documented in association with congenital localized absence of skin: junctional EB [25], dystrophic EB of both the recessive [26] and dominant [27] forms, and Bart's syndrome [28–30].

In dystrophic EB, the skin defect is usually limited in severity and extent. The lower leg and foot are most commonly involved, although the hands and arms may occasionally be affected. Involvement is usually unilateral, but may be bilateral (Figure 16.6). When biopsies have been done, they have shown a partial thickness defect in the skin with dermis and dermal appendages in the

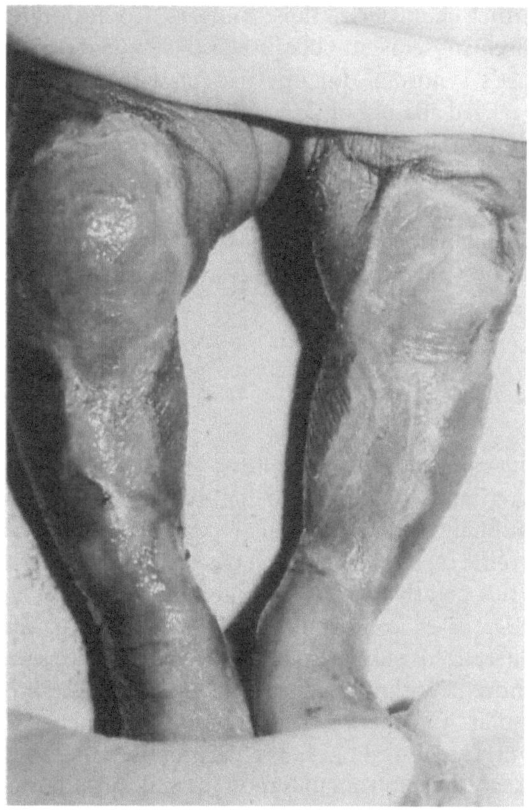

Figure 16.6 Congenital absence of skin is present bilaterally on the shins, knees and feet of a patient with epidermolysis bullosa dystrophica-recessive.

floor of the skin defect which distinguishes this abnormality from true aplasia cutis congenita [30]. A similar defect was recognized in a foetus with recessive EBD at 18 weeks gestation and suggests that this defect may result from *in utero* blistering [31]. The location on the extremities in areas subject to *in utero* movement further support this possibility. Usually, the defect heals relatively well without the necessity for skin grafting and leaves only a residual atrophic scar.

Bart's syndrome remains something of an enigma. Originally described in a large kindred with apparent autosomal dominant inheritance, this syndrome manifested congenital localized absence of skin in association with blistering, particularly of the hands and feet and, less commonly, of the arms and legs. Oral mucosal lesions, minimal residual scarring of the blistered lesions and marked improvement after puberty further characterize those patients. Confusion has arisen subsequently because of the tendency to use Bart's syndrome for any patient with congenital localized absence of skin and a blistering disease. In addition, it is uncertain whether the original Bart's patients should be classified as variants of EB simplex or dominant dystrophic EB. The best current evidence indicates that Bart's syndrome fits best in the dominant dystrophic EB category [32, 33].

16.3 GENETICS

All forms of EBD follow simple Mendelian inheritance patterns being either autosomal dominant or autosomal recessive. In general, specific types of EBD breed true. Although severity varies greatly in different kindreds with recessive EBD, cases conforming to localized and severe generalized subtypes rarely occur in the same kindred. Within a kindred, the disease tends to be similar. On the basis of clinical and inheritance data, Gedde-Dahl [34, 35] has proposed that these diseases result from mutations at multiple different gene loci: *D-EBD*-Pasini and *D-EBD*-CT loci for the dominantly inherited diseases and at least two loci, *EBD*-HS and *EBD*-I, corresponding to the recessively inherited generalized (Hallopeau–Siemens) and inversa subtypes. *EBD*-I probably results from a mutation of a different gene locus from *EBD*-HS [36, 37]. On the basis of his pedigree studies, Gedde-Dahl proposes that the localized and generalized recessive EBD are due to different mutations at the same gene locus [35].

Linkage studies have been of limited value in dystrophic EB. No specific HLA antigen associations have been demonstrated in any form of EBD.

16.4 DIFFERENTIAL DIAGNOSIS

The diagnosis of EBD depends on careful assessment of the clinical, genetic and pathological data. In general, with these data in hand, a correct diagnosis can be reached in the majority of cases. Eady and Tidman suggest that as many as a quarter of the patients do not conform to the classic types of EBD described above [38]. We are in general agreement with this position.

Diagnosis of bullous diseases in the newborn period is a special challenge. EB presents with bullae that arise on previously normal skin whereas most other blistering conditions of the neonatal period arise on erythematous and/or infiltrated abnormal skin. These conditions include bullous congenital ichthyosiform erythroderma (epidermolytic hyperkeratosis), toxic epidermal necrolysis, congenital herpes simplex, bullous mastocytosis and congenital prophyria. These conditions can usually be separated from epidermolysis bullosa by biopsy or special studies such as viral cultures or porphyrin determinations.

Differentiation among the various forms of epidermolysis bullosa may be difficult. This is especially true in sporadic cases in the absence of a family history of EB. Ultrastructural or antigen mapping studies to define the level of blister separation are required to classify the case in question into one of the major subdivisions, i.e. junctional, simplex or dermolytic EB [39–53]. Predictions of prognosis based on these findings must be guarded without a family history for guidance. Absence of anchoring fibrils correlates with more severe generalized EBD-R. Monoclonal antibody studies, in which localization with monoclonal antibodies AF1, AF2 and LH 7:2 is absent, have a similar interpretation.

Sporadic cases of apparent EBD without a family history, whether encountered in infancy or later, present problems of distinguishing recessive inheritance or spontaneous mutation in a dominantly inherited disease. This problem is most difficult in patients with a mechanobullous disease and dystrophic scarring in a relatively localized distribution where the differential diagnosis is between EBD-dominant or localized EBD-R. Ultrastructural pathology is of little help since anchoring fibrils are reduced in both diseases. Recent studies with the monoclonal antibody LH 7:2 suggest that this antibody discriminates between these cases [53].

16.5 INVESTIGATIONS

Routine light microscopic histopathology shows a non-inflammatory subepidermal blister in all forms of dystrophic epidermolysis bullosa, but is of limited usefulness. Non-inflammatory subepidermal blister separation is seen in a variety of conditions including porphyria, pseudoporphyria, bullous amyloid and others [54]. Moreover, a distinction between junctional and dystrophic EB is not possible by routine histopathology even with the use of special basement membrane stains. In EB simplex, an intraepidermal blister is usually evident, but, in the generalized form of EB simplex, cytolytic changes may be confined to the basal cells and result in a cleavage through this layer, leaving only fragments of basal keratinocytes at the base of the blister. It is easy to confuse this picture with a subepidermal cleavage plane.

Electron microscopy remains the gold standard by which the pathological lesions in EB are defined. Determination of the level of separation in the basement membrane zone is paramount in distinguishing among the major types of EB, i.e. EB simplex, junctional and dystrophic EB. In addition, specific abnormalities of anchoring fibrils have been recognized in the subtypes of both dominant and recessive EBD at the ultrastructural level.

General agreement exists that the level of separation in all forms of EBD is in the dermis beneath the lamina densa, so called dermolytic separation (Figure 16.1). In severe generalized recessive EBD, experimental blister separation can be induced with relative ease, whereas in the localized recessive or dominant forms of EBD, blisters are difficult to produce. Biopsy of the margin of a fresh (less than 12 h old) spontaneously induced lesion may be necessary to determine the level of separation. The cleavage plane is found beneath the lamina densa so that the intact lamina densa, lamina lucida and plasma membrane form the roof of the blister. Sometimes amorphous fragments of dermis may be attached to the lamina densa on the roof of the blister. Collagen degeneration (collagenolysis) may be seen in varying degrees from minimal in unblistered skin to extensive in blistered areas. Collagenolysis appears to be more a feature of the recessive than the dominant diseases.

Specific abnormalities of anchoring fibrils have been reported in both dominant and recessive types of EBD, although differences of opinion exist regarding the frequency and significance of these findings. Briggaman and Wheeler reported the absence of anchoring fibrils in the non-blistered and previously never-blistered skin of patients with severe generalized EBD [39]. Subsequently, Hashimoto *et al.* reported some patients with generalized EBD-R that showed normal anchoring fibrils, although most patients had a moderate to marked reduction in numbers of anchoring fibrils [40]. Hanna *et al.* also reported absence of anchoring fibrils in their patients with severe generalized EBD-R [41]. In a recent systematic quantitative study, Tidman and Eady showed that anchoring fibrils were totally absent from their patients with generalized severe EBD-R [42]. The weight of evidence indicates that the absence of anchoring fibrils in generalized severe EBD is a specific structural abnormality at least in the majority of these patients. The Hashimoto study may indicate that there is genetic heterogeneity within the group of patients clinically defined as having severe generalized dystrophic EB.

In localized forms of EBD-R, there is general agreement that anchoring fibrils are reduced in number, although no specific qualitative abnormalities are found [42]. The ultrastructural pathology in the inverse subtype of EBD-R is thought to be identical with the generalized type [40].

Specific ultrastructural alterations have been reported in the two subtypes of autosomal dominant EBD. In the albopapuloid type, anchoring fibrils have been reported to be qualitatively abnormal and reduced in number in both blister-prone and non-blister-prone skin [43, 44]. In the hyperplastic subtype, anchoring fibrils were diminished in number and/or abnormal only in the blister-prone areas, but not in the uninvolved areas [45]. In their quantitative morphometric study, Tidman and Eady confirmed the decrease in number of anchoring fibrils in both forms, but did not recognize a qualitative abnormality of anchoring fibrils or clearly distinguish an ultrastructural difference between patients with and without albopapuloid lesions [42].

An ultrastructural distinction between localized recessive and dominant EBD is not possible since a reduction of anchoring fibrils is found in both [42].

Immunohistochemical approaches show promise in the diagnosis of epidermolysis bullosa. These procedures offer some advantage over electron microscopy in their potentially greater availability, rapidity and lower costs. Immunofluorescence mapping studies may be useful in determining the level of blister separation analogous to what can be achieved ultrastructurally. Immunofluorescence mapping involves the use of well-characterized antibodies to basement membrane zone antigens whose localization is known, for example, bullous pemphigoid antibody localized in the plasma membrane and hemidesmosomes [46, 47], laminin within the lower portion of the lamina lucida and type IV collagen within the lamina densa [48]. Indirect immunofluorescent techniques using these antigens can be applied to skin biopsies from patients with EB [50]. For example, in EBD, where blister separation is beneath the lamina densa, all of the antigens appear in the roof of the blister. All of these antigens are normally expressed in epidermolysis bullosa with a possible exception of BP antigen which may be reduced in junctional EB. Antigen mapping is most useful in those types of EB associated with more marked mechanical fragility, i.e. junctional EB and severe generalized EBD where separation is frequently induced in the biopsy specimens by the biopsy procedure itself.

During the last several years, a series of monoclonal antibodies have been developed that show abnormal binding to the basement membrane zone in various forms of EB. Although these studies are still experimental and incomplete at this time, these novel antibodies are potentially diagnostic markers in various forms of EBD. AF1 and AF2 recognize anchoring-fibril-associated antigens that are presently uncharacterized. AF1 and AF2 binding is absent in severe generalized EBD and present in dominant EBD (albopapuloid type) [51]. KF-1 is a mouse monoclonal antibody that recognizes an uncharacterized antigen in the lamina densa. It is absent or markedly diminished in recessive dystrophic EB and reduced in dominant EBD [52]. LH 7:2 is another mouse monoclonal antibody that recognizes an antigen in the lamina densa, probably the C-terminus of type VII collagen [53]. This antibody is particularly useful, since it is absent or markedly diminished in severe generalized EBD, reduced in localized recessive EBD and present in normal amounts in dominant EBD [53]. It appears that this antibody can distinguish localized recessive from dominant EBD which cannot be done ultrastructurally. Clearly more work needs to be done in this area particularly with the use of batteries of antibodies on a large number of patients with various forms of EBD to support and extend these preliminary observations (see Chapter 12).

16.6 SYSTEMIC MANIFESTATIONS AND ASSOCIATED DISEASES

Secondary bacterial infections are a problem in all forms of EBD due to the disruption of skin integrity. As might be expected, skin infections are more extensive in the more severe forms of EBD. *Staphylococcus aureus* and beta-haemolytic streptococci are the most commonly encountered organisms. Although skin infection is generally tolerated in most infected patients, systemic symptoms such as fever and malaise may occur. Overwhelming infection and sepsis are surprisingly uncommon, but may occur, especially in the neonatal and infancy periods. Poststreptococcal glomerulonephritis may be a rare complication of the frequent beta-haemolytic streptococcal infections.

Squamous cell carcinoma may develop in any of the dystrophic forms of EB although it is most common in the more severe recessive forms [55–58]. The more severely scarred areas of skin are the predominant sites of involvement (Figure 16.7). In addition to the skin, mucosal sites have also been involved including the mouth, oesophagus [59] and bronchi [60]. Multiple carcinomas at different sites are common. The age of onset is usually in the thirties and forties but skin cancers have been seen as early as the mid-teens. These tumours vary histologically from well-differentiated squamous cell carcinomas to poorly differentiated or spindle-cell types. Regardless of histological type, they tend to behave aggressively amd metastasize frequently. Local recurrences are common owing to the difficulty in distinguishing tumour margins in the abnormal scarred skin as well as to their inherent biological aggressiveness. Death has resulted in an unusually high proportion of these cases [55].

Anaemia is common in the generalized gravis EBD-R. Severe symptomatic anaemia is sometimes seen. The mechanism of the anaemia is multifactorial involving iron deficiency due to cutaneous blood loss and the anaemia of chronic illness with its attendant partial marrow failure.

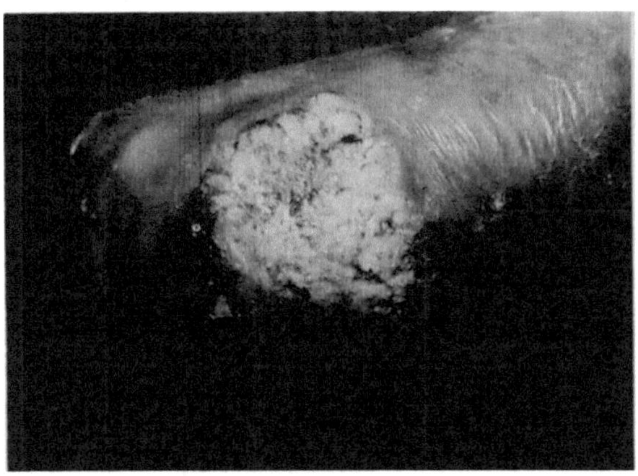

Figure 16.7 A squamous cell carcinoma involves the scarred area of the hand of a patient with epidermolysis bullosa dystrophic-recessive.

The nutritional status of the patients with generalized severe EBD-R may be compromised throughout life. In infancy, failure to gain weight is common. These patients experience growth retardation and are ultimately small and frail of stature. Nutritional intake is limited early by extensive oral erosions and difficulty in feeding. Later this is further compromised by oral scarring, dental problems and dysphagia from oesophageal stenosis (see Chapter 13).

16.7 PATHOGENESIS AND RECENT ADVANCES

Significant advances have been made in understanding the pathological mechanisms involved in EBD, although we are still a long way away from a complete understanding. Conceptually, destruction of or faulty synthesis and formation of structures responsible for epidermal–dermal adherence might produce these diseases. The characteristic level of separation seen in these diseases indicates that disadherence occurs somewhere between the lamina densa and the underlying connective tissue. Prime candidates are anchoring fibrils and the collagen fibres found in this area.

Following the observation by Pearson [1] that collagenolysis was a prominent feature in EBD-R, Eisen [61] found increased human skin collagenase activity in the skin of patients with EBD-R as well as other types of epidermolysis bullosa. These observations were confirmed and extended by others [62–64]. Cultured skin fibroblasts from patients with recessive EBD are unique in their ability to synthesize markedly increased amounts of collagenase [65–67]. Enhanced synthesis of collagenase is a marker for the disease in perhaps as many as 80% of patients [65]. In some patients, an aberrant, possibly mutant, enzyme was identified which remained functionally active [68, 69]. Abnormalities in collagenase regulation have been demonstrated [70]. Nevertheless, the manner by which human skin collagenase injures the skin and the precise structures that are damaged remain somewhat uncertain. Human skin collagenase is known to cleave both type I and type III collagen, but not type IV collagen. Recent studies indicate that type VII collagen which composes anchoring fibrils can be degraded by human skin collagenase [71].

Recently Ehrlich and his colleagues have shown that EBD-R fibroblasts exhibit abnormal cell growth in culture [72, 73]. These cells have an abnormal morphology and do not contract a collagen lattice as do normal fibroblasts. This defect was postulated to be related to enhanced synthesis of prostaglandin E_2 by the EBD-R fibroblasts. Indomethacin, an inhibitor of prostaglandin synthesis, reverses the defect in the EBD-R fibroblasts. The degree to which these observations may be unique to EBD-R fibroblasts and the relationship of these findings to the pathogenesis of EBD-R are not yet fully defined.

In dominant EBD, it is attractive to postulate that a primary anchoring fibril defect produces the disease. This would be in keeping with the association of primary structural protein abnormalities in dominantly inherited disorders. However, as indicated previously, some controversy exists regarding the specific anchoring fibril defect present in various forms of dominant EBD. A specific molecular defect has not been defined as yet in any form of dominant EBD, although an abnormality in glycosaminoglycan metabolism has been identified in the albopapuloid type. Increased amounts of chondroitin sulphates were found in both skin and urine from these patients. In addition, increased synthesis of sulphated glycosaminoglycans was found in cultured fibroblasts from these patients [73]. The manner by which this defect translates into decreased epidermo–dermal adherence is unclear at this time.

16.8 TREATMENT

Specific therapy capable of significantly reducing blister formation is now available in recessive EBD. Eisenberg and his colleagues suggested from *in vitro* studies that phenytoin inhibited human skin collagenase and used this agent successfully to treat patients with EBD-R [74]. They found a substantial decrease in blistering with the use of the drug. More extensive trials undertaken by Bauer *et al.* showed that phenytoin was effective in decreasing blister formation when administered in doses sufficient to maintain a level of 8 μg/ml or more [75, 76]. Their patients appeared to segregate into responder and non-responder groups. The responders experienced significant inhibition of their blisters and erosions. Direct suppression of human skin collagenase activity could not be demonstrated, but Bauer and his colleagues did show a decrease in the synthesis of human skin collagenase *in vitro* by fibroblasts from the EBD-R patients. Some preliminary evidence suggested that the clinical response to phenytoin could be predicted by *in vitro* response to phenytoin in culture. Further studies continue to show a favourable response in many, but not all, patients [77, 79]. See also Chapter 13.

Both retinoids and corticosteroids inhibit human skin collagenase synthesis in fibroblasts derived from EBD-R and normal subjects [80, 81]. Some preliminary evidence indicates that they may be of benefit in treatment of EBD-R [81–83], but their general use cannot be advocated at this time.

No specific therapy is presently available for the treatment of dominant EBD.

Local skin care is an important part of the management of patients with EBD and was until recently all that could be offered. Local skin care is aimed at facilitating healing of blisters and erosions, minimizing infection, and decreasing mechanical trauma to the skin.

16.9 PRENATAL DIAGNOSIS

Prenatal diagnosis has been successfully performed in severe generalized EBD [31, 84–87] and is a contribution to the management of this disease in selected situations. This procedure is best reserved for families with a proven genetic risk in whom a well-documented diagnosis of EBD-R has been made. Severe generalized recessive EBD is of such severity as to justify the interruption of pregnancy and the risk of foetoscopy which is estimated to be 5% foetal loss, 10% prematurity and the possibility of foetal injury. A foetal skin biopsy is obtained between 18 weeks gestation when sufficient amniotic fluid is present to allow the procedure until as late as 23 weeks. By 18 weeks, the epidermo–dermal junction is sufficiently well developed [87] for a morphological diagnosis to be made based on dermolytic separation in the affected foetus. Recently, a combination of biochemical, as well as of morphological markers, has been employed to make a prenatal diagnosis in a foetus at risk [87]. In addition, prenatal exclusion has been accomplished in several instances on the basis of the lack of the characteristic dermolytic separation plane in the biopsied foetal skin [31]. The finding of normal unsplit skin by foetal biopsy allows the disease to be excluded, but with less confidence than is the case with prenatal diagnosis.

REFERENCES

1. Pearson, R.W. (1962) Studies on the pathogenesis of epidermolysis bullosa. *J. Invest. Dermatol.*, **39**, 551–75.
2. Pearson, R.W. (1971) The mechanobullous diseases (epidermolysis bullosa). In *Dermatology in General Medicine* (eds T.B. Fitzpatrick, K.A. Arndt, W. Clark, *et al.*), McGraw-Hill, New York, pp. 621–43.
3. Gedde-Dahl, T. (1981) Sixteen types of epidermolysis bullosa: on their clinical discrimination, therapy and prenatal diagnosis. *Acta Dermatovenereol. (Stockholm), (Suppl.)*, **95**, 74–87.
4. Cooper, T.W., Bauer, E.A. and Briggaman, R.A. (1987) The mechanobullous diseases (epidermolysis bullosa). In *Dermatology in General Medicine* (eds. T.B. Fitzpatrick, A.Z. Eisen, K. Wolff, *et al.*, McGraw-Hill, New York, pp. 610–26.
5. Cooper, T.W. and Bauer, E.A. (1984) Epidermolysis bullosa: a review. *Pediatr. Dermatol.*, **1**, 181–8.
6. Briggaman, R.A. (1983) Hereditary epidermolysis bullosa with special emphasis on newly recognized syndromes and complications. *Dermatol. Clin.*, **1**, 263–80.
7. Haber, R.M., Hanna, W., Ramsey, C.A., *et al.* (1985) Hereditary epidermolysis bullosa. *J. Amer. Acad. Dermatol.*, **13**, 252–78.
8. Fine, J.D. (1986) Epidermolysis bullosa: clinical aspects, pathology, and recent advances in research. *Int. J. Dermatol.*, **25**, 143–57.
9. Tabas, M., Gibbons, S. and Bauer, E.A. (1987) The mechanobullous diseases. *Dermatol. Clin.*, **5**, 123–36.
10. Gedde-Dahl, T. Jr (1978) Classification of epidermolysis bullosa. In *Pädiatrische Dermatologie* (ed. J.J. Herzbert), F.K. Shattauer-Verlag, Stuttgart, pp. 65–91.
11. Davidson, B. (1965) Epidermolysis bullosa. *J. Med. Genet.*, **2**, 233–42.
12. Crawford, E.G., Jr, Burkes, J. and Briggaman, R. (1976) Hereditary epidermolysis bullosa: oral manifestations and dental therapy. *Oral Surg.*, **42**, 490–500.
13. Gorlin, R.J. (1971) Epidermolysis bullosa. *Oral Surg.*, **32**, 760–6.
14. Hitchin, A.D. (1973) The defects in cementum in epidermolysis bullosa dystrophica. *Brit. Dent. J.*, **135**, 437–42.
15. Nix, T.E., Jr and Christianson, H.B. (1965) Epidermolysis bullosa of the esophagus: report of two cases and review of literature. *South. Med. J.*, **58**, 612–20.
16. Becker, M. and Swinyard, C. (1968) Epidermolysis bullosa dystrophica in children. *Radiology*, **90**, 124–8.
17. Bergenholtz, A., Olsson, O. and Arwill, T. (1965) Epidermolysis bullosa hereditaria: II. Esophageal changes in epidermolysis bullosa hereditaria dystrophica. *Pract. Otorhinolaryngol.*, **27**, 219–24.
18. Berkmen, Y. (1974) Esophageal involvement in epidermolysis bullosa. *Amer. J. Gastroenterol.*, **62**, 145–7.
19. Orlando, R.C., Bozymski, E.M., Briggaman, R.A., *et al.* (1974) Epidermolysis bullosa: gastrointestinal manifestations. *Ann. Intern. Med.*, **81**, 203–6.
20. Warren, R., Warner, T., Gilbert, E., *et al.* (1980) Acquired double-barrel exophagus in epidermolysis bullosa dystrophica. *Thorax*, **35**, 472–6.
21. Hillemeir, C., Touloukian, R., McCallum, R., *et al.* (1981) Esophageal web: a previously unrecognized complication of epidermolysis bullosa. *Pediatrics*, **67**, 678–82.
22. Marsden, R., Sambrook Gowar, F., MacDonald, A., *et al.* (1974) Epidermolysis bullosa of the esophagus with esophageal web formation. *Thorax*, **29**, 287–95.
23. Hill, J.C. and Rodrique, D. (1971) Cicatricial, ectropion in epidermolysis bullosa and in congenital ichthyosis: its plastic repair. *Can. J. Ophthalmol.*, **6**, 89–97.
24. Shackelford, G., Bauer, E., Graviss, E.R., *et al.* (1982) Upper airway and external genital involvement in epidermolysis bullosa dystrophica. *Radiology*, **143**, 429–32.
25. Skoren, I. and Drzewiecki, K. (1979) Congenital localized skin defect and epidermolysis bullosa hereditaria letalis. *Acta Dermatovenereol. (Stockholm)*, **59**, 533–7.
26. Wojnarowska, F., Eady, R. and Wells, R. (1981) Recessive epidermolysis bullosa dystrophica with congenital localized absence of skin: Bart's syndrome. *Brit. J. Dermatol.*, **105**, 94–5.

27. Joensen, H.D. (1973) Epidermolysis bullosa dystrophica dominans in two families in the Faroe Islands. *Acta Dermatovenereol. (Stockholm)*, **53**, 53–60.
28. Bart, B.J., Gorlin, R.J., Anderson, V.E. and Lynch, F.W. (1966) Congenital localized absence of skin and associated abnormalities resembling epidermolysis bullosa. A new syndrome. *Arch. Dermatol.*, **93**, 296–304.
29. Bart, B.J. (1970) Epidermolysis bullosa and congenital localized absence of skin. *Arch. Dermatol.*, **101**, 78–82.
30. Smith, S.Z. and Cram, D.L. (1978) A mechanobullous disease of the newborn. Bart's syndrome. *Arch. Dermatol.*, **114**, 81–4.
31. Anton-Lamprecht, I. and Arnold, M-L. (1987) Prenatal diagnosis of inherited epidermolyses. *Curr. Probl. Dermatol.*, **16**, 146–57.
32. Butler, D.F., Berger, T.G., James, W.D., *et al.* (1986) Bart's syndrome: microscopic, ultrastructural and immunofluorescent mapping features. *Pediatr. Dermatol.*, **3**, 113–18.
33. Bavinick, J., vanHaeringen, A., Ruiter, D. and Van der Schroeff, J.G. (1987) Autosomal dominant epidermolysis bullosa dystrophica: are the Cockayne-Touraine, the Pasini and the Bart-types different expressions of the same mutant gene? *Clin. Genet.*, **31**, 416–24.
34. Gedde-Dahl, T., Jr (1971) *Epidermolysis Bullosa: A Clinical, Genetic and Epidemiological Study*, The Johns Hopkins University Press, Baltimore.
35. Gedde-Dahl, T., Jr (1986) Clinical heterogeneity in epidermolysis bullosa: speculations on causation and consequences for research. *J. Invest. Dermatol.*, **86**, 91–3.
36. Gedde-Dahl, T. and Anton-Lamprecht, I. (1983) Epidermolysis bullosa. In *Principles and Practice of Medical Genetics* (eds A.E.H. Emery and D.L. Rimoin), Churchill Livingstone, Edinburgh, London, Melbourne and New York, pp. 672–87.
37. Kero, M. (1984) Epidermolysis bullosa in Finland. Clinical features, morphology and relation to collagen metabolism. *Acta Dermatovenereol. (Stockholm) Suppl.*, **110**.
38. Eady, R.A.J. and Tidman, M.J. (1983) Diagnosing epidermolysis bullosa. *Brit. J. Dermatol.*, **108**, 621–6.
39. Briggaman, R.A. and Wheeler, C.E. (1975) Epidermolysis bullosa dystrophica-recessive: a possible role of anchoring fibrils in the pathogenesis. *J. Invest. Dermatol.*, **65**, 203–11.
40. Hashimoto, I., Schnyder, U.W., Anton-Lamprecht, I., *et al.* (1976) Ultrastructural studies in epidermolysis bullosa hereditaria: III. Recessive dystrophic types with dermolytic blistering (Hallopeau–Siemens types and inverse type). *Arch. Dermatol. Res.*, **256**, 137–50.
41. Hanna, W., Silverman, E., Boxall, L., *et al.* (1983) Ultrastructural features of epidermolysis bullosa. *Ultrastruct. Pathol.*, **5**, 29–36.
42. Tidman, M.J. and Eady, R.A.J. (1985) Evaluation of anchoring fibrils and other components of the dermal–epidermal junction in dystrophic epidermolysis bullosa by a quantitative ultrastructural technique. *J. Invest. Dermatol.*, **84**, 374–7.
43. Anton-Lamprecht, I. and Schnyder, U.W. (1973) Epidermolysis bullosa dystrophica dominans. Ein defekt der anchoring fibrils? *Dermatologica*, **147**, 289–98.
44. Hashimoto, I., Anton-Lamprecht, I., Gedde-Dahl, T., *et al.* (1975) Ultrastructural studies in epidermolysis bullosa hereditaria: I. Dominant dystrophic type of Pasini. *Arch. Dermatol. Forsch.*, **252**, 167–78.
45. Hashimoto, I., Gedde-Dahl, T., Schnyder, U.W., *et al.* (1976) Ultrastructural studies in epidermolysis bullosa: II. Dominant dystrophic type of Cockayne and Touraine. *Arch. Dermatol. Res.*, **255**, 285–95.
46. Westgate, G.E., Weaver, A.C. and Couchman, J.R. (1985) Bullous pemphigoid antigen localization suggests an intracellular association with hemidesmosomes. *J. Invest. Dermatol.*, **84**, 218–24.
47. Mutasim, D.F., Takahashi, Y., Labib, R.S., *et al.* (1985) A pool of bullous pemphigoid antigen(s) is intracellular and associated with the basal cell cytoskeleton–hemidesmosome complex. *J. Invest. Dermatol.*, **84**, 47–53.
48. Yaoita, H., Foidart, J-M. and Katz, S.I. (1978) Localization of the collagenous component in skin basement membrane. *J. Invest. Dermatol.*, **70**, 191–3.
49. Hintner, H., Stingl, G., Schuler, G., *et al.* (1981) Immunofluorescence mapping of antigenic determinants within the dermal–epidermal junction in mechanobullous diseases. *J. Invest. Dermatol.*, **76**, 113–18.
50. Fine, J.D. (1987) Altered skin basement membrane antigenicity in epidermolysis bullosa. *Curr. Probl. Dermatol.*, **17**, 111–26.
51. Goldsmith, L.A. and Briggaman, R.A. (1983) Monoclonal antibodies to anchoring fibrils for the diagnosis of epidermolysis bullosa. *J. Invest. Dermatol.*, **81**, 464–6.
52. Fine, J.D., Breathnach, S.M., Hintner, H. and Katz, S.I. (1984) KF-1 monoclonal antibody defines a specific basement membrane antigen defect in dystrophic forms of epidermolysis bullosa. *J. Invest. Dermatol.*, **82**, 35–8.
53. Heagerty, A.H.M., Kennedy, A.R., Leigh, I.M., *et al.* (1986) Identification of an epidermal basement membrane defect in recessive forms of dystrophic epidermolysis bullosa by LH7:2 monoclonal antibody: use in diagnosis. *Brit. J. Dermatol.*, **115**, 125–31.
54. Briggaman, R.A. (1988) Non-inflammatory

subepidermal blisters. In *Dermatopathology* (eds E. Farmer and A. Hood), in press.

55. Reed, W.B., College, J., Francis, M.J.O., *et al.* (1974) Epidermolysis bullosa dystrophica with epidermal neoplasms. *Arch. Dermatol.*, **110**, 894–902.
56. Reed, W., Roenigk, H., Dorner, W., *et al.* (1975) Epidermal neoplasms with epidermolysis bullosa dystrophica with the first report of carcinoma with the acquired type. *Arch. Dermatol. Res.*, **253**, 1–14.
57. Didolkar, M., Gerner, R. and Moore, G. (1974) Epidermolysis bullosa dystrophica and epithelioma of the skin. *Cancer*, **33**, 198–202.
58. Schwartz, R.A., Birnkrant, A.P., Rubenstein, D.J., *et al.* (1981) Squamous cell carcinoma in dominant type epidermolysis bullosa dystrophica. *Cancer*, **47**, 615–20.
59. Wetteland, P. and Höuding, G. (1956) Squamous cell carcinoma in epidermolysis bullosa. *Acta Dermatovenereol. (Stockholm)*, **36**, 27–36.
60. Almeyda, J. (1972) Epidermolysis bullosa associated with neoplasm of the bronchus. *Brit. J. Dermatol.*, **87**, 70–1.
61. Eisen, A.Z. (1969) Human skin collagenase: relationship to the pathogenesis of epidermolysis bullosa dystrophica. *J. Invest. Dermatol.*, **52**, 449–53.
62. Lazarus, G.S. (1972) Collagenase and connective tissue metabolism in epidermolysis bullosa. *J. Invest. Dermatol.*, **58**, 242–8.
63. Bauer, E.A., Gedde-Dahl, T., Jr and Eisen, A.Z. (1977) The role of human skin collagenase in epidermolysis bullosa. *J. Invest. Dermatol.*, **68**, 119–24.
64. Eisenberg, M., Williams, J.F., Stevens, L. and Schofield, P.J. (1971) Mammalian collagenase and peptidase estimation in normal skin and in the skin of patients suffering from epidermolysis bullosa. *J. Int. Res. Commun.*, **2**, 1732.
65. Bauer, E.A. and Eisen, A.Z. (1978) Recessive dystrophic epidermolysis bullosa: evidence for increased collagenase as a genetic characteristic in cell culture. *J. Exp. Med.*, **148**, 1378–87.
66. Valle, K-J. and Bauer, E.A. (1980) Enhanced biosynthesis of human skin collagenase in fibroblast cultures from recessive dystrophic epidermolysis bullosa. *J. Clin. Invest.*, **66**, 176–87.
67. Bauer, E.A. (1982) Abnormalities of collagenase expression as *in vitro* markers for recessive dystrophic epidermolysis bullosa. *J. Invest. Dermatol.*, **75** (suppl), 105s–108s.
68. Bauer, E.A. (1977) Recessive dystrophic epidermolysis bullosa: evidence for an altered collagenase in fibroblast cultures. *Proc. Natl. Acad. Sci. USA*, **74**, 4646–50.
69. Stricklin, G.P., Welgus, H.G. and Bauer, E.A. (1982) Human skin collagenase in recessive dystrophic epidermolysis bullosa. Purification of a mutant enzyme from fibroblast cultures. *J. Clin. Invest.*, **69**, 1373–83.
70. Bauer, E.A., Valle, K-J. and Esterly, N. (1982) Colchicine-induced modulation of collagenase in human skin fibroblast cultures. II. A probe for defective regulation in epidermolysis bullosa. *J. Invest. Dermatol.*, **79**, 403–7.
71. Seltzer, J.C., Eisen, A.Z., Bauer, E.A. and Burgeson, R.E. (1989) Cleavage of type VII collagen by interstitial collagenase and type IV collagenase (gelatinase) derived from human skin. *J. Biol. Chem.*, **264**, 3822–6.
72. Ehrlich, H.P., Buttle, D., Trelstad, R. and Hayashi, K. (1983) Epidermolysis bullosa dystrophica recessive fibroblasts altered behavior within a collagen matrix. *J. Invest. Dermatol.*, **80**, 56–60.
73. Ehrlich, H.P. and White, M. (1983) Effects of increased concentrations of prostaglandin E levels with epidermolysis bullosa dystrophica recessive fibroblasts within a populated collagen lattice. *J. Invest. Dermatol.*, **81**, 572–5.
74. Bauer, E.A., Fiehler, W.K. and Esterly, N.B. (1979) Increased glycosaminoglycan accumulation as a genetic characteristic in cell cultures of one variety of dominant dystrophic epidermolysis bullosa. *J. Clin. Invest.*, **64**, 32–9.
75. Eisenberg, M., Stevens, L.H. and Schofield, P.J. (1978) Epidermolysis bullosa: new therapeutic approaches. *Austr. J. Dermatol.*, **19**, 1–8.
76. Bauer, E.A., Cooper, T.W., Tucker, D.R. and Esterly, N.B. (1980) Phenytoin therapy of recessive dystrophic epidermolysis bullosa. Clinical trial and proposed mechanism of action on collagenase. *New Engl. J. Med.*, **303**, 776–81.
77. Bauer, E.A. and Cooper, T.W. (1981) Therapeutic considerations in recessive dystrophic epidermolysis bullosa. *Arch. Dermatol.*, **117**, 529–30.
78. Cooper, T.W. and Bauer, E.A. (1984) Therapeutic efficacy of phenytoin in recessive dystrophic epidermolysis bullosa. A comparison of short- and long-term treatment. *Arch. Dermatol.*, **120**, 490–5.
79. Wirth, H., Nesch, A., Ostapowicz, B. and Anton-Lamprecht, I. (1982) Phenytoin therapy of recessive dystrophic epidermolysis bullosa (epidermolysis bullosa dystrophica Hallopeau-Siemens and epidermolysis bullosa dystrophica inversa). *Z. Hautkr.*, **58**, 555–74.
80. Bauer, E.A., Seltzer, J.L. and Eisen, A.Z. (1983) Retinoic acid inhibition of collagenase and gelatinase expression in human skin fibroblast cultures. Evidence for a dual mechanism. *J. Invest. Dermatol.*, **81**, 162–9.
81. Koob, T.J., Jeffrey, J.J. and Eisen, A.Z. (1974) Regulation of human skin collagenase activity by hydrocortisone and dexamethasone in organ culture. *Biochem. Biophys. Res. Commun.*, **61**, 1083–8.

82. Fritsch, P., Klein, G., Aubock, J. and Hintner, H. (1983) Retinoid therapy of recessive dystrophic epidermolysis bullosa. *J. Amer. Acad. Dermatol.*, 9, 766–7.
83. Moynahan, E.J. (1982) The treatment and management of epidermolysis bullosa. *Clin. Exp. Dermatol.*, 7, 665–72.
84. Anton-Lamprecht, I., Jovanovic, V., Arnold, M.L., *et al.* (1981) Prenatal diagnosis of epidermolysis bullosa dystrophica Hallopeau–Siemens with electron microscopy of fetal skin. *Lancet*, **ii**, 1077–9.
85. Eady, R.A.J., Gunner, D.B., Tidman, M.J., *et al.* (1985) Prenatal diagnosis of genetic skin disease by fetoscopy and electron microscopy: report on 5 years' experience. *Brit. J. Dermatol.* **113** (Suppl. 29), 45.
86. Heagerty, A.H.M., Kennedy, A.R., Gunner, D.B. and Eady, R.A.J. (1986) Rapid prenatal diagnosis and exclusion of epidermolysis bullosa using novel antibody probes. *J. Invest. Dermatol.*, **86**, 603–5.
87. Bauer, E.A., Ludman, M.D., Goldberg, J.D., *et al.* (1986) Antenatal diagnosis of recessive dystrophic epidermolysis bullosa: collagenase expression in cultured fibroblasts as a biochemical marker. *J. Invest. Dermatol.*, 87, 597–601.

Seventeen
Exogenous triggers

Jean-Claude Roujeau

17.1 BULLOUS ERYTHEMA MULTIFORME

17.1.1 Introduction

Erythema multiforme (EM) is an acute self-limiting disease defined by characteristic clinical skin lesions. It is generally separated into two subsets: EM major or Stevens–Johnson syndrome (SJS) and EM minor. The distinction between these two forms relies, by arbitrary definition, on the involvement of at least two mucous membranes in addition to skin lesions in EM major [1–3]. It would be an oversimplification to consider bullous EM as a synonym for EM major. Bullous skin lesions, which are always present in EM major, also occur in up to 60% of inpatients with EM minor [4].

All forms are considered to be a reaction pattern to many exogenous agents, the most common being infection with herpes virus and drugs [1–3]. Post-herpetic EM may present as a recurrent disabling disease, and acyclovir is a significant advance in the management of these forms.

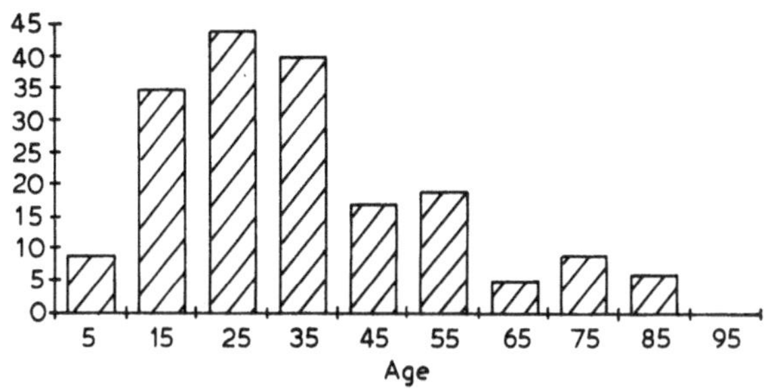

Figure 17.1 Histogram of age of onset of Stevens–Johnson syndrome. From an unpublished French epidemiological study (184 cases).

17.1.2 Presentation

(a) Age

EM occurs at all ages, but mainly in young adults, with a peak of incidence in the third decade with a mean age around 25–30 years in recent series [4–10] (Figure 17.1).

(b) Sex

Textbooks state that males are affected three to four times as frequently as females [2]. This was not the case in all recent series where both sexes were equally represented [4–10]. A slight male preponderance (1.5 : 1) remained only for cases classified as EM major or Stevens–Johnson syndrome [1, 4, 6] (Figure 17.2).

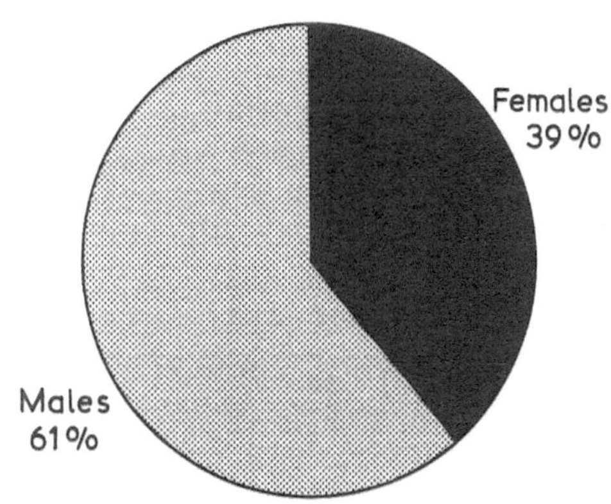

Figure 17.2 Sex ratio observed for Stevens–Johnson syndrome, taken from the same French study as in Figure 17.1 (189 cases).

(c) Frequency

EM is diagnosed in 0.1–1% of inpatients in dermatology wards [4, 8]. In Canada, the incidence of EM calculated from inpatients was 0.017% per year [10]; as many patients with minor forms were not hospitalized, the real incidence is certainly higher. Among inpatients, 20–60% of cases are EM major [4, 7–9].

17.1.3 Cutaneous distribution

The cutaneous lesions of EM are characterized by symmetric involvement of the extremities, mainly on extensor surfaces (knees, elbows, back of hands), palms and soles [1–3] (Figure 17.3). This distribution is less obvious in disseminated forms. A photodistribution is sometimes evident [3].

17.1.4 Mucous membrane involvement

It is present in 50–60% of inpatients [4–10], but is probably less common in outpatients. Mouth involvement is the most frequent, followed by ocular and genital lesions [6]. Pharynx, larynx and oesophagus are rarely involved. Oral lesions may possibly occur as the sole manifestation, for example in drug reactions [8], but it is difficult to call them oral EM, as EM is defined by the clinical aspect of the skin lesions [3]. The bullous lesions soon become erosive and lead to their own complications and sequelae. Mucosal surfaces are coated by grey pseudomembranes and crusts. Pain makes eating difficult or impossible and hypersalivation is usual.

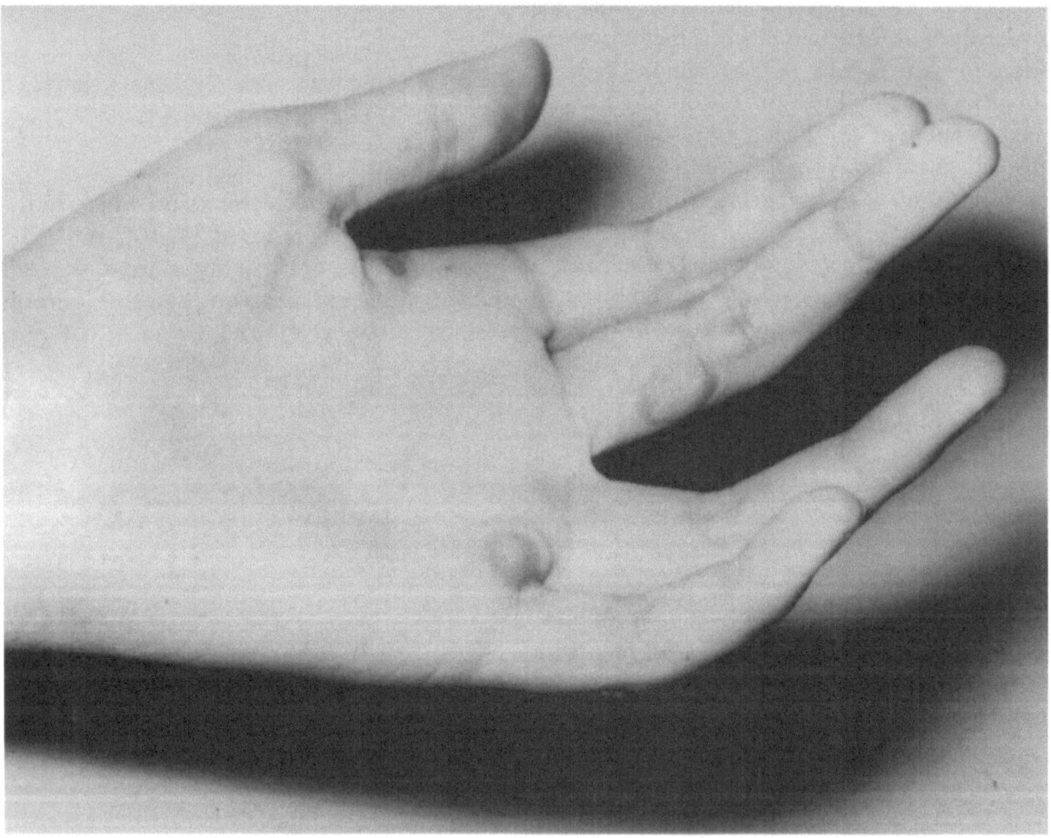

Figure 17.3 Central blisters in typical target lesions of post-herpetic erythema multiforme.

17.1.5 Morphology of lesions

Tense bullae, clear or haemorrhagic, arise in the centre of target or iris lesions (Figure 17.3). They are usually less than 1 cm in diameter. Their confluence may lead to large post-bullous erosions. Monomorphic lesions with typical concentric colour changes around the blisters are more suggestive of post-herpetic EM, while drug-induced cases are often atypical and polymorphic [1] (Figure 17.4). Lesions heal in 1–3 weeks without atrophy but usually with post-inflammatory hyperpigmentation, most marked on dark skins.

17.1.6 Genetics

Two independent teams from Ireland and from the USA found a significant association of histocompatibility antigen HLA-B15 with EM, mainly post-herpetic [11, 12]. In a small German population post-herpetic EM was associated with HLA-A9 [13]. Ocular lesions from SJS of various causes were linked to HLA-B44 (a subgroup of HLA-B12) [14]. In patients with drug-induced SJS and toxic epidermal necrolysis (TEN) we observed an increased frequency of HLA-B12 [15]. In a family with several sulphonamide-related cases SJS was associated with HLA-B12 [16].

It is therefore tempting to surmise that post-herpetic and drug-induced EM are associated with different genetic backgrounds, HLA-B15 for post-herpetic and HLA-B12 for drug-induced cases.

17.1.7 Differential diagnosis

(a) *SJS/TEN*

The question of whether SJS and TEN are two different diseases or two degrees of the same

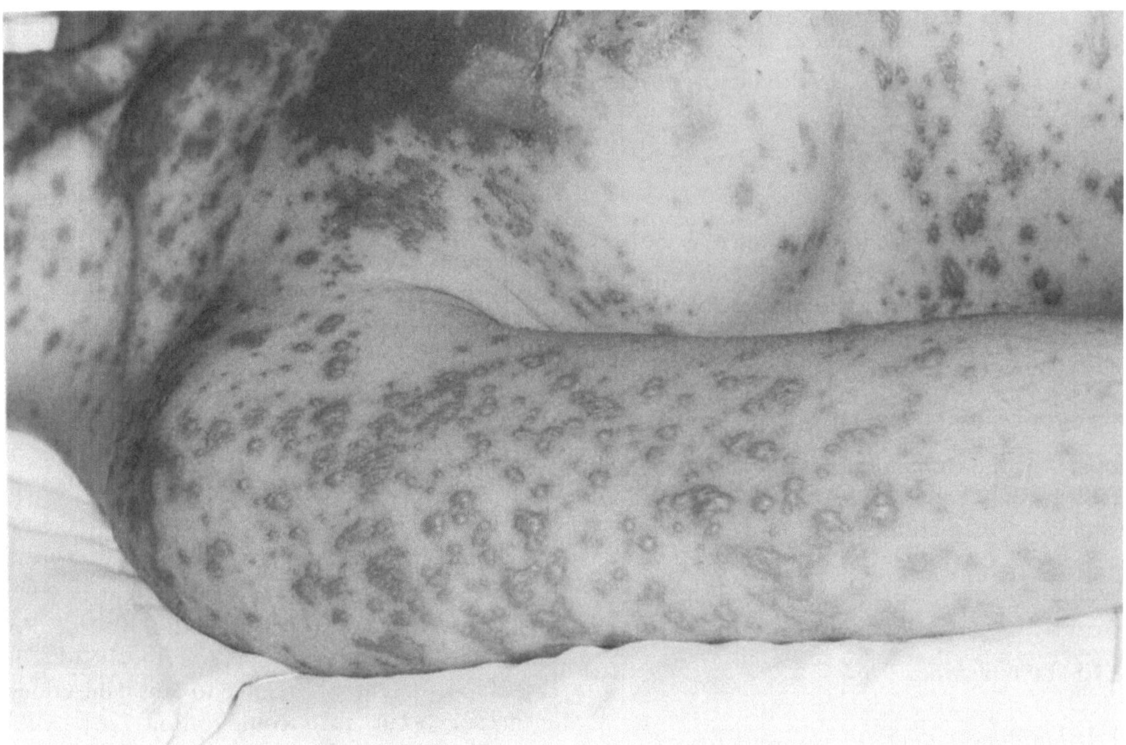

Figure 17.4 Disseminated blisters in oxyphenbutazone-induced Stevens–Johnson syndrome.

process is still controversial. The answer will require more information on their pathogenesis. Differences in sex ratios, ages of occurrence and relative frequencies of cause (Figures 17.1, 17.2, 17.5, 17.6, 17.7 and 17.11) suggest that they may be different diseases, but observations of cases that progress from SJS to TEN suggest the opposite. My own guess is that post-herpetic and drug-induced cases behave differently and that the real boundary is between post-herpetic SJS on one hand and drug-induced disease (SJS or TEN) on the other. While awaiting a better classification, we suggest keeping a practical distinction between those diseases that are life-threatening and those that are not. When more than 10–20% of the skin surface is denuded, the risk of death is present and we call the condition TEN.

(b) Sweet's syndrome

Bullous-like lesions of acute febrile neutrophilic dermatosis (Sweet's syndrome) may be confused with atypical EM. The intense infiltrate of polymorphonuclear leucocytes in the dermis, characteristic of Sweet's syndrome, is never a feature of EM.

(c) Cutaneous vasculitis

When cutaneous vasculitis manifests as blisters there are usually also polymorphic purpuric and necrotic lesions. The histological features of leucocytoclastic angeitis are not observed in EM.

(d) Autoimmune bullous diseases

Biopsy with immunofluorescent studies will establish the diagnosis in occasional cases of pemphigoid, dermatitis herpetiformis or linear IgA disease (see Chapters 5, 11 and 8 respectively) resembling EM.

17.1.8 Investigations

(a) Laboratory findings

There is no specific laboratory finding in EM. There is usually a mild neutrophilia and raised ESR [5].

(b) Histopathology

The pathology of EM is still controversial. The changes involve the dermis with accumulation of mononuclear cells around the blood vessels and the epidermis with degeneration of basal cells and necrosis of individual keratinocytes. Some authorities separate dermal and epidermal types of EM [17, 18], while others state that both patterns are always present in different sites or at different times in an individual lesion [19]. Blisters may be due to subepidermal separation with necrotic basal cells in the blister roof or to intraepidermal splitting, spongiosis and degeneration of higher keratinocytes [18, 19].

Tentative clinicopathological correlations linking drug-induced cases to the 'epidermal' type and post-herpetic cases to the 'dermal' variant need confirmation [20].

Immunofluorescence examination, if very early, may show vascular deposits of IgM and C3 in the upper dermis and sometimes granular C3 along the basement membrane zone, mainly in post-herpetic cases [21–24].

(c) Search for aetiological factors

The history of recent recurrence of herpes simplex, of other infectious disease and of drug exposure within the previous month should be sought. Chest X-ray, full blood count, liver tests and serological studies may help in determining the aetiology.

17.1.9 Systemic manifestations and associated diseases

A prodromal flu-like illness is frequent 2–7 days before the skin eruption. Fever is present in 90% of EM major cases [6] and in about 30% of EM minor. In SJS, pneumonia is observed in 10–30% of cases [3, 4, 6]. It may be related to causal infectious agents or occur as a complication [25]. Mild hepatitis is often present in drug-induced cases. Rare renal or gastrointestinal complications have been reported [26].

17.1.10 Pathogenesis and recent advances

(a) Causes of EM

In recent series about one-third of EM or SJS cases were post-infectious (herpes simplex virus being the most frequent single cause), one-third were attributed to drugs and one-third were idiopathic [4–10] (Figure 17.5).

More than one hundred different causes of EM have been reported [1–3]. Viral infections include herpes simplex, infectious mononucleosis, vaccinia, hepatitis B and orf. Bacterial infections include mycoplasma pneumoniae, yersinia, tularaemia, legionnaire's disease, *Klebsiella* and tuberculosis. Other causes include vaccinations, neoplasms, radiotherapy, sarcoidosis and lupus erythematosus.

Herpes-associated EM The relationship between herpes virus (HSV) and EM is well documented [27]. Post-herpetic cases account for 15–63% of EM [3]. HSV1 and HSV2 can both induce EM. Herpetic recurrence precedes EM by 1–3 weeks, with a mean of 10–11 days and a constant delay for each patient [28]. Every herpetic outbreak is not always followed by EM. The great majority of cases are EM minor, the mouth being usually the only mucous membrane involved [9]. The causal relationship between HSV and EM is supported by: finding of HSV [29] or HSV antigen [30] in EM lesions, the presence of HSV antigen in immune complexes detected at the beginning of EM [31]; reproduction of EM by intradermal injection of inactivated HSV in a patient with recurrent post-herpetic EM [27]; concomitant suppression of herpetic and post-herpetic EM outbreaks by acyclovir [32–34].

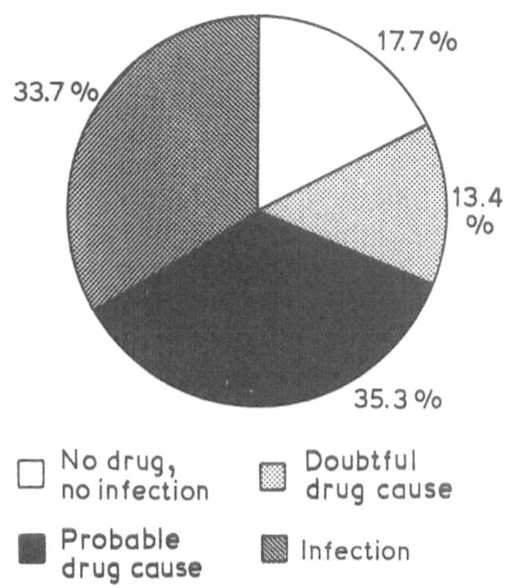

Figure 17.5 Aetiology of Stevens–Johnson syndrome (119 cases).

Recurrent cases represent 20–30% of EM [3], herpetic infection being the main cause. Herpes labialis preceded EM in 65% of recurrent cases in a recent series [28]. Finding HSV containing immune complexes in idiopathic cases of EM [31] supports the hypothesis that some 'idiopathic' cases may also be related to subclinical herpetic outbreaks.

Mycoplasma pneumoniae. Mycoplasma-associated EM is usually of the major type [3]. Any age may be affected, with a peak before 20 years of age. SJS occurs in 1–4% of patients infected with *Mycoplasma pneumoniae*, 1–3 weeks after the beginning of infection [35]. Fever, cough, myalgia, atypical pneumonia on chest X-ray, high titre of cold agglutinin (with or without haemolysis) and rising antibody titre to the organism are characteristic of mycoplasma infection [35]. This infection is documented in about 5% of cases of SJS [4–10].

Drugs. Drugs are more often involved in SJS than in EM minor (Figure 17.5). The main drugs responsible for SJS are sulphonamides, barbiturates and anticonvulsants, non-steroidal anti-inflammatory agents (NSAIDs) and antibiotics [36]. New indications for long-acting sulphonamides (prophylaxis of chloroquine-resistant malaria, management of toxoplasmosis and pneumocystosis in AIDS patients) have resulted in many cases of SJS [37–39]. Several NSAIDs recently withdrawn from the market (benoxaprofen, oxyphenbutazone, isoxicam) had a high rate of occurrence of SJS or TEN [40, 41]. SJS occurs as a rule 1–3 weeks after the beginning of drug intake, even if the therapy has been stopped. Topical medications or chemical contactants may also induce EM, after skin absorption or inhalation [42, 43]. Atypical skin lesions, extensive bullae and prominent mucous membrane involvement are suggestive of drug-induced cases.

(b) Pathogenesis

In recent years many studies have implicated humoral immune mechanisms. Deposits of immune reactants are almost universal in early lesions in the vessel walls and sometimes along the dermal–epidermal junction [20–24]. Immune complexes, cryoglobulins and breakdown products of C3 activation [44] are found in the serum of patients with acute EM. Occasionally *Mycoplasma pneumoniae* [45], complete herpes virus [29] and more often herpes antigens [30] have been detected in EM lesions. Intradermal injection of HSV antigens reproduced bullous EM in a patient with recurrent post-herpetic EM [27]. Herpes simplex antigen is part of circulating immune complexes [31]. These findings led to the concept of EM as an immune complex disease.

There are two major criticisms of this concept. First vasculitis is not a histological feature of EM [17–19]. Second most findings suggestive of humoral immune mechanisms are restricted to the very early phase of herpes-associated EM. As discussed in Section 17.2 we never found immune deposits or complement activation in drug-induced SJS or TEN where a T-cell-mediated hypersensitivity reaction is more probably involved. An immunohistochemical study of EM showed that most inflammatory cells were T lymphocytes, mainly with CD4 phenotype in the dermis and with CD8 phenotype in the epidermis. These changes, associated with Langerhans cell redistribution suggest a cellular immune mechanism [46].

17.1.11 Treatment

(a) Corticosteroids

The usefulness of corticosteroids in EM is the subject of prolonged controversy among dermatologists. The rationale for their use is founded on the hypothesis of an immunologically mediated reaction. There are anecdotal observations of dramatic improvements [1–3] as well as of occurrences of EM in spite of previous therapy with high doses of corticosteroids [47]. All studies comparing patients treated with or without corticosteroids showed no benefits and increased rates of complications in steroid-treated patients [10, 48–50]. Though uncontrolled and retrospective, these studies argue against the use of corticosteroids in EM.

(b) Acyclovir

Many authors have tried to suppress EM related to recurrent herpes simplex using acyclovir as antiviral therapy. When acyclovir is begun after the outbreak of herpes simplex, EM is not prevented [32]. Conversely continuous oral therapy is effective in preventing recurrences of both herpes and subsequent EM [32–34].

(c) Symptomatic therapy

Severe forms of EM major require topical antiseptics, parenteral fluids, electrolytes and calories, and management by specialized teams as for TEN.

17.1.12 Prognosis and sequelae

Lesions of EM heal in 2–4 weeks. The only significant complication of EM minor is the risk of recurrences. EM major on the other hand may be life-threatening. If cases with extensive epidermal loss are classified as TEN the death rate in SJS is below 5%. Sequelae include skin pigmentation disorders, weight loss, mucous membrane scarring, mainly ocular lesions, and rare cases of oesophageal stenosis [51]. Ocular sequelae of SJS include disorders of tear production and drainage, trichiasis, metaplasia of the conjunctiva, corneal chronic erosions and synechiae [52]. Such lesions may remain active for years and severely impair the vision.

References

1. Elias, P.M. and Fritsch, P.O. (1987) Erythema multiforme. In *Dermatology in General Medicine*

(eds T.B. Fitzpatrick, A.Z. Eisen, K. Wolff, I.M. Freedberg and K.F. Austen), McGraw-Hill, New York, pp. 559–63.
2. Champion, R.H. (1986) Erythema multiforme. In *Textbook of Dermatology* (eds A. Rook, D.S. Wilkinson, F.J.G. Ebling, R.H. Champion and J.L. Burton), Blackwell, Oxford, pp. 1085–8.
3. Huff, J.C., Weston, W.L. and Tonnesen, M.G. (1983) Erythema multiforme: a critical review of characteristics, diagnosis criteria, and causes. *J. Amer. Acad. Dermatol.*, **8**, 763–75.
4. Ting, H.C. and Adam, B.A. (1984) Erythema multiforme: epidemiology, clinical characteristics and natural history in fifty-nine patients. *Austr. J. Dermatol.*, **25**, 83–8.
5. Hellgren, L. and Hersle, K. (1965) Erythema multiforme. Statistical evaluation of clinical and laboratory data in 224 patients and matched healthy controls. *Acta Allergol.*, **21**, 45–51.
6. Yetiv, J.Z., Bianchine, J.R. and Owen, J.A. (1980) Etiologic factors of the Stevens–Johnson syndrome. *South. Med. J.*, **73**, 599–602.
7. Maleville, J., Massicot, P., Ponge, A., *et al.* (1983) Aspects cliniques et étiologiques de l'érythème polymorphe. A propos de quarante observations. *Semin. Hôp., Paris*, **59**, 671–5.
8. Gebel, K. and Hornstein, O.P. (1984) Drug-induced oral erythema multiforme, results of a long-term retrospective study. *Dermatologica*, **168**, 35–40.
9. Howland, W.W., Golitz, L.E., Weston, W.L. and Huff, J.C. (1984) Erythema multiforme: clinical, histopathologic and immunologic study. *J. Amer. Acad. Dermatol.*, **10**, 438–46.
10. Nethercott, J.R. and Choi, B.C.K. (1985) Erythema multiforme (Stevens–Johnson syndrome) – chart review of 123 hospitalized patients. *Dermatologica*, **171**, 383–96.
11. Middleton, M., Hutchison, T.H. and Lynd, J. (1983) HLA antigen frequency in erythema multiforme and in recurrent herpes simplex. *Tissue Antigens*, **21**, 264–7.
12. Duvic, M., Reisner, E.G., Dawson, D.V. and Ciftan, E. (1983) HLA-B15 association with erythema multiforme. *J. Amer. Acad. Dermatol.*, **8**, 493–6.
13. Simon, M., Djawari, D. and Schönberger, A. (1984) HLA-typisierung bei patienten mit herpes simplex recidivans und postherpetishem erythema exsudativum multiforme. *Z. Hautkr.*, **59**, 1087–9.
14. Mondino, B.J., Brown, S.I. and Biglan, A.W. (1982) HLA antigens in Stevens–Johnson syndrome with ocular involvement. *Arch. Ophthalmol.*, **100**, 1453–4.
15. Roujeau, J-C., Bracq, C., Huyn, N.T., *et al.* (1986) HLA phenotypes and bullous reactions to drugs. *Tissue Antigens*, **28**, 251–4.
16. Fisher, P.R. and Shigeoka, A.O. (1983) Familial occurence of Stevens–Johnson syndrome. *Amer. J. Dis. Child*, **137**, 914–16.
17. Orfanos, C.E., Schaumburg-Lever, G. and Lever, W.F. (1974) Dermal and epidermal types of erythema multiforme. *Arch. Dermatol.*, **109**, 682–8.
18. Lever, W.F. (1985) My concept of erythema multiforme. *Amer. J. Dermatopathol.*, **7**, 141–2.
19. Ackerman, A.B. and Ragaz, A. (1985) Erythema multiforme. *Amer. J. Dermatopathol.*, **7**, 133–9.
20. Finan, M.C. and Schroeter, A.L. (1984) Cutaneous immunofluorescence study of erythema multiforme: correlation with light microscopic patterns and etiologic agents. *J. Amer. Acad. Dermatol.*, **10**, 497–506.
21. Kazmierowski, J. and Wuepper, K.D. (1978) Erythema multiforme: immune complex vasculitis of the superficial cutaneous microvasculature. *J. Invest. Dermatol.*, **71**, 366–9.
22. Wuepper, K.D., Watson, P.A. and Kazmierowski, J.A. (1980) Immune complexes in erythema multiforme and Stevens Johnson syndrome. *J. Invest. Dermatol.*, **74**, 368–71.
23. Bushkell, L.L., Mackel, S.E. and Jordon, R.E. (1980) Erythema multiforme: direct immunofluorescence studies and detection of circulating immune complexes. *J. Invest. Dermatol.*, **74**, 372–4.
24. Huff, J.C., Weston, W.L. and Carr, I. (1980) Mixed cryoglobulinemia, IC1q binding and skin immunofluorescence in erythema multiforme. *J. Invest. Dermatol.*, **74**, 375–7.
25. Virant, F.S., Redding, G.J. and Novack, A.H. (1984) Multiple pulmonary complications in a patient with SJS. *Clin. Pediatr.*, **23**, 412–14.
26. Zweiban, B., Cohen, H. and Chandrasoma, P. (1986) Gastrointestinal involvement complicating Stevens–Johnson syndrome. *Gastroenterology*, **91**, 469–74.
27. Shelley, W.B. (1967) Herpes simplex virus as a cause of erythema multiforme. *J. Amer. Med. Assoc.*, **201**, 153–6.
28. Leigh, I.M., Mowbray, J.F., Levene, G.M. and Sutherland, S. (1985) Recurrent and continuous erythema multiforme, a clinical and immunological study. *Clin. Exp. Dermatol.*, **10**, 58–67.
29. Strom, J. (1969) Herpes simplex virus as a cause of allergic mucocutaneous reactions (ectodermosis erosiva pluriorificialis, Stevens–Johnson syndrome, etc.) and generalized infection. *Scand. J. Infect. Dis.*, **1**, 3–10.
30. Orton, P.W., Huff, J.C., Tonnesen, M.G. and Weston, W.L. (1984) Detection of a herpes simplex viral antigen in skin lesions of erythema multiforme. *Ann. Intern. Med.*, **101**, 48–50.
31. Kazmierowski, J.A., Peizner, D.S. and Wuepper, K.D. (1982) Herpes simplex antigen in immune complexes of patients with erythema multiforme. *J. Amer. Med. Assoc.*, **247**, 2547–50.
32. Green, J.A., Spruance, S.L., Wenerstrom, G. and Piepkorn, M.W. (1985) Post-herpetic erythema

multiforme prevented with prophylactic oral acyclovir. *Ann. Intern. Med.*, **102**, 632–3.
33. Lemak, M.A., Duvic, M. and Bean, S.F. (1986) Oral acyclovir for the prevention of herpes-associated erythema multiforme. *J. Amer. Acad. Dermatol.*, **15**, 50–4.
34. Morel, P. and Barth, P. (1986) Traitement prophylactique par l'acyclovir per os de l'érythème polymorphe récidivant, associé ou non à une infection herpétique. Etude préliminaire. *Ann. Dermatol. Venereol.*, **113**, 269–70.
35. Ali, N.J., Sillis, M., Andrews, B.E., Jenkins, P.F. and Harrison, B.D. (1986) The clinical spectrum and diagnosis of *Mycoplasma pneumoniae* infection. *Q. J. Med.*, **58**, 241–51.
36. Kauppinen, K. and Stubb, S. (1984) Drug eruptions: causative agents and clinical types. A series of inpatients during a 10-year period. *Acta Dermatovenereol. (Stockholm)*, **64**, 320–4.
37. Hernborg, A. (1985) Stevens–Johnson syndrome after mass prophylaxis with sulfadoxine for cholera in Mozambique. *Lancet*, **ii**, 1072–3.
38. Miller, K.D., Lobel, H.O., Satriale, R.F., *et al.* (1986) Severe cutaneous reactions among American travelers using pyrimethamine-sulfadoxine (Fansidar) for malaria prophylaxis. *Amer. J. Trop. Med. Hyg.*, **35**, 351–8.
39. Pearson, R.D. and Hewlett, E.L. (1987) Use of pyrimethamine-sulfadoxine (Fansidar) in prophylaxis against chloroquine-resistant *Plasmodium falciparum* and *Pneumocystis carinii*. *Ann. Intern. Med.*, **106**, 714–18.
40. Bigby, M. and Stern, R. (1985) Cutaneous reactions to nonsteroidal anti-inflammatory drugs. A review. *J. Amer. Acad. Dermatol.*, **12**, 866–76.
41. Guillaume, J.C., Roujeau, J.C., Chevais, M., *et al.* (1985) Syndrome de Lyell et ectodermose pluriorificielle au cours de traitements par les oxicams: 11 observations. *Ann. Dermatol. Venereol.*, **112**, 807–12.
42. Phoon, W.H., Chan, M.O.Y., Rajan, V.S., *et al.* (1984) Stevens–Johnson syndrome associated with occupational exposure to trichlorethylene. *Contact Dermatitis*, **10**, 270–6.
43. Fisher, A.A. (1986) Erythema multiforme-like eruptions due to topical miscellaneous compounds. Part III. *Cutis*, **37**, 262–4.
44. Wansbrough-Jones, M.H., Collas, D.M. and Bishop, S. (1986) Complement activation and spleen function in erythema multiforme associated with herpes simplex virus reactivation. *J. Clin. Lab. Immunol.*, **21**, 83–5.
45. Meseguer, M.A., de Rafael, L. and Vidal, M.L. (1986) Stevens–Johnson syndrome with isolation of *Mycoplasma pneumoniae* from skin lesions. *Eur. J. Clin. Microbiol.*, **5**, 167–8.
46. Margolis, R.J., Tonnesen, M.G., Harrist, T.J., *et al.* (1983) Lymphocyte subsets and Langerhans cells/indeterminate cells in erythema multiforme. *J. Invest. Dermatol.*, **81**, 403–6.
47. Leititis, J.U., Burghard, R., Rietschel, E., Rieger, C.H. and Brandis, M. (1985) Stevens–Johnson syndrome during an immunosuppressive therapy with cyclophosphamide and prednisone. *Clin. Pediatr.*, **197**, 441–2.
48. Rasmussen, J.E. (1976) Erythema multiforme in children. *Brit. J. Dermatol.*, **95**, 181–6.
49. Ginsburg, C.M. (1982) Stevens–Johnson syndrome in children. *Pediatr. Infect. Dis.*, **1**, 155–8.
50. Ting, H.C. and Adam, B.A. (1984) Erythema multiforme: response to corticosteroids. *Dermatologica*, **169**, 175–8.
51. Peters, M.E., Gourley, G. and Mann, F.A. (1983) Esophageal stricture and web secondary to Stevens–Johnson syndrome. *Pediatr. Radiol.*, **13**, 290–1.
52. Wright, P. and Collin, J.R. (1983) The ocular complications of erythema multiforme (Stevens–Johnson syndrome) and their management. *Trans. Ophthalmol. Soc. UK*, **103**, 338–41.

17.2 TOXIC EPIDERMAL NECROLYSIS (LYELL'S SYNDROME)

17.2.1 Introduction

Although previously recognized [1], toxic epidermal necrolysis (TEN) was described in 1956 by Alan Lyell [2] as a syndrome including staphylococcal scalded-skin syndrome (SSSS) and generalized fixed drug eruptions which are now separated from TEN [3, 4]. TEN is the best available term for a disease with necrosis and detachment of the complete epidermis (necrolysis), toxic applying to the severe constitutional symptoms and complications as well as to the drug origin of most if not all cases. Most authors classify TEN as the extreme form of erythema multiforme (EM) [5, 6]. The boundary between TEN and Stevens–Johnson syndrome is not clearly defined. TEN is the most severe blistering disease, with a death rate around 30% and potentially disabling ocular sequelae in survivors [4–7].

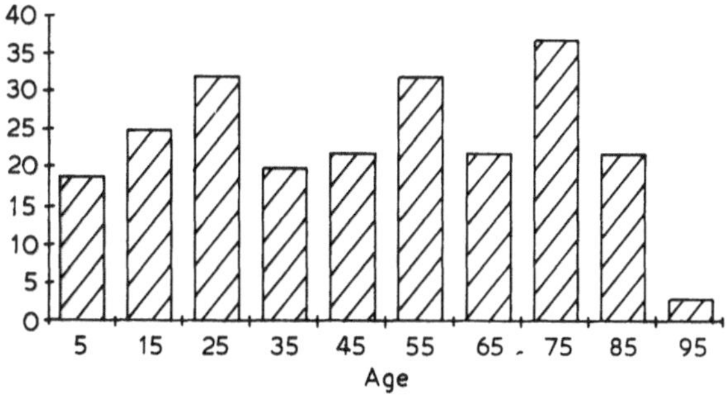

Figure 17.6 Histogram of age of onset of toxic epidermal necrolysis. From an unpublished French study (242 cases).

17.2.2 Presentation

(a) Age

TEN occurs in all ages [4, 7], including children, infants and even neonates. The incidence increases with age, probably reflecting the use of drugs (Figure 17.6).

(b) Sex

There is a female to male ratio of 3 : 2 to 2 : 1 [4, 7], as for most adverse drug reactions (Figure 17.7). More frequent drug intake by women is only one of the possible explanations.

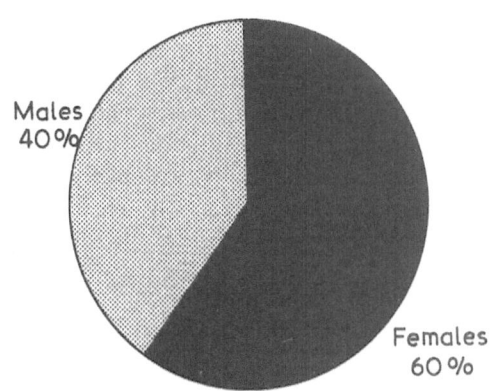

Figure 17.7 Sex ratio observed for toxic epidermal necrolysis (242 cases).

(c) Frequency

An epidemiological study of TEN in France and Germany from 1981 to 1985 gave an incidence of 1 to 1.5 cases per million per year, without seasonal variation (unpublished data). The incidence of TEN in Sweden was 0.5 per million per year in 1964–1969 [8], suggesting an increasing occurrence in recent years.

(d) Geographical distribution

Cases of TEN have been observed world wide and among all races [9–12].

17.2.3 Cutaneous distribution

The lesions begin symmetrically in the upper part of the body and progress quickly over all the body surface, usually in 2 or 3 days, sometimes in a few hours. Occasionally extension may last for a week. Only the hairy portion of the scalp is never involved [4–7].

17.2.4 Mucous membrane involvement

It is nearly universal (85–95% of cases [7], usually in several sites, heralding the disease in about one-third of cases. The order of frequency is mouth, eyes and genitalia (Figure 17.8). Widespread painful erosions, identical to those of SJS, lead to increased salivation, impaired eating, photophobia and painful micturition. Ocular lesions need specific attention since they carry a high risk of sequelae.

17.2.5 Morphology of lesions

The characteristic pattern of TEN is a widespread sheet-like loss of epidermis [1–4] (Figure 17.9). In involved areas the skin is painful, erythematous and the epidermis is raised by flaccid blisters (Figure 17.10). The Nikolsky sign is positive. Detachment of full-thickness epidermis on pressure areas (top of the back and buttocks) or on traumatic sites (for example adhesive electrodes for electrocardiogram monitoring) (Figure 17.9) leaves a dark-red oozing dermis. In other places the necrotic epidermis

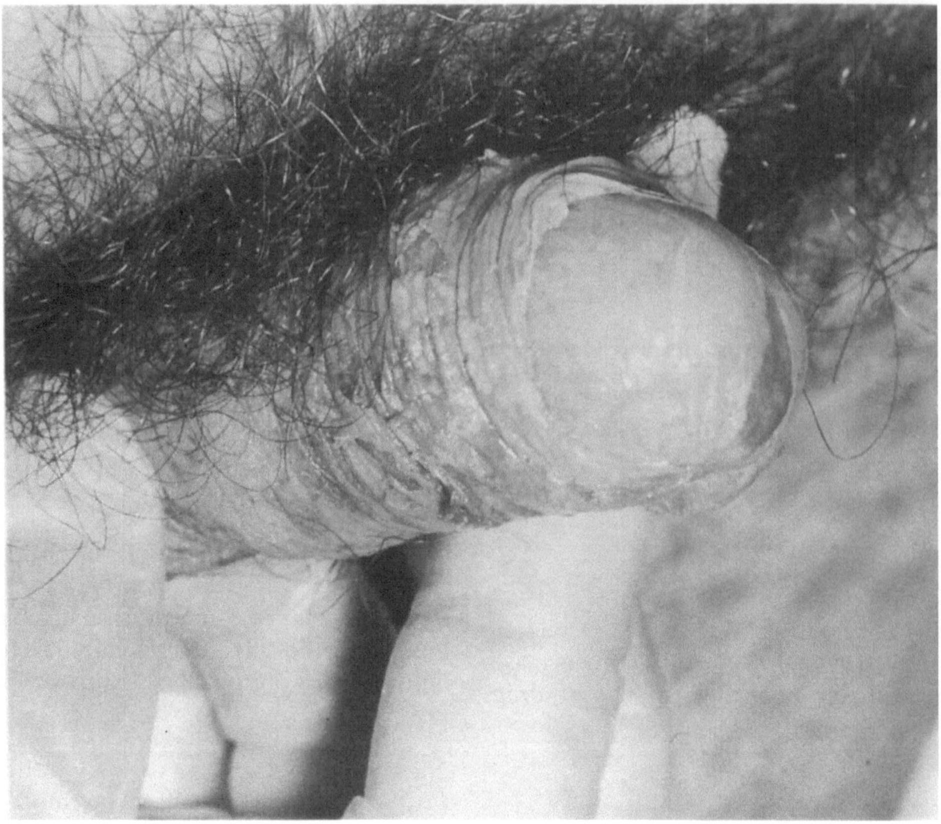

Figure 17.8 Genital involvement observed in toxic epidermal necrolysis.

remains over the dermis with a wrinkled appearance similar to a pleated tight-fitting garment. In less than 20% of cases this is the only pattern of skin lesions ('TEN d'emblée') [7]. In most cases areas of necrolysis are associated with disseminated small round erythema multiforme-like lesions [4, 7, 12] (Figure 17.10). In these cases the lesions appear as distinct EM-like papules and bullae and progress to TEN by confluence. The entire skin surface may also be involved with up to 100% of the epidermis sloughing off. These two clinical patterns often overlap in a given patient, and have the same pathology, aetiology, complications and prognosis [7].

17.2.6 Genetics

In 45 patients with TEN we found a significant increase in HLA-B12. Sulphonamide-induced TEN cases were linked to HLA-A29, -B12 and -DR7, while cases attributed to the oxicam class of non-steroidal anti-inflammatory drugs (NSAIDs) were linked to HLA-A2, -B12 and -DR4 [13]. These results, if confirmed in other series, would suggest that different genetic backgrounds related to the major histocompatibility complex might predispose to severe skin reactions to different drugs.

17.2.7 Differential diagnosis

(a) Staphylococcal scalded-skin syndrome (SSSS)

SSSS afflicts mainly infants and children and rarely adults with severe underlying disease [6]. A faint erythematous rash extends in a few hours, on which

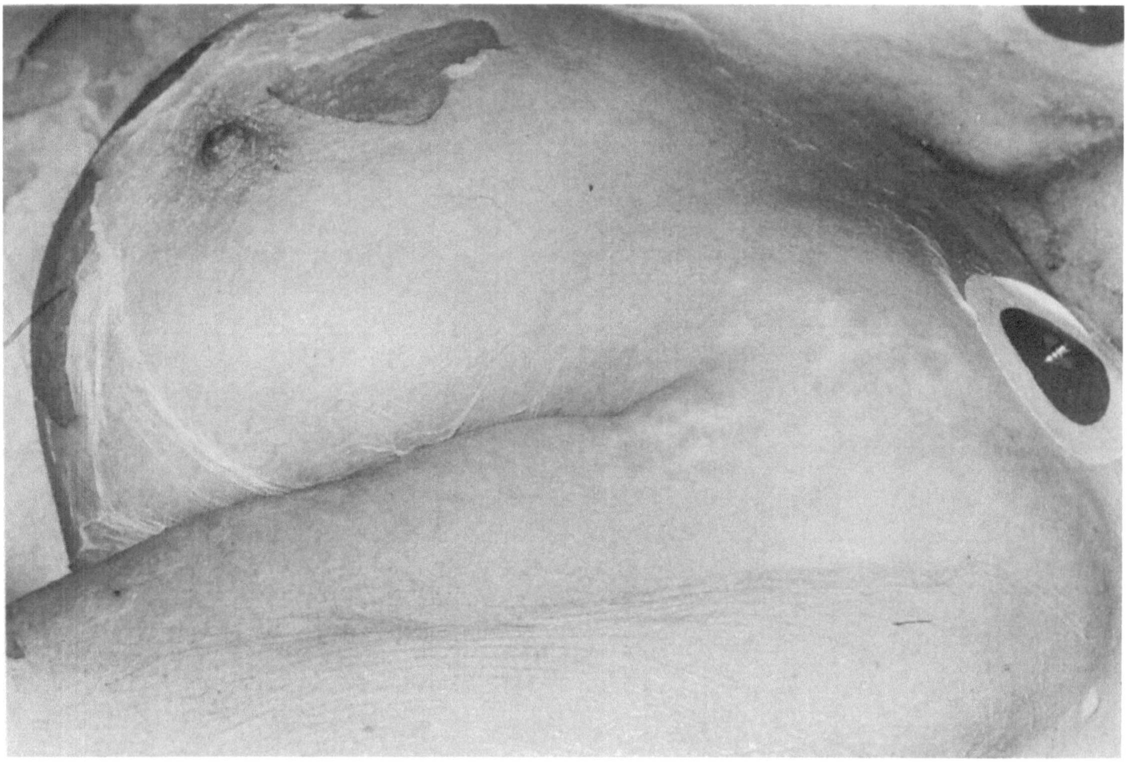

Figure 17.9 Classical pattern of widespread epidermal loss observed in toxic epidermal necrolysis.

arise large flaccid blisters with positive Nikolsky sign. Mucous membranes are spared (except for conjunctivitis) and erosions are much more superficial with little or no oozing. Histologically the separation lies within and beneath the stratum granulosum. Microscopic examination of a frozen section of detached epidermis permits emergency diagnosis [14]. SSSS is provoked by toxins [15] (epidermolysins) from some groups of *Staphylococcus aureus* (mainly phage group 2). Staphylococci are usually not present in skin lesions but in a purulent focal infection, often of the upper respiratory tract. Antibiotics stop the process in a few hours and healing follows in a few days.

(b) Toxic shock syndrome

The usual cutaneous manifestations of TSS (erythema and desquamation) are quite different from TEN. Only exceptional cases of TSS with blisters could be confused with TEN [16].

(c) Stevens–Johnson syndrome

There is no consensus to date on the relationship between SJS and TEN. Are they two variants of the same process or two different diseases? Without more knowledge on the pathogenesis the discussion is endless. We have made the arbitrary choice of a prognosis boundary [7], calling TEN the cases with necrolysis above 10% of the body surface and a significant risk of death and SJS the cases with skin blisters below 10% of the body area and a good prognosis (no death in our experience).

(d) Generalized bullous fixed drug eruption

Fixed drug eruption, when generalized, may closely mimic TEN. The well-demarcated round lesions,

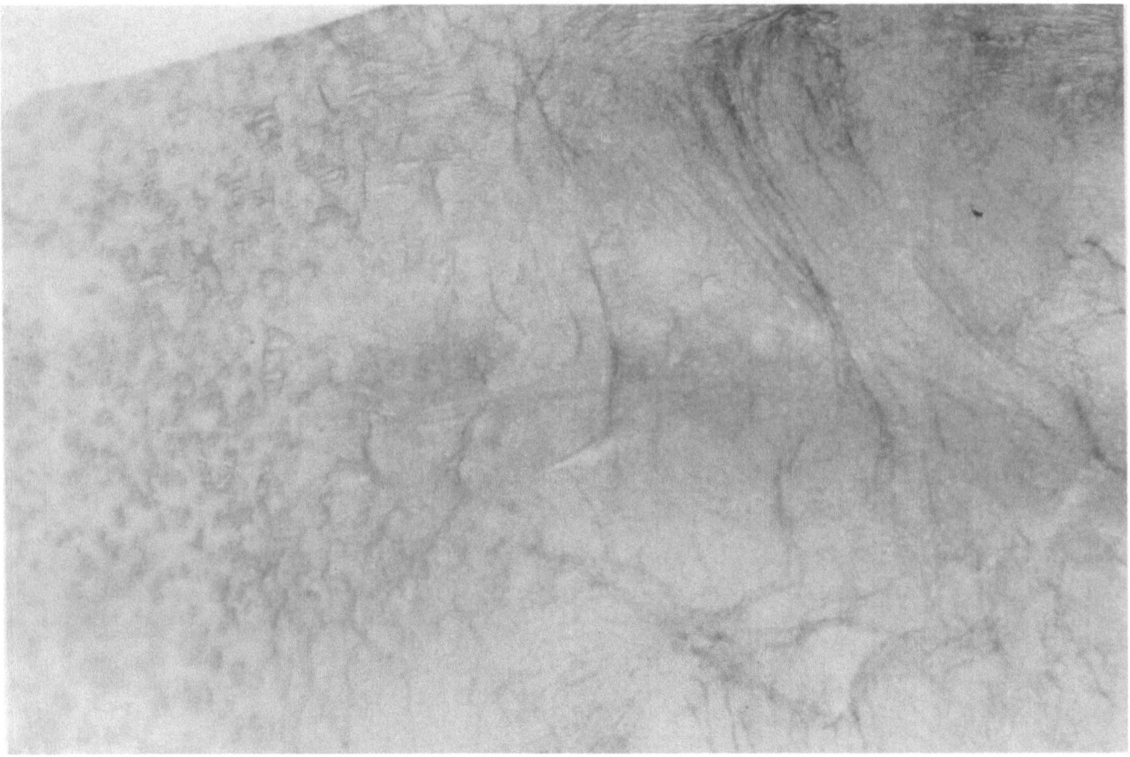

Figure 17.10 Association of large areas of epidermal sloughing with erythema multiforme-like lesions seen in toxic epidermal necrolysis.

the rarity of mucous membrane erosions and a history of previous eruption with the same drug are indicative of that rare disease, probably often confused with TEN [17].

(e) Disseminated pustular eruptions

Acute pustular psoriasis, drug-induced or post-viral pustular eruptions may look like TEN when pustules are confluent on a generalized erythroderma [18]. The histology is distinctive.

(f) Burns and bullae in comatose patients

Second-degree burns, especially chemical ones, and bullae occurring in comatose patients may resemble TEN [4]. Mucous membranes are usually spared and the distribution of the lesions is limited to exposed areas or to pressure areas.

17.2.8 Investigations

(a) Laboratory findings

Laboratory tests are not diagnostic but are needed at least daily to monitor visceral involvement and complications.

(b) Histopathology

The lesions of TEN are indistinguishable from those of the 'epidermal type' of EM [19]. The upper dermis shows a mild infiltration by mononuclear cells without vascular alterations. Epidermal changes begin in the basal cell layer as intercellular oedema with a sparse exocytosis of mononuclear cells further involving all the Malpighian layer. Close contacts between dyskeratotic and mononuclear cells ('satellite cell necrosis') are occasionally observed [20, 21]. At a more advanced stage the necrosis extends from basal cells to the whole epidermis. The lamina densa remains in the floor of the blister [19].

Direct immunofluorescence is always negative [22], apart from a single case report of immune deposits around the basal cells [23].

TEN is clinically distinct, and experienced dermatologists do not need a pathological study to make the diagnosis. However, we recommend obtaining a skin biopsy in every case in which drug(s) may be involved to avoid subsequent controversies.

(c) Tests for assessing drug responsibility

There is no reliable test to link a case to a specific drug. Drug challenge, which may be potentially life-threatening, must not be performed [4–7]. The lymphocyte transformation test has no value in TEN [24]. Other *in vitro* tests have not been adequately studied. The utility and safety of skin tests remain to be proven [25–27].

The determination of the 'culprit' drug relies on the timing of the reaction and on the knowledge of other accidents attributed to the same or related drugs [28]. The severity of TEN causes a few cases to have profound implications on the development of a drug. Each case of TEN must be reported to regulatory agencies and to the drug company involved after a strict drug inquiry.

17.2.9 Systemic manifestations and associated diseases

(a) Systemic manifestations and complications

Fever and flu–like symptoms often precede the occurrence of mucocutaneous lesions by 1–3 days [4–7]. High fever usually persists up to complete skin healing, even in the absence of superinfection [7]. A sudden drop in temperature is more indicative of severe sepsis than fever. Asthenia, skin pain and anxiety are extreme.

Destruction of the cutaneous barrier produces important loss of fluids, electrolytes and proteins, and carries the risk of sepsis, as in second-degree burns of similar extent. Weight loss, oliguria and pre-renal azotaemia are customary as a consequence of fluid losses reaching 4–5 litres a day when 50% of the body surface is involved. Sepsis is the main cause of death [7]. The skin lesions are always colonized by pathogens, *Staphylococcus aureus* in the first days, followed by Gram-negative rods especially *Pseudomonas aeruginosa*. These two rods are the main causes of severe sepsis [7, 29]. However, TEN carries a worse prognosis than burns of the same surface area because of multisystemic involvement.

Hepatic involvement is present in half of the patients, ranking from slight elevation of transaminases to frank hepatitis in 10% [7, 30]. Stress, infection and possibly pancreatitis cause glycosuria in half of the cases [31].

Haematological abnormalities are frequent [32, 33] with anaemia and lymphopenia in 90% of cases, neutropenia in 30% and thrombocytopenia in 15%. Eosinophilia is very unusual. Disseminated intravascular coagulation has been reported [34], but we have never observed it.

Nephropathy, acute tubular necrosis and, rarely, glomerulonephritis have been observed in half of the cases in a post-mortem series of TEN cases [5]. Such observations are very difficult to attribute to TEN itself rather than to infection or fluid balance problems. We observed heavy proteinuria in only two cases, both with septicaemia.

Lung involvement is the most severe complication. Our team noticed that subclinical interstitial oedema was often present on early chest X rays, with frequent (30%) development of frank pulmonary oedema due to increased alveolo-capillar permeability (unpublished observations). In 10–20% of cases pulmonary function is so compromised as to require artificial ventilation.

Other visceral manifestations reported in a few cases include gastrointestinal erosions [35] and bleeding [29], and pulmonary embolism [7].

(b) Associated diseases

Since TEN is related to drugs, patients usually have an underlying disease. Many authors have emphasized the frequency of pre-existent infections [4–6], even in cases not related to antimicrobial drugs. Initial infections, usually not documented, seem to be viral rather than bacterial.

Several cases of TEN have been reported in patients suffering from systemic lupus erythematosus [36, 37].

AIDS patients given sulphonamides for opportunistic infections have many more cutaneous reactions (including SJS and TEN) than expected [38].

17.2.10 Pathogenesis and recent advances

(a) Causes of TEN

Drugs In a consensus workshop (Créteil, 1985) it was agreed that, apart from graft-versus-host disease, 'reaction to drugs was to date the only documented cause of TEN' (Figure 17.11). This conclusion was derived more from 'accumulation of clinical experience' (Lyell) than based on scientific evidence. The proof of a drug reaction is usually lacking. There are only a few published cases of recurrence of TEN after drug rechallenge [3, 17, 28, 39, 40]. However, cases occurring without any drug exposure are so rare as to cast doubt on the reliability of the drug inquiry. In our own series of 87 patients, only three had received no drug before the onset of TEN [28] (Figure 17.11).

The term drugs must be taken in a broad sense since foods [3] and fumigants [41] have also been implicated in a few cases. Drugs implicated in the literature are mainly sulphonamides [8, 9, 17], anticonvulsants [40], analgesics and less frequently NSAIDs [42]. In our experience [28] a drug was identified in 77% (67 of 87) of patients (Table 17.1). NSAIDs (mainly phenylbutazone and oxicam derivatives) were the most common cause of TEN in this series with 29 cases (43%), followed by sulphonamides with 17 cases (25%). Seven cases only were attributed to anticonvulsants (10%). Although aspirin and various antipyretics, analgesics and antibiotics are frequently cited in the literature, they were notably infrequently implicated in our series. These drugs are often given for the early manifestations of TEN such as the flu-like symptoms, or given with more likely suspects and so can often be excluded as the cause of TEN.

The mean time from first drug administration to onset of TEN was 14 days for all drugs [28]. Although longer or shorter times do not completely exclude the drug, one should consider as 'prime

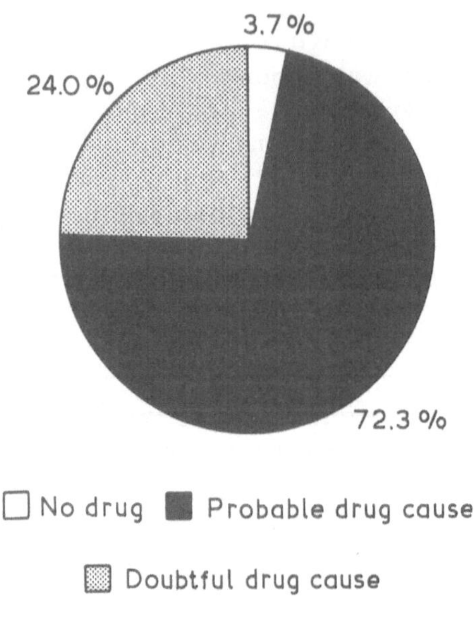

Figure 17.11 Aetiology of toxic epidermal necrolysis (242 cases).

Table 17.1 Drugs considered to be responsible for TEN in 67 out of 87 patients (68 drugs) [28]

NSAIDS	29
Oxyphenbutazone	11
Phenylbutazone	5
Isoxicam	5
Piroxicam	5
Other	3
Sulphonamides	18
Cotrimoxazole	12
Other	6
Anticonvulsants	7
Carbamazepine	3
Miscellaneous	14
Allopurinol	4
Chlormezanone	3
Noramidopyrine	2
Acetylsalicylic acid	1
Buzepide–clocinizine–norephedrine	1
Erythromycin	1
Rifampicin	1
Pyritinol	1

suspect(s)' drug(s) introduced within 1–3 weeks before the onset of TEN.

Acute graft-versus-host disease (aGVHD) TEN has been described in an animal model of cutaneous acute graft-versus-host disease (aGVHD) [43]. A few cases of TEN have been reported in man following bone marrow transplantation (BMT) [44, 45] and are then considered the most severe cutaneous manifestation of aGVHD. In our own experience of nine cases of TEN occurring after BMT four were clearly drug induced and five more probably related to aGVHD [46].

(b) Pathogenesis of TEN

TEN is generally considered as a hypersensitivity reaction to drugs [4]. Most drugs, and/or their reactive metabolites, that induce TEN can behave as haptens capable of eliciting immune reactions after combination with appropriate 'carrier' proteins. Indirect arguments supporting an immune reaction in TEN include: an animal model of TEN in hamsters undergoing cutaneous aGVHD [43]; the occurrence of TEN in man after bone marrow transplantation [44, 45]; the time intervals between drug intake and the reaction (14 days for the first occurrence, less than 2 days in the rare recurrences) [28]; the Sjögren-like syndrome following TEN [47]; and finally the imbalance of T lymphocyte subsets during TEN [48]. In fact direct evidence for an immunological mechanism is still lacking [49].

Antibodies are probably not involved. Direct immunofluorescence studies are usually negative. Serum antibodies reacting with the cytoplasm of epidermal cells, occasionally found after TEN [50], are non-specific and probably a consequence of the disease [49]. There is no evidence of complement activation in the acute phase of TEN [22]. The observation of antibodies reacting with epidermis or mononuclear cells only in presence of the culprit drug [51] has not yet been confirmed.

Cell-mediated cytotoxic reactions against epidermal cells would more easily explain the pathological findings of 'satellite cell necrosis' [20, 21]. Immunohistological studies have shown that keratinocytes express HLA-DR antigens (personal observation) and that most lymphocytes invading the epidermis are T cells with a CD8 phenotype [52]. Both findings are consistent with a hypersensitivity reaction.

Many authors claimed that they have demonstrated a hypersensitivity to drugs in TEN patients by skin testing or *in vitro* reactions. Unfortunately adequate controls (for example patients who took the drug without adverse reaction) were usually missing. With such controls we were unable to find any specific reaction of patients' lymphocytes to the culprit drug *in vitro* [24]. Furthermore the occurrence of TEN in patients receiving high doses of steroids or in patients with AIDS challenges the concept of a classic type of delayed hypersensitivity to drugs.

The extreme rarity of the disease is probably best explained on the basis of several concomitant factors including genetic background, viral infection, altered immune reactivity and drugs (Lyell's 'jackpot hypothesis'). These factors might either liberate autocytotoxic cells or enhance a specific immunological reaction against keratinocytes modified by drug or metabolite(s). Interleukin 1/ETAF released by lysed epidermal cells and other lymphokines may contribute to fever and general symptoms.

17.2.11 Treatment

Management of TEN should be undertaken in specialized wards.

(a) 'Specific' therapy

Corticosteroids For 30 years corticosteroids had been held to be the specific therapy for TEN. Not only was proof of their effectiveness lacking, but many cases occurred in patients receiving high doses of corticosteroids for pre-existent diseases. Fifteen years ago an uncontrolled retrospective study found that TEN patients treated with corticosteroids had a higher death rate [53]. More recently in a unit specializing in the management of severe TEN the death rate fell from 66 to 33% after withdrawal of steroid therapy as the only change [29, 54]. Although uncontrolled, these data suggest that corticosteroids may be detrimental to TEN patients and must be avoided.

Plasma exchange Plasma exchange, performed with the aim of removing offending drugs and/or unknown pathogenic factors, induced 'dramatic' arrest of disease progression in a few patients [55]. We used plasma exchange in the initial phase in six cases matched with six 'untreated' patients and observed more disease extension.

(b) Symptomatic management

Since venous access across skin lesions carries a high risk of septicaemia, central lines must be avoided. As far as possible we give fluids by a nasogastric tube. Some prescribed prophylactic systemic antibiotics while others use them only in the presence of definite infection. Skin disinfection is of paramount importance and the pathogens colonizing the skin must be carefully monitored.

(c) Local treatment

Patients are best managed on an air fluidized bed. Recently hyperbaric oxygen [56], or biological dressings such as porcine cutaneous xenografts, cutaneous allografts, amnion or collagen-based skin substitute have been proposed to improve healing [57, 58]. Ocular lesions require daily examination by an ophthalmologist. Antiseptic or antibiotic eye drops are instilled every 2 h and ongoing synechiae must be disrupted by a blunt instrument.

17.2.12 Prognosis and sequelae

The death rate for drug-induced TEN can reach 60 or 70% [29,59] but is usually around 30%. All patients with TEN and aGVHD bar one died. In our series of 87 patients (excluding aGVHD) the death rate was 25%. Infection was the cause of death in half of the fatal cases. Age, area of necrolysis and rise in blood urea were the main prognostic factors [7].

Among survivors, long-lasting pigmentary disturbances are common, with either hyperpigmented or depigmented areas. Occurrence of naevi have been reported [60]. Nails are frequently shed and regrowth may be abnormal. Mucosal erosions lasting for months are not uncommon. Phimosis may require surgery. Oesophageal strictures have been observed. Persistent ocular lesions are the most disabling, affecting 40% of survivors [61]. A Sjögren-like sicca syndrome, inturned eyelashes, epithelial proliferation on conjunctiva and cornea contribute to an active 'post-TEN' ocular syndrome. Blindness may result from these lesions.

References

1. Debré, R., Lamy, M. and Lamotte, M. (1939) Un cas d'érythrodermie avec épidermolyse chez un enfant de douze ans. *Bull. Soc. Pediat.*, **37**, 231–8.
2. Lyell, A. (1956) Toxic epidermal necrolysis: an eruption resembling scalding of the skin. *Brit. J. Dermatol.*, **68**, 355–61.
3. Lyell, A. (1967) A review of toxic epidermal necrolysis in Britain. *Brit. J. Dermatol.*, **79**, 662–71.
4. Lyell, A. (1979) Toxic epidermal necrolysis (the scalded skin syndrome): a reappraisal. *Brit. J. Dermatol.*, **100**, 69–86.
5. Rasmussen, J.E. (1980) Toxic epidermal necrolysis. *Med. Clin. North Amer.*, **64**, 901–20.
6. Snyder, R.A. and Elias, P.M. (1983) Toxic epidermal necrolysis and staphylococcal scalded skin syndrome. *Dermatol. Clin.*, **1**, 235–48.
7. Revuz, J., Penso, D., Roujeau, J.-C., *et al.* (1987) Toxic epidermal necrolysis : clinical findings and prognosis factors in 87 patients. *Arch. Dermatol.*, **123**, 1160–5.
8. Bôttiger, L.E., Strandberg, I. and Westerholm, B. (1975) Drug induced febrile mucocutaneous syndrome. *Acta Med. Scand.*, **198**, 229–33.
9. Bergoend, H., Löefler, A., Amar, R. and Maleville, J. (1968) Réactions cutanées survenues au cours de la prophylaxie de masse de la méningite cérébro-spinale par un sulfamide long-retard. *Ann. Dermatol. Syphil.*, **95**, 481–90.
10. Strobel, M., Ndiaye, B., Padonou, F. and Marchand, J.P. (1980) Le syndrome de Lyell à Dakar. *Dakar Med.*, **25**, 261–7.
11. Chan, H.L. (1984) Observations on drug-induced toxic epidermal necrolysis in Singapore. *J. Amer. Acad. Dermatol.*, **10**, 973–8.
12. Ruiz-Maldonado, R. (1985) Acute disseminated epidermal necrosis types 1, 2 and 3: study of sixty cases. *J. Amer. Acad. Dermatol.*, **13**, 623–35.
13. Roujeau, J.-C., Huyn, N.T., Bracq, C., *et al.* (1987). HLA antigens and toxic epidermal necrolysis. *Arch. Dermatol.*, **123**, 1171–3.
14. Amon, R.B. and Dimond, R.L. (1975) TEN, rapid differentiation between staphylococcal and drug-induced disease. *Arch. Dermatol.*, **11**, 986–90.

15. Melish, M.E. and Glasgow, L.A. (1970) The staphylococcal scalded skin syndrome: development of an experimental model. *New Engl. J. Med.*, **282**, 1114–19.
16. Elbaum, D.J., Wood, C., Abuabara, F. and Morhenn, V.B. (1984) Bullae in a patient with toxic shock syndrome. *J. Amer. Acad. Dermatol.*, **10**, 267–72.
17. Kauppinen, K. (1972) Cutaneous reactions to drugs with special reference to severe bullous mucocutaneous eruptions and sulphonamides. *Acta, Dermatovenereol.* (Stockholm)., **52**, (Suppl. 68), 1–89.
18. Rouchouse, B., Bonnefoy, M., Pallot, B., *et al.* (1986) Acute generalized exanthematous pustular dermatitis and viral infection. *Dermatologica*, **133**, 180–4.
19. Orfanos, C.E., Schaumburg-Lever, G. and Lever, W.F. (1974) Dermal and epidermal types of erythema multiforme. *Arch. Dermatol.*, **109**, 682–8.
20. Breathnach, S.M., McGibbon, D.H., Ive, F.A. and Black, M.M. (1982) Carbamazepine ("Tegretol") and toxic epidermal necrolysis: Report of three cases with histopathological observations. *Clin. Exp. Dermatol.*, **7**, 585–91.
21. Roujeau, J.-C., Dubertret, L., Moritz, S., *et al.* (1985) Involvement of macrophages in toxic epidermal necrolysis. *Brit. J. Dermatol.*, **113**, 425–30.
22. Revuz, J. and Typhagne, F. (1978) Immune complexes, complement and immunofluorescence in Lyell syndrome. In *Immunopathologie Cutanée* (eds J. Thivolet and D. Schmitt), Edition INSERM, Paris, pp. 373–6.
23. Stein, K.M., Schlappner, O.L.A., Heaton, C.L. and Decherd, J.W. (1972) Demonstration of basal cell immunofluorescence in drug-induced toxic epidermal necrolysis. *Brit. J. Dermatol.*, **86**, 246–52.
24. Roujeau, J.-C., Albengres, E., Moritz, S., *et al.* (1985) Lymphocyte transformation test in toxic epidermal necrolysis. *Int. Arch. Allergy Appl. Immunol.*, **78**, 22–4.
25. Schöpf, E., Schulz, K.H., Kessler, R., *et al.* (1975) Allergologische Untersuchungen beim Lyell-Syndrom. *Z. Hautkr.*, **50**, 865–73.
26. Tagami, H., Tatsuta, K., Iwatski, K. and Yamada, M. (1983) Delayed hypersensitivity in ampicillin-induced toxic epidermal necrolysis. *Arch. Dermatol.*, **119**, 910–13.
27. Roujeau, J.-C., Bagot, M., Revuz, J. and Touraine, R. (1984) Delayed hypersensitivity in drug induced toxic epidermal necrolysis. *Arch. Dermatol.*, **120**, 1418.
28. Guillaume, J.-C., Roujeau, J.-C., Penso, D., Revuz, J. and Touraine, R. (1987) The culprit drugs in 87 cases of toxic epidermal necrolysis (Lyell syndrome). *Arch. Dermatol.*, **123**, 1166–70.
29. Halebian, P.H., Corder, V., Herndon, D. and Shires, G.T. (1983) A burn center experience with toxic epidermal necrolysis. *J. Burn Care Rehabilit.*, **4**, 176–83.
30. Klein, S.M. and Khan, M.A. (1983) Hepatitis, toxic epidermal necrolysis and pancreatitis in association with sulindac therapy. *J. Rheumatol.*, **10**, 512–13.
31. Revuz, J., Roujeau, J.-C., Guillaume, J.-C., Penso, D. and Touraine, R. (1987) Treatment of toxic epidermal necrolysis, Créteil's experience. *Arch. Dermatol.*, **123**, 1156–8.
32. Bombal, C., Roujeau, J.-C., Kuentz, M., Revuz, J. and Touraine, R. (1983) Anomalies hématologiques au cours du syndrome de Lyell. *Ann. Dermatol. Venereol.*, **110**, 113–19.
33. Goens, J., Song, M., Fondu, P., Blum, D. and Achten, G. (1986) Haematological disturbances and immune mechanisms in toxic epidermal necrolysis. *Brit. J. Dermatol.*, **114**, 255–9.
34. Kvasnicka, J., Rezac, J., Svejda, J., *et al.* (1979) Disseminated intravascular coagulation associated with toxic epidermal necrolysis (Lyell's syndrome). *Brit. J. Dermatol.*, **100**, 551–8.
35. Roupe, G., Ahlmen, M., Fagerberg, B. and Suurküla, M. (1986) Toxic epidermal necrolysis with extensive mucosal erosions of the gastrointestinal and respiratory tracts. *Int. Arch. Allergy Appl. Immunol.*, **80**, 145–51.
36. Burge, S.M. and Dawber, R.P.R. (1985) Stevens–Johnson syndrome and toxic epidermal necrolysis in a patient with systemic lupus erythematosus. *J. Amer. Acad. Dermatol.*, **13**, 665–6.
37. Sayag, J., Mongin, M., Weiller, P.J., *et al.* (1980) Nécrolyse épidermique toxique au cours d'un lupus érythémateux disséminé. *Ann. Dermatol. Venereol. (Paris).*, **107**, 1077–81.
38. Jaffe, H.S., Amman, A.J., Abrams, D.I., Lewis, B.J. and Golden, J.A. (1983) Complication of cotrimoxazole in treatment of AIDS associated pneumocystis *Carinii pneumonia* in homosexual men. *Lancet*, **ii**, 1109–11.
39. Pegram, P.S., Mountz, J.D. and O'Bar, P.R. (1972) Ethambutol-induced toxic epidermal necrolysis. *Arch. Intern. Med.*, **141**, 1677–8.
40. Schmidt, D. and Kluge, W. (1983) Fatal toxic epidermal necrolysis following reexposure to phenytoin: a case report. *Epilepsia*, **24**, 440–3.
41. Radimer, G.F., Davis, J.H. and Ackerman, A.B. (1974) Fumigant induced toxic epidermal necrolysis. *Arch. Dermatol.*, **110**, 103–4.
42. Stern, R.S. and Bigby, M. (1984) An expanded profile of cutaneous reactions to nonsteroidal anti-inflammatory drugs. *J. Amer. Med. Assoc.*, **252**, 1433–7.
43. Billingham, R.E. and Streilein, J.W. (1968) Toxic epidermal necrolysis and homologous disease in hamsters. *Arch. Dermatol.*, **98**, 528–39.

44. Peck, G.L., Herzig, G.P. and Elias, P.M. (1972) Toxic epidermal necrolysis in a patient with graft-vs-host reaction. *Arch. Dermatol.*, **105**, 561–9.
45. Saurat, J.H. and Piguet, P.F. (1984) Human and murine cutaneous graft-vs-host disease. Potential models for the study of immunologically mediated skin disease. *Brit. J. Dermatol.*, **111**, (Suppl. 27), 213–18.
46. Villeda, G., Roujeau, J.-C., Cordonnier, C., *et al.* (1986) Toxic epidermal necrolysis following bone marrow transplantation (9 cases): GvHD or drug reaction? *Bone Marrow Transplant.*, **1**, 72.
47. Roujeau, J.-C., Phlippoteau, C., Koso, M., *et al.* (1985) Sjögren-like syndrome following toxic epidermal necrolysis. *Lancet*, **i**, 609–11.
48. Roujeau, J.-C., Moritz, S., Guillaume, J.-C., *et al.* (1985) Lymphopenia and abnormal balance of T lymphocyte subpopulations in toxic epidermal necrolysis. *Arch. Dermatol. Res.*, **277**, 24–7.
49. Merot, Y. and Saurat, J.H. (1985) Clues to pathogenesis of toxic epidermal necrolysis. *Int. J. Dermatol.*, **24**, 165–8.
50. Van Joost, T. (1974) Incidence of circulating antibodies reactive with basal cells of skin in drug reactions. *Acta Dermatovenereol. (Stockholm)*, **54**, 183–8.
51. Veermer, B.J. and Claas, F.J.H. (1985) Toxic epidermal necrolysis. *Arch. Dermatol.*, **121**, 715–16.
52. Merot, Y., Gravallese, E., Guillen, F.J. and Murphy, G.F. (1986) Lymphocyte subsets and Langerhans' cells in TEN. Report of a case. *Arch. Dermatol.*, **122**, 455–8.
53. Garabiol, B. and Touraine, R. (1976) Syndrome de Lyell de l'adulte éléments de pronostic et déductions thérapeutiques. Etude de 27 cas. *Ann. Med. Intern. (Paris).*, **127**, 670–2.
54. Halebian, P.H., Corder, V.J., Madden, M.R., *et al.* (1986) Improved burn center survival of patients with toxic epidermal necrolysis managed without corticosteroids. *Ann. Surg.*, **204**, 503–12.
55. Kamanabroo, D., Schmitz-Langraf, W. and Czarnetzki, B.M. (1985) Plasmapheresis in severe drug-induced toxic epidermal necrolysis. *Arch. Dermatol.*, **121**, 1548–9.
56. Ruocco, V., Bimonte, D., Luongo, C. and Florio, M. (1986) Hyperbaric oxygen treatment of toxic epidermal necrolysis. *Cutis*, **38**, 267–71.
57. Heimbach, D.M., Engrav, L.H., Marvin, J.A., Harnar, T.J. and Grube, B.J. (1987) Toxic epidermal necrolysis. A step forward in treatment. *J. Amer. Med. Assoc.*, **257**, 2171–5.
58. Pruitt, B.A. (1987) Burn treatment for the unburned. *J. Amer. Med. Assoc.*, **257**, 2207–8.
59. Westly, E.D. and Wechsler, H.L. (1984) Toxic epidermal necrolysis, granulocytic leukopenia as a pronostic indicator. *Arch. Dermatol.*, **120**, 721–6.
60. Kopf, A.W., Grupper, C., Baer, R.L., *et al.* (1977) Eruptive melanocytic nevi after severe bullous disease. *Arch. Dermatol.*, **113**, 1080–4.
61. Roujeau, J.-C., Phlippoteau, C., Koso, M., *et al.* (1985) Sequelles oculaires et syndrome sec au decours du syndrome de Lyell. *Ann. Dermatol. Venereol.*, **112**, 883–8.

17.3 FIXED DRUG ERUPTION (FDE)

17.3.1 Introduction

Fixed drug eruption is the only skin condition always provoked by drugs or chemicals. The first observation was reported by Brocq [1] and attributed to antipyrine. These are usually one or a few rounded lesions typically evolving as erythema, blister and residual pigmentation. Recurrences on the same site(s) after each ingestion of the offending drug are a hallmark of the disease. Local immunological memory is probably involved. Rare generalized bullous forms may be difficult to differentiate from TEN.

17.3.2 Presentation

(a) Age and sex

FDE occurs at all ages, most patients being between 20 and 40 years old [2–4]. A male preponderance is noted in some series [2, 4, 5], but the real sex ratio is unknown.

(b) Frequency and geographical distribution

Incidence of FDE varies widely between countries. It is relatively common in Northern Europe, Africa and India but quite rare in France. Negroids may be more susceptible to FDE than Caucasoids [2]. In Finland FDE is the second most common type of cutaneous drug reaction accounting for 21% of patients hospitalized for skin drug reactions [6].

17.3.3 Cutaneous distribution

Fixed drug eruption may occur anywhere on the skin and mucous membranes [2, 7]. Extremities are more often involved than the trunk, the most common sites being the face, the arms and the genitalia. A solitary lesion is usual at first, new lesions occurring sometimes with repeated attacks. Most patients have less than five lesions. Occasionally large and numerous lesions may involve a significant part of the body surface (16 out of 92 cases in Kauppinen's recent series [8]).

17.3.4 Mucous membrane involvement

It occurs, alone or together with skin lesions, in 30–50% of cases. Lips and genitalia are the favourite sites, often in continuity with skin involvement. Acute lesions of mucous membranes are well-defined erosions sometimes surrounded by an erythematous halo.

17.3.5 Morphology of lesions

Lesions begin 15 min to 2 h after ingestion of the drug with localized itching or a burning sensation, followed by the appearance in 1–8 h of round or oval oedematous red patches of varying size (usually a few centimetres). Blisters occur on the patches in about 30% of cases [3] (Figure 17.12), other cases showing eczematous changes or desquamation. The lesions resolve in 1–3 weeks, usually leaving a well-demarcated ashy-grey hyperpigmentation (Figure 17.13). A new drug challenge will induce inflammatory changes on the previously involved sites with occasional appearance of new lesions.

17.3.6 Genetics

No genetic predisposition is known.

17.3.7 Differential diagnosis

Pigmented patches following erythema and/or blisters are often due to phototoxic reactions from

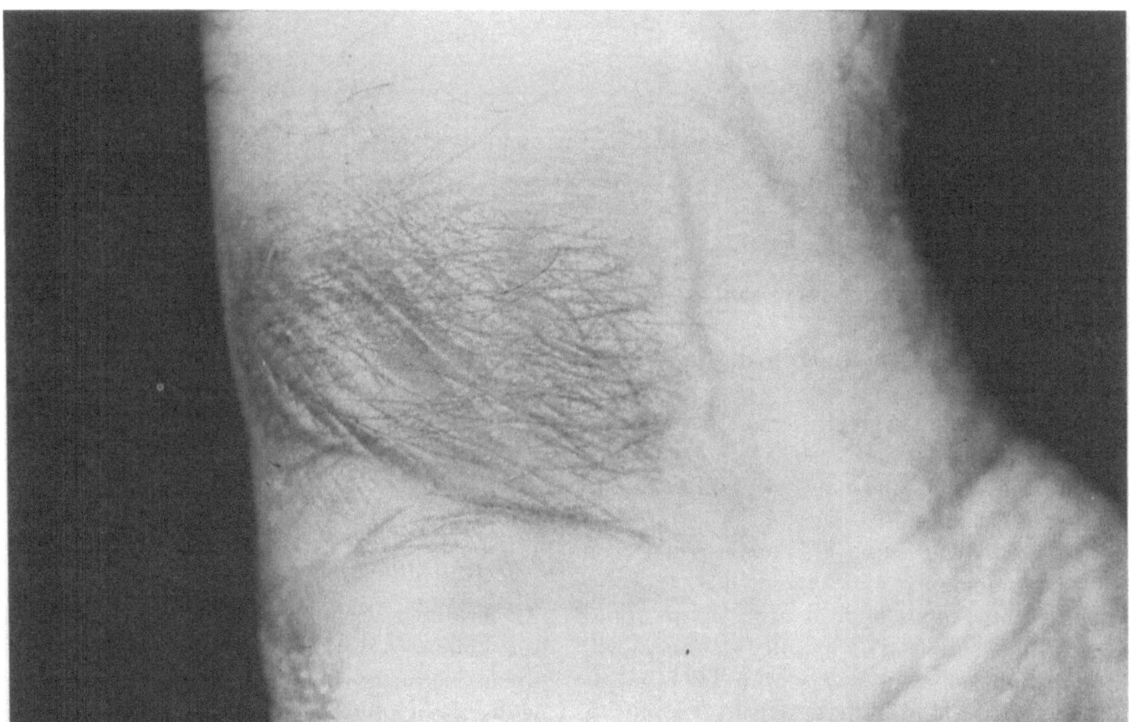

Figure 17.12 Active lesion of fixed drug eruption.

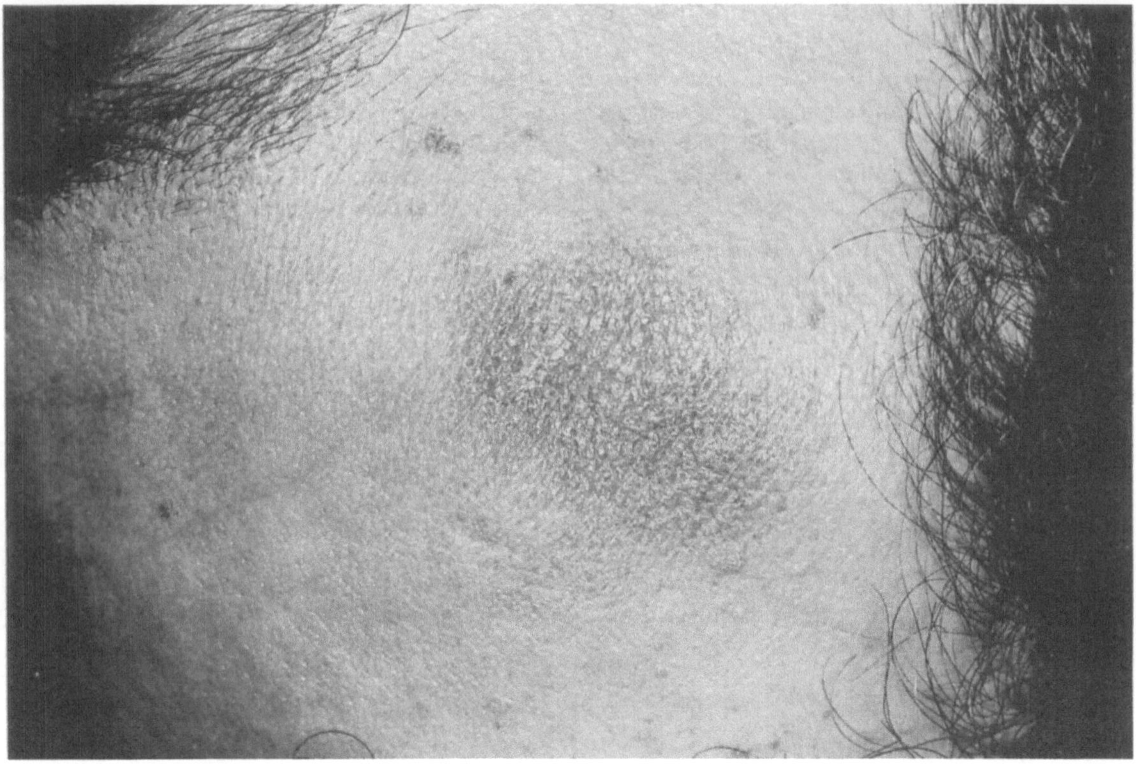

Figure 17.13 Residual pigmentation after fixed drug eruption.

contact with plants or bergamot containing perfumes. The flowing or bizarre distribution is different from the well-demarcated round or oval pattern of FDE.

Drug-induced hyperpigmentation (phenothiazines, amiodarone etc.) is not as well demarcated as FDE and a history of inflammatory flare-up is lacking.

The history will help to differentiate FDE from the post-inflammatory hyperpigmentation of lichen planus, lupus erythematosus or morphea. Generalized bullous FDE is often confused with Stevens–Johnson syndrome or with TEN, but the history of previous blisters, paucity of mucous membrane erosions, good general health and absence of erythema multiforme-like skin lesions support a diagnosis of FDE [3].

17.3.8 Investigations

(a) Laboratory findings

A mild to moderate leucocytosis, occasional hypereosinophilia and hypergammaglobulinaemia are the only changes [7].

(b) Histopathology

The histological pattern of FDE is not specific and very similar to those of EM or TEN [3, 7]. During the active phase the upper dermis is oedematous with a slight infiltrate, mainly of mononuclear cells. Most changes occur within the epidermis with exocytosis, appearance of dyskeratotic cells and degeneration of basal cells resulting in epidermal cleavage. Pigmentary incontinence is usual and in the late phases melanin-loaded macrophages are found in the upper dermis. Immunofluorescence microscopy studies are negative or non-specific [7, 9].

(c) Tests for assessing drug responsibility

With the exception of the potentially life-threatening generalized bullous forms, oral challenge is widely considered as harmless and as the best proof of the drug responsible [3–8]. A refractory period may follow acute exacerbations for a few weeks [2, 7]. Doses equivalent to one-quarter or one-half of a single therapeutic dose are often enough to elicit the eruption. If the test is negative after 24 h a larger dose may be given. Oral challenge is positive in more than 95% of cases [3–8].

Skin tests have given less consistent results [7, 10]. They are always negative on uninvolved skin. On the sites of previous eruptions, patch tests are often positive, with erythema occurring from 30 min to 18 h after testing [11]. The percentage of positive reactions is increased to 75% by using vehicles that increase penetration of the drug [11].

Lymphocytes from FDE patients underwent blast transformation when both the causative drugs and autologous sera were added to the culture medium [12]. The diagnostic value of such *in vitro* testing has not been further assessed.

17.3.9 Systemic manifestations and associated diseases

Systemic manifestations are unusual. Fever occurs in 10–20% of localized forms, more frequently in generalized bullous forms, sometimes with general malaise, abdominal cramps or diarrhoea, but without severe systemic symptoms [7]. There is no reported association with other diseases.

17.3.10 Pathogenesis and recent advances

(a) Drugs causing FDE

More than 70 substances have been blamed for causing FDE [7]. The most common are barbiturates, phenazones, sulphonamides, cyclines, dapsone, phenolphthalein, aspirin and paracetamol [2–5, 8, 13]. The relative frequency of these drugs varies in the main series, probably reflecting geographical variations in prescribing habits. In a recent series phenazones had ranked first with 42% of cases, and barbiturates second with 26% [8]. Cross-reactivity is not uncommon within the same class of drugs (cyclines or phenazones). Sensitization to several drugs may occur, occasionally each inducing a flare-up in different sites [14].

(b) Pathogenesis

FDE is generally held to be an immunological reaction to drugs, as suggested by the 'memory' evidenced by oral or local challenge tests. In fact its pathogenesis remains unclear [7, 10]. Several autotransplantation studies between normal and involved skin have given variable responses to the question of whether the 'memory' for the reaction stays in the epidermis or in the dermis. Autoradiographic studies have failed to detect persistent drug in post-lesional skin.

Recent immunohistochemical studies [9] showed that both CD4- and CD8- positive T lymphocytes were represented among the dermal mononuclear cells, CD8-positive cells appearing to be more active in exocytosis, and that keratinocytes expressed HLA DR in some lesions. The most distinctive observation was the finding of a remnant suprabasal band of CD8-positive lymphocytes in healed skin 3 weeks after challenge [9]. These cells could be responsible for the 'memory' function.

In addition to these findings, pointing to a probable role for T lymphocytes, previous studies have suggested involvement of serum factors. Maximal lymphocyte proliferation *in vitro* in the presence of the causative drug required the addition of autologous serum obtained during the acute phase [12]. 'Acute phase serum' also induced inflammatory changes when subsequently injected into healed lesions, but not in normal skin [15]. The serum factors (metabolites of the drug, mediators, lymphokines etc.) responsible have not been identified.

17.3.11 Treatment

Corticosteroid therapy has been proposed for the severe forms. However, oral corticosteroids failed to prevent recurrence in some cases and did not help patients with generalized FDE [8].

17.3.12 Prognosis and sequelae

The only sequelae are long-lasting pigmented patches. Even generalized bullous FDE carries a good prognosis in contrast with TEN. Fatalities have occurred but are exceptional [3]. It is hard to understand how a widespread destruction of the epidermis can have so good a prognosis, unless fatal cases are classified as TEN rather than as FDE.

References

1. Brocq, L. (1894) Eruption érythémato-pigmentée fixe due à l'antipyrine. *Ann. Dermatol. Syphil. (Paris)*, **5**, 308–13.
2. Browne, S.G. (1964) Fixed eruption in deeply pigmented subjects: clinical observations on 350 patients. *Brit. Med. J.*, **2**, 1041–4.
3. Kauppinen, K. (1972) Cutaneous reactions to drugs with special reference to severe bullous mucocutaneous eruptions and sulphonamides. *Acta. Dermatovenereol. (Stockholm)*, **52** (Suppl. 68).
4. Sehgal, V.N. (1974) Causes of fixed drug eruptions. *Dermatologica*, **148**, 120–3.
5. Kanwar, A.J., Bharija, S.C. and Belhaj, M.S. (1986) Fixed drug eruptions in children; a series of 23 cases with provocative tests. *Dermatologica*, **172**, 315–18.
6. Kauppinen, K. and Stubb, S. (1984) Drug eruptions: causative agents and clinical types. *Acta Dermatovenereol.*, **64**, 320–4.
7. Korkij, W. and Soltani, K. (1984) Fixed drug eruption, a brief review. *Arch. Dermatol.*, **120**, 520–4.
8. Kauppinen, K. and Stubb, S. (1985) Fixed eruptions: causative drugs and challenge tests. *Brit. J. Dermatol.*, **112**, 575–8.
9. Hindsen, M., Christensen, O.B., Gruic, V. and Löfberg, H. (1987) Fixed drug eruption: an immunohistochemical investigation of the acute and healing phase. *Brit. J. Dermatol.*, **116**, 351–60.
10. Ackroyd, J.F. (1985) Fixed drug eruptions. *Brit. Med. J.*, **290**, 1533–4.
11. Alanko, K., Stubb, S. and Reitamo, S. (1987) Topical provocation of fixed drug eruption. *Brit. J. Dermatol.*, **116**, 561–7.
12. Gimenez-Camarasa, J.M., Garcia-Calderon, P. and De Moragas, J.M. (1975) Lymphocyte transformation test in fixed drug eruption. *New Engl. J. Med.*, **292**, 819–21.
13. Pasrisha, J.S. (1979) Drugs causing fixed eruptions. *Brit. J. Dermatol.*, **100**, 183–5.
14. Pasrisha, J.S. and Shukla, S.R. (1979) Independent lesions of fixed eruption due to two unrelated drugs in the same patient. *Brit. J. Dermatol.*, **101**, 361–2.
15. Wyatt, E., Greaves, M. and Søndergaard, J. (1972) Fixed drug eruption (phenolphthalein): evidence for a blood-borne mediator. *Arch. Dermatol.*, **106**, 671–3.

Eighteen
Bullous eruption of systemic lupus erythematosus

W. Ray Gammon and Robert A. Briggaman

18.1 INTRODUCTION

Chronic vesiculobullous eruptions are relatively uncommon in systemic lupus erythematosus (SLE). Their incidence among patients with skin lesions has been estimated at less than 5% [1–3]. Blistering eruptions in SLE can be divided into three categories. The first includes a number of primary blistering diseases that have been reported in association with SLE. These include bullous pemphigoid (BP) [4–9], dermatitis herpetiformis (DH) [10–14], pemphigus vulgaris/foliaceous [15–20], epidermolysis bullosa acquisita (EBA) [21, 22], erythema multiforme [23, 24], porphyria cutanea tarda [25], toxic epidermal necrolysis [26] and dystrophic epidermolysis bullosa [27]. Each of these diseases has its own diagnostic features and the association with SLE is generally regarded as fortuitous and not a specific manifestation of SLE. Many of the primary blistering diseases are associated with autoimmune features that may be difficult to distinguish from the cutaneous immunological features of SLE. These similarities may cause problems in establishing the diagnosis of a primary blistering eruption in a patient with SLE.

A second category includes blisters that occur within specific LE skin lesions. Specific LE lesions demonstrate characteristic histopathological changes that include vacuolization of basal keratinocytes and a mononuclear leucocyte infiltrate in the upper dermis [28]. Morphological examples of these lesions include: maculopapular and plaque-like erythemas, e.g. malar erythema, discoid LE, and the papulosquamous and annular erythemas, characteristic of subacute cutaneous LE. Although specific LE lesions typically do not vesiculate, microscopic dermo–epidermal separation and less often clinically apparent blistering may occur [28]. This category of blisters is regarded as an uncommon but specific manifestation of SLE. The blisters do not have the diagnostic features of primary bullous diseases and do not appear to arise on skin that is not simultaneously affected by specific LE lesions.

Recently a third, relatively distinctive, type of blistering eruption has been described. Names that have been used for the eruption include bullous eruption of SLE, bullous SLE, vesiculobullous SLE and SLE with herpetiform blisters. Blisters in this disorder do not arise within specific LE lesions but, as in the primary blistering diseases, arise *de novo* on clinically normal appearing skin.

The disorder is defined by its clinical, pathological and immunopathological features which include: a diagnosis of SLE by criteria of the American Rheumatism Association; a chronic widespread blistering eruption; a subepidermal blister with acute neutrophil-predominant inflammation in the upper dermis; immunoglobulin (Ig) and complement deposits at the basement membrane zone (BMZ) by direct immunofluorescence and immune deposits on and/or beneath the lamina densa by immunoelectron microscopy [29, 30]. In addition, the eruption in most patients appears to respond dramatically to the sulphone compound, dapsone [29]. Although some features of the eruption are seen in some primary blistering diseases, the combination is relatively unique and not typical of any of the primary bullous diseases. For this reason, bullous eruption of SLE has been regarded as a specific manifestation of SLE rather than the coexistence of SLE and a primary bullous disease.

Although all patients share diagnostic clinical, pathological and immunopathological features, there are differences in the immunohistology that suggest the disorder may be heterogeneous. Furthermore, recent studies have shown that some patients have immunological features that are indistinguishable from those found in patients with EBA.

18.2 CLINICAL FEATURES

18.2.1 Presentation: age, sex, frequency

The first case of bullous eruption of SLE was reported in 1973 by Pedro and Dahl [31]. They described a 17-year-old female who presented with a widespread bullous eruption and subsequently developed clinical and serological features of SLE. The blisters did not arise within specific skin lesions of SLE. A biopsy of one of the blisters did not show histopathological features of specific LE lesions but showed a subepidermal blister and neutrophilic microabscesses in dermal papillae similar to the histological features of DH. Direct immunofluorescent studies showed a heavy band of granular IgG and IgA deposits along the BMZ and not granular–fibrillar deposits of IgA in dermal papillae typical of DH. Other features that were atypical for DH included a response to steroids and oral blisters.

Since the report by Pedro and Dahl, 19 additional cases have been reported [29–38]. Among these 20 cases, the mean age is 22 years with a range of 15–51 years. Over half the cases have been in patients less than 30 years old and about one-third have been in patients age 20 or less. Approximately 75% of patients have been female and 70% have been black. One oriental patient has been reported. The age, sex and ethnic distribution appears to be the same as in SLE in general.

Although the disease appears to be relatively rare, it is probably not as rare as the small number of reported cases suggests. In our experience, it has been the most common cause of a chronic blistering eruption in SLE. The disorder has only recently been recognized and since it shares a number of features with BP and DH, it is likely that cases have been reported as the coexistence of SLE and either BP or DH.

18.2.2 Cutaneous distribution, mucous membrane involvement and morphology of lesions

The clinical features of the eruption are not diagnostic. Primary lesions include vesicles, bullae and maculopapular erythemas (Figure 18.1) Blisters may arise on clinically normal appearing (non-erythematous) skin but are often preceded by erythema. Blisters tend to be tense and not easily ruptured but when they do, leave erosions and crusts. Healing may be associated with temporary postinflammatory hyper- or hypo-pigmentation but scarring is not a typical feature. Skin fragility which may accompany pemphigus or EBA is not a feature.

Variability in the distribution of lesions is a feature. In most cases blisters are widespread. In some cases, they are more numerous on sun-exposed sites but in no case are they confined to those sites [30]. Some patients have grouped vesicles over extensor surfaces similar to the morphology and distribution of lesions in DH. In most of these cases blisters have also been present on non-extensor surfaces. In other cases, the clinical picture is dominated by relatively large blisters (bullae) on the trunk and flexural surfaces. The size and distribution of lesions in these cases closely mimic BP. Involvement of oral mucous membranes has been described in about one-third of patients. The most prominent symptom is pruritus which may be severe.

Interestingly most patients do not have other cutaneous manifestations of SLE. Malar erythema, non-scarring alopecia and photosensitivity have been noted in only a few cases. Discoid LE lesions and the annular and papulosquamous erythemas associated with subacute cutaneous LE have not been reported.

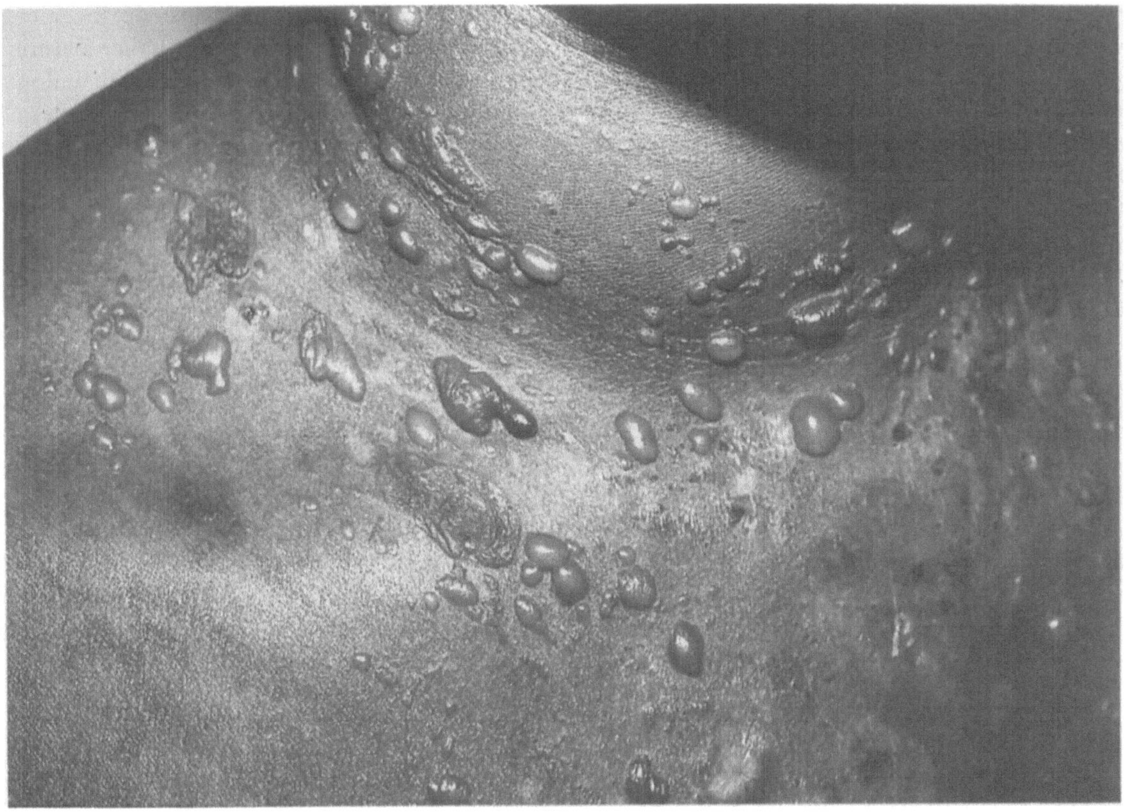

Figure 18.1 Neck and upper chest showing tense vesiculobullous lesions in a patient with SLE.

18.3 DIFFERENTIAL DIAGNOSIS

Making the diagnosis of bullous eruption of SLE generally does not present serious difficulties if the patient meets diagnostic criteria for SLE and the cutaneous eruption is evaluated by histological, direct immunohistological, serological and immunoelectron microscopic methods. In patients with a linear pattern of immune reactant deposition at the BMZ, the major differential consideration is the coexistence of SLE and BP. Although this association has never been proven, it has been reported [4–9]. If the patient has a circulating anti-BMZ antibody, it can be tested by indirect immunofluorescence on NaCl-separated skin to determine whether it has the binding features of BP or EBA antibodies. In the absence of a circulating antibody, direct immunoelectron microscopy is required to determine if the immune deposits are located on and beneath the lamina densa as in bullous eruption of SLE or in the lamina lucida as in BP.

In patients with a granular pattern of deposits containing IgA, the major differential consideration is DH [29]. Exclusion of coexistent DH and SLE may be difficult and requires careful consideration of the clinical, pathological, and immunological features of both diseases. Dermatitis herpetiformis is characterized clinically by pruritic grouped vesicles on an erythematous base distributed over extensor skin surfaces. Flexural skin lesions, mucosal lesions and large bullae which are frequent in bullous eruption of SLE are rare in DH. Both diseases may respond dramatically to dapsone but the response is not as consistent in bullous eruption of SLE. Dermatitis herpetiformis invariably re-activates when dapsone is withdrawn and probably persists for life, while bullous eruption of SLE is a more limited disease and may not recur after cessation of dapsone therapy. Cutaneous histology may not be helpful since both diseases are characterized by sub-epidermal blisters and neutrophilic micro-abscesses in the papillary dermis. Most patients with DH have a granular pattern of IgA deposits in the papillary dermis but in some cases the deposits may be distributed along the length of the BMZ. In bullous eruption of SLE the deposits are always distributed along the BMZ. Immunoglobulins other than IgA are rarely seen in DH while they are always seen in bullous eruption in SLE. The presence of other Igs with granular IgA deposits would not exclude a diagnosis of coexistent DH and SLE since deposits due to both diseases could be present simultaneously and overlap the same region of the basement membrane. Other features of DH which are not found in patients with bullous eruption of SLE include gluten-sensitive entero-pathy and dermopathy and a very high incidence of the HLA phenotypes, B8 and DR3.

18.4 INVESTIGATIONS

18.4.1 Histology

One of the most consistent features of the eruption is the cutaneous histopathology. It is remarkable both for its similarity to the histology of DH and linear IgA disease and its dissimilarity to the histology of non-bullous LE lesions [29]. The changes described in early lesions include dermo–

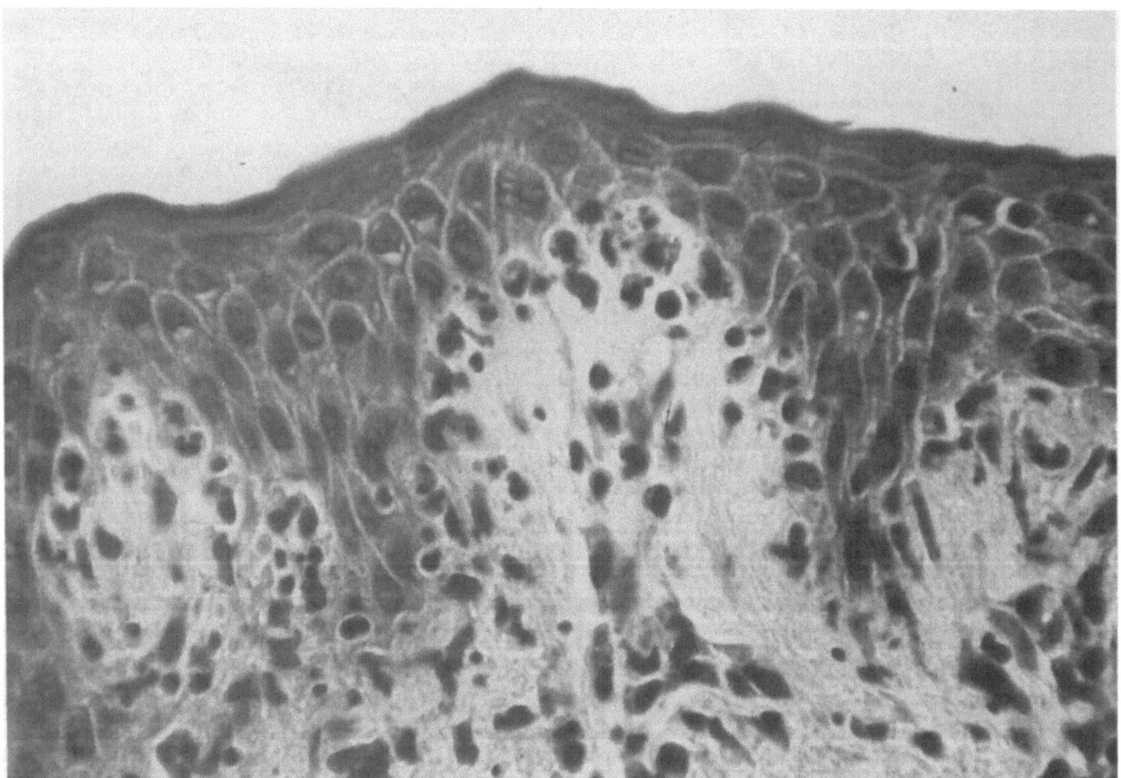

Figure 18.2 Routine histology of an early lesion showing neutrophils beneath the BMZ in dermal papillae (× 400).

epidermal separation at the BMZ with a relatively intact epidermis and an acute inflammatory infiltrate mainly composed of neutrophils in the upper dermis and at the BMZ. In many cases the inflammatory infiltrate is accentuated in dermal papillae similar to DH (Figure 18.2). In some cases, the infiltrate is more evenly distributed along the BMZ similar to lesions in linear IgA disease. In addition to neutrophils, the infiltrate may include mononuclear cells and eosinophils. The histological features characteristic of non-bullous LE lesions, i.e. basal keratinocyte vacuolization and mononuclear cell-predominant inflammation, are not characteristic of bullous eruption of SLE. In a few cases, vasculitis characterized by neutrophils invading vessel walls, leucocytoclasis and fibrin deposition has been described in papillary venules and in the upper dermal venular plexus [29]. This is not a consistent finding and it appears unlikely that the eruption is due to a vasculitis. The typical clinical features of vasculitis such as purpura, dermal necrosis and ulceration are not features of bullous eruption of SLE. To date there are no reports on the ultrastructural changes in lesions by scanning electron microscopy.

18.4.2 Direct immunofluorescence

Direct immunofluorescent studies show that deposits of Ig and complement proteins at the BMZ are a characteristic feature of the eruption. The deposits have been described in lesional or perilesional skin in all cases and at sites distant from lesions in all but one case. All the major Ig classes (IgG, IgA and IgM) have been detected. In most cases the deposits consist of more than one Ig class

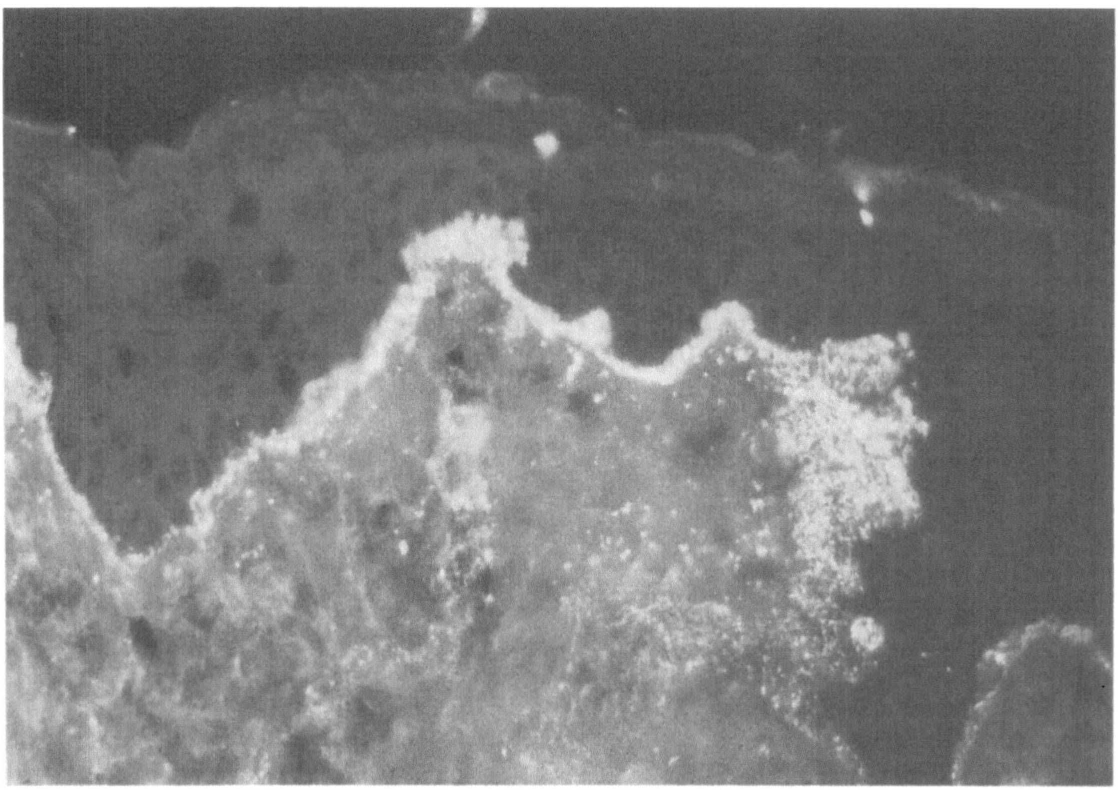

Figure 18.3 Direct immunofluorescence of perilesional skin showing granular IgG deposits in the upper dermis and at the BMZ (× 400).

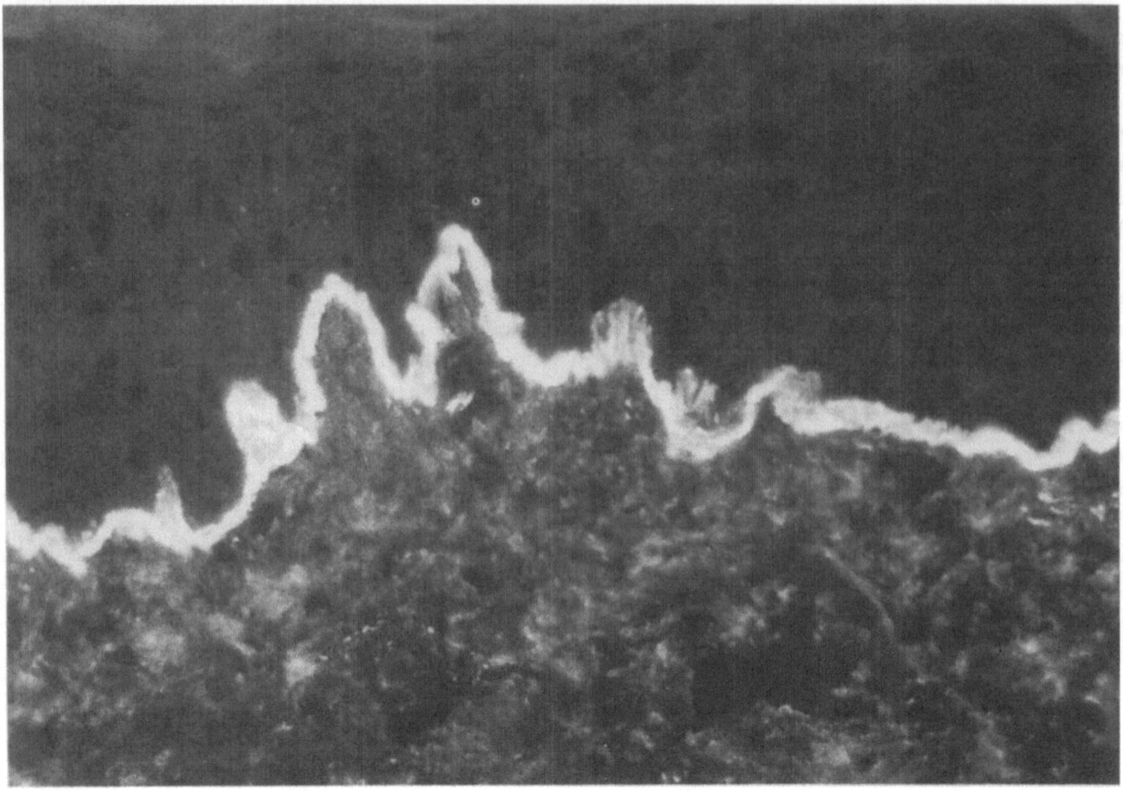

Figure 18.4 Direct immunofluorescence of perilesional skin showing linear IgG deposits at the BMZ (× 400).

and in many cases they consist of all three. Immunoglobulin G has been detected in all cases, IgA in two-thirds and IgM in half.

Two major patterns of immune reactant deposition are described. In about 40% of cases, the pattern is granular, fibrillar or thready and indistinguishable from the pattern seen in most SLE patients without blisters (Figure 18.3). In the majority, the pattern is linear-homogeneous (Figure 18.4). This pattern is characterized by a relatively broad band in most cases. In some the band is narrow and ribbon-like, resembling the pattern in primary bullous diseases associated with anti-BMZ autoantibodies (bullous and cicatricial pemphigoid, herpes gestationis, EBA). Interestingly, IgG has been the predominant Ig in all patients with the linear-homogeneous pattern of deposits.

An important question is whether the deposits are a primary feature of the bullous eruption or a consequence of SLE. Undoubtedly, some of the deposits in some patients are present as a consequence of SLE since most patients with that disease are characterized by cutaneous immune reactants. However, several lines of evidence suggest deposits are also due to the blistering eruption. There is a very high incidence of deposits in patients with bullous eruption of SLE compared to patients with SLE alone. The observation that all patients with the bullous eruption have deposits in lesional and/or perilesional skin and all but one have deposits in skin sites distant from lesions contrasts with the incidence (50–75%) of cutaneous immune deposits in clinically normal appearing skin in the general SLE population [39–47]. In addition, there is a higher incidence of IgG and IgA deposits among patients with the bullous eruption. Immunoglobulin G and IgA occur in 100% and 67% respectively of patients with the bullous eruption. Data compiled from 239 patients with non-bullous SLE show that the incidence of IgG varies from 28 to 85% with a mean of 42% and the incidence of IgA varies from 0 to 28% with a mean of 14% [39–47]. Additional evidence is the finding that most patients have a linear pattern of immune reactant deposition. That pattern has rarely been reported in non-bullous SLE [48, 49]. The most convincing evidence is the recent finding that circulating anti-BMZ antibodies are a feature in some patients (*infra vide*).

18.4.3 Direct immunoelectron microscopy

The results of immunoelectron microscopy have been reported in a few patients with linear immune deposits [29, 32, 34, 35, 37]. These studies show that the deposits in most patients are located on and just beneath the lamina densa (Figure 18.5). In two patients, the reactants were found in the upper dermis just beneath the lamina densa [29]. In neither case can the deposits be distinguished from those in EBA and those reported in some patients with cutaneous and systemic forms of non-bullous LE, but they can easily be distinguished from the lamina lucida deposits in patients with pemphigoid [50–52].

18.4.4 Anti-BMZ antibodies

In recent studies, we detected circulating anti-BMZ antibodies in sera of four of five

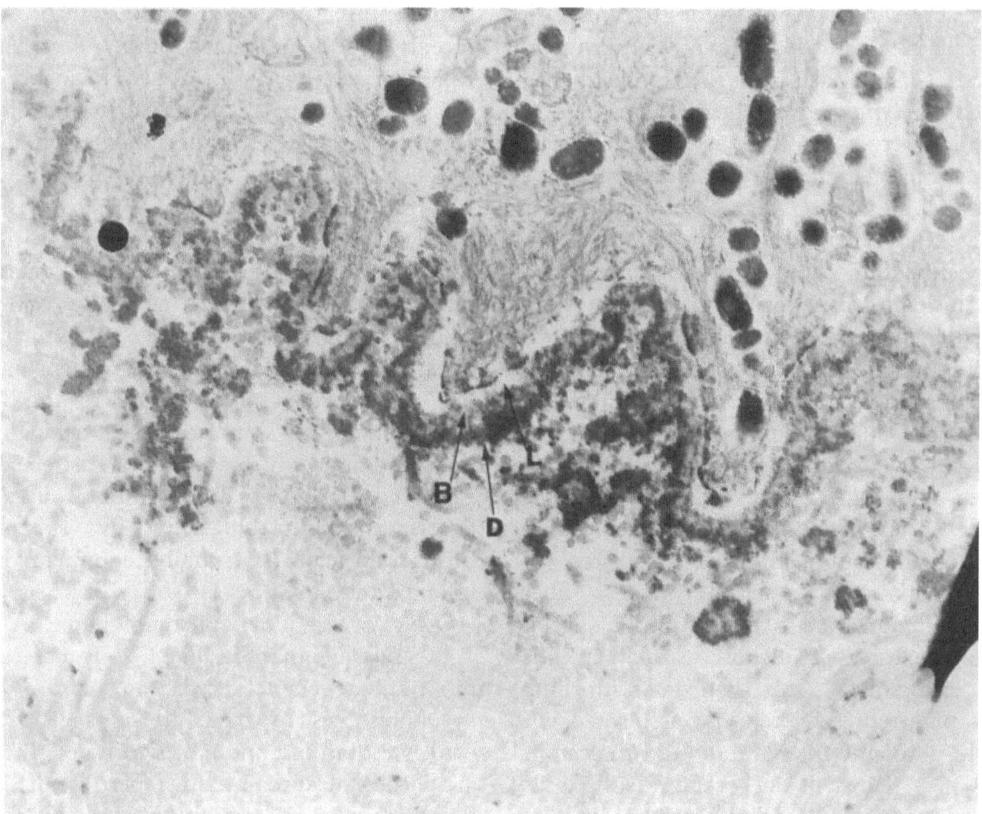

Figure 18.5 Immunoelectron micrograph of perilesional skin showing IgG deposits (D) on and just beneath the lamina densa (B). No deposits are in the lamina lucida (L) (× 22 000).

patients using modified indirect immunofluorescent techniques [35]. When the sera were examined by indirect immunofluorescence on cryostat sections of fresh frozen normal human skin, antinuclear staining of keratinocytes and fibroblasts was observed but no staining of the BMZ was seen. However, when the sera were examined on skin in which the BMZ had been separated through the lamina lucida by incubation in 1.0 M NaCl (NaCl-separated skin), IgG bound to the dermal side of the BMZ. The titres of IgG anti-BMZ antibodies in the sera ranged from 1:40 to 1:160.

In studies using indirect immunoelectron microscopy and immunoblotting, we found that the anti-BMZ autoantibodies bound on and just beneath the lamina densa and reacted with 290- and 145-kDa autoantigens extracted from normal human dermis–lamina densa. These findings were the same as previously reported for EBA antibodies [35–53]. The 290- and 145- kDa proteins extracted from dermis-lamina densa have subsequently been identified as type VII collagen suggesting that autoantibodies to type VII collagen are a feature of EBA and some patients with bullous eruption of SLE and that the linear pattern of immune deposits at the BMZ may be a marker for those patients [54]. We have now found autoantibodies with features indistinguishable from EBA antibodies in six of seven patients with bullous eruption of SLE who had linear immune deposits at the BMZ.

Several patients with granular deposits have been examined for circulating anti-BMZ antibodies, including one examined by us using NaCl-separated skin, and the antibodies could not be detected. This finding, coupled with the observation that bullous diseases associated with anti-BMZ antibodies generally have a linear pattern of immune deposits at the BMZ, suggests there may be at least two subsets of patients with bullous eruption of SLE. Patients with linear deposits may represent a subset associated with anti-BMZ autoantibodies and those with granular deposits may represent one or more subsets not associated with those antibodies. However, the possibility that some or all patients with the granular pattern might also have anti-BMZ autoantibodies cannot be excluded simply on the basis of immunofluorescent pattern. Several studies have reported eluting anti-BMZ antibodies of undefined antigenic specificity from the cutaneous deposits in a number of patients with non-bullous SLE and most of those patients had a granular pattern of immune reactant deposition [55–57]. In addition, there is evidence that some patients with non-bullous SLE and granular immune deposits have circulating anti-BMZ antibodies [58, 59].

Patients with bullous eruption of SLE and anti-BMZ autoantibodies can be viewed as the coexistence of SLE and EBA. They have the diagnostic features of EBA including a chronic acquired blistering eruption involving skin and mucous membranes, a subepidermal blister histologically, linear deposits of Ig (predominantly IgG) and complement proteins at the BMZ, immune deposits on and beneath the lamina densa and circulating and tissue deposited autoantibodies with features of EBA antibodies [50]. We have recently shown that both disorders are characterized by an increased incidence of the class II HLA antigen, DR2, suggesting that both share common genetic traits that may predispose to the development of autoimmunity to the BMZ [60].

If one assumes the disease is the coexistence of SLE and EBA, then it would appear that SLE influences the expression of EBA. Patients with bullous eruption of SLE are generally younger than those with EBA, have an eruption of much shorter duration, respond dramatically to dapsone which has not been observed in EBA, and are not characterized by skin fragility and healing with scars and milia which are characteristic features of EBA. Furthermore, although both diseases are characterized histologically by subepidermal blisters, the acute neutrophil-predominant DH-like inflammation which is so typical of bullous eruption of SLE is very uncommon in EBA.

It is possible that SLE like EBA is a disease with an immunogenetic predisposition to develop autoantibodies to type VII collagen. There is evidence that autoantibodies to type VII collagen are part of the autoantibody repertoire of SLE [35]. Furthermore, it has been shown that the ultrastructural location of BMZ immune deposits in some patients with non-bullous LE is indistinguishable from that seen in patients with

EBA and bullous eruption of SLE with anti-BMZ antibodies [51]. It is conceivable that under circumstances of abnormal immune regulation which is characteristic of SLE, some patients produce anti-type VII collagen autoantibodies which in turn cause a bullous eruption that shares immunological features with EBA but which is expressed differently due to factors peculiar to the host or SLE.

18.5 PATHOGENESIS

The pathogenesis of blisters in bullous eruption of SLE is unclear. The histology would suggest that inflammation is responsible. The cause of inflammation is not known. One reasonable hypothesis is that inflammation may be due to activation of the complement system by immune complexes at the BMZ. It is well known that immune complex activation of the complement system generates a number of complement by-products that can mediate several inflammatory responses [61]. One of those products, C5a, is derived from activation of C5 and can mediate directed migration (chemotaxis) and recruitment of leucocytes, and activate those cells to generate and release reactive oxygen intermediates and proteinases.

It has not been possible to demonstrate a direct cause and effect relationship between BMZ complex-mediated complement activation and inflammation in bullous eruption of SLE; however, in patients with the linear pattern of immune deposits, it has been possible to obtain quantitative data concerning the functional ability of the cutaneous complexes to activate complement at the BMZ and generate C5-derived inflammatory activity. This has been done using a method called complement-dependent neutrophil attachment [37]. When cryostat sections of fresh frozen skin containing complement-activating BMZ immune complexes are incubated with a source of complement (fresh normal human serum) and normal human peripheral blood neutrophils for 45 min at 37° C, neutrophils migrate and attach to the BMZ. After washing and staining, attachment is quantified by counting the number of cells along the BMZ. A number of control studies have shown that the number of cells migrating and attaching to the BMZ is proportional to the amount of complement activating immune complex at the BMZ and the dose of C5 in the system.

Using the method, we have examined complement-dependent neutrophil attachment in skin from normal humans and lesional and perilesional skin from several diseases with immune deposits at the BMZ including bullous eruption of SLE, non-bullous SLE, EBA patients with and without neutrophil-predominant inflammation and BP [37, 62, 63]. The results of those studies have shown that complexes in patients with bullous eruption of SLE generate high levels of complement-dependent neutrophil-attachment activity compared to complexes in patients with non-bullous SLE, EBA patients without neutrophil-predominant inflammation and BP (Figure 18.6). The only complexes that generate levels of activity equivalent to those in bullous eruption of SLE are those from EBA patients whose lesions show neutrophil-predominant inflammation. Although these studies do not prove that immune-complex-mediated complement activation and generation of

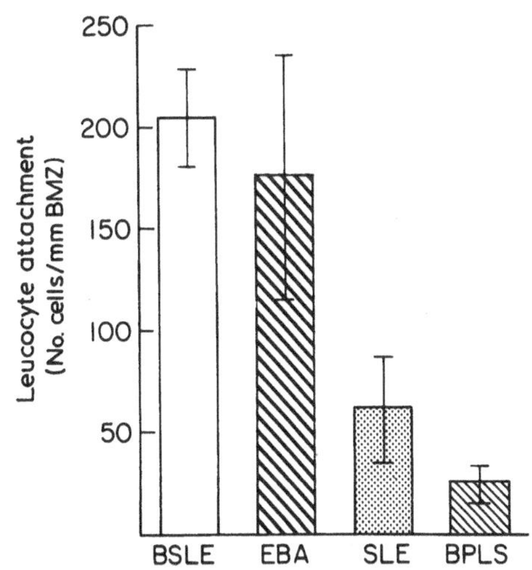

Figure 18.6 Comparison of leucocyte attachment mediated by BMZ immune complexes in perilesional skin from four patients with bullous eruption of SLE (BSLE), six patients with EBA, ten patients with non-bullous LE (SLE) and ten patients with bullous pemphigoid (BPLS). Results are means ± S.E.M.

C5-derived activity is responsible for inflammation in bullous eruption of SLE, they do show that the complexes are capable of expressing that function and that there is a strong relationship between complement-dependent neutrophil attachment and the presence of neutrophils in skin lesions.

In other studies, we have shown that incubating viable histologically normal split-thickness skin from a patient with active bullous eruption of SLE with complement and normal human neutrophils generates activity that causes neutrophils to penetrate the dermis and migrate to and accumulate at the BMZ [37]. With prolonged incubation the neutrophils cause separation of the BMZ.

Using similar methods we treated viable normal human skin with EBA autoantibodies in tissue culture and then incubated those tissues with neutrophils and complement [64]. In those cases, neutrophils migrated to the BMZ and caused dermo–epidermal separation.

Together, the above studies provide strong indirect evidence that in bullous eruption of SLE, anti-BMZ autoantibodies form complexes at the BMZ, activate the complement system and generate C5-derived chemotactic activity that subsequently recruits and activates neutrophils that contribute to blister formation.

18.6 TREATMENT

On the basis of the results of relatively few reported cases, the most consistently effective therapy is considered to be dapsone. The response is usually rapid and complete and patients may remain in remission after the drug is discontinued. The dosage and precautions regarding dapsone use in bullous eruption of SLE are the same as in DH; however, in the former, there should be intermittent attempts to discontinue the drug since a sustained drug-free remission may occur. In a few cases dapsone therapy has not been successful and may have made the systemic disease worse. Systemic glucocorticosteroids in doses of 1–2 mg/kg body weight have been reported as being either effective, partially effective or ineffective.

18.7 PROGNOSIS

The prognosis of the bullous eruption in patients with bullous eruption of SLE is good. The duration is variable but generally shorter than that of most chronic acquired bullous diseases. In some cases, it has lasted for only several weeks to a few months; in others, it has persisted for more than a year. The course may be characterized by spontaneous exacerbations and remissions.

In general, the patient's prognosis is influenced more by the systemic disease than the bullous eruption. For that reason, it is important to follow closely systemic disease activity. The relationship between the activity of the bullous disease and the systemic disease has been inconsistent. In a few cases, a close correlation has been reported, but in a number of others, no correlation has been seen. Although there may not be a close temporal correlation between the activities of the cutaneous and systemic disease, it appears that bullous eruption of SLE is often associated with more severe forms of SLE. This is suggested by the very high incidence of clinically significant glomerulonephritis (more than 90% of cases), antibodies to native DNA and hypocomplementaemia. Interestingly bullous eruption of SLE has not been reported in the milder forms of LE such as subacute cutaneous LE and chronic cutaneous LE.

ACKNOWLEDGEMENTS

This work was supported by NIH grants AR 30475 and AM 10546.

REFERENCES

1. Armas-Cruz, R., Harnecker, J., Ducach, G., Jalil, J. and Gonzalez, F. (1958) Clinical diagnosis of systemic lupus erythematosus. *Amer. J. Med.*, **25**, 409–19.
2. Tuffanelli, D.L. and Dubois, E. L. (1964) Cutaneous manifestations of systemic lupus erythematosus. *Arch. Dermatol.*, **90**, 377–86.
3. Rothfield, N. and Weissman, G. (1961) Bullae in systemic lupus erythematosus. *Arch. Int. Med.*, **107**, 174–80.
4. Jordan, R.E., Muller, S.A., Hale, W.L. and Beutner,

E.H. (1969) Bullous pemphigoid associated with systemic lupus erythematosus. *Arch. Dermatol.*, **99**, 17–25.

5. Miller, J.F., Downham, T.F., II and Chapel, T.A. (1978) Coexistent bullous pemphigoid and systemic lupus erythematosus. *Cutis*, **21**, 368–73.
6. Kumar, V., Binder, W.L., Schotland, E., Beutner, E.H. and Chorzelski, T.P. (1978) Coexistence of bullous pemphigoid and systemic lupus erythematosus. *Arch. Dermatol.*, **114**, 1187–90.
7. Szabó, E., Husz, S. and Kovács, L. (1981) Coexistent atypical bullous pemphigoid and systemic lupus erythematosus. *Brit. J. Dermatol.*, **104**, 71–5.
8. Clayton, C.A. and Burnham, T.K. (1982) Systemic lupus erythematosus and coexisting bullous pemphigoid: Immunofluorescent investigations. *J. Amer. Acad. Dermatol.*, **7**, 236–45.
9. Stoll, D.M. and King, L.E., Jr (1984) Association of bullous pemphigoid with systemic lupus erythematosus. *Arch. Dermatol.*, **120**, 362–6.
10. Moncada, B. (1974) Dermatitis herpetiformis. An association with systemic lupus erythematosus. *Arch. Dermatol.*, **109**, 723–5.
11. Meyer, A., Jenni, C. and Krebs, A. (1976) Diagnostische probleme beim gleichzeitgen auftreten von bullösen dermatosen and lupus erythematodes visceralis. *Dermatologica*, **153**, 57–64.
12. Davies, M.G., Marks, R. and Waddington, E. (1976) Simultaneous systemic lupus erythematosus and dermatitis herpetiformis. *Arch. Dermatol.*, **112**, 1292–4.
13. Aronson, A.J., Soltani, K., Aronson, I.K. and Ong, R.T. (1979) Systemic lupus erythematosus and dermatitis herpetiformis. *Arch. Dermatol.*, **115**, 68–70.
14. Thomas, J.R., III and Su, W.P.D. (1983) Concurrence of lupus erythematosus and dermatitis herpetiformis. A report of nine cases. *Arch. Dermatol.*, **119**, 740–5.
15. Blanchet, P.H., Auffret, N., Fauchard, J., *et al.* (1981) Association of thymoma with pemphigus foliaceous, nephrotic syndrome and lupus biology. *Ann. Dermatol. Venereol.*, **108**, 471.
16. Chorzelski, T.P., Jablonska, S. and Blaszezyk, M. (1968) Immunopathologic investigation on the Senear–Usher syndrome (coexistence of pemphigus and lupus erythematosus). *Brit. J. Dermatol.*, **80**, 211.
17. Kough, E. H. and Barnes, W.Y. (1964) Thymoma associated with erythroid aplasia, bullous skin eruption at the LE cell phenomenon. *Ann. Intern. Med.*, **61**, 308.
18. Somorin, A.O., Agbakwu, S.N. and Nwaefuna, A. (1981) Systemic lupus erythematosus and pemphigus vulgaris preceded by depressive psychosis. *Central Afr. J. Med.*, **27**, 12.
19. Ngo, A.W., Straka, C. and Fretzin, D. (1986) Pemphigus erythematosus: A unique association with systemic lupus erythematosus. *Cutis*, **38**., 160–3.
20. Cruz, P.D., Jr, Coldiron, B.M. and Sontheimer, R.D. (1987) Concurrent features of lupus erythematosus and pemphigus erythematosus following myasthenia gravis and thymoma. *J. Amer. Acad. Dermatol.*, **16**, 472–80.
21. Dotson, A.D., Raimer, S.S., Pursky, T.V. and Tschen, J. (1981) Systemic lupus erythematosus occurring in a patient with epidermolysis bullosa acquisita. *Arch. Dermatol.*, **117**, 422–6.
22. Palestine, R.F., Kossard, S. and Dicken, C.H. (1981) Epidermolysis bullosa acquisita: a heterogeneous disease. *J. Amer. Acad. Dermatol.*, **5**, 43–53.
23. Jablonska, S., Blaszczyk, M. and Jarzabek, M. (1971) Bullous erythema multiforme concomitant with lupus erythematosus in the light of immunofluorescent studies. *Polish Med. J.*, **10**, 773–81.
24. Rowell, N.R., Beck, J.S. and Anderson, G.R. (1963) Lupus erythematosus and erythema multiforme-like lesions. *Arch. Dermatol.*, **88**, 176.
25. Cram, D.L., Epstein, J.H. and Tuffanelli, D.L. (1973) Lupus erythematosus and porphyria. Coexistence in seven patients. *Arch. Dermatol.*, **108**, 779–84.
26. Braverman, I.M. (1981) in *Skin Signs of Systemic Disease*, 2nd edn, W.B. Saunders, Philadelphia, p. 287.
27. Archibald, G.C. (1976) Epidermolysis bullosa dystrophica and systemic lupus erythematosus. *Proc. R. Soc. Med.*, **69**, 881–3.
28. Gilliam, J.N. and Sontheimer, R.D. (1982) Subacute cutaneous lupus erythematosus. *Clin. Rheum. Dis.*, **8**, 343–52.
29. Hall, R.P., Lawley, T.J., Smith, H.R. and Katz, S.I. (1982) Bullous eruption of systemic lupus erythematosus. Dramatic response to Dapsone therapy. *Ann. Intern. Med.*, **197**, 165–70.
30. Camisa, C. and Sharma, H.M. (1983) Vesiculobullous systemic lupus erythematosus. *J. Amer. Acad. Dermatol.*, **9**, 924–33.
31. Pedro, S.D. and Dahl, M.V. (1973) Direct immunofluorescence of bullous systemic lupus erythematosus. *Arch. Dermatol.*, **107**, 118–20.
32. Olansky, A.J., Briggaman, R.A., Gammon, W.R., Kelly, T.F. and Sams, W.M., Jr. (1982) Bullous systemic lupus erythematosus. *J. Amer. Acad. Dermatol.*, **7**, 511–20.
33. Penneys, N.S. and Wiley, H.E., III (1979) Herpetiform blisters in systemic lupus erythematosus. *Arch. Dermatol.*, **115**, 1427–8.
34. Tani, M., Shimizu, R., Ban, M., Murata, Y. and Tamaki, A. (1984) Systemic lupus erythematosus with vesiculobullous lesions. Immunoelectron

microscopic studies. *Arch. Dermatol.*, **120**, 1497–501.
35. Gammon, W.R., Woodley, D.T., Dole, K.C. and Briggaman, R.A. (1985) Evidence that anti-basement membrane zone antibodies in bullous eruption of systemic lupus erythematosus recognize epidermolysis bullosa acquisita autoantigen. *J. Invest. Dermatol.*, **84**, 472–6.
36. Jacoby, R.A. and Abraham, A.A. (1979) Bullous dermatosis and systemic lupus erythematosus in a 15-year-old boy. *Arch. Dermatol.*, **115**, 1094–7.
37. Barton, D.D., Fine, J.D., Gammon, W.R. and Sams, W.M., Jr (1986) Bullous systemic lupus erythematosus: An unusual clinical course and detectable circulating autoantibodies to the epidermolysis bullosa acquisita antigen. *J. Amer. Acad. Dermatol.*, **15**, 369–73.
38. Gammon, W.R., Briggaman, R.A., Inman, A.O., III, Merritt, C.C. and Wheeler, C.E., Jr (1983) Evidence supporting a role for immune complex-mediated inflammation in the pathogenesis of bullous lesions of systemic lupus erythematosus. *J. Invest. Dermatol.*, **81**, 320–5.
39. Dantzig, P.I., Mauro, J., Rayhanzadeh, S. and Rudofsky, U.H. (1975) The significance of a positive cutaneous immunofluorescence test in systemic lupus erythematosus. *Brit. J. Dermatol.*, **93**, 531–7.
40. Morris, R.J., Guggenheim, S.J., McIntosh, R.M., Rubin, R.L. and Kohler, P.F. (1979) Simultaneous immunologic studies of skin and kidney in systemic lupus erythematosus. *Arthr. Rheum.*, **22**, 864–70.
41. Wertheimer, D. and Barland, P. (1976) Clinical significance of immune deposits in the skin in SLE. *Arthr. Rheum.*, **19**, 1249–55.
42. Noel, L.H., Droz, D. and Rothfield, N.F. (1978) Clinical and serologic significance of cutaneous deposits of immunoglobulins, C3, and Clq in SLE patients with nephritis. *Clin. Immunol. Immunopathol.*, **10**, 381–8.
43. Sontheimer, R.D. and Gilliam, J.N. (1979) a reappraisal of the relationship between subepidermal immunoglobulin deposits and DNA antibodies in systemic lupus erythematosus: A study using the Crithidai Luciliae immunofluorescence anti-DNA assay. *J. Invest. Dermatol.*, **72**, 29–32.
44. Halevy, S., Ben-Bassat, M., Joshua, H., Hazaz, B. and Feuerman, E.J. (1979) Immunofluorescent and electron-microscope findings in the uninvolved skin of patients with systemic lupus erythematosus. *Acta Dermatovenereol. (Stockholm)*, **59**, 427–33.
45. Brown, M.M. and Yount, W.J. (1980) Skin immunopathology in systemic lupus erythematosus. *J. Amer. Med. Assoc.*, **243**, 38–42.
46. Halberg, P., Ullman, S. and Jørgensen, F. (1982) The lupus band test as a measure of disease activity in systemic lupus erythematosus. *Arch. Dermatol.*, **118**, 572–6.
47. Bernstein, J.E., Soltani, K., Cristancho, N. and Aronson, A.J. (1983) Prognostic implications of cutaneous immunoglobulin deposits in systemic lupus erythematosus. *Int. J. Dermatol.*, **22**, 29–34.
48. Monroe, E.W. (1977) Lupus band test. *Arch. Dermatol.*, **113**, 830–4.
49. Harrist, T.J. and Mihm, M.C., Jr (1980) The specificity and clinical usefulness of the lupus band test. *Arthr. Rheum.*, **23**, 479–90.
50. Briggaman, R.A., Gammon, W.R. and Woodley, D.T. (1985) Epidermolysis bullosa acquisita of the immunopathological type (dermolytic pemphigoid). *J. Invest. Dermatol.*, **85**, 79s–84s.
51. Albini, B., Holubar, K., Shu, S. and Wolff, K. (1979) Enzyme antibody methods in immunodermatopathology. In *Immunopathology of the Skin* (eds E.H. Beutner, T.P. Chorzelski and S.F. Bean), John Wiley and Sons, New York, pp. 103–9.
52. Horiguchi. Y. and Imamura, S. (1986) Discrepancy between the localization of *in vivo* bound immunoglobulins in the skin and *in vitro* binding sites of circulating anti-BMZ antibodies in bullous pemphigoid: Immunoelectron microscopic studies. *J. Invest. Dermatol.*, **87**, 715–19.
53. Woodley, D.T., Briggaman, R.A., O'Keefe, E.J., Inman, A.O., Queen, L.L. and Gammon, W.R. (1984) Identification of the basement membrane autoantigen in epidermolysis bullosa acquisita. *New Engl. J. Med.*, **310**, 1007–13.
54. Woodley, D.T., Burgeson, R.E., Lunstrum, G.P., *et al.* (1987) The epidermolysis bullosa acquisita antigen is type VII procollagen. *Clin. Res.*, **35**, 726A.
55. Landry, M. and Sams, W.M., Jr (1973) Systemic lupus erythematosus: Studies of the antibodies bound to skin. *J. Clin. Invest.*, **52**, 1871–80.
56. Wierchowiecki, M.O., Quismorio, F.P. and Friou, G.J. (1975) Immunoglobulin deposits in skin in systemic lupus erythematosus. *Arthr. Rheum.*, **18**, 77–82.
57. Begrin, A.J. and Thivolet, J. (1971) Les globulines fixes a la junction dermoepidermigna dans le lupus erythemateux sont-elle des anticorps anti-membrane basale? *Presse Med.*, **79**, 1070–6.
58. Nicholes, B.K. and Gilliam, J.N. (1981) Isolation and characterization of an epidermal basement membrane zone antigen which may be involved in antibody binding at the dermal–epidermal junction in systemic lupus erythematosus. *Fed. Proc.*, **40**, 198.
59. Nicoles, B.K. and Gilliam, J.N. (1982) Counter immunoelectrophoretic detection of epidermal basement membrane antibody in systemic lupus erythematosus serum. *Clin. Res.*, **30**, 600.
60. Gammon, W.R., Heise, E.R., Burke, W.A., *et al.* (1988) Increased frequency of HLA-DR2 in patients with autoantibodies to epidermolysis bullosa acquisita antigen: evidence that the expression of

autoimmunity to type VII collagen is HLA class II allele associated. *J. Invest. Dermatol.*, **91**, 228–32.
61. Fearon, D.T. and Wong, W.W. (1983) Complement ligand–receptor interactions that mediate biological responses. *Annu. Rev. Immunol.*, **1**, 243–72.
62. Gammon, W.R., Merritt, C.C., Lewis, D.M., *et al.* (1982) Functional evidence for complement-activating immune complexes in the skin of patients with bullous pemphigoid. *J. Invest. Dermatol.*, **78**, 52–7.
63. Gammon, W.R. and Briggaman, R.A. (1987) Functional heterogeneity of immune complexes in epidermolysis bullosa acquisita. *J. Invest. Dermatol.*, **89**, 478–83.
64. Gammon, W.R., Inman, A.O., III and Wheeler, C.E., Jr (1984) Differences in complement-dependent chemotactic activity generated by bullous pemphigoid and epidermolysis bullosa acquisita immune complexes: demonstration by leukocyte attachment and organ culture methods. *J. Invest. Dermatol.*, **83**, 57–61.

Nineteen

Porphyrias

David R. Bickers

19.1 INTRODUCTION

The synthesis of haem is obligatory for all aerobic cells because of the importance of this prosthetic group for a variety of metabolic processes. It is an iron-chelated tetrapyrrole that facilitates electron-transfer reactions vital for energy exchange and also catalyses the introduction of molecular oxygen into a broad range of endogenous and exogenous substrates which assists in diminishing their biological activity and enhancing their rate of excretion from the body.

Normally, haem synthesis is regulated by a series of enzymes (Figure 19.1), the activity or synthesis of which can be altered by the metabolic demands of the cell. Furthermore, it is generally believed that once haem is produced it binds to its various haemoproteins, and, with degradation of the protein, the haem is catabolized by the enzyme haem oxygenase to bile pigments. This necessitates the existence of a biochemical pathway that is continuously capable of synthesizing haem, and the ongoing nature of this process amplifies the possibility of significant derangements in the cell should an aberration occur in the regulation of its synthesis.

It is generally believed that haem regulates its own synthesis by directly inhibiting or indirectly repressing the production of the mitochondrial enzyme known as 5-aminolaevulinate synthase. This enzyme catalyses the conversion of succinate and glycine to the aminoketone 5-aminolaevulinate. When excessive amounts of 5-aminolaevulinic acid are added to cultured cells, much of it is converted to haem, suggesting that 5-aminolaevulinate synthase is the rate-limiting enzyme for the haem pathway.

The compartments in the body with major requirements for haem are the bone marrow and the liver. Since, in general, haem cannot be reutilized and since the daily demand for haemoglobin production in the marrow and for various haemoproteins in the liver is quite high,

Succinate
+
Glycine
↓ 5-Aminolaevulinate synthetase
5-Aminolaevulinate
↓ 5-Aminolaevulinate hydratase
Porphobilinogen
↓ Porphobilinogen deaminase
Hydroxymethylbilane
↓ Uroporphyrinogen III synthase
Uroporphyrinogen III
↓ Uroporphyrinogen decarboxylase
Coproporphyrinogen III
↓ Coproporphyrinogen oxidase
Protoporphyrinogen IX
↓ Protoporphyrinogen oxidase
Protoporphyrin IX
Fe^{2+} ↓ Ferrochelatase
↓
Haem

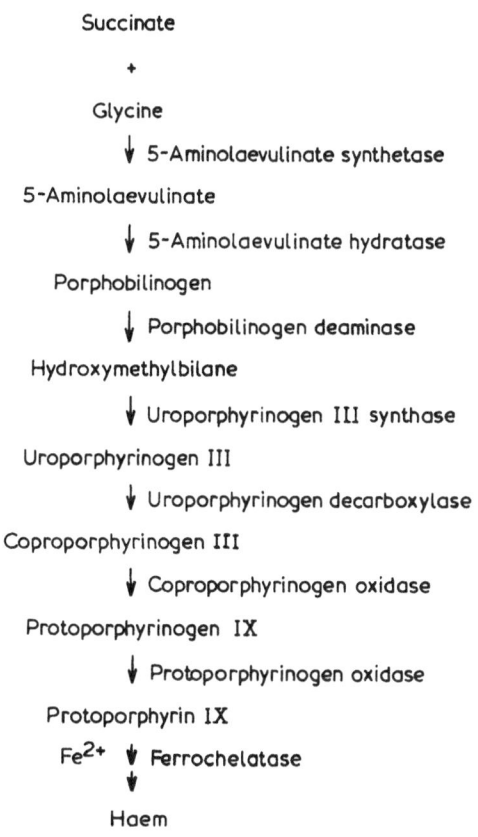

Figure 19.1 Pathway of haem synthesis.

there is a need for continuous production of this tetrapyrrole. In the marrow, the demand for haem synthesis is met by enhanced activity of 5-aminolaevulinate synthase and other enzymes in the pathway, whereas in the liver, it is generally agreed that the activity of this enzyme is the primary driving force for haem production [1].

Since haem is generated in stepwise fashion and since the steps themselves are dependent upon enzyme proteins that are genetically regulated, it has become clear that a family of human diseases exists, known as the porphyrias, that are the result of derangements in this otherwise precisely controlled process. The porphyrias are of two broad types: erythropoietic and hepatic and at least ten types have been described [2].

In this chapter, only those porphyrias in which blistering may occur will be discussed. These include certain types of the erythropoietic and the hepatic porphyrias. Of the hepatic porphyrias, porphyria cutanea tarda (PCT) (sporadic and familial), and variegate porphyria are most often accompanied by a vesiculobullous eruption. Of the porphyrias of bone marrow origin, such lesions occur only in congenital erythropoietic porphyria (CEP; Gunther's disease) whereas in erythropoietic protoporphyria these are rarely manifest. Hepatoerythropoietic porphyria (HEP) appears to be a homozygous variant of PCT, although its biochemical manifestations suggest abnormal marrow haem synthesis. The disease also manifests vesicles and bullae.

It is generally agreed that the vesiculobullous lesions appear in the human cutaneous porphyrias as a result of a photosensitizing process. This cutaneous photosensitization is believed to relate to the ability of porphyrins to absorb incident radiant energy in the visible portion of the photobiological action spectrum and to transfer that energy to vital cellular structures, thereby producing tissue injury.

The explanation for the accumulation of these photosensitizing porphyrins in the body of patients with porphyria lies in the abnormally regulated haem synthesis that accompanies the aberrant enzyme activity of the haem pathway in each of these diseases. Porphyrins are oxidized tetrapyrroles with resonating structures that can absorb radiant energy. With the exception of protoporphyrin, only reduced porphyrins (porphyrinogens) are intermediates in haem synthesis. Porphyrinogens are not photosensitizers. When one of the enzymes crucial for haem production is deficient, the pathway attempts to compensate for the diminshed production of haem by derepressing the synthesis of 5-aminolaevulinate synthase, the rate-limiting enzyme for haem production. This compensatory mechanism is vitally important since loss of cellular haem is incompatible with life. One side effect of the increased 5-aminolaevulinate synthase activity is to generate larger amounts of substrate for the defective enzyme, thereby ultimately enhancing haem production. Unfortunately, however, the altered kinetic behaviour of the defective enzyme precludes it from converting all of this substrate to haem. Inevitably, some of the substrate (porphyrinogen/porphyrin) begins to accumulate in the tissue of origin and then spills over into the circulation where it is transported intravascularly (largely bound to plasma proteins) and into the skin where it is capable of absorbing incident radiant energy, particularly in the visible spectrum (400–410 nm Soret band and between 600–650 nm). Although the absorption in the Soret band is most intense, the longer wavelengths penetrate the skin more efficiently.

The type of photosensitizing response to different porphyrins varies considerably for reasons that remain unclear. The polarity of the side-chain constituents greatly influences the lipid-water partition coefficient. For example, the 8-carboxyporphyrin, uroporphyrin, is highly water-soluble and largely excreted in the urine; the 4-carboxyporphyrin, coproporphyrin, has partial water and lipid solubility and is excreted in both urine and stool; and the 2-carboxyporphyrin, protoporphyrin, is highly lipid-soluble and excreted only in the stool. These solubility differences may alter the transport pathways of these porphyrins and influence the type of structural damage they evoke following excitation with appropriate wavelengths of energy [3].

Studies on the pathogenesis of the cutaneous manifestations of the vesiculobullous porphyrias have focused on the photosensitizing properties of the porphyrins. The electronic configuration of porphyrins enhances their capacity to absorb incident radiation which converts the stable ground state molecule to metastable excited states by promoting electrons from their ground-state orbitals to higher energy orbitals. These are known as singlet (antiparallel spin) and triplet (parallel spin) states and are capable of dissipating their absorbed energy as fluorescence (singlet decay) and phosphorescence (triplet decay), the latter of which is long-lived (10^{-4} s). Transfer of energy to a substrate directly (Type I) or indirectly by means of excited oxygen (Type II) is crucial for photosensitization. Singlet oxygen as well as superoxide anions, hydrogen peroxide and hydroxyl radicals have each been implicated in porphyrin photosensitization, and multiple vulnerable cellular (mast cells and polymorphonuclear neutrophils) and subcellular (lipid-rich membranes, proteins, cholesterol and intracellular organelles) targets have been identified [4–6]. Activation of the complement pathway with diminution of total haemolytic complement and with the generation of potent chemotactic factors has also been demonstrated [7].

Using murine ear swelling as a model system for the study of porphyrin sensitization [8], we have shown that superoxide anions as well as hydrogen peroxide and hydroxyl radicals are generated, and that activation of xanthine oxidase and a calcium-dependent protease may be a fundamental component of porphyrin photosensitization in the skin [9].

It is important to emphasize that photoexcited porphyrins could produce tissue injury in multiple ways. Thus, as mentioned, it has been shown that irradiated porphyrins can activate the complement pathway *in vitro* and that sera obtained from patients whose skin was irradiated with appropriate wavelengths of light demonstrates diminution of certain complement components [7]. The activation of complement may result in the release of pro-inflammatory mediators such as the anaphylotoxins C3a and C5a which have potent chemotactic effects on polymorphonuclear leucocytes, and the latter may be the direct cause of tissue injury. These two hypotheses (reactive oxygen species and complement activation) are not mutually exclusive and their respective roles in the development of the vesiculobullous lesions seen in certain cutaneous porphyrias remain to be elucidated.

19.2 ERYTHROPOIETIC PORPHYRIAS

Since congenital erythropoietic porphyria is the only disorder in which vesiculobullous lesions are prominent, this type of porphyria of erythropoietic origin will be discussed as a prototype.

19.2.1 Congenital erythropoietic porphyria

(a) Clinical features

Presentation This disease generally is manifest at or shortly after birth and may affect both sexes. It is extremely rare with perhaps less than 100 reported cases in the world literature [10]. The disease was first described by Schultz in the late 19th century and was studied extensively by Gunther for whom the disease is named.

Cutaneous findings The initial manifestation of CEP is pinkish-red to brown discoloration of the nappies (diapers) in infants. The first dermatological features are acute erythema and swelling with associated vesicles and bullae on sun-exposed skin [11]. The bullous lesions contain fluid that may exhibit the reddish-pink fluorescence characteristic of porphyrins if excited with a Woods lamp. The extent of tissue injury in this disease is extraordinary and repeated episodes of blistering lead to chronic scarring changes with scleroderma-like acral mutilation that may culminate in the loss of digits and grossly deformed ears and nose. Affected individuals bear a striking resemblance to patients with severe systemic sclerosis or with recessive dystrophic epidermolysis bullosa. Additional cutaneous features include mottled pigmentary change (hypo- and hyper-pigmentation), hypertrichosis and scarring alopecia.

Mucous membrane involvement There is no characteristic mucous membrane involvement in this disease; however, there is a unique red to brown staining discoloration of the deciduous and permanent teeth know as erythrodontia. This is due to deposition of excessive porphyrins in the dentine which may become more apparent upon examination of the teeth with a Woods light.

(b) Genetics

CEP is an autosomal recessive disorder in which two mutant alleles result in deficient uroporphyrinogen III synthase activity [12]. There is also increased activity of porphobilinogen deaminase activity which is probably secondary to the haemolysis-induced erythropoietic hyperactivity seen in these patients [13]. Affected individuals have 10–30% of the normal uroporphyrinogen III synthase activity, and presumed heterozygotes have activity between that of patients and normals [14]. The abnormal activity of the enzyme may be due to a coding defect in the gene that regulates its synthesis.

(c) Differential diagnosis

The pattern of vesiculobullous lesions in infancy with dark urine and chronic scarring is quite characteristic of CEP. The major type of porphyria that can be confused with this disease is HEP in which severe photosensitivity with increased skin fragility, vesiculobullous lesions, hypertrichosis and scleroderma-like changes can all occur. Generally, however, this is less severe than that occurring in CEP. Furthermore, there are distinctive biochemical features of HEP that help to distinguish the two disorders.

Additional diagnostic considerations include recessive dystrophic epidermolysis bullosa in which blistering, severe multilation and scarring can occur. However, the involved areas in such patients are not limited to sun-exposed sites and there are characteristic abnormalities of fibroblast collagenase that can be detected by research investigation [15].

(d) Investigations

The basic genetic defect is diminished uroporphyrinogen III synthase activity in the marrow and this can be detected in cultured skin fibroblasts from affected individuals [16]. These patients excrete enormous amounts of uroporphyrin and lesser amounts of coproporphyrin in their urine (I isomer >80%). Stool porphyrin excretion is also elevated and consists primarily of coproporphyrin I and smaller amounts of uroporphyrin I. Plasma and erythrocytes both contain increased uroporphyrin I and coproporphyrin I.

(e) Systemic manifestations

The major systemic feature of CEP is splenomegaly which is probably secondary to the marked haemolysis that occurs in these patients. Interestingly, it has been emphasized that the intermittent nature of the haemolytic process is a striking and specific feature of CEP and this may be due to the increased intracellular porphyrin concentrations [10]. Some believe that this is predominantly a 'photohaemolytic' process, but this is controversial [17]. There may also be intrinsic abnormalities of the erythrocytes themselves independent of the porphyrin overload since patient's cells have decreased survival when administered to normal individuals, and normal erythrocytes do not exhibit a shortened half-life when transfused into patients with CEP [18].

(f) Pathogenesis and recent advances

The pathogenesis relates to a primary gene defect and secondary photosensitization due to the large increases in tissue porphyrin concentration. Recent studies from Desnick's laboratory have characterized the gene defect in CEP [19].

(g) Treatment

There is currently no satisfactory treatment for CEP. Preventive measures such as avoidance of sun exposure and minimizing trauma of the skin are only slightly helpful.

Beta-carotene Oral administration of this free-radical scavenger is clearly helpful in diminishing the cutaneous photosensitivity of erythropoietic protoporphyria and has been recommended in

CEP, although it is at best only partially effective [20].

Splenectomy Some have advocated this procedure as an approach to diminishing the haemolytic anaemia and the cutaneous photosensitivity [21]. Unfortunately, this procedure is not clearly effective in either regard and should be reserved for patients with severe hypersplenism in whom decreased haemolysis may be desirable [10].

Induced polycythaemia/hypertransfusion/haematin infusions These approaches are designed to reduce marrow porphyrin production by diminishing the demand for haem synthesis, and there have been sporadic case reports suggesting that these approaches may be useful in selected patients [22–24].

Agents to diminish enteral absorption of porphyrins Enterohepatic recirculation of porphyrins cleared through the liver can be a detriment to effective faecal excretion of these compounds. This has led to the use of orally administered sorbents such as charcoal and cholestyramine which can bind porphyrins in the gut and enhance their excretion by precluding their reabsorption [25, 26]. In one study, transfusion with packed red blood cells was performed in one patient at sufficient intervals to maintain haematocrit at 40%. This resulted in a 50% decrease in plasma porphyrins, and an 80% decrease in urine and stool porphyrins with substantial improvement in the severity and the rate of healing of the affected skin. Oral charcoal (30 g every 3 h for 36 h) reduced plasma porphyrin concentration to normal levels by 20 h and was more effective than either cholestyramine or transfusion therapy. Skin porphyrin concentration was reduced more than 90% by oral charcoal therapy. In further studies, chronic oral charcoal administration (60 g three times per day for 9 months) was shown to result in a sustained decrease in plasma porphyrin levels near the normal range and to obviate cutaneous photosensitivity. The only side effect of the chronic charcoal therapy was decreased levels of vitamin B_{12}, vitamin D and folate which returned to normal with appropriate supplementation. This approach may prove useful and needs to be assessed in additional patients.

(h) *Prognosis and sequelae*

To date, patients with early onset of the disease have rarely survived beyond the age of 40 due either to repeated infections or to marrow failure. The mutilating skin changes secondary to scarring are quite debilitating.

(i) *Genetic counselling and prenatal diagnosis*

Genetic counselling is an important component of the management of this disease. Heterozygotes have blood uroporphyinogen III synthase levels intermediate between affected individuals and normal controls and can be identified. Prenatal diagnosis is also possible by assaying amniotic fluid porphyria, porphyrin synthesis by amniotic cells or by measuring uroporphyrinogen III synthase [27].

19.3 HEPATIC PORPHYRIAS

19.3.1 Introduction

The hepatic porphyrias are the most common of the human porphyrias, and patients with these disorders manifest a vesiculobullous eruption on sun-exposed skin that is generally characteristic. It is not as severe as that occurring in CEP, but can be a significant cause of morbidity. There are four major categories of porphyria cutanea tarda (PCT) known as (1) familial or inherited, (2) sporadic, symptomatic or acquired, (3) toxic and (4) hepatoerythropoietic porphyria (HEP) [28]. The photocutaneous manifestations of these categories are similar and in this chapter they will be discussed together.

19.3.2 Clinical features

(a) Presentation

Familial PCT generally begins in the first two decades of life whereas sporadic PCT is a disease of middle-aged to older adults. In aggregate, PCT is by far the most common type of porphyria seen in dermatological practice. These disorders occur world wide, although there have been clusters of cases in certain geographical areas. For example, large numbers of cases of toxic porphyria were identified in Turkey in the 1950s and 60s as a consequence of the ingestion of wheat seed that had been treated with the fungicide, hexachlorobenzene [29]. It is now known that this chemical is capable of inhibiting the enzyme uroporphyrinogen decarboxylase which is essential for the conversion of uroporphyrinogen to coproporphyrinogen [30]. A second cluster of cases has been reported in South African Bantus and is thought to be due to the excessive ingestion of iron that occurs in these individuals as a consequence of their chronic drinking of 'kaffir' beer, a brew that is concocted in iron-containing pots [31]. It is believed that large amounts of iron leached out from the brewing vessels contribute to the excessive PCT seen in these individuals. Indeed, there is evidence that iron may influence uroporphyrinogen decarboxylase, both directly by inhibiting its activity and indirectly by influencing its susceptibility to inhibition by halogenated hydrocarbons or reactive oxygen species [32].

(b) Cutaneous distribution

The major cutaneous features of all types of PCT include vesiculobullous lesions, facial hypertrichosis, mottled pigmentary change on light-exposed areas and scleroderma-like induration on both light-exposed and light-protected areas. Most patients demonstrate increased skin fragility and are generally unaware that sunlight is playing a role in their skin disorder. Patients often complain that the most trivial injury to the affected skin results in either blister formation or in shearing away of the skin leaving moist eroded areas which slowly heal with scars and milia.

The hypertrichosis that occurs is usually in a unique pattern predominantly affecting the periorbital areas of the face with growth around the lateral edge of the eyes up onto the forehead. This is distinct from androgen-dependent hirsutism which is present in the 'beard' region.

Pigmentary changes are also common and generally resemble chloasma with a mottled pattern of hypo- and hyper-pigmentation that is exaggerated by sun exposure. Some affected individuals may become quite dark in colour.

The scleroderma-like pattern of induration occurs most commonly on the trunk and develops insidiously with gradual hardening and diminished pigmentation of affected areas. There is often a striking resemblance to scleroderma although acrosclerosis and Raynaud's phenomenon do not develop.

Mucous membranes

No involvement is known.

19.3.3 Genetics

The major enzymic abnormality in all types of PCT is deficient activity of uroporphyrinogen decarboxylase. It is important to emphasize that diminished enzyme activity can only be detected in the liver of patients with sporadic and toxic PCT and in all tissues of patients with the familial variant and with HEP [33–35].

Enzyme activity in familial PCT is about half normal, and the gene dosage suggests that this activity represents full expression of a normal gene that is allelic to a 'silent' mutant gene [36]. Mutations producing familial PCT appear to be cross-reactive material (CRIM)-negative when assessed with polyclonal antisera raised against uroporphyrinogen decarboxylase; no CRIM-positive families have been identified [36, 37]. Homozygous deficiency of uroporphyrinogen decarboxylase is thought to be present in patients with HEP [38]. No gene deletions or rearrangements could be detected, and the half-life of the abnormal protein was 12 times shorter than that of the normal enzyme. Cloning and sequencing of a complementary DNA for the mutated gene revealed a single amino acid change at position 281 (glutamate for glycine) [39]. In another patient with this disease, a mutant isozyme of uroporphyrinogen decarboxylase was detected using an immunochemical approach [40]. Finally, studies in an affected family with this disease have shown that it is the result of homozygous inheritance of a defect in the gene for uroporphyrinogen decarboxylase, that the severity of clincal signs and symptoms relates to the level of residual enzyme activity and that expression of the gene defect can be heterogeneous [41].

In the sporadic or symptomatic form of PCT, there is diminished uroporphyrinogen decarboxylase activity which is apparently limited only to the liver. During active periods of the disease, diminished activity of the enzyme (up to 70%) occurs with no associated change in the amount detectable in the hepatocyte by immunochemical methods which may even be elevated. Enzyme activity seems to remain low after induction of remission by phlebotomy and/or chloroquine therapy, but then may gradually rise to normal levels.

The cause of sporadic PCT is unknown, although a history of alcohol and/or oestrogen ingestion is present in many patients. There is, however, no evidence for an inherited enzyme deficiency.

19.3.4 Differential diagnosis

The cutaneous manifestations of familial, sporadic and toxic PCT as well as HEP are strikingly similar and the specific disease can usually be identified by measurement of urine, stool and erythrocyte porphyrins and/or porphyrin precursors or by enzyme assay procedures. The specific abnormalities are beyond the scope of this discussion, but can be found elsewhere [42]. The major porphyria that needs to be distinguished is variegate porphyria, since the cutaneous manifestations are identical to those occurring in the various types of PCT.

Other dermatological disorders that need to be considered include pseudoporphyria and epidermolysis bullosa acquisita. Pseudoporphyria mimics the bullous skin lesions of PCT and the histological and ultrastructural features of the lesions may closely resemble those of PCT, but there is no evidence for any aberration of porphyrin–haem synthesis [43]. This syndrome is associated with the ingestion of a number of drugs including furosemide, nalidixic acid, tetracycline and naproxen [44–47]. Bullous dermatosis of haemodialysis has many of the features of pseudoporphyria, but may occur with or without drug ingestion and may well be related to changes secondary to dialysis itself [48]. (See Chapter 21.)

The second major differential diagnosis is the acquired form of epidermolysis bullosa (see Chapter 10) in which blisters form over pressure points particularly in acral areas after trivial trauma followed by healing with scarring and milia formation. Linear deposits of IgG and C_3 occur at the basement membrane zone of affected skin. Recent studies indicate that the antigen in this disease is type VII collagen [49], and ultrastructural studies reveal reduced numbers of anchoring fibrils in lesional and normal-appearing skin which does not occur in PCT [50]. These patients have totally normal porphyrin and porphyrin precursor excretion which rules out cutaneous porphyria.

19.3.5 Investigations

PCT is a subepidermal blistering process. Careful studies have shown that there is a continuum of change in the skin of patients with this disease.

The histopathological features of PCT include epidermal hyperkeratosis, hypergranulosis, acanthosis and a homogeneous thickening of the upper dermal blood vessel walls in involved skin [51]. The latter may be associated with positive staining for glycosaminoglycans and periodate–Schiff-positive diastase-resistant material in the vessel walls.

Immunofluorescent studies reveal homogeneous deposition of IgG in and adjacent to blood vessels and to a lesser extent at the dermo–epidermal zone in involved but generally not in uninvolved skin. IgM is seen sporadically and all indirect immunofluorescent studies have been negative.

Electron microscopic changes consist of extensive reduplication of the basal lamina of the small upper dermal blood vessels [52]. Widened perivascular spaces are seen with finely fibrillar material which extends beyond the basal lamina and may be small collagen fibrils [53]. Discrete electron-lucent membrane-limited vacuoles are present in a perivascular location [54].

In areas adjacent to blisters, these vacuoles are greatly increased in number and some tend to coalesce. Coated vesicles are often fused with the membranes of the vacuoles. The membrane-limited vacuoles are also present in the superficial dermis close to the basal lamina that separates dermis and epidermis.

In the blisters themselves, the superficial dermis takes on a netlike appearance due to the apparent fusion of the vacuolar limiting membranes. Interruption of the basal lamina occurs in certain areas where epidermal basal cells have formed vacuoles as well. These ultrastructural changes are probably the result of porphyrin photosensitization which then produces the characteristic sub-epidermal blister.

Klein *et al.* employed an indirect immuno-fluorescence technique to examine the basal membrane zone with antisera to type IV collagen and laminin and with bullous pemphigoid sera [55]. Bullae were judged to be junctional if pemphigoid antigen was present on the roof and type IV collagen and laminin were present at the base, and were judged to be dermolytic if all three reagents were in the blister roof. In PCT, small vesicles are dermolytic and large bullae are junctional. Dermolytic cleavage has also been reported by Pearson and Wolff *et al.* [51, 56].

The major test procedures to be performed in the cutaneous porphyrias include quantitative measurement of urine, stool and blood porphyrins. In PCT, the major excretion abnormalities include increased urinary uroporphyrin, 7-carboxy-porphyrin and to a much lesser extent copro-porphyrin (uroporphyrin and 7-carboxyporphyrin: coproporphyrin ratio >5:1) and increased faecal isocoproporphyrin. Plasma porphyrins are increased and erythrocyte porphyrins are normal. The pattern of excretion in urine and faeces of patients with HEP closely resembles that seen in PCT, but differs in that uroporphyrin and iso-coproporphyrin excretion is higher in the faeces and there is elevated erythrocyte zinc proto-porphyrin [57]. In CEP, there is elevated urine uroporphyrin and 7-, 6- and 5-carboxyporphyrins as well as coproporphyrin (predominantly isomer I whereas III is predominant in PCT and HEP). In variegate porphyria, urinary uroporphyrin and coproporphyrin excretion are marginally increased whereas stool protoporphyrin and coproporphyrin are usually elevated substantially.

The most direct method of defining the type of porphyria present in a patient suspected of having one of these disorders is to measure the activity of the enzyme involved. In the case of familial PCT and HEP, measurement of uroporphyrinogen decarboxylase in erythrocytes will confirm the diagnosis [58]. In familial PCT (autosomal dominant) enzyme activity is approximately half-normal and in HEP (homozygous defect) it is between 5 and 15% of normal [59]. In variegate porphyria, measurement of mitochondrial proto-porphyrinogen oxidase in fibroblasts or lympho-blasts will confirm the diagnosis [60, 61]. In CEP, uroporphyrinogen III synthase is decreased in erythrocytes [62].

19.3.6 Systemic manifestations and associated diseases

In sporadic and familial PCT, increased hepatic iron stores occur which may have a direct inhibitory effect upon uroporphyrinogen decarboxylase, although this is controversial [58]. The inhibitory effect of iron on the enzyme has been explained in two ways: (1) direct inhibition by the metal and (2) indirect inhibition due to the generation of free radicals in the presence of oxygen and an electron donor such as cysteine [63].

Abnormal liver function tests, increased serum iron, increased liver parenchymal iron as well as needle-like crystals in the hepatocytes may occur [64]. Autopsy studies of patients with PCT have revealed foci of hepatocellular carcinoma in 39% and 47% of patients studied [65, 66]. Screening of 96 patients with PCT by measuring alpha-foetoprotein and radioisotopic liver scans did not reveal any hepatic neoplasms [66].

Diabetes mellitus has been identified in 15% of patients and as many as 50% may have an abnormal glucose tolerance test [67]. Lupus erythematosus has occurred in a small number of patients with PCT but the significance of the association is unclear [68].

The major systemic manifestation of variegate porphyria is the acute attack that includes varying combinations of abdominal pain with neuro-psychiatric and/or neurological involvement [69]. Variegate porphyria and PCT may coexist in the same individual [70].

19.3.7 Pathogenesis and recent advances

The pathogenesis of PCT and variegate porphyria is directly related to the hepatic overproduction of porphyrins which circulate in the plasma to the skin where they can absorb incident solar radiation and evoke cutaneous photosensitization. Thus, the skin is attacked as an innocent bystander by a disease process that originates in the liver.

The major recent advances in the porphyrias relate to more precise characterization of the enzyme abnormalities that are responsible for these diseases and their genetic regulation. This has been discussed in Section 19.3.3 above.

19.3.8 Treatment

Effective management is based upon diminishing hepatic overproduction of photosensitizing porphyrins and includes phlebotomy therapy and/or low-dose oral chloroquine or hydroxy-chloroquine [71–73]. Prior to initiating specific therapy, it is essential to advise the patient to discontinue the ingestion of ethanol or oestrogenic hormones as well as iron supplements or other potential porphyrinogenic drugs. Phlebotomy is generally conducted at weekly or biweekly intervals by removing 500 cc of whole blood at each visit until the haemoglobin falls into the mildy anaemic range (10–11 g%). These can then be discontinued after which gradual clinical and biochemical improvement will ensue usually over a period of 6–18 months assuming the patient does not become re-exposed to the porphyrinogenic agents mentioned above [74]. The effectiveness of phlebotomy seems to correlate with the depletion of body iron stores although this is controversial [75, 76].

The use of antimalarials was initially difficult because of the severe hepatotoxicity that developed in patients with PCT who received high doses of these drugs [76, 77]. However, it was soon appreciated that intermittent low-dose therapy even at doses as low as 125 mg twice weekly was effective while obviating the hepatotoxic response [78–80]. The mechanism of action of the anti-malarials is controversial, but may involve the formation of drug–porphyrin complexes in the liver or enhanced iron excretion [81, 82]. Combinations of phlebotomy and antimalarials have also been recommended [83].

There is no effective treatment for the cutaneous photosensitivity that accompanies variegate porphyria except the avoidance of porphyrinogenic drugs and even this is effective primarily if not exclusively for the acute attacks. No effective therapy exists for HEP.

19.3.9 Prognosis and sequelae

Sporadic and familial PCT usually responds to phlebotomy and/or chloroquine therapy with resolution of the vesiculobullous lesions within 6–12 months and of the other changes over a period of several years. Scarring, however, is generally permanent. Toxic porphyria generally improves slowly with elimination of exposure to the offending agent. Skin changes may persist for years and in the case of hexachlorobenzene poisoning in Turkey, these have remained for more than 25 years. Long-range follow-up of patients with HEP is not yet available.

19.3.10 Genetic counselling

This has not been explored in detail, but is now possible with the molecular characterization of uroporphyrinogen decarboxylase.

REFERENCES

1. Bickers, D.R. (1986) Porphyria: basic science aspects. *Dermatol. Clin. North Amer.*, **4**, 277–90.
2. Elder, G.H. (1986) Metabolic abnormalities in the porphyrias. *Semin. Dermatol.*, **5**, 88–98.
3. Kohn, K. and Kessel, D. (1979) On the mode of cytotoxic action of photoactivated porphyrins. *Biochem. Pharmacol.*, **28**, 2465–70.
4. Poh-Fitzpatrick, M.B. (1986) Molecular and cellular mechanisms of porphyrin photosensitization. *Photodermatology.*, **3**, 148–57.
5. Kerdel, F.A., Soter, N.A. and Lim, H.W. (1987) *In vivo* mediator release and degranulation of mast cells in hematoporphyrin derivative-induced phototoxicity in mice. *J. Invest. Dermatol.*, **88**, 277–80.
6. Pigatto, P., Altomare, G., Polenghi, M.M., *et al.* (1985) Role of the polymorphonuclear neutrophils

in the phototoxic reaction in porphyria cutanea tarda. *Photodermatology*, **2**, 372–6.

7. Lim. H.W., Perez, H.D., Poh-Fitzpatrick, M.B., *et al.* (1981) Generation of chemotactic activity in serum from patients with erythropoietic protoporphyria and porphyria cutanea tarda. *New Eng. J. Med.*, **304**, 212–16.
8. Hawkins, C.W., Bickers, D.R., Mukhtar, H., *et al.* (1986) Cutaneous porphyrin photosensitization: Murine ear swelling as a marker of the acute response. *J. Invest. Dermatol.*, **86**, 638–42.
9. Athar, M., Elmets, C.A., Bickers, D.R. and Mukhtar, H. (1989) A novel mechanism for the generation of superoxide anion in hematoporphyrin derivative-mediated cutaneous photosensitization activation of the xanthine oxidase pathway. *J. Clin. Invest.*, **83**, 1137–43.
10. Nordmann, Y. and Deybach, J.C. (1986) Congenital erythropoietic porphyria. *Semin. Dermatol.*, **5**, 106–14.
11. Murphy, G. M., Hawk, J.L.M., Nicholson, D.C., *et al.* (1987) Congenital erythropoietic porphyria (Gunther's disease). *Clin. Exp. Dermatol.*, **12**, 61–5.
12. Romeo, G. and Levin, E.Y. (1969) Uroporphyrinogen III cosynthetase in human congenital erythropoietic porphyria. *Proc. Natl. Acad. Sci. U.S.A.*, **63**, 856–63.
13. Kramer, S., Viljoen, E., Meyer, A.M., *et al.* (1965) The anemia of erythropoietic porphyria with the first description of the disease in an elderly patient. *Brit. J. Haematol.*, **11**, 666–75.
14. Romea, G., Glenn, B.L. and Levin, E.Y. (1970) Uroporphyrinogen cosythetase in asymptomatic carriers of congenital erythropoietic porphyria. *Biochem. Genet.*, **4**, 719–26.
15. Eisen, A.Z. (1969) Human skin collagenase: Relationship to pathogenesis of epidermolysis bullosa dystrophica. *J. Invest. Dermatol.*, **52**, 449–53.
16. Grandchamp, B., Deybach, J.C., Grelier, M., *et al.* (1980) Studies of porphyrin synthesis in fibroblasts of patients with congenital erythropoietic porphyria and of a case of homozygous coproporphyria. *Biochim. Biophys. Acta*, **629**, 577–86.
17. Sassa, S. and Kappas, A. (1981) in *Advances in Human Genetics, Vol. 11* (eds H. Harris and K. Hirschorn), Plenum Press, New York, pp. 121–231.
18. Haining, R.C., Cowger, M.C., Shurtleff, D.B., *et al.* (1968) Congenital erythropoietic porphyria I. Case report, special studies and therapy. *Amer. J. Med.*, **45**, 624–37.
19. Tsai, S.F., Bishop, D.F. and Desnick, R.J. (1987) Coupled-enzyme and direct assays for uroporphyrinogen III synthase activity in human erythrocytes and cultures lymphoblasts. Enzymatic diagnosis of heterozygotes and homogygotes with congenital erythropoietic porphyria. *Anal. Biochem.*, **166**, 120–33.
20. Sneddon, I.B. (1978) β-carotene in congenital porphyria. *Arch. Dermatol.*, **114**, 1242–3.
21. Aldrich, R.A., Hawkinson, V., Grinstein, M., *et al.* (1951) Photosensitive or congenital porphyria with hemolytic anemia. I. Clinical and fundamental studies before and after splenectomy. *Blood*, **6**, 685–98.
22. Haining, R.C., Lowger, M.L., Labbe, R.F., *et al.* (1970) Congenital erythropoietic porphyria II. The effects of induced polycythemia. *Blood*, **36**, 297–309.
23. Piomelli, S., Poh-Fitzpatrick, M.B., Seaman, C., *et al.* (1986) Complete suppression of the symptoms of congenital erythropoietic porphyria by long-term treatment with high-level transfusions. *New Engl. J. Med.*, **314**, 1029–31.
24. Watson, C.J., Bossenmaier, I., Cardinal, R., *et al.* (1974) Repression by hematin of porphyrin biosynthesis in erythrocyte precursors in congenital erythropoietic porphyria. *Proc. Natl. Acad. Sci. U.S.A.*, **71**, 278–82.
25. Lischner, H.W. (1966) Cholestryamine and porphyrin binding. *Lancet*, **ii**, 1079–80.
26. Pimstone, N.R., Gandhi, S.N. and Mukerji, S.K. (1987) Therapeutic efficacy of oral charcoal in congenital erythropoietic porphyria. *New Engl. J. Med.*, **316**, 390–3.
27. Deybach, J.C., Grandchamp, B., Gselier, M., *et al.* (1980) Prenatal exclusion of congenital erythropoietic porphyria (Gunther's disease) in a fetus at risk. *Hum. Genet.*, **53**, 217–21.
28. Mascaro, J.M., Herrero, C., Lecho, M., *et al.* (1986) Uroporphyrinogen-decarboxylase deficiencies: Porphyria cutanea tarda and related conditions. *Semin. Dermatol.*, **5**, 115–24.
29. Cam, C. and Nigogosyan, G. (1963) Acquired toxic porphyria cutanea tarda due to hexachlorobenzene. Report of 348 cases caused by this fungicide. *J. Amer. Med. Assoc.*, **183**, 88–91.
30. Elder, G.H. (1976) The effect of the porphyrinogenic compound hexachlorobenzene, on the activity of hepatic uroporphyrinogen decarboxylase in the rate. *Clin. Sci. Mol. Med.*, **51**, 71–80.
31. Cripps, D.J. (1987) Diet and alcohol effects on the manifestation of hepatic porphyrias. *Fed. Proc.*, **46**, 1894–1900.
32. Mukerji, S.K., Pimstone, N.R. and Burns, M. (1984) Dual mechanism of inhibition of rat liver uroporphyrinogen decarboxylase activity by ferrous iron: its potential role in the genesis of porphyria cutanea tarda. *Gastroenterology*, **87**, 1248–54.
33. Elder, G.H. and Lee, G.B., (1978) Decreased hepatic uroporphyrinogen decarboxyase in porphyria cutanea tarda. *New Engl. J. Med.*, **299**, 274–8.
34. Verneuil, H. de, Aitken, G. and Nordmann, Y.

(1978) Familial and sporadic porphyria cutanea: Two different diseases. *Hum. Genet.*, **42**, 145–51.
35. Elder, G.H. (1986) Metabolic abnormalities in the porphyrias. *Semin. Dermatol.*, **5**, 88–98.
36. Elder, G.H., Sheppard, D.M., Tovey, J.A., *et al.* (1983) Immunoreactive uroporphyrinogen decarboxylase in porphyria cutanea tarda. *Lancet,* i, 1301–4.
37. Verneuil, H. de, Beaumont, C., Deybach, J.C., *et al.* (1984) Enzymatic and immunological studies of uroporphyrinogen decarboxylase in familial porphyria cutanea tarda and hepatoerythropoietic porphyria. *Amer. J. Hum. Genet.*, **36**, 613–22.
38. Verneuil, H. de, Grandchamp, B, Romeo, P.H., *et al.* (1986) Molecular analysis of uroporphyrinogen decarboxylase deficiency in a family with two cases of hepatoerythropoietic porphyria. *J. Clin. Invest.*, **77**, 431–5.
39. Verneuil, H. de, Grandchamp, B., Beaumont, C., *et al.* (1986) Uroporphyrinogen decarboxylase structural mutant (Gly^{281}-Glu) in a case of porphyria. *Science,* **234**, 732–4.
40. Fujita, H., Sassa, S., Toback, A.C., *et al.* (1987) Immunochemical study of uroporphyrinogen decarboxylase in a patient with mild hepatoerythopoietic porphyria. *J. Clin. Invest.*, **79**, 1533–7.
41. Toback, A.C., Sassa, S., Poh-Fitzpatrick, M.B., *et al.* (1987) Hepatoerythropoietic porphyria: Clinical, biochemical, and enzymatic studies in a three-generation family lineage. *New Engl. J. Med.*, **316**, 645–50.
42. Bickers, D.R. and Pathak, M.A. (1987) in *Dermatology in General Medicine* (eds T.B. Fitzpatrick, A. Eisen, K. Wolff, *et al.*), McGraw-Hill, New York, pp. 1666–715.
43. Judd, L.E., Henderson, D.W. and Hill, D.C. (1986) Naproxen-induced pseudoporphyria. A clinical and ultrastructural study. *Arch. Dermatol.*, **122**, 451–4.
44. Burry, J.N. and Lawrence, J.R. (1976) Phototoxic blisters from high frusemide dosage. *Brit. J. Dermatol.*, **94**, 495–9.
45. Ramsay, C.A. and Obreshkova, E. (1974) Photosensitivity from nalidixic acid. *Brit. J. Dermatol.*, **91**, 523–8.
46. Epstein, J.H., Tuffanelli, D.L., Subert, J.S., *et al.* (1976) Porphryia-like cutaneous changes induced by tetracycline hydrochloride photosensitization. *Arch. Dermatol.*, **112**, 661–6.
47. Howard, A.M., Dowling, J. and Varigos, G. (1985) Pseudoporphyria due to naproxen. *Lancet,* i, 819–20.
48. Lamkin, B.C. and Bickers D.R. (1983) Porphyria cutanea tarda: A metabolic human blistering disease. *Dermatol. Clin.* **1**, 249–62.
49. Woodley, D.T., Burgeson, R.E., Lungstrum, G.P., *et al.* (1988) The epidermolysis bullosa acquisita antigen in the globular carboxyl terminus of Type VII procollagen. *J. Clin. Invest.*, **81**, 683–7.
50. Yaoita, H., Briggaman, R.A., Lawley, T.J., *et al.* (1981) Epidermolysis bullosa acquisita: Ultrastructural and immunological studies. *J. Invest. Dermatol.*, **76**, 288–92.
51. Wolff, K., Honigsmann, H., Rauschmeier, W., *et al.* (1982) Microscopic and fine structural aspects of porphyrias. *Acta Dermatovenereol. Suppl.*, **100**, 17–28.
52. Caputo, R., Berti, E. and Gasparini, G. (1983) The morphologic events of blister formation in porphyria cutanea tarda. *Int. J. Dermatol.*, **22**, 467–72.
53. Kint, A. (1970) Comparative electron microscopic study of the perivascular hyaline from porphyria cutanea tarda and from lipoid proteinosis. *Arch. Klin. Exp. Dermatol.*, **239**, 203–17.
54. Epstein, J.H., Tuffanelli, D.L. and Epstein, W.L. (1973) Cutaneous changes in the porphyrias. *Arch. Dermatol.*, **107**, 689–98.
55. Klein, G.F., Hintner, H.F., Schuler, G., *et al.* (1983) Junctional blisters in acquired bullous disorders of the dermal/epidermal junction zone: Role of the lamina lucida as the mechanical locus minoris resistentiae. *Brit. J. Dermatol.*, **109**, 499–508.
56. Pearson, R.W. (1967) in *Ultrastructure of Normal and Abnormal Skin* (ed. A.S. Zelickson), Lea and Febiger, Philadelphia, pp. 320–34.
57. Smith, S.G. (1986) Hepatoerythropoietic porphyria. *Semin. Dermatol.*, **5**, 125–37.
58. Verneuil, H. de, Sassa, S. and Kappas, A. (1983) Purification and properties of uroporphyrinogen decarboxylase from human erythrocytes. A single enzyme catalyzing the four sequential decarboxylations of uroporphyinogens I and III. *J. Biol. Chem.*, **258**, 2454–60.
59. Elder, G.H., Smith, S.G., Herrero, C., *et al.* (1981) Hepatoerythropoietic porphyria: A new irp [pr] jurompgem decarboxylase defect or homozygous porphyria cutanea tarda. *Lancet,* **1**, 916–19.
60. Brenner, D.A. and Bloomer, J.R. (1980) The enzymatic defect in variegate porphyria. Studies with cultured human skin fibroblasts. *New Engl. J. Med.*, **302**, 765–9.
61. Deybach, J.C., de Vernueil, H. and Nordmann, Y. (1981) The inherited enzymatic defect in porphyria variegata. *Hum. Genet.*, **58**, 425–8.
62. Nordmann, Y. and Deybach, J.C. (1982) Congenital erythropoietic porphyria. *Semin. Liver Dis.*, **2**, 154–63.
63. Mukerji, S.K., Pimstone, N.R. and Burns, M, (1984) Dual mechanism of inhibition of rat liver uroporphyrinogen decarboxylase activity by ferrous iron: Its potential role in the genesis of porphyria cutanea tarda. *Gastroenterology,* **87**, 1248–54.
64. Bruguera, M. (1986) Liver involvement in porphyria. *Semin. Dermatol.*, **5**, 178–85.

65. Grossman, M.E. and Bickers, D.R. (1978) Porphyria cutanea tarda: A rare manifestation of hepatic tumors. *Cutis*, **21**, 782–4.
66. Topi, G.C., Gandolfo, L.D., De Costanza, F., *et al.* (1980) Porphyria cutanea tarda and hepatocellular carcinoma. *Int. J. Biochem.*, **12**, 883–5.
67. Muhlbauer, J.E. and Pathak, M.A. (1979) Porphyria cutanea tarda. *Int. J. Dermatol.*, **18**, 767–80.
68. Hetherington, G.W., Jelton, R.L., Know, J.M., *et al.* (1970) The association of lupus erythmatosus and porphyria. *Brit. J. Dermatol.*, **82**, 118–24.
69. Day, R.S. (1986) Variegate porphyria. *Semin. Dermatol.*, **5**, 138–54.
70. Day, R.S., Eales, L. and Meissner, D. (1982) Coexistent variegate porphyria and porphyria cutanea tarda. *New Engl. J. Med.*, **307**, 36–41.
71. Ippen, H. (1961) Allgemeinsymptome der spaten Hautporphyrie (PCT) als Hinweise fur deren Behandlung. *Dtsch. Med. Wschr.*, **86**, 127–33.
72. Cripps, D.J. and Curtis, A.C. (1962) Toxic effect of chloroquine on porphyria hepatica. *Arch. Dermatol.*, **86**, 575–81.
73. Bickers, D.R. and Merk, H. (1986) The treatment of porphyrias. *Semin. Dermatol.*, **5**, 186–97.
74. Ramsay, C.A., Magnus, I. A., Turnbull, A., *et al.* (1974) The treatment of porphyria cutanea tarda by venesection. *Q. J. Med.*, **43**, 1–13.
75. Lundvall, O. (1971) The effect of replenishment of iron stores after phlebotomy therapy in porphyria cutanea tarda. *Acta Med. Scand.*, **1–2**, 51–63.
76. Malina, L. (1986) Treatment of chronic hepatic porphyria (PCT). *Photodermatology.*, **3**, 113–21.
77. Felscher, B.F. and Redeker, A.G. (1966) Effect of chloroquine or hepatic uroporphyrin metabolism in patients with porphyria cutanea tarda. *Medicine*, **45**, 575–82.
78. Kowertz, M. (1973) The therapeutic effect of chloroquine. Hepatic recovery in porphyria cutanea tarda. *J. Amer. Med. Assoc.*, **223**, 515–19.
79. Saltzer, E., Redeker, A.G. and Wilson, J.W. (1968) PCT remission following chloroquine without adverse effects. *Arch. Dermatol.*, **98**, 496–8.
80. Kordac, V. and Semradova, M. (1974) Treatment of porphyria cutanea tarda with chloroquine. *Brit. J. Dermatol.*, **90**, 95–100.
81. Scholnick, P.L., Epstein, J.H. and Marver, H.S. (1973) The molecular basis of the action of chloroquine in porphyria cutanea tarda. *J. Invest. Dermatol.*, **61**, 226–32.
82. Taljaard, J.J.F., Shanley, B.C., Stewart-Wynne, E.G., *et al.* (1972) Studies on low dose chloroquine therapy and the action of chloroquine in symptomatic porphyria. *Brit. J. Dermatol.*, **87**, 261–9.
83. Swanbeck, G. and Wennersten, G. (1977) Treatment of porphyria cutanea tarda with chloroquine and phlebotomy. *Brit. J. Dermatol.*, **97**, 77–82.

Twenty
Bullous Amyloidosis

Stephen Michael Breathnach

20.1 INTRODUCTION

Amyloidosis refers to the abnormal extracellular deposition of one of a series of unrelated proteins which show green birefringence on alkaline Congo Red staining of tissue sections viewed under polarized light microscopy, and share a characteristic fibrillar ultrastructure [1, 2]. Amyloidosis, including cutaneous varieties, may broadly be classified into systemic and localized types, all of which are comparatively rare conditions [2]. Bullous amyloidosis, which should be distinguished from reactive amyloidosis secondary to congenital epidermolysis bullosa, has been reported almost exclusively in association with primary and myeloma-associated systemic amyloidosis. Clinically evident mucocutaneous involvement in these conditions occurs in up to 40% of cases [2]. Bullous lesions in systemic amyloidosis are exceptional, and have been the subject of very few case reports.

20.2 CLINICAL FEATURES

20.2.1 Presentation

In a large series of 182 patients with primary and 47 patients with myeloma-associated systemic amyloidosis the mean age of onset was 65 years, and there was a slight male preponderance [3]. In the 15 cases (eight male, seven female) of plasma cell dyscrasia-related bullous amyloidosis reviewed in this section (twelve primary, three myeloma-associated), the mean age was 62 years (range 51–82) [4–12]. The duration of blistering prior to presentation, where stated, ranged from 6 months to 10 years.

20.2.2 Distribution and morphology of the lesions

Widespread bullae and erosions occurring with or without associated ecchymoses were present in six of the 15 cases of primary or myeloma-associated bullous amyloidosis [5, 8–12]. In two cases, involvement was confined to the hands or feet [6, 10], in one case to the dorsa of the hands, (Figure 20.1), forehead and temples [7], in another case to the arms and back [6], and in a further case to the legs [4]. In each case, bullae were induced by minor trauma; their size ranged from a few mm up to 3 cm in diameter. Scarring with milia formation was noted in three cases [5, 7, 8] (Figure 20.2). In five cases, bullae were the presenting and only cutaneous sign [7, 10–12]. In two other cases, bullae were confined to the tongue and buccal mucosa [6]. The other signs of amyloid are usually present, i.e. purpura and ecchymoses occurring spontaneously or after minor trauma are the commonest signs, whilst the most characteristic lesions consist of waxy smooth amber-coloured papules, nodules and plaques distributed in flexural areas. Other cutaneous findings have been diffuse scleroderma-like involvement, alopecia, cutis verticis gyrata and nail dystrophy.

20.2.3 Miscellaneous

An unusual case of bullous amyloidosis in a 45-year-old female with a 12-year history of

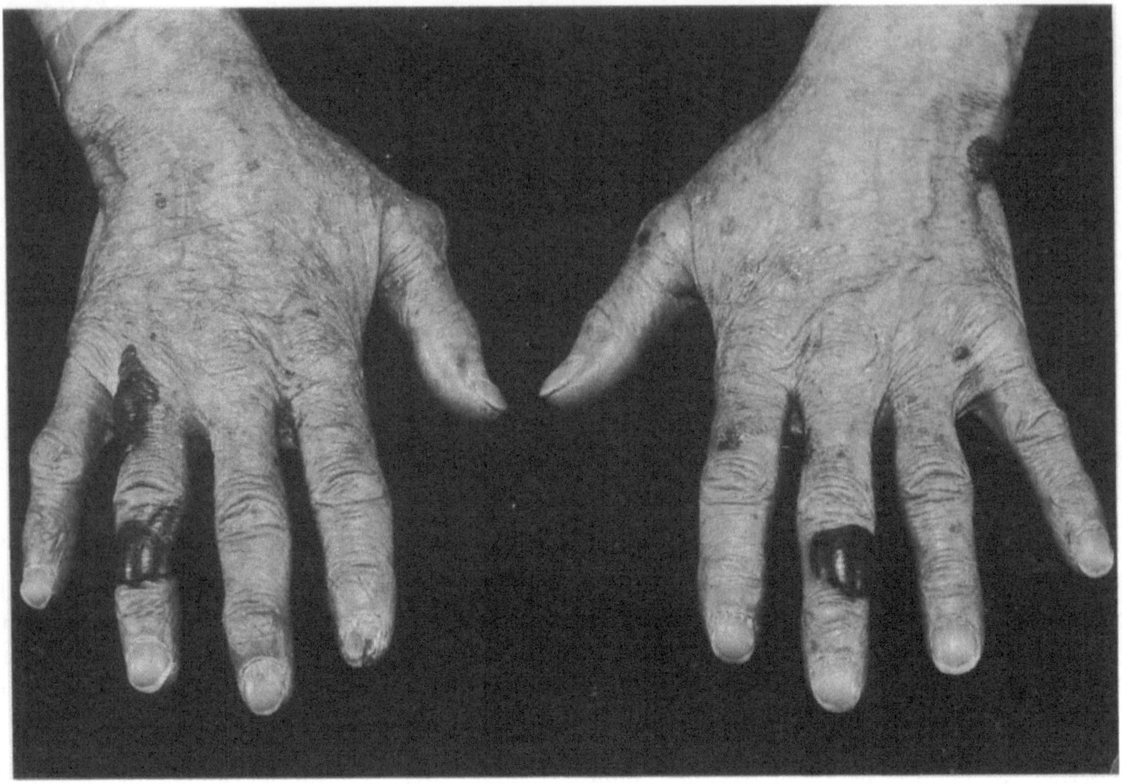

Figure 20.1 Bullous amyloid: blistering on the hands (St John's Hospital for Diseases of the Skin, London).

relapsing widespread pruritic migratory urticated erythematous plaques located especially on buttocks and thighs, surmounted by grouped and isolated vesicles with occasional large 3 cm bullae, has been described [13]. The eruption was associated with pigmentary changes and ichthyosiform hyperkeratosis, but no systemic involvement. Amyloid deposits were in the uppermost dermis, and ultrastructurally the split was at the level of the lamina lucida. The eruption was also atypical for its response to prednisolone.

20.3 DIFFERENTIAL DIAGNOSIS

The differential diagnosis of bullous amyloidosis includes bullous pemphigoid, bullous drug eruptions and (especially in the context of adult onset of cutaneous fragility, haemorrhagic subepidermal bullae and milia formation) porphyria cutanea tarda and epidermolysis bullosa acquisita (see Chapters 5, 10, 17, 19).

20.4 INVESTIGATIONS

Blistering is usually subepidermal in bullous amyloidosis, and occurs within extensive dermal amyloid deposits well below the basement membrane zone [4–10]. In three cases splitting occurred at the dermo–epidermal junction [11, 12]; in two this was associated with contiguous amyloid deposits [11], but in the other amyloid was seen only in deep blood vessels [12]. Skin biopsies reveal amyloid as an amorphous homogeneous eosinophilic material in the dermis, usually unassociated with an inflammatory infiltrate. Special stains for amyloid include Methyl Violet

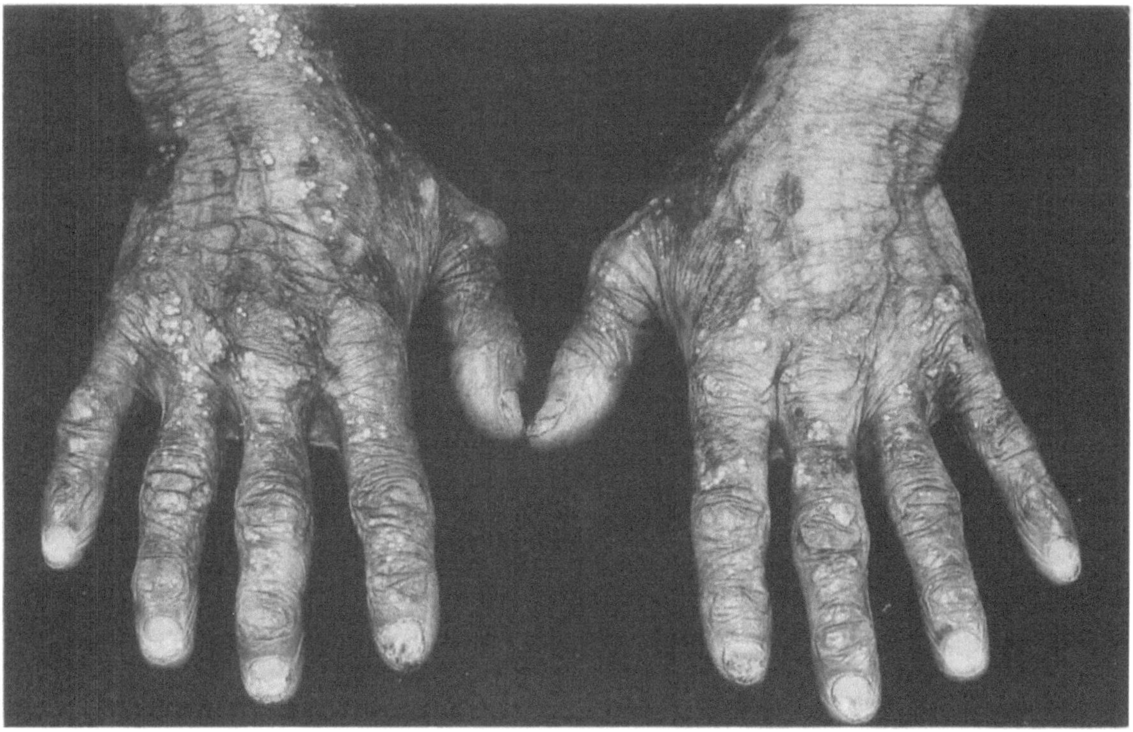

Figure 20.2 Bullous amyloid: scarring and milia formation (later stage of same patient in Figure 20.1).

and Cresyl Violet, periodic acid-Schiff, alkaline Congo Red with polarized light microscopy (Figure 20.3) and fluorescence with thioflavine T. Specific antisera directed against various types of amyloid fibril protein are also used. Occasionally ultrastructural examination for the presence of the characteristic fibrils is necessary.

Biopsy of subcutaneous abdominal fat, sural nerve, rectum, stomach, jejunum, liver, kidney, spleen, bone marrow or endomyocardium may be diagnostic. Routine haematological, hepatic, cardiac and renal function tests should be performed. Distinction between primary and myeloma-associated amyloidosis may be aided by bone marrow biopsy and radiological survey. Serum protein electrophoresis, urine Bence-Jones protein screen and immunoelectrophoresis of both serum and concentrated urine usually (but not always) demonstrate a paraprotein.

20.5 SYSTEMIC MANIFESTATIONS OF AMYLOIDOSIS

Patients may present with features of myeloma, or with carpal tunnel syndrome, macroglossia, hepatomegaly, or ascites and oedema, resulting from cardiac failure or the nephrotic syndrome. Cardiovascular involvement may cause angina, infarction, arrhythmias, orthostatic hypotension or claudication. Gastrointestinal amyloidosis may cause haemorrhage or malabsorption. Peripheral neuropathy, lymphadenopathy, lacrimal and parotid gland infiltration and amyloid deposition in joints have been recorded. Haematological complications include isolated Factor X deficiency, disseminated intravascular coagulation and fibrinolysis with severe bleeding. Cardiac and renal failure are the major causes of death.

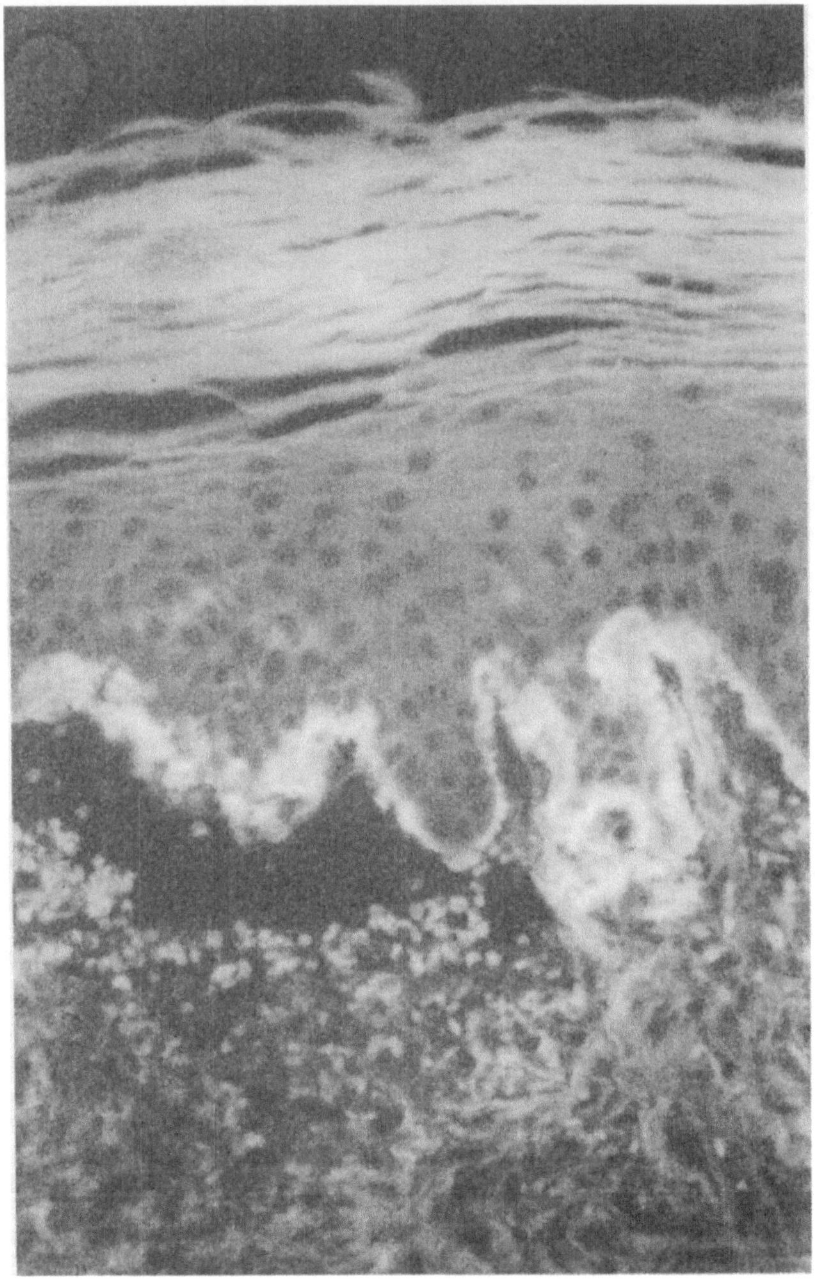

Figure 20.3 Deposition of Congo Red positive material in the roof of the blister in bullous amyloid.

20.6 PATHOGENESIS

Amyloid deposition in primary and myeloma-associated systemic amyloidosis occurs as a result of plasma cell dyscrasia [1]. Abnormal light chains are almost always present in the serum or urine even in so-called primary systemic amyloidosis. The amyloid fibrils are derived from these circulating (usually lambda class) precursors, and are composed of intact immunoglobulin light chains, light chain fragments (particularly the variable –terminal region) or both (protein AL) [1, 14]. Amyloid P component, a glycoprotein constantly associated with tissue amyloid, may be involved in the deposition and maintenance of amyloid deposits [15]. In bullous amyloidosis, trauma-induced blisters are thought to occur as a result of intradermal splitting caused by shearing forces acting on amyloid deposits.

20.7 THERAPY

There is currently no effective therapy for patients with plasma cell dyscrasia-related systemic amyloidosis [2]. Although occasional patients respond partially to chemotherapy, overall survival figures for patients treated with combined melphalan and prednisone, or with placebo, are not substantially different [16], and colchicine therapy seems not to be beneficial either [17].

20.8 PROGNOSIS

The lack of effective therapy is reflected in the prognosis. In some series no patient with AL amyloid survived for longer than 1 [18] or 2 years [19] from the time of diagnosis. In other series, the median survival of patients with primary systemic amyloidosis without myeloma is up to 14.7 months, compated with 5 months for patients with myeloma-associated amyloidosis, and 13–20 months for patients with myeloma not complicated by amyloid [3, 20, 21]. Survival does depend on response to therapy and the extent of disease; the median survival of patients with primary amyloidosis with response to chemotherapy was 28 months, compared to 7.5 months in non-responders and 6 months in patients with congestive cardiac failure [3, 22].

REFERENCES

1. Glenner, G.G. (1980) Amyloid deposits and amyloidosis. The β-fibrilloses. *New Engl. J. Med.*, **302**, 1283–92.
2. Breathnach, S.M. (1988) Amyloid and amyloidosis. *J. Amer. Acad. Dermatol.*, **18**, 1–16.
3. Kyle, R.A. and Greipp, P.R. (1983) Amyloidosis (AL): Clinical and laboratory features in 229 cases. *Mayo Clin. Proc.*, **58**, 665–83.
4. Chow, C. and Burns, R.E. (1967) Bullous amyloidosis. A case report. *Arch. Dermatol.*, **95**, 622–5.
5. Muller, S.A., Sams, W.M. Jr and Dobson, R.L. (1969) Amyloidosis masquerading as epidermolysis bullosa acquisita. *Arch. Dermatol.*, **99**, 739–47.
6. Northover, J.M.A., Pickard, J.D., Murray-Lyon, I.M., *et al.* (1972) Bullous lesions of the skin and mucous membranes in primary amyloidosis. *Postgrad. Med. J.*, **48**, 351–3.
7. Hunter, J.A.A. (1976) Primary systemic amyloidosis imitating porphyria cutanea tarda. *Proc. R. Soc. Med.*, **69**, 235–6.
8. Bluhm, J.F. III., Johnson, S.C. and Norback, D.H. (1980) Bullous amyloidosis. Case report with ultrastructural studies. *Arch. Dermatol.*, **116**, 1164–8.
9. Trump, D.L., Allen, H., Olson, J., *et al.* (1980) Epidermolysis bullosa acquisita. Association with amyloidosis and multiple myeloma. *J. Amer. Med. Assoc.*, **243**, 1461–2.
10. Westermark, P., Ohman, S., Domar, M. and Sletten, K. (1981) Bullous amyloidosis. *Arch. Dermatol.*, **117**, 782–4.
11. Holden, C.A., Weston, M.J. and MacDonald, D.M. (1982) Trauma-induced bullae; the presenting feature of systemic amyloidosis associated with plasma cell dyscrasia. *Brit. J. Dermatol.*, **107**, 701–6.
12. Walton, S., MacDonald, K.J.S., Marks, J. and Callaghan, J. (1983) Trauma-induced bullae: the presenting feature of systemic amyloidosis associated with plasma cell dyscrasia. *Brit. J. Dermatol.*, **108**, 628.
13. Ruzicka, T., Schmoeckel, C., Ring, J., *et al.* (1985) Bullous amyloidosis. *Brit. J. Dermatol.*, **113**, 85–95.
14. Glenner, G.G., Terry, W., Harada, M., *et al.* (1971) Amyloid fibril proteins: Proof of homology with immunoglobulin light chains by sequence analyses. *Science*, **172**, 1150–1.

15. Breathnah, S.M. (1985) The cutaneous amyloidoses. Pathogenesis and therapy. *Arch. Dermatol.*, **121**, 470–5.
16. Kyle, R.A. and Greipp, P.R. (1978) Primary systemic amyloidosis: Comparison of melphalan and prednisone versus placebo. *Blood*, **52**, 818–27.
17. Kyle, R.A., Greipp, P.R., Garton, J.P. and Gertz, M.A. (1985) Primary systemic amyloidosis. Comparison of melphalan/prednisone versus colchicine. *Amer. J. Med.*, **79**, 708–16.
18. Pick, A.I., Frohlichmann, R., Lavie, G., *et al.* (1981) Clinical and immunochemical studies of 20 patients with amyloidosis and plasma cell dyscrasia. *Acta Haematol.*, **66**, 154–67.
19. Brandt, K., Cathcart, E.S. and Cohen, A.S. (1968) A clinical analysis of the course and prognosis of forty-two patients with amyloidosis. *Amer. J. Med.*, **44**, 955–69.
20. Kyle, R.A. and Bayrd, E.D. (1975) Amyloidosis: Review of 236 cases. *Medicine*, **54**, 271–99.
21. Barth, W.F., Willerson, J.T., Waldmann, T.A. and Decker, J.L. (1969) Primary amyloidosis. Clinical, immunochemical and immunoglobulin metabolism studies in fifteen patients. *Amer. J. Med.*, **47**, 259–73.
22. Fielder, K. and Durie, B.G.M. (1986) Primary amyloidosis associated with multiple myeloma. Predictors of successful therapy. *Amer. J. Med.*, **80**, 413–18.

Twenty-one

Bullous dermatoses associated with renal disease

Vanessa A. Venning

21.1 INTRODUCTION

A blistering disorder resembling porphyria cutanea tarda has been reported in haemodialysis patients as well as in uraemic patients while receiving frusemide. Furthermore glomerulonephritis has occurred in association with a variety of blistering diseases including dermatitis herpetiformis, bullous pemphigoid and linear IgA disease. These various associations are discussed.

21.2 BULLOUS DISORDERS ASSOCIATED WITH HAEMODIALYSIS

In 1975 Gilchrest *et al.* [1] and Korting [2] independently described a bullous eruption, clinically and histologically indistinguishable from porphyria cutanea tarda (PCT), occurring in patients with chronic renal failure (CRF) undergoing haemodialysis. In all but one patient, porphyrin estimations in urine and stool were normal and the terms 'bullous dermatosis of haemodialysis' (BDH) [1] or 'pseudoporphyria' were coined. Since then several similar cases with normal levels of urinary and stool porphyrins have been reported [3–9]. However, one of Korting's original cases had elevated urinary porphyrins [2] and later Poh-Fitzpatrick and her colleagues reported three further cases in which PCT-like skin changes in haemodialysis patients were accompanied by elevated plasma porphyrins, and a porphyrin profile consistent with PCT [10, 11]. Subsequent reports have confirmed the existence of a variety of porphyrin abnormalities in similar patients [1, 13–22]; the overall incidence of such PCT-like eruptions in haemodialysis patients has been estimated to be from 1 [5] to 16% [7].

21.2.1 Clinical findings

Clinically, the skin changes are indistinguishable from porphyria cutanea tarda. Bullae of the backs of the hands and face, skin fragility, atrophic scars, milia, pigmentary and sclerodermatous changes have all been described [1–22] following the onset of haemodialysis by 2 months [5] to 6 years [17].

21.2.2 Histological findings

Histologically, the bullae are subepidermal, with slightly oedematous dermal papillae projecting into the blister space. The small blood vessels are thickened with periodate–Schiff-positive material [1, 2, 5, 6], and while there is only scant infiltration by monocytes and polymorphs, there are large numbers of degranulated mast cells, particularly near vessels. The dermal collagen shows elastotic change, and homogeneous basophilic material among the disorganized collagen bundles. On electron microscopy the vessels are seen to be sheathed by concentric basal laminae and granular deposits. Away from the vessels there are extensive sheets of granulofilamentous material and active secretory fibroblasts. The basement membrane is thickened and sub-basal deposits of granular or homogeneous material infiltrate the collagen [23].

21.2.3 Immunofluorescence findings

Immunofluorescence studies have either been negative [5, 15] or have shown immune deposits (usually IgG, less frequently IgA and IgM) around dermal blood vessels [1–3] or in the basement membrane zone [3]. Although usually absent, C3 has been reported accompanying immunoglobulin deposits [3].

21.2.4 Porphyrin estimations

Although most of the early cases of bullous dermatosis of haemodialysis were associated with normal porphyrin levels, these estimations were performed on urine and faeces and not plasma [1, 3, 5, 6, 8, 9]. Subsequently cases with high levels of urinary uroporphyrin have occurred [10, 11, 17], though it is now recognized that urinary clearance of porphyrins in uraemic patients is depressed and does not accurately reflect body porphyrin content [13, 17], and that biliary excretion is also unpredictable. Hence, increasing reliance is placed on plasma porphyrin estimation and there are several reports of patients with BDH with raised plasma uroporphyrin levels [10–13, 18], although in other cases plasma levels have been normal [10]. Furthermore it has now been shown that patients with CRF (whether dialysed or not) may have raised plasma uroporphyrin levels even in the absence of skin changes [13, 17, 20, 24]. Hyperporphyrinaemia was present in 60% of haemodialysis patients in one series [17]; Poh-Fitzpatrick found porphyrin levels in CRF patients overlapping with the lower end of the range found in true symptomatic PCT [24]. In general, CRF patients with bullae have higher plasma porphyrin levels than those without [13, 20]. The accumulation of uroporphyrin in plasma in CRF is not simply due to reduced urinary clearance. The isomer composition is also altered and this probably reflects interference with hepatic uroporphyrin decarboxylase activity [13]. The precursors of uroporphyrin (aminolaevulinic acid and porphobilinogen) do not accumulate in CRF [13]. Erythrocyte uroporphyrin decarboxylase activity has been normal in some patients [16, 21] though others have had depressed enzyme activity, suggesting a pre-existing genetically determined PCT in these cases [14, 17]. Underlying familial PCT has been confirmed by family studies in one of these cases [17]. Erythrocyte protoporphyrin levels may be moderately raised in CRF, and this probably reflects chronic anaemia [13, 19].

21.2.5 Predisposing factors

Apart from mild chronic hyperporphyrinaemia of chronic renal failure, little is known of the additional factors predisposing a small proportion of these patients to develop PCT-like skin changes. Exposure to intense sunlight has been a clear precipitating factor in some [1, 6, 9] but results of phototesting have been negative [1]. Alcohol consumption or iron overload may have been contributory factors in a few cases [10–13, 24] and some patients have been receiving known phototoxic drugs, e.g. frusemide [5, 6]. Aluminium toxicity has been suggested [5] as aluminium administration to rats causes chronic liver intoxication and porphyria [25] and because hepatic accumulation of aluminium is known to occur in some dialysed patients. Photosensitizing chemicals eluted from dialysis tubing have also been postulated but not documented [3].

21.2.6 Treatment

Treatment is unsatisfactory. Uroporphyrin is largely protein bound and poorly dialysable [10, 11, 16]. Even when porphyrin levels have been partially reduced, this failed to produce clinical remission [14]. Neither sunscreens [1] nor chloroquine [14] have proved helpful. Phlebotomy is capable of inducing remission [9, 16], but it is generally contraindicated in these patients. Plasma exchange has been successfully employed in one patient [22].

21.2.7 Prognosis

The clinical course is variable, some patients having a brief self-limiting eruption [19] while others experience recurrent relapses, frequently after exposure to sun [1, 9]. A patient reported by Topi *et al.* with familial PCT and CRF [17] had bullae followed by rapidly progressive sclerodermatous change in exposed skin, appearing over a few months. In some patients whose bullae developed whilst taking frusemide, the eruption has subsided in spite of continuing the drug.

21.3 BULLOUS DERMATOSES, CHRONIC RENAL FAILURE AND FRUSEMIDE

There are now many reports of bullous eruptions on sun-exposed skin occurring in patients with CRF while receiving frusemide [5, 6, 26–31]. Some of these have occurred in haemodialysis patients [27,30], while other cases have had advanced renal failure, not yet requiring dialysis [26–31]. A similar eruption has also occurred in a patient on frusemide with only mildly impaired renal function (creatinine clearance 62 ml/min) [29]. Histologically the bullae have been indistinguishable from those seen in PCT, though clinically scarring and milia have not been reported. The doses of frusemide implicated have generally been high (0.5–2.0 g/day) [6, 27, 29–31] though in one case the dose was only 40 mg/day [26]. Bullae have usually occurred after several months of treatment and have also spontaneously remitted in spite of continuation of the drug [29]. In a study of 56 CRF patients receiving frusemide Heydenreich *et al.* found no differences between the frusemide levels, the urinary and plasma porphyrins, or in the HL-A type, between the 12 patients with bullae and those without [20]. Phototesting in three patients with CRF who developed bullae while taking frusemide showed low minimal erythema doses to UV-A but normal thresholds to UV-B [31]. A widespread bullous eruption, with histological and immunofluorescence findings typical of bullous pemphigoid, has also occurred in a CRF patient on frusemide [32].

A single case of bullae occurring on sun-exposed skin has been reported in a CRF patient receiving nalidixic acid [33], a drug that is also phototoxic in non-uraemic subjects [34].

In view of the similarity between drug-associated bullous eruptions in CRF, and those reported in dialysis patients not receiving such medication, and in the light of the knowledge that porphyrin metabolism and excretion is altered in uraemic patients [13], it appears likely that potentially phototoxic drugs act as just one of several predisposing factors in the causation of bullae in CRF patients.

21.4 BULLOUS DISORDERS AND GLOMERULONEPHRITIS

21.4.1 Dermatitis herpetiformis (DH)

Glomerular disease has been reported in 11 patients with dermatitis herpetiformis [35–45], four with proliferative [36, 38], two with mesangio-proliferative and three with membranous glomerulonephritis. In all reported cases there have been significant deposits of IgA in glomerular structures and most have also had deposits of IgG, IgM and C3. A further three cases of nephrotic syndrome (without renal biopsy findings) associated with DH have also been reported [45]. However, the incidence of clinical nephritis in patients with DH is low. Davies *et al.* [46] screened 42 DH patients for glomerulonephritis by creatinine clearance, 24 h urinary protein and routine urinalysis. Only one patient (who also had systemic lupus erythematosus) had evidence of glomerulonephritis and this patient had a linear deposit of IgA and other immunoreactants and would not now be regarded as having DH. However, subclinical glomerular deposition of immune complexes may occur more frequently. In an electron microsopic study of eight DH patients, Reunala *et al.* [47] found evidence of immune complex deposition in the glomeruli of five.

Glomerulonephritis may either precede or follow the onset of DH [38] and in one case the diseases showed a remarkably parallel course [42], with gluten exclusion apparently inducing remission of both skin lesions and the nephrotic syndrome, as well as coexisting coeliac disease. Furthermore, nephrotic relapses were preceded on two occasions by flare ups of DH.

The nature of the immune complexes deposited in the skin and glomerulus in patients with coexistent DH and glomerulonephritis is unknown. HLA studies suggest that some persons are genetically predisposed to the development of immune complex diseases. The HLA haplotype B8 and DRW3 are known to be associated with DH and coeliac disease [38, 48]. DRW3 is also associated with idiopathic membranous glomerulonephritis [49], some cases of which have recently been associated with mesangial deposits of IgA [50]. Furthermore, the HLA-B8/DRW3 haplotype has been associated with an impaired ability to clear immune complexes [51] and this haplotype has been reported in one of the patients with coexistent DH and glomerulonephritis [42] though not in all [44].

21.4.2 Bullous pemphigoid (BP)

Sporadic case reports have appeared in the literature of BP occurring in association with immune complex glomerulonephritis [52–59]. The glomerular lesions reported include minimal change [52], membranous [53, 54, 57, 58], diffuse proliferative [55] and mesangioproliferative [59] glomerulonephritis. Most were associated with granular glomerular deposits of IgG and C3 [54, 55, 58] or IgG, IgA, C3 and Clq [57]. Von Joost *et al.* comment on a strikingly linear deposit of IgG, IgA, IgM and C3 along the glomerular basement membrane in one patient [59].

BP may either precede or follow the onset of glomerulonephritis [57]. In two cases a somewhat parallel clinical course has occurred with both skin lesions and proteinuria remitting on prednisolone [55]. In others, the glomerulonephritis has been unremitting in spite of steroids [56, 59]. BP sera do not normally cross-react with glomerular basement membrane [60], and some patients with coexistent BP and glomerulonephritis have had multiple diseases of an autoimmune nature [56, 57], suggesting generally aberrant immune responses to a variety of autoantigens. Several of the reported cases have had circulating anti-skin BMZ antibodies [52–55, 57–59]. However, with the exception of a single case of BP associated with Goodpasture's Syndrome [61], anti-glomerular antibodies have been absent [53, 58, 59]. Glomerulonephritis is associated with immune complex deposition [62], and although circulating immune complexes are known to occur in some BP patients [63], they have not so far been detected in patients with coexistent BP and glomerulonephritis [57, 59].

21.4.3 Other bullous disorders

Linear IgA disease [59] and chronic bullous dermatosis of childhood (CBDC) [64] have each been associated in single case reports with glomerulonephritis (membranous and membrano-proliferative respectively). In the former, both IgA and IgG were deposited in the glomeruli, whereas the child with CBDC had IgG, IgM and C3 (but not IgA) in the kidney, and hypergammaglobulinaemia and low serum complement were additional findings. Davies *et al.* have reported a case of mesangioproliferative glomerulonephritis in a patient believed to have DH, but whose immuno-fluorescence findings were consistent with linear IgA disease [46]. Pemphigus foliaceus has occurred with immune complex glomerulonephritis in a patient receiving penicillamine for severe rheumatoid arthritis [65] as well as in a 16-year-old boy without exposure to penicillamine [66].

A severe bullous eruption with histological features suggestive of toxic epidermal necrolysis has been reported in association with glomerulonephritis and chronic active hepatitis in a single patient [67].

21.4.4 Miscellaneous associations of bullous disorders and kidney disease

Renal amyloidosis has occurred as a complication of dystrophic epidermolysis bullosa in both adults [68–70] and children [71], presumably as a result of chronic sepsis [71].

REFERENCES

1. Gilchrest, B., Rowe, J.W. and Mihm, M.C. (1975) Bullous dermatosis of haemodialysis. *Ann. Intern. Med.*, 83, 480–3.

2. Korting, G.W. (1975) Über Porphyria-cutanea-tarda-artige Hautver-Änderungen bei langzeit-hämodialysepatienten. *Dermatologica,* **150,** 58–61.
3. Thivolet, J., Euvrard, S., Perrot, H., *et al.* (1977). La pseudo-porphyrie cutanée des haemodialyses. *Ann. Dermatol. Vénereol.,* **104,** 12–17.
4. Perrot, H., Germain, D., Euvrard, S. and Thivolet, J. (1977). Porphyria cutanea tarda-like dermatosis by haemodialysis; ultrastructural study of exposed skin. *Arch. Dermatol. Res.,* **259,** 177–85.
5. Brivet, F., Drüke, T., Guillermette, J., Zingraff, J. and Crosnier, J. (1978). Porphyria cutanea tarda-like syndrome in haemodialysed patients. *Nephron,* **20,** 258–66.
6. Rotstein, H. (1978) Photosensitive bullous eruption associated with chronic renal failure. *Aust. J. Dermatol.,* **19,** 58–64.
7. Giffron-Euvrard, S., Thivolet, J., Laurat, G., *et al.,* (1977). Recherche de la pseudo-porphyrie cutanée tardive chez 100 hémodialysés. *Dermatologica,* **155,** 193–9.
8. Webster, S.B., and Dahlberg, R.J. (1980). Bullous dermatosis of haemodialysis, case report and review of the dermatologic changes in chronic renal failure *Cutis,* **25,** 322–6.
9. Olmstead, C.B., and Clack, W.E. (1981). Bullous dermatosis of haemodialysis. *Cutis,* **27,** 614–18.
10. Poh-Fitzpatrick, M.B., Bellet, N., DeLeo, V.A., Grossman, M.E. and Bickers, D.R. (1978). Porphyria cutanea tarda in two patients treated with haemodialysis for chronic renal failure. *New Engl. J. Med.,* **299,** 292–4.
11. Poh-Fitzpatrick, M.B., Masullo, A.S. and Grossman, M.E. (1980) Porphyria cutanea tarda associated with chronic renal disease and haemodialysis. *Arch. Dermatol.,* **116,** 191–5.
12. Fisher, D.G. (1979). Bullous dermatosis and chronic renal failure differential diagnosis. *Dermatology,* **2,** 15–21.
13. Day, R.S. and Eales, L. (1980). Porphyrins in chronic renal failure. *Nephron,* **26,** 90–5.
14. García-Parilla, J., Ortega, R. and Pena, M.L. (1980). Porphyria cutanea tarda during maintenance haemodialysis. *Brit. Med. J.,* **280,** 1358–60.
15. Wilkin, J.K., Kaplan, R.J. and Acchiardo, S.R. (1980). Porphyria cutanea tarda in a chronic haemodialysis patient. *South. Med. J.,* **73,** 1066–7.
16. Lichenstein, J.R., Babb, E.J. and Felsher, B.F. (1981). Porphyria cutanea tarda in a patient with chronic renal failure on haemodialysis. *Brit. J. Dermatol.,* **104,** 575–8.
17. Topi, G.C., D'Alessandro, G.L., Cancarini, G.C., *et al.* (1981). Porphyria cutanea tarda in a haemodialysed patient. *Brit. J. Dermatol.,* **104,** 579–80.
18. Hanno, R. and Callen, J.P. (1981). Porphyria cutanea tarda as a cause of bullous dermatosis of haemodialysis; a case report and review of the literature. *Cutis,* **28,** 261–3.
19. Kron, J. and Linß, G. (1983). Porphyria-cutanea-tarda-artige Hautveränderungen bei chronischen hämodialysepatienten. *Z. Ges. Inn. Med. Jahrg.,* **38,** 242–8.
20. Seubert, S., Seubert, A., Wolfgang, K. and Kiffe, H. (1985). A porphyria cutanea tarda-like distribution of porphyrins in plasma, haemodialysate, hemofiltrate, and urine of patients on chronic hemodialysis. *J. Invest. Dermatol.,* **85,** 107–9.
21. Harlan, S.L. and Winkelmann, R.K. (1983). Porphyria cutanea tarda and chronic renal failure. *Mayo Clin. Proc.,* **58,** 467–71.
22. Disler, P., Day, R., Burman, N., Blekkenhorst, G. and Eales, L. (1982). Treatment of haemodialysis-related porphyria cutanea tarda with plasma exchange. *Amer. J. Med.,* **72,** 989–93.
23. Poh-Fitzpatrick, M.B., Sosin, A.E. and Bemis, J. (1982). Porphyrin levels in plasma and erythrocytes of chronic haemodialysis patients. *J. Amer. Acad. Dermatol.,* **7,** 100–4.
24. Kushner, J.P. (1982). The enzymatic defect in porphyria cutanea tarda. *New Engl. J. Med.,* **306,** 799–800.
25. Berlyne, G.M. (1976). Aluminium intoxication. *New. Engl. J. Med.,* **294,** 1130.
26. Keczkes, K. and Farr, M. (1976). Bullous dermatosis of chronic renal failure. *Brit. J. Dermatol.,* **95,** 541–6.
27. Burry, J.N. and Lawrence, J.R. (1976). Phototoxic blisters from high dose frusemide. *Brit. J. Dermatol.,* **94,** 495–9.
28. Coles, G.A. and Verrier Jones, K. (1976). Uraemic Bullae. *Brit. Med. J.,* **ii,** 525–6.
29. Kennedy, A.C. and Lyell, A. (1976). Acquired epidermolysis bullosa due to high dose frusemide. *Brit. Med. J.,* **i,** 1509–10.
30. Heydenreich, G., Pindborg, T. and Schmidt, H. (1977). Bullous dermatosis in patients with chronic renal failure on high dose frusemide. *Acta Med. Scand.,* **202,** 61–4.
31. Anderson, C.D., Larsson, L. and Skogh, M. (1985). UVA photosensitivity in photosensitive bullous disease of chronic renal failure. *Photodermatology,* **2,** 111–14.
32. Ingber, A., David, M. and Feuerman, E.J. (1986). Haemorrhagic bullous pemphigoid following frusemide treatment – an unusual case. *Z. Hautkr.,* **61,** 1554–6.
33. Susskind, W. and Lyell, A. (1965). Suspected reaction to nalidixic acid. *Brit. Med. J.,* **i,** 316.
34. Ramsay, C.A. and Obreshkova, E. (1974). Photosensitivity from nalidixic acid. *Brit. J. Dermatol.,* **91,** 523–7.
35. De Coteau, W.E., Gerrard, J.W. and Cunningham, T.A. (1973). Glomerulitis in dermatitis herpetiformis. *Lancet,* **ii,** 679–80.

36. Pape, J.F., Mellbye, O.J., Øystese, B. and Brodwall, E.K. (1978). Glomerulonephritis in dermatitis herpetiformis. *Acta Med. Scand.*, **203**, 445–8.
37. Moorthy, A.V., Zimmerman, S.W. and Maxim, P.E. (1978). Dermatitis herpetiformis and coeliac disease. *J. Amer. Med. Assoc.*, **239**, 2019–20.
38. Davies, M.G. and Davies, P.G. (1979). Dermatitis herpetiformis glomerulonephritis and HLA DRW3. *Lancet*, **ii**, 911.
39. Tan, C.Y., Davies, M.G. and Marks, R. (1980). Coexisting dermatitis herpetiformis and membranous glomerulonephritis. *Clin. Exp. Dermatol.*, **5**, 177–9.
40. Combs, R.C. and Haxelrigg, D.E. (1980). Dermatitis herpetiformis and membranous glomerulonephritis. *Cutis*, **25**, 660–1.
41. Helin, H., Mustonen, J., Reunala, T. and Pasternak, A. (1983). IgA nephropathy associated with coeliac disease and dermatitis herpetiformis. *Arch. Pathol. Lab. Med.*, **107**, 324–7.
42. Gaboardi, F., Perletti, L., Cambie, M. and Mihatsch, M.J. (1983). Dermatitis herpetiformis and nephrotic syndrome. *Clin. Nephrol.*, **20**, 49–51.
43. Bartoli, E., Bosincu, L., Costanzi, G., *et al.* (1982). IgA pseudo linear deposits in glomerular basement membranes in dermatitis herpetiformis. *Amer. J. Clin. Pathol.*, **78**, 377–80.
44. Heironimus, J.D. and Perry, E.L. (1986). Dermatitis herpetiformis and glomerulonephritis. *Amer. J. Med.*, **80**, 508–10.
45. El-Hafnawi, H., Gawad, Z.A. and El-Marsafy, M.K. (1964). Nephrotic syndrome as a complication in dermatitis herpetiformis. *Arch. Klin. Exp. Dermatol.*, **218**, 429–34.
46. Davies, M.G., Marks, R. and Nuki, G. (1978). Dermatitis herpetiformis – a skin manifestation of a generalized disturbance in immunity. *Q. J. Med.*, **47**, 221–48.
47. Reunala, T., Helin, H., Pasternak, A., Linder, E. and Kalimo, K. (1983). Renal involvement and circulating immune complexes in dermatitis herpetiformis. *J. Amer. Acad. Dermatol.*, **9**, 219–23.
48. Pehamberger, H., Holubar, K. and Mayr, W.R., (1981). HLA-DR3 in dermatitis herpetiformis. *Brit. J. Dermatol.*, **104**, 321–4.
49. Klouda, P.T., Acheson, E.J., Goldby, F.S., *et al.* (1979). Strong association between idiopathic membranous nephropathy and HLA-DRw3. *Lancet*, **ii**, 770.
50. Doi, T., Kanatsu, K., Nagai, H., Kohrogi, N. and Hamashimi, T. (1983). An overlapping syndrome of IgA nephropathy and membranous nephropathy. *Nephron*, **35**, 24–30.
51. Lawley, T.J., Hall, R.P., Fauci, A.S., *et al.* (1981). Defective F_c-receptor function associated with HLA-B8/DRW3 haplotype. *New. Engl. J. Med.*, **304**, 185–92.
52. Bean, S.F., Good, R.A. and Windhorst, D.B. (1970). Bullous pemphigoid in an 11-year-old boy. *Arch. Dermatol.*, **102**, 205–8.
53. Esterly, N.B., Gotoff, S.P., Lolekha, S., *et al.* (1973). Bullous pemphigoid and membranous glomerulonephropathy in a child. *J. Pediatr.*, **83**, 467–70.
54. Glasson, P., Pfister, G., Poffet, D., Chatelnat, F. and Favre, H. (1982). Glomerular lesions in a patient with bullous pemphigoid. *Kidney Int.*, **21**, 123.
55. Mérot, Y., Poffet, D., Glasson, P., Chatelnat, F. and Saurat, J.H. (1983). Glomérulonéphrite et pemphigoïde bulleuse: deux observations. *Ann. Dermatol. Venerol.*, **110**, 739–40.
56. Singhal, P.C. and Scharschmidt, L.A. (1985). Membranous nephropathy associated with primary biliary cirrhosis and bullous pemphigoid. *Ann. Allergy.*, **55**, 484–5.
57. Simon, C.A. and Winkelmann, R.K. (1986). Bullous pemphigoid and glomerulonephritis; report of 4 cases. *J. Amer. Acad. Dermatol.*, **14**, 456–63.
58. Kida, K., Takaya, Y. and Makino, H. (1981). Membranous glomerulonephritis associated with bullous pemphigoid. *Nippon Jinzo Gakkai Shi*, **23**, 799–805.
59. Van Joost, T., Mutendam, J., Heule, F., *et al.* (1986). Subepidermal bullous autoimmune disease associated with immune nephritis. *J. Amer. Acad. Dermatol.*, **14**, 214–20.
60. Pothupitiya, G.M., Wojnarowska, F., Bhogal, B.S. and Black, M.M. (1988). Distribution of the antigen in adult linear IgA disease and chronic bullous dermatosis of childhood suggests that it is a single and unique antigen. *Brit. J. Dermatol.*, **118**, 175–82.
61. Davenport, A., Verbov, J.L. and Goldsmith, H.J. (1987). Circulating anti-skin basement membrane zone antibodies in a patient with Goodpastures. *Brit. J. Dermatol.*, **117**, 125–7.
62. Wilson, C.B. (1980). Immunopathologic evaluation of renal disease. In *Renal Disease*, 4th edn (eds D. Black and N.F. Jones), Blackwell. Scientific Publications, Oxford, pp. 139–68.
63. Tappenheiner, G., Heine, K.G., Kahl, J.C. and Jordon, R.E. (1977). C_{1q} binding substances in pemphigus and bullous pemphigoid. *Clin. Exp. Immunol.*, **28**, 40–8.
64. Chappe, S.G., Esterly, N.B., Furey, N.L., Hurley, J.K. and Hsueh, K. (1981). Subepidermal bullous diseases and glomerulonephritis in a child. *J. Amer. Acad. Dermatol.*, **5**, 280–9.
65. Sparrow, G.P. (1979). Penicillamine, pemphigus and the nephrotic syndrome occurring simultaneously. *Brit. J. Dermatol.*, **98**, 103–5.
66. Janssens, M., de Muynck, M., Verresen, L. and Missotten, L. (1985). An unusual association of subacute sclerosing glomerulonephritis, pemphigus foliaceous and infiltration of the deep corneal layers. *Bull. Soc. Belge. Ophthal.*, **215**, 95–100.

67. Breathnach, S.M., Dutt, M.K. and Black, M.M. (1980). A severe bullous eruption occurring in a patient with chronic active hepatitis and glomerulonephritis. *Arch. Dermatol.*, **116**, 1061–3.
68. Brownstein, M.H. and Helwig, E.G. (1974). Systemic amyloidosis complicating dermatosis. *Arch. Dermatol.*, **102**, 1–7.
69. Miescher, G. (1937). Epidermolysis bullosa vegetans mit Amyloid *Dermatol. Z.*, **76**, 1–5.
70. Thivolet, J. (1965). Epidermolyse bulleuse dystrophique compliquée d'amyloïdose viscérale. *Bull. Soc. Franc. Dermatol. Syphil.*, **72**, 315–19.
71. Malága, S., Fernández Toral, J., Santos, F., Riesgo, I. and Crespo, M. (1983). Renal amyloidosis complicating a recessive epidermolysis bullosa in childhood. *Helv. Paediatr. Acta*, **38**, 167–70.

Index